CANCER

Proceedings of the
1980 International Symposium on Cancer

Presented by
Memorial Sloan-Kettering Cancer Center

Cosponsored by
the National Cancer Institute and
the American Cancer Society

September 14–18, 1980

Grune & Stratton Rapid Manuscript Reproduction

CANCER
Achievements, Challenges, and Prospects for the 1980s
Volume 2

Edited by

Joseph H. Burchenal, M.D.
Memorial Sloan-Kettering Cancer Center
New York, New York

Herbert F. Oettgen, M.D.
Memorial Sloan-Kettering Cancer Center
New York, New York

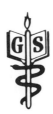

Grune & Stratton
A Subsidiary of Harcourt Brace Jovanovich, Publishers
New York   London   Toronto   Sydney   San Francisco

Grune & Stratton, Inc.
111 Fifth Avenue
New York, New York 10003

Distributed in the United Kingdom by
Academic Press Inc. (London) Ltd.
24/28 Oval Road, London NW 1

Library of Congress Catalog Number 80-85158
International Standard Book Number 0-8089-1357-3
Printed in the United States of America

Contents

Preface

Much has been achieved in the years since the Panel on Cancer of the United States Senate began the deliberations that led to the National Cancer Act, passed in 1971, and the subsequent development of the National Cancer Program, a unique event in the history of biology and medicine in this country. Knowledge about the epidemiology, etiology and prevention of cancer has increased, many types of disseminated cancer are no longer completely incurable and great strides have been made in the area of multidisciplinary therapy, particularly adjuvant chemotherapy. At the ten-year mark it seemed appropriate to assess the acomplishments of the past decade, to define current challenges and to gauge the prospects of meeting them during the next decade. To that end, an international conference, presented by Memorial Sloan-Kettering Cancer Center and cosponsored by the National Cancer Institute and the American Cancer Society, entitled "Cancer 1980: Achievements, Challenges, Prospects," was held September 14–18, 1980, in New York City.

The Program Committee, composed of members from the sponsoring institutions, selected 26 major basic and clinical topics for discussion. Leading experts from all over the world were asked to present overviews of these topics in plenary sessions and to select additional speakers to develop important aspects of their particular area in more detail in complementary symposia. The response to these invitations was most gratifying. Up-to-date manuscripts of the presentations were received at the time of the conference, and they have been arranged so that each overview paper is followed by the corresponding symposium papers.

We are grateful to Dr. Edward J. Beattie, Jr., General Chairman, and Dr. William S. Howland, Vice Chairman, for conceiving this conference, to the members of the Program Committee for shaping it, to the speakers who made it a success, to Ms. Leslie Anton for coordinating the entire program, to Steven K. Herlitz, Inc., for organizing the conference, and to the staff at Grune & Stratton for assembling these volumes for rapid publication.

Joseph H. Burchenal
Herbert F. Oettgen

Contributors

Miriam Adams, M.D.
Director, Office of Cancer Communications
Memorial Sloan-Kettering Cancer Center
New York, New York

James Anderson, M.D.
Children's Cancer Study Group
Los Angeles, California

Zalmen Arlin, M.D.
Hematology/Lymphoma Service
Department of Medicine
Memorial Sloan-Kettering Cancer Center
New York, New York

Kerry Atkinson, M.D.
Assistant Professor of Medicine
Division of Oncology
University of Washington School of Medicine
Fred Hutchinson Cancer Research Center
Seattle, Washington

Edward J. Beattie, Jr., M.D.
General Director
Memorial Hospital
New York, New York

J. B. Belasco, M.D.
Department of Pediatrics
The University of Pennsylvania
The Children's Cancer Research Center
Children's Hospital of Pennsylvania
Philadelphia, Pennsylvania

Costan W. Berard, M.D.
Chairman, Division of Pathology
St. Jude Children's Research Hospital
Memphis, Tennesee

Jean Bernard, M.D.
Institut de Recherches sur les Leucémies et les Maladies du Sang
Hopital Saint-Louis
Paris, France

Gerald P. Bodey, M.D.
Department of Developmental Therapeutics
The University of Texas System Cancer Center
M.D. Anderson Hospital and Tumor Institute
Houston, Texas

Gianni Bonadonna, M.D.
Director, Division of Medical Oncology
Istituto Nazionale Tumori
Milan, Italy

Vivien H. C. Bramwell, M.D.
Senior Registrar
Cancer Research Campaign
Department of Medical Oncology
Manchester University, Christie Hospital and Holt Radium Institute
Manchester, England

R. W. Brockman, Ph.D.
Head, Biological Chemistry Division
Southern Research Institute
Birmingham, Alabama

Joseph H. Burchenal, M.D.
Member, Sloan-Kettering Institute
Director, Clinical Investigation
Memorial Sloan-Kettering Cancer Center
New York, New York

Lawrence D. Burke, M.D.
Program Director for Rehabilitation
Division of Cancer Control and Rehabilitation
National Cancer Institute
National Institutes of Health
Silver Spring, Maryland

Patrick J. Byrne, M.D.
Instructor in Medicine
Georgetown University School of Medicine
Vincent T. Lombardi Cancer Research Center
Washington, D.C.

Fernando Cabanillas, M.D.
The University of Texas System Cancer Center
M.D. Anderson Hospital and Tumor Institute
Houston, Texas

George P. Canellos, M.D.
Chief, Division of Medical Oncology
Sidney Farber Cancer Institute
Boston, Massachusetts

Graziano C. Carlon, M.D.
Clinical Chief
Department of Critical Care
Memorial Sloan-Kettering Cancer Center
New York, New York

Stephen K. Carter, M.D.
Director, Northern California Cancer Program
Palo Alto, California

Bruce A. Chabner, M.D.
Clinical Pharmacology Branch
Division of Cancer Treatment
National Cancer Institute
National Institutes of Health
Bethesda, Maryland

A. Philippe Chahinian, M.D., F.A.C.P.
Associate Professor
Department of Neoplastic Diseases
Mount Sinai School of Medicine
City University of New York
New York, New York

Constance Cirrincione, M.S.
Department of Biostatistics
Memorial Sloan-Kettering Cancer Center
New York, New York

R. Lee Clark, M.D.
President Emeritus
The University of Texas System Cancer Center
M.D. Anderson Hospital and Tumor Institute
Texas Medical Center
Houston, Texas

Bayard Clarkson, M.D.
Hematology/Lymphoma Service
Department of Medicine
Memorial Sloan-Kettering Cancer Center
New York, New York

G. J. D'Angio, M.D.
Department of Radiation Therapy
The University of Pennsylvania
The Children's Cancer Research Center
Children's Hospital of Philadelphia
Philadelphia, Pennsylvania

Noorbibi K. Day
Head, Laboratory of Complement and Effector Biology
Memorial Sloan-Kettering Cancer Center
New York, New York

Vincent T. DeVita, Jr., M.D.
Acting Director
National Cancer Institute
National Institutes of Health
Bethesda, Maryland

Ross C. Donehower, M.D.
Clinical Pharmacology Branch
Division of Cancer Treatment
National Cancer Institute
National Institutes of Health
Bethesda, Maryland

Monroe Dowling, M.D.
Hematology/Lymphoma Service
Department of Medicine
Memorial Sloan-Kettering Cancer Center
New York, New York

Peggy Dufour, M.A.
Department of Biostatistics
Memorial Sloan-Kettering Cancer Center
New York, New York

Bo Dupont, M.D.
Member and Professor
Human Immunogenetics Section
Memorial Sloan-Kettering Cancer Center
New York, New York

Peter H. Ellims, M.D.
Clinical Pharmacology Branch
Division of Cancer Treatment
National Cancer Institute
National Institutes of Health
Bethesda, Maryland

Gabriel Fernandes, M.D.
Associate, Laboratory of Developmental Immunobiology
Sloan-Kettering Institute for Cancer Research
New York, New York

Isaiah J. Fidler, M.D., Ph.D.
Director, Cancer Metastasis and Treatment Laboratory
Frederick Cancer Research Center
National Cancer Institute
National Institutes of Health
Frederick, Maryland

Emil Frei III, M.D.
Director and Physician-in-Chief
Sidney Farber Cancer Institute
Boston, Massachusetts

Emil J Freireich, M.D.
Department of Developmental Therapeutics
The University of Texas System Cancer Center
M.D. Anderson Hospital and Tumor Institute
Houston, Texas

Timothy Gee, M.D.
Hematology/Lymphoma Service
Department of Medicine
Memorial Sloan-Kettering Cancer Center
New York, New York

Edmund Gehan, Ph.D.
Department of Biomathematics
The University of Texas System Cancer Center
Houston, Texas

Arvin S. Glicksman, M.D.
Department of Radiation Oncology
Rhode Island Hospital and
Section of Radiation Medicine
Brown University
Providence, Rhode Island

Robert B. Golbey, M.D.
Chief, Solid Tumor Service
Memorial Sloan-Kettering Cancer Center
New York, New York

Robert A. Good, M.D., Ph.D.
Vice President
Memorial Sloan-Kettering Cancer Center
New York, New York

Alexander A. Green, M.D.
Department of Hematology/Oncology
St. Jude Children's Research Hospital
Memphis, Tennessee

Denman Hammond, M.D.
Director, Kenneth Norris, Jr., Cancer Research Institute
Comprehensive Cancer Center
University of Southern California and
Chairman, Children's Cancer Study Group
Los Angeles, California

John A. Hansen, M.D.
Associate Professor
Division of Oncology
Department of Medicine, University of Wisconsin
Puget Sound Blood Center
The Fred Hutchinson Cancer Research Center
Seattle, Washington

F. Ann Hayes, M.D.
Department of Hematology/Oncology
St. Jude Children's Research Hospital
Memphis, Tennessee

Jane E. Henney, M.D.
National Cancer Institute
National Institutes of Health
Bethesda, Maryland

W. Michael Hogan, M.D.
Medicine Branch
National Cancer Institute
National Institutes of Health
Bethesda, Maryland

James F. Holland, M.D.
Professor and Chairman
Department of Neoplastic Diseases
Mount Sinai Medical Center
New York, New York

Jimmie C. Holland, M.D.
Chief, Psychiatry Service
Department of Neurology
Memorial Sloan-Kettering Cancer Center
New York, New York

Susan M. Hubbard, M.D.
National Cancer Institute
National Institutes of Health
Bethesda, Maryland

Claude Jacquillat, M.D.
Institut de Recherches sur les Leucémies et les Maladies du Sang
Hopital Saint-Louis
Paris, France

Derek Jenkin, M.D.
Children's Cancer Study Group
Los Angeles, California

Stephen E. Jones, M.D.
Professor of Medicine
Chief, Section of Hematology-Oncology
University of Arizona Cancer Center
Tucson, Arizona

Herbert Kaizer, M.D.
Johns Hopkins University Oncology Center
Baltimore, Maryland

Henry S. Kaplan, M.D.
Maureen Lyles D'Ambrogio Professor of Radiology
Director, Cancer Biology Research Laboratory
Department of Radiology
Stanford University Medical Center
Stanford, California

Neena Kapoor, M.D.
Memorial Sloan-Kettering Cancer Center
New York, New York

Michael Keating, M.D.
Department of Developmental Therapeutics
The University of Texas System Cancer Center
Houston, Texas

Sanford Kempin, M.D.
Hematology/Lymphoma Service
Department of Medicine
Memorial Sloan-Kettering Cancer Center
New York, New York

Irwin H. Krakoff, M.D.
Director, Vermont Regional Cancer Center
University of Vermont
Burlington, Vermont

Awtar Krishan, M.D.
Professor and Chief
Division of Cytokinetics
Comprehensive Cancer Center for the State of Florida
University of Miami School of Medicine
Miami, Florida

Ti Li Loo, Ph.D.
Professor of Therapeutics
Chief, Pharmacology Branch
Department of Developmental Therapeutics
M.D. Anderson Hospital and Tumor Institute
Houston, Texas

Lawrence G. Lum, M.D.
Assistant Professor of Pediatrics
Division of Oncology
University of Washington School of Medicine
Fred Hutchinson Cancer Research Center
Seattle, Washington

Linda S. Martin, R.N.
The University of Texas System Cancer Center
M.D. Anderson Hospital and Tumor Institute
Houston, Texas

Paul J. Martin, M.D.
Associate in Medical Oncology
University of Washington
Fred Hutchinson Cancer Research Center
Seattle, Washington

Alvin M. Mauer, M.D.
Director, St. Jude Children's Research Hospital
Memphis, Tennessee

Harold M. Maurer, M.D.
Professor and Chairman
Department of Pediatrics
Medical College of Virginia
Virginia Commonwealth University
Richmond, Virginia

Kenneth B. McCredie, M.D.
Department of Developmental Therapeutics
The University of Texas System Cancer Center
M.D. Anderson Hospital and Tumor Institute
Houston, Texas

Robert J. McKenna, M.D.
Clinical Professor of Surgery, USC
Director of Regional Activities
LAC-USC Comprehensive Cancer Center
Los Angeles, California

Roland Mertelsmann, M.D.
Hematology/Lymphoma Service
Department of Medicine
Memorial Sloan-Kettering Cancer Center
New York, New York

E. Mihich, M.D.
Director, Grace Cancer Drug Center, and
Department of Experimental Therapeutics
Roswell Park Memorial Institute
Buffalo, New York

Denis R. Miller, M.D.
Enid A. Haupt Professor and Chairman
Department of Pediatrics
Memorial Sloan-Kettering Cancer Center
New York, New York

John A. Montgomery, Ph.D.
Vice President
Southern Research Institute
Birmingham, Alabama

John Neefe, M.D.
Assistant Professor of Medicine
Georgetown University School of Medicine
Washington, D.C.

Richard J. O'Reilly, M.D.
Director, Marrow Transplantation Program
Memorial Sloan-Kettering Cancer Center
New York, New York

Joseph T. Painter, M.D.
Vice President and Professor of Medicine
The University of Texas System Cancer Center
M.D. Anderson Hospital and Tumor Institute
Houston, Texas

Thomas Pajak, Ph.D.
Cancer and Leukemia Group B
Scarsdale, New York

H. M. Pinedo, M.D.
Head, Division of Biochemical Pharmacology
Head, Department of Oncology
Netherlands Cancer Institute and Free University Hospital
Amsterdam, The Netherlands

George Poste, M.D.
Principal Cancer Research Scientist
Department of Experimental Pathology
Roswell Park Memorial Institute
Buffalo, New York

Yair Reisner, Ph.D.
Memorial Sloan-Kettering Cancer Center
New York, New York

Victorio Rodriguez, M.D.
The University of Texas System Cancer Center
M.D. Anderson Hospital and Tumor Institute
Houston, Texas

Hon. Paul G. Rogers
Hogan and Hartson
Washington, D.C.

Gerald Rosen, M.D.
Attending Physician
Departments of Pediatrics and Medicine
Memorial Sloan-Kettering Cancer Center
New York, New York

Saul A. Rosenberg, M.D.
Professor of Medicine and Radiology
Stanford University
Stanford, California

Sydney E. Salmon, M.D.
Professor of Medicine
Director, Cancer Center
University of Arizona
Tucson, Arizona

George W. Santos, M.D.
Professor of Oncology and Medicine
Johns Hopkins University Oncology Center
Baltimore, Maryland

F. M. Schabel, Jr., M.D.
Director, Chemotherapy Research
Southern Research Institute
Birmingham, Alabama

Peter Schauer, M.D.
Hematology/Lymphoma Service
Department of Medicine
Memorial Sloan-Kettering Cancer Center
New York, New York

Philip S. Schein, M.D.
Professor of Medicine and Pharmacology
Georgetown University School of Medicine
Vincent T. Lombardi Cancer Research Center
Washington, D.C.

William R. Shapiro, M.D.
Head, George C. Cotzias Laboratory of Neuro-oncology
Memorial Sloan-Kettering Cancer Center
New York, New York

Paul Sherlock, M.D.
Memorial Sloan-Kettering Cancer Center
New York, New York

Maurice E. Shils, M.D., D. Sc.
Director, Clinical Nutrition
Attending Physician, Department of Medicine
Memorial Sloan-Kettering Cancer Center and
Professor of Medicine
Cornell University Medical College
New York, New York

Stuart E. Siegal, M.D.
Head, Division of Hematology-Oncology
Children's Hospital of Los Angeles and
Associate Professor of Pediatrics
University of Southern California School of Medicine
Children's Cancer Study Group
Los Angeles, California

Frederick P. Smith, M.D.
Assistant Professor of Medicine
Georgetown University School of Medicine
Washington, D.C.

Rainer Storb, M.D.
Professor of Medicine
Division of Oncology
University of Washington School of Medicine
Fred Hutchinson Cancer Research Center
Seattle, Washington

Keith M. Sullivan, M.D.
Assistant Professor of Medicine
Division of Oncology
University of Washington School of Medicine
Fred Hutchinson Cancer Research Center
Seattle, Washington

H. J. Tagnon, M.D.
Emeritus Professor of Medicine and Oncology
University of Brussels Medical School and
Former Chief of Clinical Investigation
Institut Jules Bordet and
Past President, E.O.R.T.C.
Brussels, Belgium

E. Donnall Thomas, M.D.
Professor and Head
Division of Oncology
Department of Medicine
University of Washington School of Medicine
Fred Hutchinson Cancer Research Center
Seattle, Washington

Tsoi Mang-so, M.D.
Research Associate Professor of Medicine
Division of Oncology
University of Washington School of Medicine
Fred Hutchinson Cancer Research Center
Seattle, Washington

Pinuccia Valagussa, B.S.
Consultant Statistician
Istituto Nazionale Tumori
Milan, Italy

Manuel Valdivieso, M.D.
The University of Texas System Cancer Center
M.D. Anderson Hospital and Tumor Institute
Houston, Texas

Umberto Veronesi, M.D.
Chairman, World Health Organization International Melanoma Group
General Director
Istituto Nazionale Tumori
Milan, Italy

Paul L. Weiden, M.D.
Associate Professor of Medicine
Division of Oncology
University of Washington School of Medicine
Fred Hutchinson Cancer Research Center
Seattle, Washington

Marise Weil, M.D.
Institut de Recherches sur les Leucémies et les Maladies du Sang
Hopital Saint-Louis
Paris, France

Jack Wilson, M.D.
Children's Cancer Study Group
Los Angeles, California

Robert P. Witherspoon, M.D.
Assistant Professor of Medicine
Division of Oncology
University of Washington School of Medicine
Fred Hutchinson Cancer Research Center
Seattle, Washington

Steven S. Witkin, M.D.
Associate, Laboratory of Complement and Effector Biology
Memorial Sloan-Kettering Cancer Center
New York, New York

Robert E. Wittes, M.D.
Associate Attending Physician
Solid Tumor Service
Department of Medicine
Memorial Sloan-Kettering Cancer Center
New York, New York

Paul V. Woolley III, M.D.
Associate Professor of Medicine and Pharmacology
Georgetown University School of Medicine
Washington, D.C.

Alan Yagoda, M.D.
Associate Attending Physician
Department of Medicine
Memorial Sloan-Kettering Cancer Center
New York, New York

Omar C. Yoder, Ph.D.
Division of Cancer Treatment
National Cancer Institute
National Institutes of Health
Bethesda, Maryland

Charles W. Young, M.D.
Chief, Developmental Chemotherapy Service
Department of Medicine
Memorial Sloan-Kettering Cancer Center
New York, New York

Robert C. Young, M.D.
Medicine Branch
National Cancer Institute
National Institutes of Health
Bethesda, Maryland

C. Gordon Zubrod, M.D.
Director, Comprehensive Cancer Center of the State of Florida
University of Miami School of Medicine
Miami, Florida

Developmental Therapy

Development of Anti-Cancer Therapy

C. Gordon Zubrod

Director
Comprehensive Cancer Center of the State of Florida
University of Miami School of Medicine
Miami, Florida

The determination to cure cancer is a goal of society that dates back to the beginnings of medical history(27). After 3500 years, the average cure rate is 41%(9) -- an improvement of about 1% every hundred years. Because almost all of the cures have been effected in the last 100 years, the rate of improvement is really 1% every 2½ years and there is evidence that the pace quickens(9). Everyone recognizes that prevention of cancer is a much more desirable goal than the treatment of established disease. The inability of society to eliminate cigarette smoking or to alter other circumstances that lead to cancer, means that prevention of cancer is remote. The improved treatment of established cancer will therefore remain a goal of high priority for at least several generations. It is my purpose to trace the evolution of anti-cancer therapy, to provide a setting for the remaining 2½ days of our program in which our speakers will review the evidence for the accelerating rate of cancer cures. Improvement in cancer treatment was based upon changing concepts of the pathogenesis of cancer, and I hope to show the influence of concept to treatment of the past and present, and then to use emerging perceptions of cancer pathogenesis to guess at the therapeutic strategy of tomorrow.

Until fairly recently, most cancers were thought to be localized diseases that metastasized only after the tumor had grown to a rather large size. Early attempts at cure were based on simple surgical removal of the tumor. Beginning about a hundred years ago, the concept of local tissue spread followed by lymphatic invasion and trapping of tumor cells in regional lymph nodes led to en bloc dissection for cancers of the breast, rectum, head and neck, and for melanomas(32). Spread to distant organs by way of the blood was thought to be delayed for a considerable period. Failures were considered as resulting from inadequate surgery, and super-radical surgery developed for cancer of the pancreas, stomach, breast, and lower extremities and pelvic areas(32).

With the discovery of the curative effects of ionizing radiation for skin cancer in 1899, another modality for local treatment became available, and by the 1920's, experience and radiation biology theory had sufficiently developed to show five-year survivals for head and neck cancers(17). Megavoltage and many refinements in dosage techniques led to the ability to treat a local tumor and its regional tissues and lymph nodes, much in the style of en bloc resection. In the lymphomas which, even when they advance beyond the regional area, often stay within the lymphatic system, cures of fairly wide-spread disease by total lymph node irradiation became common.

The concept of cancer as a localized/regional disease and the use of modern surgery and/or radiation to rid the body of the regionally contained cancer have certainly led to the cure of many patients. However, even when the surgeon and the radiation oncologist have done their best in patients who seem to have localized/regional disease, many patients die of metastatic cancer. A measure of the present failure rate for some of the common carcinomas is shown in Table I.

TABLE I
Early Hematogenous Spread Of The Common Carcinomas
As Roughly Estimated From Failure Rates* Of
Current (Local/Regional) Therapy

Cancer	New Cases	Deaths	% Failures
LUNG	117,000	101,000	86
STOMACH	23,000	14,000	60
COLO-RECTAL	114,000	53,000	47
BREAST	108,000	36,000	33

*Calculated from Cancer Facts and Figures 1980, American Cancer Society.

This failure rate is a rough approximation of the degree to which cancer is not a localized/regional disease at the time of diagnosis. The flaw in this concept of regional lymphatic containment began to be recognized in the mid-1950's, when tumor cells were demonstrated in the circulating blood(12). Animal studies of drugs given very briefly during and after surgery suggested that such adjuvant chemotherapy could prevent surgically induced hematogenous spread,(8,2,26) but clinical application through the early 1960's was ineffective. Gradually the concept gained acceptance, that hematogenous spread early in the course of many tumors was part of the natural history of cancer(20). This meant that even though many tumors seemed to be contained in their region of origin, there existed clinically inapparent micrometastases in distant organs. Thus, no matter how complete the loco-regional eradication, many patients would still die because their cancers had become systemic, early in their growth history. Thus by the late 1950's the concept that many cancers were metastatic early in their course required that they be treated not only loco-regionally, but also with drugs that could reach and kill all tumor cells in the body

Drugs that could cause remission of clinical cancer have been known for at least two millenia(7). It was not until the 1940's that the highly active drugs, nitrogen mustard, antifolates and cortisone, were discovered(36). Although these and most other anti-tumor agents became of biologic interest for reasons other than their effects on cancer, it was their high activity in rodent tumors that led to their trial in man. Their effects were first demonstrated in cancers that were unquestionably systemic -- the lymphomas and the acute leukemias. Trials in the solid tumors showed much less dramatic effects than in the hematologic neoplasms. Because of the important role of mouse tumors in signalling activity in man, the techniques of chemotherapeutic screening developed in the 1930's by Boyland, Furth, Lettré, and Yoshida were made part of combined experimental-clinical efforts by Haddow, Shear, Yoshida and Gellhorn, and especially by Rhoads and Farber and their colleagues(34). Arrangements were made to receive new drugs from industrial and university sources, but it soon became apparent that in order to develop new agents a more systematic scheme was needed. Pharmaceutical houses had helped with these early efforts, but because of the then perceived limited usefulness of anti-tumor drugs, development was not economically feasible within the industry. In 1952, the National Advisory Cancer Council began discussing these problems, and they too decided it unwise to support drug development. In 1954 Congress directed NCI to start a program and in the following year the Cancer Chemotherapy National Service Center (CCNSC) was born. Over a period of ten years, NCI with the help of many scientists from the scientific community and from industry, gradually set in motion all the elements of a drug development program -- screening, toxicology, pharmacology, formulation, clinical trials and supportive care. Its purpose was not so much the discovery of new drugs, but the quantitative evaluation of candidate anti-cancer agents. The major contribution of the first ten years was two-fold: the development of the clinical trial and of the backup for moving drugs active in mouse systems into trial. In the mid-1960's the CCNSC was merged with relevant intramural activities in chemotherapy in order to use the growing availability of active drugs and knowledge of chemotherapeutic principles to bring about drug cures.

Although highly active drugs first became recognized in the 1940's, it was not until the late 1950's that it was shown that systemic cancer could be cured by drugs. In 1956, Li, Hertz and Spencer began their studies of methotrexate in metastatic choriocarcinoma(18). Although it seemed apparent to those on the scene that a new era had arrived, the claim of cure was received sceptically, but by 1962 there was no doubt of the significance(16). It is a little ironic that after the intense interest in the chemotherapy of the acute leukemias since 1947, the cure of systemic cancer should first be demonstrated in a solid tumor. The implications were not lost, and in 1962 NCI founded the Acute Leukemia Task Force, which, working in concert with cooperative groups and the Southern Research Institute and many other scientists laid out a curative strategy for acute lymphocytic leukemia(36). The key observations were beautifully quantitative trials by Leukemia B(13), the VAMP program of Freireich, Frei and Karon(14), and the treatment of CNS leukemia by Pinkel and his colleagues at St. Jude(1).

A number of basic principles of drug cure came out of the experience with acute leukemia, and these were applied widely to other tumors. I do not wish to steal the thunder of later speakers, but it is essential to my theme to point out that about a dozen cancers can be cured because of the ability of drugs to get rid of systemic cancer(35). It is also necessary to recognize that all of these cancers occur in young people and are characterized by rapid growth. This rapid growth is due to the high percentage of cancer cells that are dividing(21,29). In turn, this high growth fraction is one of the main determinants making these tumors so drug susceptible. The Acute Leukemia Task Force used the data of cell population kinetics in devising curative regimens. The attempts during the 1970's to apply cell kinetic theory to the treatment of the slowly growing common carcinomas was a vast disappointment.

By the mid 1960's, the two conceptual threads of this story were woven together. The need for systemic treatment of micrometastases met up with the proof of the concept that drugs could cure metastases. This principle was quickly applied to Wilms' tumor by both Leukemia groups, and by 1968 shown to be spectacularly effective(4,33). However, this was accomplished in a high growth fraction tumor, so drug sensitive that even clinically apparent metastatic disease could be cured. Some hope that a common slowly growing tumor could yield to adjuvant chemotherapy now emerged. In 1968 Dr. Bernie Fisher and his colleagues published a 10 year followup of the 1957 study of breast cancer based on the chemotherapy of cells supposedly spread hematogenously by the surgeon and showed a slight but significant survival in those receiving 3 days of thiotepa (11). A rigorous experimental examination at the Southern Research Institute of the principles involved gave great encouragement. Linda Simpson-Herren and colleagues showed that micrometastases had kinetic features making them highly susceptible to drugs(28). Frank Schabel demonstrated in many animal models that high cure rates of the micrometastases could be obtained by surgery plus post-operative chemotherapy(25). Long, Donegan and Evans in 1962 began studies of adjuvant thiotepa given for 7 months following radical mastectomy(19). Nissen-Meyer and his colleagues in Scandinavia undertook in 1965 a study of the effects of one course of cyclophosphamide on breast cancer(23). In the early 1960's Paul Carbone was treating breast cancer with prolonged post-operative 5-fluorouracil and phenylalanine mustard in a small pilot study. His discussions with both Bernie Fisher and Gianni Bonadonna led to their classic adjuvant trials in breast

cancer(2,10). Dr. Bonadonna will speak to these areas in
detail, so I shall only say that at this time his study
and that of Nissen-Meyer both show significant increases
in percent of patients surviving at five and ten years
respectively. So both the theory of drug treatment of
micrometastases, and its application to this one common
carcinoma give hope that systemic disease can be cured
when drugs are given for a prolonged period after surgery.
In some situations, at least, preoperative chemotherapy
might provide the further advantage of slightly earlier
drug treatment of the systemic disease(24). The extension
of such adjuvant chemotherapy to other types of the common
carcinomas has the difficulty that, to be effective, the
drug regimen must be highly active, and at the present
time disease such as cancers of gastrointestinal tract,
lung, head and neck, and cervix, are insufficiently drug
susceptible to predicate cure of micrometastases(5,35).
      The goal for the future of adjuvant chemotherapy of
the common carcinomas must be the discovery of more active
drugs and the use of known drugs more efficiently. The
inability to cure 100% of the highly drug sensitive
cancers of the young also calls for better drugs or drug
regimens. Although a majority of these rapidly growing
cancers are cured, there is still a substantial proportion
who die of their cancer, and this calls attention to a new
concept of cancer that will alter future management.
Clinical trials demonstrating cures of the rapidly growing
tumors of the young were based on histologic similarities
of the tumors included in the study. Actually, these
tumors are very heterogeneous mixtures. The ability to
study surface antigens of cancer cells, through the
techniques provided by hybridomas and their monoclonal
antibodies, has shown how mixed a bag are such diseases as
"acute lymphocytic leukemia"(6) or "histiocytic
lymphoma"(3). And of course refinements in histologic
classification give rise to even more complex
heterogeneity(31). So when we are looking at drug
sensitivity, we must ask how curable is a specific subset
within the heterogeneous mixture thrown together by the
inadequacies of morphology. Of course future drug trials
must be reorganized so that they are based upon the anti-
genically diagnosed subsets. And what of the animal
screens? Should there not be a one to one match between
the cell type of the mouse and the patient?
      If we assume that eventually all histologic cancer
entities can be redefined in terms of more realistic

antigenic subsets, what then should be the strategy for the future? The objective is the discovery of drug regimens sufficiently active to cure systemic disease whether amongst the young or the old. To date this discovery depends upon the use of mouse tumors for screening and other preclinical studies, and ultimate correlation with clinical trial. This strategy is slow, indirect and imprecise, but as Dr. Schabel will point out, it is the best means we have. The new goal becomes the initial study of drugs and regimens in human tumors that are homogeneous clones. Smith and colleagues(30) and Hamburger and Salmon(15) have made substantial beginnings toward that goal with studies of drug sensitivity in tissue cultures of human tumors in soft agar. While there are many problems, ultimately, I believe, the use of cloned human tumors should replace murine tumors for screening. Similarly, the study of cell kinetics and all the other elements determining the most efficient drug schedules, should take place -- not in a transplanted mouse tumor system, but against the human tumor grown in the athymic mouse. There of course remains the problem of the predictability of animal pharmacokinetics for man, and I think this can be solved only by moving early into pharmacokinetic studies in patients. One would also hope that immunotherapy and hyperthermia would add to the control of systemic cancer, but because they have yet to influence cures, I have omitted them from the discussion.

In summary, then, I have traced the development of cancer treatment by showing its dependence upon the evolution of concepts of cancer pathogenesis. As of today, cancer is thought of as resulting from a transformed cell which doubles itself at varying rates and that remains localized to the site of origin for varying periods. Cells break away from the original clone and soon get into the lymphatics of the regional drainage area. As long as the cells remain thus contained, modern surgery and/or ionizing radiation has a good chance of cure. Once hematogenous spread occurs, and clearly this may happen early in a cancer's growth, curative chemotherapy is required. Chemotherapy has been proved to cure systemic disease but only sometimes; and new concepts of homogeneous subsets and new technical advances give promise of extending these gains to many more patients.

REFERENCES

1. Aur RJA, Simone J, Hustu O, et al.: Central nervous system therapy and combination chemotherapy of childhood lymphocytic leukemia. Blood 37:272-281, 1971.
2. Bonadonna G, Valagussa P, Rossi A, et al.: CMF adjuvant chemotherapy in operable breast cancer. Jones SE, Salmon SE (eds): Adjuvant Therapy of Cancer II. New York, Grune and Stratton, 1979.
3. Brouet JC, Labaume S, Seligmann M: Evaluation of T and B lymphocyte membrane markers in human non-Hodgkin malignant lymphomata. Brit J Cancer 31(suppl 2):121-127, 1975.
4. Burgert EO, Glidewell O: Dactinomycin in Wilms' tumor. J Am Med Assn 199:464-468, 1967.
5. Carter SK, Bakowski MT, Hellman K: Chemotherapy of Cancer. New York, John Wiley and Sons, 1980.
6. Chessells JM, Hardisty RM, Rapson NT, Greaves MF: Actue lymphoblastic leukemia in children: classification and prognosis. Lancet 2:1207-1309, 1977.
7. Creasey WA: Anti-neoplastic and immunosuppressive agents, Sartorelli AC, Johns DG (eds): Handbook of Exp Pharmacology XXXVIII/2. Berlin, Springer-Verlag, 1975, pp 670-694.
8. Cruz EO, McDonald GO, Cole WH: Prophylactic treatment of cancer. The use of chemotherapeutic agents to prevent tumor metastases. Surgery 40: 291-296, 1956.
9. DeVita V, Henney J, Stonehill E: Introduction - Cancer mortality: the good news, in Jones SE, Salmon SE (eds):Adjuvant Therapy of Cancer II. New York, Grune and Stratton, 1979, pp 3-674.
10. Fisher B, Carbone P, Economou SG, et al.: L-phenylalanine mustard in the management of primary breast cancer. A report of early findings. New Eng J Med 292:117-122, 1975.
11. Fisher B, Slack N, Katrych D, et al.: Ten year followup results of patients with carcinoma of breast in a cooperative clinical trial evaluating surgical adjuvant chemotherapy. Surg Gynecol and Obstet 140:528-534, 1975.
12. Fisher DR, Turnbull RB Jr: The cytologic demonstration and significance of tumor cells in the mesenteric venous blood in patients with colorectal carcinoma. Surg Gynecol Obstet 100:102-108, 1955.

13. Frei E III, Freireich EJ, Gehan E, et al.: Studies of sequential and combination anti metabolite therapy in acute leukemia: 6-mercaptopurine and methotrexate. Blood 18:431-454, 1961.
14. Freireich EJ, Karon M, Frei E III: Quadruple combination therapy (VAMP) for acute lymphocytic leukemia of childhood. Proc Am Assoc Cancer Res 5:20(abst), 1964.
15. Hamburger AW, Salmon SE: Primary bioassay of human tumor stem cells. Science 197:461-463, 1977.
16. Hertz R, Lewis L, Lipsett MB: Five years experience with the chemotherapy of metastatic trophoblastic disease in women. Am J Obstet Gynecol 86:808-814, 1963.
17. Kaplan HS: Historic milestones in radiobiology and radiation therapy. Seminars in Oncol 6:479-489, 1979.
18. Li MC, Hertz R, Spencer DB: Effect of methotrexate upon choriocarcinoma and chorioadenema. Proc Soc Exper Biol and Med 93:361-366, 1956.
19. Long RTL, Donegan WL, Evans AM: Extended surgical adjuvant chemotherapy for breast carcinoma. Am J Surg 117;701-704, 1969.
20. Martin DS: An appraisal of chemotherapy as an adjuvant to surgery for cancer. Am J Surg 97:685-686, 1959.
21. Mendelsohn ML: Autoradiographic analysis of cell proliferation in spontaneous breast cancer of C_3H mouse III. The growth fraction. J Natl Cancer Inst 28:1015-1029, 1962.
22. Moore GE, Kondo T: Study of adjuvant chemotherapy by model experiments. Surgery 44:199-209, 1958.
23. Nissen-Meyer R, Kjellgren K, Malmio K, et al.: Surgical adjuvant chemotherapy. Results with one short course with cyclophosphamide after mastectomy for breast cancer. Cancer 41:2088-2098, 1977.
24. Rosen G, Marcove RC, Caparros B, et al.: Primary osteogenic sarcoma: the rationale for preoperative chemotherapy and delayed surgery. Cancer 43:2163-2177, 1979.
25. Schabel FM Jr: Concepts for systemic treatment of micrometastases. Cancer 35:15-24, 1975.
26. Shapiro D, Fugmann RA: A role for chemotherapy as an adjunct to surgery. Cancer Res 17:1098-1101, 1957.

27. Shimkin MB: Contrary to nature. DHEW Publication (NIH) 76-720. Washington DC, US Government Printing Office, 1977, pp 1-498.
28. Simpson-Herren L, Sanford AH, Holmquist JP: Cell population kinetics of transplanted and metastatic Lewis lung cancer. Cell Tissue Kinetics 7:349-361, 1974.
29. Skipper HE, Schabel FM Jr, Wilcox WS: Experimental evaluation of potential anti cancer agents. XIII. On the criteria and kinetics associated with the "curability" of experimental leukemia. Cancer Chemotherapy Repts 35:3-111, 1964.
30. Smith IE, Courtenay VD, Gordon MY: A colony forming assay for human tumour xenografts using agar in diffusion chambers. Brit J Cancer 34:476-483, 1976.
31. Strauchen JA, Young RC, DeVita VT Jr, et al.: Clinical relevance of the histopatholgoical subclassification of diffuse "histiocytic" lymphoma. N Engl J Med 299:1382-1387, 1978.
32. Sugarbaker EV, Ketcham AS, Zubrod CG: Interdisciplinary cancer therapy. Current Prob in Surg 14(6): 3-69, 1977.
33. Wolff J, Krivit W, Newton WA jr, et al.: Single versus multiple dose dactinomycin therapy of Wilms' tumor. New Eng J Med 279:290-294, 1968.
34. Zubrod CG, Schepartz S, Leiter J, et al.: The chemotherapy program of the National Cancer Institute: history, analysis and plans. Cancer Chmotherapy Report 50:349-550, 1966.
35. Zubrod CG: Selective toxicity of anticancer drugs: Presidential address. Cancer Res 38:4377-4384, 1978.
36. Zubrod, CG: Historic milestones in curative chemotherapy. Seminars in Oncology 6:490-505, 1979.

Laboratory Methods for the Detection and Development of Clinically Useful Anticancer Drugs

F. M. SCHABEL, JR.

Director
Chemotherapy Research
Southern Research Institute
Birmingham, Alabama 35255

INTRODUCTION

Excluding hormonal agents, 39 anticancer drugs useful in treating cancer patients are now commercially available and 60 more are in various stages of clinical trials.[8] Animal tumors responsive to these drugs are well known. More than 100 different spontaneous or transplantable tumors of laboratory animals (primarily mice and rats) have been or are being used in different laboratories around the world to detect and develop currently available useful drugs.[30] None of these animal tumors has been shown to respond to treatment with all of the anticancer drugs useful in man and each animal tumor, when treated with drugs useful in man, has a variable treatment response correlation with one or more human tumors and an unknown response correlation with drugs that have been reported to be inactive against these animal tumor(s) but not tested against human tumors. Additionally, all human tumors do not respond to all clinically useful drugs. There are both quantitatively and qualitatively variable response rates of human tumors, of the same histologic

*Work from Southern Research Institute reported herein was supported by Contracts NO1-CM-43756 and NO1-CM-97309 from the Division of Cancer Treatment and Grant CA17303 from the National Large Bowel Cancer Project, National Cancer Institute, National Institutes of Health, Department of Health and Human Services, U.S.A.

11

type and disease staging, to treatment with clinically useful drugs. Therefore, even human tumors with apparently similar natural history up to clinical presentation are often unreliable predictors of the drug response of apparently similar human tumors.

Although man and laboratory mammals have much in common, e.g., they have vital organs that are histologically similar and that carry out the same or very similar kinds of basic anabolic and catabolic metabolism, there are many recognized and probably many unrecognized metabolic (enzymatic and biochemical) and pharmacologic differences between man and laboratory animals that doubtless influence drug metabolism (e.g., activation, degradation), and pharmacokinetics (plasma half-life, excretion rates, etc.) and, hence, anticancer activity.

Both laboratory and clinical oncologists and chemotherapists engaged in searches for and development of new anticancer drugs should always remember two facts: (1) no animal tumor system has been objectively demonstrated to be a reliable predictor for the drug response of any human tumor but (2) with few exceptions up to the present time, the acceptance of a new drug as a candidate for trial in human cancer patients has awaited the demonstration of its selective cytotoxicity for tumor cells over vital normal cells in intact, tumor-bearing experimental animals.

POSSIBLE REASONS FOR POOR DRUG ACTIVITY CORRELATION BETWEEN TUMORS IN MAN AND ANIMALS

Experimental cancer chemotherapists have often been accused of misleading clinical oncologists because they claimed anticancer activity for drugs in experimental tumor systems that was not demonstrable when these drugs were used in human cancer patients. There are many possible-to-probable reasons for this lack of demonstrated positive correlation in drug sensitivity of transplantable tumors in experimental animals and naturally occurring tumors in man. Important among these are:

(1) No common etiology between any animal and human tumor(s) has been objectively demonstrated. The greatest success in the use of animal models for the detection and development to clinical utility of chemotherapeutic agents has been with infectious diseases (bacterial, protozoal, and viral). This is due, in the main, to common etiology of these diseases in man and in the usefully predictive animal models used.

(2) With the possible exception of a requirement for asparagine by a limited number of human leukemias[27] and one subline of a transplantable murine leukemia (L5178Y),[3] no unequivocal data establishing the presence of different vital biochemical pathways in tumor cells as compared to vital normal cells in man or animals have been reported. Therefore, a biochemical basis for selecting any animal tumor, irrespective of histologic similarity, as a logical

and likely positive biochemical predictor for the drug response of any human tumor is not available.

(3) Human tumors are usually far advanced in their natural history from origin to host death when first detected and, at least to this time, relatively few experimental chemotherapy studies with advanced and grossly evident animal tumors have been reported. Very extensive and available laboratory data clearly indicate that the therapeutic (cytotoxic) activity of many, if not most, anticancer drugs is much less against large body burdens than against small body burdens of the same tumor cells, particularly solid tumors, in the same laboratory animals. At least some of the likely reasons for this usually observed tumor-mass:drug-sensitivity relationship are well recognized; e.g., (a) the growth fraction (GF)* in a given tumor site decreases as tumor mass increases and most antimetabolite anticancer drugs kill only those drug-sensitive tumor cells that they reach in lethal concentration when the cells are in the drug-sensitive phase of the cell cycle and (b) the distance to the nearest capillary or blood source of nutrients or drugs increases for a progressively larger fraction of the viable (clonogenic) tumor cells as the tumor mass increases. An otherwise cytotoxic drug, cell cycle specific or not, will not kill a tumor cell it cannot reach in lethal concentration. It follows, therefore, that at least some of the lack of positive correlation of drug response of animal tumors and human tumors may be due to vascular and mass differences as well as the total body burden of viable tumor cells at the time of drug treatment in drug-sensitive animal tumors and drug-insensitive human tumors.

(4) In the main, active anticancer agents have steep dose-response curves in tumor-bearing experimental animals and in man, and the laboratory investigator can and does employ drug doses up to the LD_{10}. Drug treatment of human tumors, even by clinical study groups, escalates drug doses up to similar toxicity with indicated caution and care; and it is likely with many experimentally active drugs, and obvious with others, that physiologically and pharmacologically similar drug doses have not been used against both the reported drug-sensitive animal tumors and the target human tumors.

(5) The last, and probably most important, reason for the lack of clearly established positive correlation between claimed response to drug treatment of animal tumors and human tumors is probably little more than semantic. Up to the present time, anticancer drug activity has had a different meaning to laboratory oncologists and clinical oncologists. In drug treatment of human leukemias, the minimum requirement for reporting clinical activity is a > 50% reduction in leukemic cells in the bone marrow.

---

*GF is the fraction of the total viable (clonogenic) tumor cell population that is in the active cell division cycle at a given point in time.

Usually this will not result in increased duration of life. To obtain normal cell counts in the peripheral blood and significant increase in duration of life usually requires >90% reduction in leukemic cells in the marrow and "cure" may require reduction in the body burden of tumor cells of as much as 11 orders of magnitude (kill of 100 billion tumor cells).[10] In humans with solid tumors, >50% reduction of measurable tumor volume is the minimal effect required to report drug activity. Until quite recently, anticancer drug activity of this magnitude was seldom seen or reported by treatment of experimental solid tumors in the laboratory. Laboratory workers have usually reported anticancer drugs as being active and, therefore, effective by inference, if the drug treatment increased the life span of leukemic mice by $\geq 25\%$ (a 25% increase in life span often correlates with a 100-fold increase in body burden of tumor cells[22]) or held growth of solid tumors under treatment to $\leq 50\%$ of that of untreated controls. To further compound the lack of communication, the body burden of viable tumor cells at start of drug treatment of experimental leukemias in the laboratory has seldom exceeded 10^5 to 10^6 and the body burden of in vivo clonogenic solid tumor cells at start of drug treatment in the laboratory often is about 10^3. The medical oncologist, on the other hand, begins treatment of human patients with clinically evident solid tumors when the body burden of tumor cells is at least $>10^8$ and may approach 10^{10} to 10^{11}. While the percent of viable clonogenic tumor cells in these human tumors is unknown, it could be, and in some cases probably is, high. In any event, advanced cancer is usually treated in man, and early and grossly inapparent disease is usually treated in experimental animals. Complete inhibition of tumor growth under treatment of either leukemias or solid tumors would be negative to the clinician, since an actual reduction of >90% of leukemic cells in the marrow or reduction of solid tumor masses of >50% is necessary before objectively established activity by drug treatment is considered to have been demonstrated. As a result, what the laboratory worker has called an "active" anticancer drug in experimental animals has often failed when tested against clinically recognized tumors in man.

It would be surprising if positive correlation between drug response of human cancer and animal models of human cancer should occur under these circumstances since such different tumor staging, drug doses, and activity endpoints are commonly used in the laboratory and the clinic. Effective drug treatment of systemic cancer is the goal of the medical oncologist, and I assume it is the goal of the experimental cancer chemotherapist. If so, it is incumbent upon the laboratory investigator to define his criteria for anticancer activity in the laboratory to the medical oncologist. If we are to attempt to make meaningful and reliable comparisons between therapeutic activity of anticancer drugs in animals and man, we must use the same endpoints for measuring activity. For example, laboratory data on drug activity should be interpreted to indicate in reliable and reproducible quantitative terms, whether the clonogenic tumor cell population increased, was static, or decreased under drug treatment. Laboratory oncologists have been in a position to make such therapeutic response evaluations with experimental leukemias and solid tumors for many years, but they usually have not done so, and, as a result, they have suffered the well-earned and to-be-expected reputation of giving medical oncologists experimental data of limited value. We cannot at present objectively approach the reasons for lack of positive correlation between drug response of animal and human tumors cited in (1) and (2) above, but (3) and (5) can and are being directly approached by some experimental cancer chemotherapists and (4) is getting increased attention and effective application by an increasing number of medical oncologists.

SEARCHES FOR NEW ANTICANCER AGENTS - SCREENING

In Vitro Screens

Searches for new anticancer drugs using tumor cells growing in culture have been used for many years and continue to be used. The greatest limitation of in vitro screens is that they contain no vital normal cell component with which to relate comparative cytotoxicity to the tumor cells. Drug doses used in vitro must be estimated from likely plasma drug levels at maximum tolerated doses in man or animals and the duration of drug exposure to be used in vitro must be estimated from only very limited knowledge of the half-life of most clinically useful drugs in the plasma, or at the tumor cell surface, in man and/or animals. Also, tumor cell cultures generally have a much higher GF than do the tumors of origin, particularly if the tumors are treated in either animals or man after they have become grossly evident or have presented clinically. Therefore, the growth kinetics of the tumor cell population, so important in determining therapeutic response of most tumors to all anticancer drugs and especially to antimetabolite drugs, is seldom similar in vitro and in the intact host. Last, but also of very great importance, cell cultures have no liver, kidneys, and/or other functional organs that are necessary to activate some, degrade others, and excrete most, if not all, useful anticancer drugs. Thus, it is impossible to effectively model the complex physiology and pharmacology of the intact tumor-bearing animal, including man, in any in vitro system. Cell culture systems will generally overestimate the cytotoxic activity of drugs that do not need to be activated to be cytotoxic and probably will miss those that do need to be activated, e.g., cyclophosphamide. For these reasons, tumor cell culture screens are of limited utility. They usually require less drug, but not appreciably less money.

Salmon and coworkers are undertaking screening for new anticancer agents using primary in vitro cultures of human tumor cells
from patients.[5] This is an important investigative activity that is
just beginning. If human tumor cells in primary culture will select
more and better clinically useful drugs than have the established
human tumor cells in vitro or animal tumors in vitro or in vivo that
have been used to this time, then a major advance in screening for
new anticancer drugs will have been made.

Drug Selection for Therapy

The use of primary cultures of human tumor cells exposed to
currently available anticancer drugs, in attempts to make pretreatment selection of optimally active drugs against a patient's own
tumor (as is commonly and effectively done in determining antibiotic sensitivity of pathogenic bacteria cultured from the infected
patient, e.g., the Bauer-Kirby procedure), is being investigated by
Salmon and associates[16] and by Von Hoff, Rosenblum, and others.[14]
One of the more interesting biological observations with these in
vitro human tumor cloning systems has been the marked
heterogeneity of response to clinically useful drugs, even among
cells from histologically similar tumors.

I will not discuss this work further here, since Dr. Salmon is
presenting it at this meeting. It goes without saying, however, that
such investigations are clearly indicated since they hold the
promise of enabling the clinician to select specific and active
drug(s) for use in individual tumor patients with systemic cancer
requiring drug treatment.

In Vivo Screens

As noted above, no animal tumor model nor, in fact, any human
tumor has been objectively demonstrated to reliably predict for the
drug response of any human tumor. That fact notwithstanding,
with few exceptions up to the present time, the acceptance of a
new drug as a candidate for trial in human cancer patients has
awaited the demonstration of its selective cytotoxicity for tumor
cells over vital normal cells in intact tumor-bearing experimental
animals.

The selection of in vivo tumor systems for screening for anticancer drugs has been and remains a highly controversial matter.
Having observed the process and participated in both the selection
and application of animal tumors for use as detection screens for
candidate anticancer drugs over the past 30 years, I can only
conclude that there are nearly as many opinions as participants. In
the United States, we have had a continuously changing spectrum
of animal tumors in our primary in vivo screens. Each new director
responsible for conducting the large primary screening program of
the National Cancer Institute (NCI), intent upon using the screening system(s) that would most effectively select the largest number

of ultimately useful anticancer drugs, has made changes in the tumor systems and testing procedures of his predecessors, always, I'm sure, after considering the recommendations of the most experienced and critical experts from within the NCI and the research community outside the NCI. This type of change in screening models and methods has been indicated. It is the essence of research in drug development, particularly if empirical screening is involved, to find and establish better methods to accomplish our purpose(s). Tumor models for screening are research tools and, if the tools we are using are not enabling us to do the best job, we had better look for better tools.

Everyone in the world who is seeking better anticancer drugs is looking for better model systems to detect them. That there is no concensus among experimental cancer chemotherapists throughout the world regarding the best screening models is documented by the compilation of the tumor models being used in 1975 to screen for and develop new anticancer drugs in the 16 countries in the world most active in this effort.[30] Over 100 different tumors of laboratory rodents were listed with only a limited overlap of commonly used tumors.

A number of laboratories throughout the world are now investigating the possibility that human tumor xenografts growing in athymic "nude" or immune-deprived mice may be better predictors of the drug response of histologically similar human tumors than animal models of human tumors. This idea is not new. It was investigated in depth about 25 years ago,[26] but without ultimate practical application. Since Dr. Krishan will be discussing human tumor xenografts, I won't discuss them further here. Whether the current models of this earlier concept will be more useful than those of 25 years ago remains to be determined. Some reasons for possible failure of human tumor xenografts in athymic "nude" mice to predict for the drug sensitivity of other histologically similar human tumors have recently been clearly stated by Giovanella:[11]

1. Anticancer drug activity in human patients is influenced by the pharmacology of the drug (plasma half-life, activation, degradation, excretion, etc.) in the patient. Human tumors growing in the athymic "nude" mouse have a mouse stroma and the metabolism of the host mouse, not of a human, and especially not of the donor (source) of the human tumor.
2. Assuming that human tumors heterotransplanted into athymic "nude" mice are identical to the corresponding tumor in the human donor in terms of sensitivity to drugs, screening with it for new clinically useful drugs or using it to predict sensitivity to available drugs will have a positive predictive correlation directly related to the percentage of human tumors of that histologic type that respond to treatment with the drug under trial. Since the response rates to clinically useful drugs of specific histologic types of human tumors are so variable and often quite low, the indication is that a sizeable panel of human tumors in athymic "nude" mice would have to be used to

effectively avoid a high rate of false negative observations with new and as yet unrecognized clinically useful drugs.

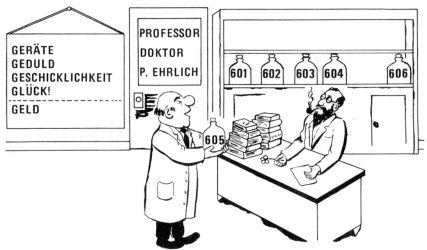

"THIS MAKES THE 605TH DRUG WE'VE TESTED WITHOUT FINDING AN EFFECTIVE CURE ; I SAY LETS CHUCK THE WHOLE THING,"

At the present time, no one knows the best laboratory models to use as in vivo screens for new anticancer agents. Paul Ehrlich, the father of effective chemotherapy and an aggressive screener, is reported to have said that in order to obtain success in research four big "G's" were needed: Geduld - patience, persistence; Geschicklichkeit - skill, ingenuity; Glück - luck; and Geld -money.[1] Cancer chemotherapists badly need at least one more: Geräte - apparatus, tools, or in this case, reliably predictive tumor models for drug sensitivity of human tumors.

DEVELOPMENT OF CLINICALLY USEFUL DRUGS

Once a new anticancer drug is discovered, two major developmental activities are indicated and usually followed:

(1) Determination of Optimal Therapeutic Activity. Extensive experimental trials are conducted in the laboratory against animal tumors to determine the best methods for using the drug. Such studies include the determination of the optimal dose and treatment schedule of the new drug when used alone in relation to:

(a) The growth cycle of individual tumor cells, i.e., schedule dependency. Is the drug cytotoxic against both resting and actively dividing tumor cells, and if cytotoxic only against actively dividing cells, is its cytotoxicity limited to one or more phases of the cell division cycle?

(b) The size of the tumor cell population, i.e., is the body burden of a large mass of viable (clonogenic) tumor cells (advanced disease) reduced less than that of a small tumor mass of viable tumor cells (early disease) under similar drug treatment?

(c) Whether aggressive (high-dose) short-term treatment is better than, equal to, or poorer than extended chronic treatment in reducing the body burden of tumor cells.

(d) Whether tumor cells selected for resistance to other anticancer drugs are sensitive or cross-resistant to the new drug.

(e) Whether the new drug shows improved therapeutic activity when used in combination with one or more other drugs. Since most drug treatment of human cancer uses two or more active drugs in combination, searches are made in vivo for drug combinations with (1) synergistic cytotoxicity for tumor cells, (2) less-than-additive toxicity for vital normal cells, and (3) with drug combinations showing either (1) or (2), whether or not simultaneous or sequential treatment with the two or more drugs in the combination is most effective.

(2) Congener Synthesis. Attempts are made to synthesize or structurally modify the new drug, a procedure that has often resulted in the development of drugs with better therapeutic activity, lesser toxicity to vital normal cells, improved pharmacologic properties, etc, than the parent drug. I won't say any more about this important aspect of anticancer drug development since Dr. Montgomery will be discussing it in detail at this meeting.

All of the developmental studies discussed above require drug-sensitive tumor systems in animals that allow reliable and reproducible quantitation of selective cytotoxic activity for tumor cells over vital normal cells in intact tumor-bearing laboratory animals. If we could conduct all anticancer drug development studies (anticancer activity, pharmacology, toxicology) in man, we would all feel more confident of the data developed as they relate to man, but in our culture the hazards to human life preclude this approach. In addition, "Good laboratory researchers can invent and exclude hypotheses within days or weeks in some cases."[5] The time factor is an important asset of carefully controlled experimental studies because therapy trials in man usually take so much longer.

If we consider the natural history of cancer from its origin to death of the patient, then almost all cancer in man is far advanced at the time of first detection and start of treatment.[9] Exceptions to this are the few patients undergoing adjuvant therapy (drug or other) shortly after surgery of grossly evident and probably metastatic primary tumors. As shown in Fig. 1, one cancer cell and all of its progeny must go through nearly 30 doublings in man, to between 10^8 and 10^9 cells, before the tumor is first detectable by x-ray or palpation and often the primary is much larger when first detected.[9,10] Useful clinical response to drug treatment requires reduction in the body burden of leukemic cells of $>90\%$ and

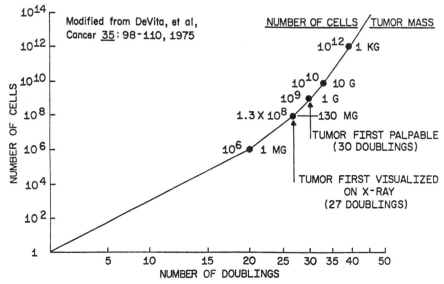

Fig. 1.   Theoretical growth curve relating the number of cell divisions that one tumor cell (at origin) and all of its progeny must go through to reach a given mass in a single tumor focus in man.[9]   (Used with permission of CANCER.)

reduction in measurable tumor masses if more than 50%. Tumor stasis or any growth under treatment, usually reported as activity by laboratory workers, would not be reported as objective response by critical and competent medical oncologists.

As previously stated, the most meaningful observation the experimental cancer chemotherapist can make and report is whether treatment with a new drug or a drug of established clinical utility, alone or in combination with other drugs or other thera- peutic modalities, results in inhibition of growth, growth stasis, or actual reduction in the body burden of viable and clonogenic tumor cells in reliable and reproducible quantitative terms. Procedures for such quantitative determinations are well established and can be easily carried out with both leukemias and solid tumors of animals in the laboratory.[19,20,22]

DeVita has recently said, "There are few cancers in animals that truly mimic the natural history of human cancers."[6] I agree with Dr. DeVita, but there are some transplantable leukemias and solid tumors of mice with which effective (sometimes curative) treatment of advanced disease with clinically useful anticancer drugs has been accomplished under conditions of tumor staging and tumor cell and population growth kinetics, which are similar in many ways to some leukemias, lymphomas, and solid tumors in man when they first present clinically. With the animal tumors, the clinicians' parameters for determining objective response, e.g., partial and complete remission or tumor regression, duration of disease-free interval, and cure, can be measured and reported.[20,22]

I believe it is this type of experimental drug treatment of advanced and grossly evident animal tumors that will enable the laboratory investigator to mimic the clinical problems with animal tumors and, hopefully, to provide medical oncologists with useful indications for improving drug treatment of advanced cancer in man.

CURE OF ADVANCED ANIMAL TUMORS BY DRUG TREATMENT

Leukemias, Lymphomas, and Plasma Cell Tumors

In Table 1 are listed the published reports of drug cure of significant numbers of animals with advanced leukemias, lymphomas, and plasma cell tumors. In the case of leukemia L1210, the body burden of viable and clonogenic tumor cells at start of treatment was objectively shown to exceed 10^8 and the advanced systemic disease could be diagnosed on the basis of elevated leukemic lymphoblasts in the peripheral blood.[18] The other examples in Table 1 had similar disease staging at start of drug treatment.

Solid Tumors

We have reported partial and complete regression of eleven and cure of seven advanced transplantable solid tumors of mice (osteosarcoma; carcinoma of the lung, colon, and breast; and melanoma) by treatment with representatives of all of the chemical and functional classes of clinically useful anticancer drugs.[18,20,21] Drug treatment was started when the primary tumors were closely staged, all were grossly evident (all ≥ 100 mg and some as large as 5 gm), many had already metastasized and all were uniformly fatal if untreated. Variable partial regression (PR), complete regression

TABLE 1

Advanced Experimental Leukemias, Lymphomas, and Plasma Cell Tumors Curable with Available Drugs

Tumor	Histologic Type	Host	Disease Staging at Start of Treatment	Treatment	"Cures"	Ref.
Transplanted						
L1210	ALL	BDF1 mouse	24 hr before death	Ara-C + CCNU	50%	17
Adj. P.C. 5	Myeloma	BALB/c mouse	2.7 g	Aniline mustard	100%	29
			Median day of death	CPA, BCNU, or Sarcolysin	90%	2
Pla 1	Plasma Cell	Hamster	1 g	CPA	90%	12
AKR Leukemia { Leukemia-Lymphoma		AKR mouse	24 hr before death	CPA + BCNU	Up to 80%	28
			72 → 48 hr before death	Amphotericin B → BCNU	10-90%	13
Spontaneous						
AKR Leukemia { Leukemia-Lymphoma		AKR mouse	Diagnostic thymoma, splenomegaly, and elevated WBC	Vincristine + Prednisone → CPA + Ara-C / CPA + MeCCNU → PalmO-ara-C	10-20%	23

CPA = Cyclophosphamide. PalmO-ara-C = 5'-palmitate of ara-C.

(CR), and cure rates were repeatedly observed using single-drug and combination-drug treatment. Combination-drug treatment was generally more effective than single-drug treatment as disease staging became more advanced.[18,20,21] In many ways, the responses of these advanced solid tumors of mice mimic those commonly seen with drug treatment of responsive human tumors originating in histologically similar organs or tissues of man. Further, I believe the variable regression and cure rates observed with these advanced animal tumors may provide some important concepts and principles of drug treatment of tumors worthy of serious consideration by medical oncologists planning drug treatment of human tumors with curative intent.

VARIABLE REGRESSION RATES OF CLOSELY STAGED ADVANCED SOLID TUMORS UNDER TREATMENT WITH THE SAME DOSE OF EFFECTIVE DRUGS

Individual primary tumor mass plots of five different advanced solid tumors in mice under treatment with effective anticancer drugs are shown in Figs. 2 and 3. Syngeneic mice and closely

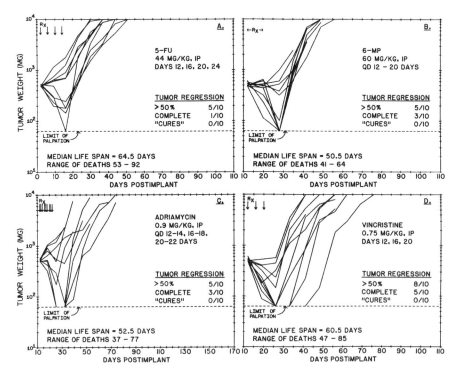

Fig. 2. Variable response of advanced (480 to 610 mg) Ridgway osteogenic sarcoma to treatment with 5-FU (A), 6-MP (B), adriamycin (C), or vincristine (D).

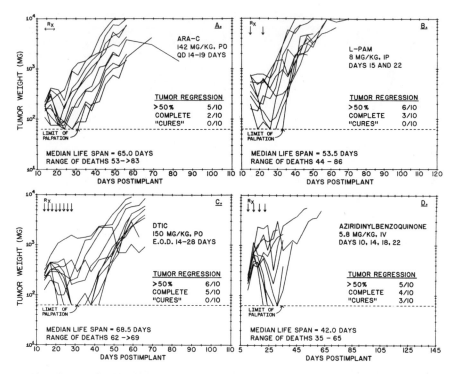

Fig. 3. Variable response of advanced (120 to 220 mg) colon adenocarcinoma 36 to treatment with ara-C (A), advanced (160 to 700 mg) mammary adenocarcinoma 16/C to treatment with L-PAM (melphalan) (B), advanced (100 to 300 mg) colon carcinoma 07 to treatment with DTIC (C), and advanced (100 to 250 mg) colon carcinoma 26 to treatment with aziridinylbenzoquinone (D).

staged (similar size) advanced tumors were selected for drug treatment. The same drug treatment ($\leq LD_{10}$) was given to each tumor-bearing animal. Each tumor implant came from the same donor source and the growth kinetics of each tumor in each mouse was considered to be the same because, with each, the interval from tumor implant to start of treatment was the same. Each animal was treated with the same dose(s) of the same drug from the same bottle at the same time and, therefore, treatment was considered to have been identical. The variable regression responses seen with a variety of histologic types of solid tumors appear to simulate the variable regression rates commonly seen in treatment of many advanced drug-sensitive solid tumors of man. Of additional interest, the drugs shown are representative of the major chemical and functional classes of clinically useful anti-cancer drugs, e.g., antimetabolites, alkylating agents, mitotic inhibitors, and drugs that bind to or intercalate with DNA.

The data in Fig. 4 indicate that these variable regression rates are drug-dose responsive. All data in Fig. 4 were from a single, internally controlled experiment. At 125 mg/kg/dose of cyclo-phosphamide (CPA), which was the LD_{30} in these mice bearing

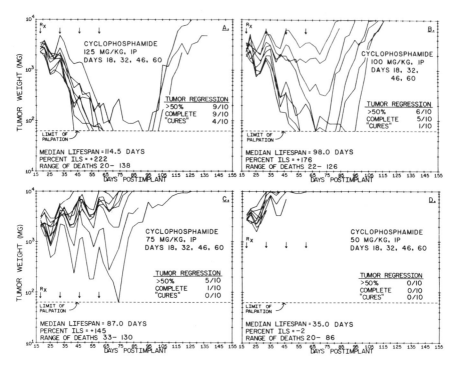

Fig. 4. Individual tumor response of advanced Ridgway osteogenic sarcoma in a dose response study with cyclophosphamide (CPA). Treatment was begun 18 days postimplant of tumor when individual tumors ranged from 2 to 3.5 gm in weight. (A) CPA treatment every 14 days x 4 at 125 mg/kg per dose. (B) 100 mg/kg per dose. (C) 75 mg/kg per dose. (D) 50 mg/kg per dose. ILS, increase in life span.[20] (Used with permission from Academic Press, New York.)

advanced Ridgway osteogenic sarcoma (ROS), regression to below palpable size (CR) occurred in all mice surviving drug treatment and four were cured. At 100 mg/kg/dose of CPA, the LD_{20} in these mice, the CR, PR, and cure rates dropped markedly; and at 75 and 50 mg/kg/dose of CPA, further reduction in CR, PR, and cure rates was seen. Similar reduction in regression and cure rates of all advanced drug-sensitive solid tumors of mice under treatment are commonly seen when drug doses are reduced.[18,20,21]

Therapeutic Synergism

Therapeutic synergism of active drugs against advanced solid tumors using the clinicians' activity parameters (PR, CR, and cure) can be convincingly demonstrated. In Fig. 5 are shown individual tumor responses of a drug-sensitive tumor (ROS) to treatment with CPA plus 6-MP. All data were from a single, internally controlled experiment. A range of doses from frankly toxic to inactive was used in each drug(s) treatment and optimal respones at $\leq LD_{10}$ doses were plotted. High CR and cure rates were obtained with

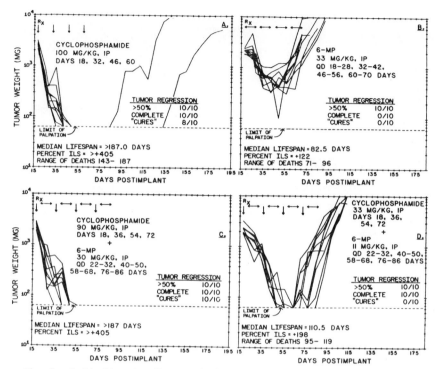

Fig. 5. Combination chemotherapy of advanced Ridgway osteogenic sarcoma with CPA plus 6-MP. Therapeutic synergism (100% cures) obtained at ≤LD10 doses with the two-drug combination. (A) Optimum tumor response in mice treated with ≤LD10 of CPA alone. (B) Treated with 6-MP alone. (C) Treated with CPA plus 6-MP. (D) Treated with less than optimum doses of CPA plus 6-MP. Note regression and regrowth during treatment with 6-MP (B) and with low-dose combination treatment (D). ILS, increase in life span.[20] (Used with permission from Academic Press, New York.)

CPA alone and a high PR rate but no cures were obtained with 6-MP. When CPA and 6-MP were used in combination, a 100% cure rate was obtained. However, when the doses of the combination of CPA plus 6-MP were dropped to about one-third of the curative dose, 100% CR but no cures were obtained. In my judgment, an important principle and concept for medical oncologists seeking curative drug treatment with effective drug combinations of drug-responsive advanced solid tumors of man illustrated by the data in Fig. 5 is: treat to dose-limiting toxicity even in cases where CR is obtained in responding patients.

Another example of therapeutic synergism of combination chemotherapy of advanced solid tumors in mice, is shown in Fig. 6. Advanced (200 to 400 mg) mammary adenocarcinoma 04/A was treated with adriamycin or 5-FU alone and in combination. Marked variation in regression responses but no CR's were obtained by treatment with adriamycin alone or 5-FU alone, but with the drug combination, a 100% PR, 50% CR, and 10% cure rate was obtained. Many similar examples with other drugs and other advanced tumors have been repeatedly observed.[18,20,21]

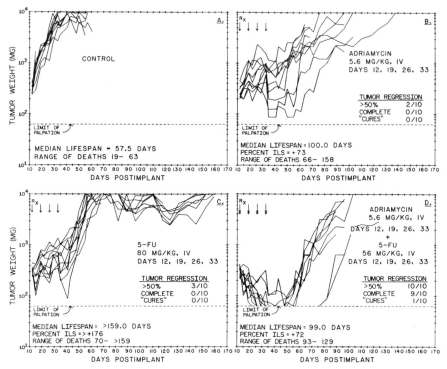

Fig. 6. Combination chemotherapy of advanced mammary adenocarcinoma (04/A) with adriamycin plus 5-FU. Therapeutic synergism based on improved partial and complete tumor regression rates at ≤LD$_{10}$ doses. (A) Individual tumor growth in untreated control mice.
(B) Same in mice treated with adriamycin. (C) Same in mice treated with 5-FU. (D) Same
in mice treated with adriamycin plus 5-FU. Optimum tumor responses were selected from a
dose response study with each treatment. ILS, increase in life span.[20] (Used with permission of Academic Press, New York.)

Sequential Versus Simultaneous Administration of Therapeutically Synergistic Drugs

The data in Fig. 7 illustrate a comparison of sequential as
compared to simultaneous administration of individually active
drugs (anguidine and 5-FU) against advanced colon adenocarcinoma
38. Neither drug at ≤LD$_{10}$ doses resulted in a high cure rate. PR,
CR, and cure rates were much better when anguidine plus 5-FU
were given simultaneously as compared to sequentially at 3- to 4-
day intervals with four courses of treatment.

Treatment Failure Due to Overgrowth of Drug-Resistant Tumor Cells

The medical oncologist usually treats advanced cancer (large
body burden of tumor cells) with drugs. Inherent in this is the
probability of having drug-resistant tumor cells as a subpopulation

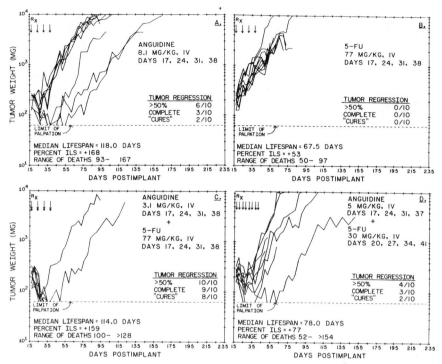

Fig. 7. Combination chemotherapy of advanced colon adenocarcinoma 38 with anguidine plus 5-FU. Therapeutic synergism (80% cures) at ≤LD10 doses of anguidine plus 5-FU given simultaneously but not with anguidine plus 5-FU given sequentially. (A) Optimum tumor response in mice treated with ≤LD10 doses of anguidine. (B) Treated with ≤LD10 doses of 5-FU. (C) Treated with ≤LD10 doses of anguidine plus 5-FU simultaneously. (D) Treated with ≤LD10 doses of anguidine plus 5-FU sequentially. Optimum tumor responses were selected from a dose response study with each treatment. ILS, increase in life span.[4] (Used with permission of CANCER.)

among the initially drug-sensitive tumor cells, and this probability increases as the size of the tumor cell population increases. Many laboratory studies, in which relatively small body burdens of tumor cells are used, either fail to see or to consider this real and major obstacle to cure with drug treatment that initially causes CR but ultimately fails when tumor reappears under continuing treatment or fails to respond after recurrence. Medical oncologists are very familiar with this common occurrence with initially effective, but ultimately failing, drug treatment of tumors of man.

Fig. 8 illustrates this phenomenon with advanced mammary adenocarcinoma 16/C treated with 5-FU alone or 5-FU plus adriamycin. Initially, drug-sensitive (high PR and CR rates) tumors resume growth under continuing treatment with initially very effective drugs, either alone or in combination. The data in Figs. 5B and D and 7C and D show other examples. Many additional examples have been commonly observed in the laboratory.[24] The examples shown in Figs. 5, 7, and 8 indicate that the clinical problem of ultimate failure of initially drug-responsive

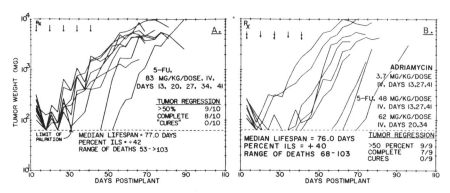

Fig. 8. Overgrowth of advanced (100 to 300 mg) mammary adenocarcinoma 16/C under initially effective (high CR rate) treatment with 5-FU (A) or 5-FU plus adriamycin (B).[24] (Used with permission of Pergamon Press, Ltd, Oxford.)

tumors which reappear under maintenance therapy can be modeled and studied with advanced solid tumors in animals. The tools to study this problem are at hand. One possible approach is to use doses of effective drugs up to dose-limiting toxicity with initially effective drugs as illustrated in Fig. 5C and D. Extensive experimental data with drug treatment of advanced murine leukemias (body burden $>10^7$ viable tumor cells at start of treatment) has shown that failure to cure with either single drugs or drug combinations is often due to overgrowth of subpopulations of tumor cells resistant to the first drug(s) used. [24,25] Cures of these advanced leukemias can be obtained by changing to other drug treatment at about the nadir of body burden of tumor cells that can be obtained by treatment with the first effective but noncurative drugs used. [24,25] Drug-resistant sublines of a variety of animal tumor cells that are initially responsive to representatives of all of the major chemical and functional classes of clinically useful anticancer drugs have been isolated and sensitivity and cross-resistance to other anticancer drugs have been determined.[24] Thus, the tools may be available to provide rational, logical, and objectively indicated guidance to medical oncologists to approach this serious obstacle to effective and curative drug treatment of advanced cancer in man.

DISCUSSION AND SUMMARY

Among the 700,000 new cases of cancer in man (exclusive of skin and in situ cervix) that occur each year in the United States, about 60% fail to be cured by surgery or radiation because there are grossly evident metastases when the disease is first detected or they develop recurrent tumor following initial treatment with curative intent.[7] The major promise for curative treatment in these patients is effective systemic treatment, primarily chemotherapy but with the possible support of immunity-related factors. Among these two, chemotherapy has clearly been more effective against cancer in man or animals than immune modulation. More than forty clinically useful anticancer drugs are commercially available and 60 or more are being evaluated for clinical utility, but no one or any group of these agents appears to be the broadly useful and markedly effective (curative) one(s) we need and seek. What are the possible methods to increase the effectiveness of cancer chemotherapy? Two approaches are indicated: (1) seek and find more effective drugs and (2) improve the therapeutic effectiveness of currently available drugs.

Seek and find: Since no animal model(s) with the objectively established and reliable ability to predict for the drug response of one or more human tumors is available, we must continue to seek better predictive models, and meanwhile continue the search for new drugs with the models we have, which have served us well up to now. We should also continue to seek animal tumors with higher probability of being reliable predictive models for treatment response in man, e.g., those with common etiology or similar biochemical deficiencies or unique functions, as one or more human tumors. The likelihood of developing a markedly improved in vivo screen for clinically useful anticancer drugs seems remote, but we must continue the search.

Improve current drugs: Here we have proven and effective tools at hand, their only serious limitation being that they use the treatment responses of animal tumors, without established predictive reliability for man, as the basis for accepting improved treatment potential. With these animal tumors we can and do: (1) Attempt to improve therapeutic effectiveness, at least for drug-sensitive animal tumor systems by congener synthesis of currently available effective drugs. This is a drug-development method with a history of improving therapeutic activity in all of chemotherapy; e.g., antibacterial, antiprotozoal, antiviral, and anticancer drugs as well as centrally active drugs, diuretics, cardiac glucosides, insulins, and other hormones, etc., etc. (2) Develop better methods of using currently available drugs. Among these are (a) proper treatment scheduling, e.g., compare high-dose short course with low-dose chronic treatment, or continuous infusion; compare iv, ip, or oral treatment; (b) determine optimal drug combinations and, with those with synergistic therapeutic activity, whether simultaneous or sequential drug delivery is better; and (c) determine the resistance and cross-resistance of drug-resistant tumor cells to new drug(s). (3) Increase the challenge to treatment with the animal model systems. Laboratory investigators working with animal models of human cancer can and should treat similarly staged disease in animals to that faced by medical oncologists in treating cancer in man and report results of therapy trials against animal tumors using the medical oncologists' parameters for drug activity in man; namely, partial regression, complete regression, duration of complete regression, and cure. If none of these are observed, the laboratory worker should at least report the body burden of viable and clonogenic tumor cells or disease staging at start of drug treatment and whether or not the body burden of tumor cells in animals increased, was static, or decreased under drug treatment, in reliable and reproducible quantitative terms, and at $\leq LD_{10}$ doses. Simple methods for making such data analyses are well known and documented. If such procedures are used in the laboratory, improved communication and understanding between the laboratory and clinical cancer chemotherapists will result. Also, laboratory data will be collected that may be (probably will be) more useful in helping medical oncologists improve the effectiveness of clinical chemotherapy of cancer in man.

REFERENCES

1. Baldry PE: The Battle Against Bacteria. London, Cambridge University Press, 1965.
2. Bergsagel DE: Personal communication.
3. Burchenal JH: Success and failure in present chemotherapy and the implications of asparaginase. Cancer Res 29:2262-2269, 1969.
4. Corbett TH, Griswold DP Jr, Roberts BJ, et al.: Evaluation of single agents and combinations of chemotherapeutic agents in mouse colon carcinomas. Cancer 40(5):2660-2680, 1977.
5. DeVita VT: The evolution of therapeutic research in cancer. N Engl J Med 298(16):907-910, 1978.
6. DeVita VT: Human models of human diseases; breast cancer and the lymphomas. Int J Radiat Oncol Biol Phys 5:1855-1867, 1979.
7. DeVita VT Jr, Henney JE, Stonehill, E: Cancer mortality: The good news, in Jones SE, Salmon SE (eds): Adjuvant Therapy of Cancer II (Proceedings of the 2nd International Conference on the Adjuvant Therapy of Cancer, Tucson, Arizona, 1979). New York: Grune and Stratton, Inc, 1979, xv-xx.
8. DeVita VT, Kershner LM: Cancer, the curable diseases. Am Pharm NS20(4):16-22, 1980.
9. DeVita VT Jr, Young RC, Canellos GP: Combination versus single agent chemotherapy: A review of the basis for selection of drug treatment of cancer. Cancer 35:98-110, 1975.
10. Frei E III, Freireich EJ: Progress and prospectives in the chemotherapy of acute leukemia, in Goldin A, Hawking F, Schnitzer RJ (eds): Advances in Chemotherapy, Vol. 2. New York, Academic Press, Inc, 1965, pp 269-298.
11. Giovanella BC: Experimental chemotherapy of human tumors heterotransplanted in nude mice, in Mihich E, Eckhardt S (eds): Antibiotics and Chemotherapy. Vol. 28. Design of Cancer Chemotherapy: Experimental and Clinical Approaches. Basel, S Karger, 1980, pp 21-27.

12. Griswold DP Jr, Schabel FM Jr, Wilcox WS, et al.: Success and failure in the treatment of solid tumors. I. Effects of cyclophosphamide (NSC-26271) on primary and metastatic plasmacytoma in the hamster. Cancer Chemother Rep 52: 345-387, 1968.

13. Medoff G, Valeriote F, Lynch RG, et al.: Synergistic effect of amphotericin B and 1,3-bis(2-chloroethyl)-1-nitrosourea against a transplantable AKR leukemia. Cancer Res 34:974-978, 1974.

14. Salmon SE (ed): Cloning of Human Tumor Stem Cells. New York, Alan R Liss, Inc, in press, 1980.

15. Salmon SE: Applications of the human tumor stem cell assay to new drug evaluation and screening, in Salmon SE (ed): Cloning of Human Tumor Stem Cells. New York, Alan R Liss, Inc, in press, 1980.

16. Salmon SE, Alberts DS, Meyskens F, et al.: Clinical correlations of in vitro drug sensitivity, in Salmon SE (ed): Cloning of Human Tumor Stem Cells. New York, Alan R Liss, Inc, in press, 1980.

17. Schabel FM Jr: In vivo leukemic cell kill kinetics and "curability" in experimental systems, in The Proliferation and Spread of Neoplastic Cells (21st Annual Symposium on Fundamental Cancer Research, 1967, The University of Texas MD Anderson Hospital and Tumor Institute at Houston). Baltimore, Williams and Wilkins Co, 1968, pp 379-408.

18. Schabel FM Jr: Animal models as predictive systems, in Cancer Chemotherapy - Fundamental Concepts and Recent Advances (19th Annual Clinical Conference on Cancer, 1974, The University of Texas MD Anderson Hospital and Tumor Institute at Houston). Chicago, Year Book Medical Publishers, Inc, 1975, pp 323-355.

19. Schabel FM Jr: Test systems for evaluating the antitumor activity of nucleoside analogues, in Walker RT, DeClercq E, Eckstein F (eds): Nucleoside Analogues: Chemistry, Biology, and Medical Applications. Vol. 26. NATO Advanced Study Institutes Series A: Life Sciences. New York, Plenum Publishing Corp, 1979, pp 363-394.

20. Schabel FM Jr, Griswold DP Jr, Corbett TH, et al.: Testing therapeutic hypotheses in mice and man: Observations on the therapeutic activity against advanced solid tumors of mice treated with anticancer drugs that have demonstrated or potential clinical utility for treatment of advanced solid tumors of man, in Busch H, DeVita V Jr (eds): Cancer Drug Development, Part B. Methods in Cancer Research, Vol. 17. New York, Academic Press, Inc, 1979, pp 3-51.

21. Schabel FM Jr, Griswold DP Jr, Corbett TH, et el.: Variable responses of advanced solid tumors of mice to treatment with anticancer drugs, in Fidler IJ, White RJ (eds): Design of Models for Screening of Therapeutic Agents for Cancer. New York, Van Nostrand Reinhold Co, in press, 1980.

22. Schabel FM Jr, Griswold DP Jr, Laster WR Jr, et al.:
     Quantitative evaluation of anticancer agent activity in
     experimental animals. Pharmac Ther A 1:411-435, 1977.
23. Schabel FM Jr, Skipper HE, Trader MW, et al.: Combination
     chemotherapy for spontaneous AKR lymphoma. Cancer
     Chemother Rep 4:53-72, 1974.
24. Schabel FM Jr, Skipper HE, Trader MW, et al.: Concepts for
     controlling drug-resistant tumor cells, in Mouridsen HT,
     Palshof T (eds): Breast Cancer. Experimental and Clinical
     Aspects. Oxford, England: Pergamon Press, Ltd, 1980, pp.
     199-212.
25. Skipper HE, Schabel FM Jr, and Lloyd HH: Experimental
     therapeutics and kinetics: Selection and overgrowth of
     specifically and permanently drug-resistant tumor cells.
     Semin Hematol 15:207-219, 1978.
26. Toolan HW: The transplantable human tumor. Ann NY Acad
     Sci 76(3):733-740, 1958.
27. Uren JR, Handschumacher RE: Enzyme therapy, in Becker
     FF (ed): Cancer: A Comprehensive Treatise, Vol. 5. New
     York, Plenum Publishing Corp, 1977, pp 457-487.
28. Valeriote FA, Bruce WR, Meeker BE: Synergistic action of
     cyclophosphamide and 1,3-bis(2-chloroethyl)-1-nitrosourea on
     a transplanted murine lymphoma. J Natl Cancer Inst 40:935-
     944, 1968.
29. Whisson ME, Connors TA: Cure of mice bearing advanced
     plasma cell tumours with aniline mustard. Nature 206(4985):
     689-691, 1965.
30. World Health Organization: Descriptions of Systems Used in
     Experimental Screening of Anticancer Preparations in
     Sixteen Countries (CAN/75.6), 1975.

Application Of The
Human Tumor Stem Cell Assay In The
Development Of Anticancer Therapy

SYDNEY E. SALMON, M. D.

Professor of Medicine and Director
Cancer Center
University of Arizona
Tucson, Arizona

INTRODUCTION

Until the present, experimental mouse tumor systems have
been the primary approach for screening new drugs for anticancer activity (1). However, the approach depends heavily
on the use of a few signal mouse tumors and may well have
missed compounds which were inactive in the L1210 or P388
leukemia prescreen. Even a broadened panel of 5-6 transplantable tumors of differing histology while better, might still
be too limited, and assumes that a few cloned murine tumors
will provide a predictive model for drug effects on human
tumors.

Increased interest has recently developed for application
of a new in vitro system for drug screening. This interest
is based on observations made with a two-layer soft agar
clonogenic assay for spontaneous human tumors, "the Human Tumor Stem Cell Assay." This Petri dish assay was reported by
Hamburger and Salmon in 1977 (2-4), and subsequently applied
by other investigative groups (e.g., 5-9). As currently
carried out, plating of single cell suspensions from human
tumors gives rise to 30 or more colonies per 500,000 cells
plated after 10-14 days in 50%-90% of specimens from tumors
of various histologies (10). Ovarian, lung and bladder cancer and neuroblastoma have some of the highest success rates
reported thus far with the clonogenic assay (4-6). Some of
the hard, solid tumors (e.g., breast, colon) are more difficult to grow, and better techniques for cell disaggregation
are needed. For measurement of standard cytotoxic drug sensitivity in this assay, cells are exposed for 1 hour to vari-

ous drug concentrations (all of which are easily achieved clinically), the cells are then washed and plated in standard fashion. When the assay has been applied to standard drug testing on tumor biopsies from patients it has proven to be predictive of the clinical response to a variety of agents (11-13). With regard to prediction response, both our group and Von Hoff's documented that the assay predicts clinical drug resistance with over ninety-five percent accuracy and drug sensitivity with 60%-70% accuracy (11-13). An important finding in these studies and those of Ozol's (8) has been evidence of significant heterogeneity in response of tumors of the same histology to a variety of cytotoxic agents. Drug sensitivity of specific tumor types to a series of standard drugs was observed at frequencies that were quite similar to the frequency of clinical activity of these agents (14). Examples of this phenomenon are shown in Table 1 which contains sensitivity of ovarian TCFUs* of some common anticancer drugs. As is apparent from the data, cis-platinum was the most active agent against TCFUs from previously untreated patients (62% sensitive), which is quite similar to its clinical activity. Similar findings have been obtained with 5-FU on colon TCFUs wherein 30% were sensitive (14); this result is quite similar to the 20%-30% clinical response rate to this agent. Patients who had received prior chemotherapy generally have lower in vitro response rates to drugs used (e.g., Table 1) and conversion of from in vitro sensitivity to resistance has been documented in patients who were tested in vitro with a specific drug, treated with that drug clinically and then retested subsequent to relapse (13). However, administration of drugs from unrelated classes did not appear to induce drug resistance (13).

TABLE 1

Percentage Of Patients With Ovarian Cancer Whose TCFUs
Were Sensitive* To Several Standard Agents

Drug	No Prior Therapy Patients	Prior Therapy Patients	P
Cis-platinum	62%	29%	.007
Doxorubicin	42%	19%	.04
Bleomycin	33%	17%	.04
Vinblastine	46%	29%	.25
	(80 tests)	(228 tests)	

* Definition of sensitive includes "sensitive" and "intermediate" categories from area-under-the-curve analysis with low concentrations of drugs (< 0.1 μg/ml for 1 hour).

* Tumor colony-forming units

While detailed computation of limits for drug sensitivity
for specific agents have been carried out in our laboratories
by measurement of the area under linear survival-concentra-
tion curves from an initial patient "training set" (15), a
simpler empirical definition of in vitro sensitivity which
appears adequate for many cytotoxic drugs is that sensitivity
is present when survival of tumor colony-forming units is reduced to 30% of control or less with a 1-hour exposure to a
drug concentration which is readily attained in vivo (e.g.,
10%-20% of the achievable concentration-time product). Thus,
most drug dosages used for standard drug testing in vitro are
0.1 µg/ml or less.

Recently, our group has initiated an investigation of the
applicability of the stem cell assay to new drug screening.
The rationale and a detailed discussion of the application of
the tumor stem cell assay for new drug screening has recently
been published (16). Two levels of screening can be considered with the assay: (a) Testing of entirely new agents as a
screen for anticancer activity, and (b) testing prospectively
known active phase I-II new agents to either prospectively
correlate in vitro results with clinical results or to select
new drugs for individual patients.

PRIMARY SCREENING OF NEW AGENTS

Our initial studies were all counted using inverted microscopy and proved to be quite time consuming. More recently,
we have used an automated and computerized image analysis system (Bausch & Lomb Omnicon series) using feature analysis and
a special series of programs to rapidly scan the Petri dishes
and count tumor colonies and exclude artifacts (17). Of importance to standardization of screening, TCFUs from many tumors can be preserved in viable fashion by cryopreservation
using techniques quite similar to those used for bone marrow
preservation. A summary of our experience with cryopreservation appears in Table 2. Comparisons of cytotoxic drug sur-
vival-concentration curves of TCFUs from fresh and viable
thawed cells from the same tumor have been quite similar, indicating maintenance of the drug sensitivity phenotype after
freezing. Thus, the investigator has the potential to "bank"
various common and rare tumor types and carry out screening
activities in an orderly and systematic manner, and repeat
specific tests at various concentrations when desirable.

TABLE 2
Experience With Cryopreservation of Human TCFUs

Tumor Type	No. of Samples	Fresh Cells percent with >30 colonies/plate	Frozen Cells percent with >30 colonies/plate
Ovarian	27	63%	48%
Lung	9	66%	55%
Colon	3	66%	33%
Melanoma	14	64%	50%
Breast	6	50%	50%
Misc.*	9	33%	11%
Total	68	59%	44%**

* Stomach, bladder, cervical, neuroblastoma, pancreas, sarcoma, etc.
** 75% of the tumors which gave rise to colonies from fresh
   cells also gave rise to adequate numbers of colonies from
   the frozen aliquot.

In order to maximize the sensitivity to identify potential
new anticancer drugs, we established a protocol wherein we
first test new agents against fresh or cryopreserved TCFUs
from human tumors by continuous contact of the drug with
cells in the agar. If a drug concentration of 10 µg/ml is
used in the initial test (and the drug is stable in vitro),
the concentration-time product achieved will be in the range
of 3300 µg hours when the cultures are incubated for 14 days
prior to counting. TCFUs which proliferate from a single
cell suspension and form tumor colonies of 30 cells or more
in the presence of such drug exposure are clearly resistant
to the agent tested. Virtually all the standard cytotoxic
drugs (which do not require bioactivation) which we have
tested are readily detected with this type of screening assay
when tested against tumors from previously untreated patients
with neoplasms of the types for which the given agent is used
clinically. For example, doxorubicin usually reduces survival of TCFUs from tumors of types known to be frequently sensitive to anthracyclines to less than 1% of control at 10 µg/
ml by continuous contact. For screening unknown agents, reduction in survival to less than 30% or 10% should be considered. This test appears to be quite sensitive, and therefore
should miss relatively few active agents if a variety of previously untreated tumors are used in the testing. Some of
the advantages of the tumor stem cell assay for new drug
screening are summarized in Table 3. If TCFU survival is
reduced to less than 30% of control, then the unknown agent
is retested at lower concentrations, and also by 1-hour exposure against a broadened panel of tumors of the same type in
which sensitivity was observed as well as other tumor types.
Use of bioactivation (e.g., with hepatic microsomes) could be
considered to detect agents which require in vivo activation.

TABLE 3
Potential Advantages Of Human Tumor Colony Assay
For New Drug Screening

1. Simple, relatively rapid assay with defined reagents, quantitative results in useful biological terms.
2. Assay directly applicable to fresh or frozen biopsies containing clonogenic human tumor cells.
3. Dose response curves for established anticancer drugs predictive of clinical response.
4. Standard panels of cryopreserved cells can be established and banked for assay use and quality control.
5. Assay has sensitivity to detect activity in submicrogram amounts in fermentation broths or with scarce compounds.
6. Automated counting permits standardization of assay results and reporting from multiple laboratories.

Some initial tests of this system in our laboratory included a series of compounds which were sent as unknowns by the Drug Evaluation Branch of NCI. These compounds were tested against TCFUs from fresh or cryopreserved tumors obtained from 29 patients (ovarian, breast, lung, melanoma, colon, pancreas, sarcoma). After testing was completed, the blind was broken and it was disclosed that all 6 compounds (Table 4) are classed as compounds of interest to the Drug Evaluation branch of NCI. All are currently of uncertain clinical value and are scheduled or in phase I-II clinical trial. The compounds which showed "some activity" in vitro in the tumor stem cell assay included the alkylating-like drug, NSC-135758 (piperazinedione), the glutamine antagonist, NSC-163501 (AT 125 or acivicin) and an alkylating agent with epoxide groups, NSC-296934 (the Henkel compound). Based on these results, it would seem reasonable to carry out further studies on NSC-135758, 163501 and 296934 particularly in breast and endometrial cancer where the most profound effects were observed. All of these agents exhibited their greatest effects on TCFUs from the same three tumor specimens suggesting that some similar mechanism for susceptibility may be present. The three agents which were inactive in the in vitro assay proved to include amygdalin (NSC-15780 or laetrile), the soluble form of ICRF-159 (ICRF 187 or NSC-167980) and dihydroxyazacytadine (NSC-264880). While the latter two compounds have some activity in murine leukemias, amygdalin has been inactive in those systems as well. Based on in vitro results, further testing of the inactive agents would be deferred unless some other result or rationale strongly suggested that further testing be carried out. Recently we initiated testing of eight new anthracycline analogs synthesized at Farmitalia. Initial tests at the 10 µg level indi-

TABLE 4
Results From Blinded Testing Of New Agents
From NCI With The Human Tumor Stem Cell Assay*

NSC No.	Other Identification	10 µg/ml: continuous contact in agar		
		Proportion of Tumors (%) with < 30% Survival of TCFUs	Proportion of Tumors (%) with < 10% Survival of TCFUs	Type of Sensitive Tumors
135758	Piperazinedione	6/29 (21%)	2/29 (7%)	Endometrial Breast Lung Pancreas
15780	d-amygdalin (laetrile)	0/29 (0%)	0/29 (0%)	
163501	AT 125 5-isoxazaleacetic acid (acivicin)	4/28 (14%)	3/28 (11%)	Endometrial Breast Lung
169780	soluble ICRF 159	0/28 (0%)	0/28 (0%)	
264880	dihydro-5-azacytidine	0/28 (0%)	0/28 (0%)	
296934	Henkel compound	3/28 (11%)	3/28 (11%)	Endometrial Breast

* 9 ovarian, 6 breast, 5 lung, 5 melanoma, 4 miscellaneous
(endometrial, colon, Ewing's sarcoma, pancreas). The
blind was broken after this testing was completed.

cate that all are active (survival < 1%) against TCFUs from
several breast and gastric carcinomas. Repeat testing at
lower dosage exposures may permit discrimination between analogs and suggest which ones might be advanced to clinical
trial. This of course assumes that the agents pass the standard toxicology screen. Following the lead of Epstein (7),
our laboratory initiated testing of human leukocyte interferon, and more recently other more highly purified interferons. Human leukocyte interferon is clearly as active as
some cytotoxic agents against TCFUs from certain patients.
While the mechanism responsible for the in vitro activity remains to be elucidated, the assay has the potential for standardization in selection of new interferon preparations for
clinical trial in relation to in vitro oncolytic activity.
Previously, such selections have been made primarily on the
basis of the antiviral activity of interferons. Based on
evidence on the in vitro assay procedure from various investigators, the Drug Evaluation Program of the Division of

Cancer Treatment of NCI has decided to launch a three-year test of the tumor stem cell assay for new drug screening that will involve a series of extramural contractors. As currently described, the program will have a one-year pilot phase during which 50 drugs will be evaluated against TCFUs from at least 10 tumors by each contractor. Subsequently, the consortium will test a total of 1,000 drugs annually for the following 2 years. The test will include both "actives" and "inactives" from the P388 murine prescreen. This evaluation of the 1,000 compounds in the in vitro test will be assessed in relationship to the 15,000 compounds tested annually through NCI's in vivo murine program. In this standard screen a P388 leukemia prescreen and a tumor panel for a limited number (500-1,000) of selected agents is carried out (limited to positives in the prescreen and compounds with other rationale) (1). Should the NCI's test of the tumor stem cell assay prove to identify new or novel structures not detected in the murine system, it is conceivable that the basic orientation of the screening program may be altered. The "proof of the pudding" is of course in the testing. This will require that some compounds which are found to be very active only in the tumor stem cell assay (and which pass toxicology) be approved for entry into clinical trials in the appropriate tumor types and dose ranges so that the validity of the predictions can be assessed. Current NCI guidelines for new drug development do in fact allow for precisely this logical sequence of events.

SECONDARY SCREENING OF NEW AGENTS

Another promising application of the in vitro assay for screening is in the area of testing of agents which have already been selected for clinical trial. In concept, a phase II in vitro trial could markedly reduce the scale of initial clinical trials wherein new agents are given to patients to determine whether they would have anti-tumor effect (16, 18). At present, much of the expense and toxicity of such agents unfortunately involves patients who achieve no benefit from the agent administered. If patients received such agents only if their TCFUs manifest sensitivity to them, then new drugs would not have to be given to patients predicted to be resistant. This policy seems justified in view of the assay's clear capability of identifying drugs which will be clinically inactive (10-13). There are three major trial designs which can be applied in relation to in vitro studies. These are summarized in Table 5 and discussed elsewhere (9, 11). We have initiated prospective correlative trials with several new agents including the new agents AMSA (19), 13-cis-retinoic acid (20), and dihydroxyanthracenedione (21).

TABLE 5
Types of Clinical Trials With The Tumor Stem Cell Assay

1. Retrospective Correlative Analysis
   (Assay done entirely independently of clinical drug
   selection and trial plan)
2. Prospective Correlative Trial
   (Assay drugs selected to encompass all agents used
   in the clinical trial plan)
3. Prospective Decision-Aiding Trials
   (Clinical trial drugs for individual patients
   selected by assay results)

Our most detailed experience with the prospective correlative
trial design has been a trial of AMSA recently presented by
Ahmann et al. (22). This pilot study for the Southwest Oncology Group, tested an every 3-week intravenous schedule of
AMSA at a dosage of 120 mg/M^2. Twenty-one of the patients
treated at the University of Arizona Cancer Center had tumor
biopsies performed for in vitro sensitivity studies. The
overall clinical response rate in this group was 7/21 or 33%.
Thirteen of the tumors had inadequate growth in vitro. The
clinical response rate in that patient cohort was 4/13 or 31%.
Among the 8 patients whose TCFUs manifest adequate in vitro
growth, the clinical response rate was 3/8 or 38%. Three
patients' TCFUs manifest in vitro sensitivity (reduction in
TCFU survival to < 30% of control at the 0.1 µg/hr. dose) and
all three responded clinically. The 5 patients whose cells
were resistant in vitro also failed to respond clinically.
Thus, while the series is small, the in vitro results were
clearcut and statistically significant (p = <.02). Based on
this promising result in a prospective correlative trial, we
have recently designed a more generalized protocol which
would permit the decision-aiding trial design to be used for
a variety of new phase I-II agents with the objective of administering such experimental compounds to only those patients whose tumors are predicted to respond to the new agent.
Should this design prove successful, the definition of the
"clinical response rate" might require some reconsideration
with some emphasis placed on the relation of clinical response to in vitro sensitivity.
    While this analysis of secondary screening has focused on
the issue of drug selection for specific patients and simpli-
fication of clinical trials, it is also clear that valuable
pharmacologic information can be gained which would be relevant to phase I studies. Specifically, for a variety of
standard agents, clinical response is associated with in
vitro sensitivity at 10%-20% of the clinically achievable

concentration-time product or less. Given this guideline,
preclinical in vitro testing could potentially project the
required clinical dosing and plasma concentration time product range which ideally should be investigated in phase I
studies. The requirement for exquisite sensitivity in vitro
is not unique to anticancer drugs; a similar phenomenon has
also been observed with antibiotics which have proven effective for difficult bacterial infections. Presumably, exquisite in vitro sensitivity can be translated into clinical
dosing schedules which overwhelm potential pharmacologic
sanctuaries, pharmacogenetic differences in drug handling and
variability in sensitivity of subclones. Drugs that are
highly active at low dosage (e.g., 0.01 µg/ml for 1 hour) are
therefore of particular interest in new drug development and
clinical trials.

SUMMARY

The in vitro soft-agar clonogenic assay for human tumor
stem cells has proven capable of supporting growth of tumor
colony-forming cells (TCFU) from a wide variety of human
tumors. Initial clinical trials of standard agents have
shown the assay to be predictive of clinical drug sensitivity
or drug resistance to a wide variety of chemotherapeutic
agents. As a result of these observations, the assay is now
being applied to two new areas which hold substantial promise:
(a) Primary Screening to detect entirely new anticancer drugs,
and (b) Secondary Screening for selection of phase I-II
agents for administration to cancer patients whose TCFUs
manifest sensitivity. These two areas of application of the
assay represent the focus of this analysis. Preliminary data
are presented which support the contention that the tumor
stem cell assay should have major utility in both of these
areas of screening. Further testing and evaluation by many
investigators is therefore clearly warranted. Broadscale application may markedly simplify and speed the development of
effective anticancer therapy.

ACKNOWLEDGEMENTS

I want to thank Drs. Anne Hamburger, Ronald Buick, Jeff-
rey Trent, Thomas Moon, H.-S. George Chen, David S. Alberts,
Frank L. Meyskens, Jr., Stephen E. Jones, F. H. Ahmann, and
Brian G. M. Durie for their major scientific and clinical input in these studies, and Ms. Barbara Soehnlen, Laurie Young,
and Rosa Liu for outstanding technical assistance. I also
wish to thank Dr. Mary Wolpert of the Drug Evaluation Branch
of NCI for sending the six unknown compounds for the testing
summarized in Table 4, and for maintaining the blind until
the data summary was prepared. These studies were supported
in part by U.S.P.H.S. grants CA-21839, CA-17094, and CA-23074
from the National Cancer Institute, and a grant from the
Lasker Foundation.

REFERENCES

1.   DeVita VT, Oliverio VT, Muggia FM, et al.: The drug development and clinical trials programs of the Division of Cancer Treatment, National Cancer Institute. Cancer Clin Trials 2:195-216, 1979.

2.   Hamburger AW, Salmon SE: Primary bioassay of human tumor stem cells. Science 197:461-463, 1977.

3.   Hamburger AW, Salmon SE: Primary bioassay of human myeloma stem cells. J Clin Invest 60:846-854, 1977.

4.   Hamburger AW, Salmon SE, Kim MB, et al.: Direct cloning of human ovarian carcinoma cells in agar. Cancer Res 38:3438-3443, 1978.

5.   Von Hoff DD, Harris GJ, Johnson G, et al.: Initial experience with the human tumor stem cell assay system: potential and problems, in Salmon S (ed): Cloning of Human Tumor Stem Cells. New York, Alan Liss, 1980, pp 113-124.

6.   Buick RN, Stanisic TH, Fry SE, et al.: Development of an agar-methyl cellulose clonogenic assay for cells in transitional cell carcinoma of the human bladder. Cancer Res 39:5051-5056, 1979.

7.   Epstein LB, Shen J-T, Abele JS, et al.: Further experience in testing the sensitivity of human ovarian carcinoma cells to interferon in an in vitro semi-solid agar culture system: comparison of solid and ascitic forms of the tumor, in Salmon S (ed): Cloning of Human Tumor Stem Cells. New York, Alan Liss, 1980, pp 277-290.

8.   Ozols RF, Wilson JKV, Grotzus KR, et al.: Cloning of human ovarian cancer cells in soft agar from malignant effusions and peritoneal washings. Cancer Res 40:2743, 1980.

9.   Salmon SE (ed): Cloning of Human Tumor Stem Cells. New York, Alan Liss, 1980, pp 360.

10.   Salmon SE, Hamburger AW, Soehnlen BJ, et al.: Quantitation of differential sensitivity of human tumor stem cells to anticancer drugs. New Engl J Med 298:1321-1327, 1978.

11.   Alberts DS, Salmon SE, Chen H-SG, et al.: In vitro clonogenic assay for predicting response of ovarian cancer to chemotherapy. Lancet 2:340-342, 1980.

12.   Von Hoff DD: Clinical correlations of drug sensitivity in tumor stem cell assay. Proc Amer Assoc Cancer Res and Amer Soc Clin Oncol 21:abst 535, p 134, 1980.

13.   Salmon SE, Alberts DS, Meyskens FL, et al.: Clinical correlations of in vitro drug sensitivity, in Salmon S (ed): Cloning of Human Tumor Stem Cells. New York, Alan Liss, 1980, pp 223-245.

14. Salmon SE, Von Hoff DD: In vitro evaluation of anti-cancer drugs with the human tumor stem cell assay. Sem in Onc, in press, 1980.

15. Moon TE: Quantitative and statistical analysis of the association between in vitro and in vivo studies, in Salmon S (ed): Cloning of Human Tumor Stem Cells. New York, Alan Liss, 1980, pp 209-221.

16. Salmon SE: Applications of the human tumor stem cell assay to new drug evaluation and screening, in Salmon S (ed): Cloning of Human Tumor Stem Cells. New York, Alan Liss, 1980, pp 291-312.

17. Kressner BE, Morton RRA, Martens AE, et al.: Use of an image analysis system to count colonies in stem cell assays of human tumors, in Salmon S (ed): Cloning of Human Tumor Stem Cells. New York, Alan Liss, 1980, pp 179-193.

18. Salmon SE: A new concept: in vitro phase II clinical trial with the human tumor stem cell assay. Proc Amer Assoc Cancer Res and Amer Soc Clin Oncol 21:abst C-41, p 329, 1980.

19. Von Hoff DD, Howser P, Gormley P, et al.: Phase I study methansulfonamide, N-(4-(9-acridinylamino)-3-methoxy-phenyl)-(m-AMSA) using a single dose schedule. Cancer Treat Rep 62:1421-1426, 1978.

20. Meyskens FM, Salmon SE: Inhibition of human melanoma colony formation by retinoids. Cancer Res 39:4055-4057, 1979.

21. Von Hoff DD, Pollard E, Kuhn J, et al.: Phase I clinical investigation of dihydroxyanthracenedione (NSC 301-739). Proc Amer Assoc Cancer Res and Amer Soc Clin Oncol 21:abst C-119, p 349, 1980.

22. Ahmann F, Meyskens F, Jones S, et al.: A broad phase II trial of AMSA with in vitro stem cell culture drug sensitivity correlation. Proc Amer Assoc Cancer Res and Amer Soc Clin Oncol 21:abst C-199, p 369, 1980.

Drug Studies in Nude Mice Xenografts

Awtar Krishan

Professor and Chief
Division of Cytokinetics
Comprehensive Cancer Center for the State of Florida
University of Miami School of Medicine
Miami, Florida

BACKGROUND

A number of systems for heterotransplantation of human tumors have been developed and include growth of tumors in immunological sanctuaries (e.g. brain, anterior eye chamber, cheek pouch,(21) renal capsule(1) or implantion of human tumor cells in neonatal, immunologically compromised or immature, animals.(2,8,29)

The discovery of the hairless mutant 'nude' mouse, which subsequently showed also an athymic condition, provided the necessary model for workers requiring heterotransplants of human cell lines and tumors in a convenient, easily reproducible host.(3,20,25) Numerous studies, includhg two international symposia and a monograph have been published on the various aspects of nude mice genetics, immunology and heterotransplantation and chemotherapy of tumor biopsies.(4,6,7,9,17)

HETEROTRANSPLANTATION OF CELL LINES, TISSUES AND TUMORS

Stiles and Kawahara(28), have concluded that 'normal diploid cells from animals or humans have never produced tumors whereas established lines of neoplastic origin have usually, though not always, produced tumors in nude mice.'

In contrast to the failure of cell lines of normal diploid origin to grow in nude mice, a variety of non-malignant tissues from various vertebrate and invertebrate sources have been successfully transplanted in nude mice. Interesting examples of successful, though bizzare, transplants include nude mice with cat fur, chicken feathers or reptilian scales.(23)

Malignancies of ectodermal, neural, endocrine, gastrointestinal, urogenital and hematopoietic origin have been successfully grown either as implants or as serially transplantable xenografts.(6,7,26) Hormone secreting tumors and tumors dependent on hormones for their continued proliferation have been relatively difficult to transplant. In most cases, the xenografts remain localized at the site of inoculation and only rarely metastasize to other areas.(24,27)

In xenografts of human gynecological tumors, we have seen stability of the aneuploid clones over the various transplantation levels.(20) In contrast, cell lines established from these tumors have shown rapid evolution of multiploid clones.(12)

EXPERIMENTAL CHEMOTHERAPY STUDIES

A number of workers have used xenografts of human solid tumors for monitoring drug sensitivity and effects on tumor growth.(7,18,22) A typical study is that by Giovanella, et al,(9) who tested the chemotherapeutic sensitivity of 15 serially transplanted human tumor xenografts in nude mice. Tumors included in this study were carcinomas of breast, lung and colon, melanomas and sarcomas. Drugs chosen were representative of the major classes including antimetabolites, alkylating agents, antitumor antibiotics and alkaloids. From these studies it was concluded that "in a majority of cases, positive responses mean only a slowing down of the growth of the tumor. Such slowing down of tumor growth does not appreciably affect survival". Tumor regression was rare and eventually the tumor regrew after cessation of therapy. However, the following important conclusions were drawn from this study: Tumors of the same histological type did not respond similarly to the same drug; response to a drug was similar in different passages of the same xenograft; response to a drug (negative or positive) was similar in the patient and the xenograft.

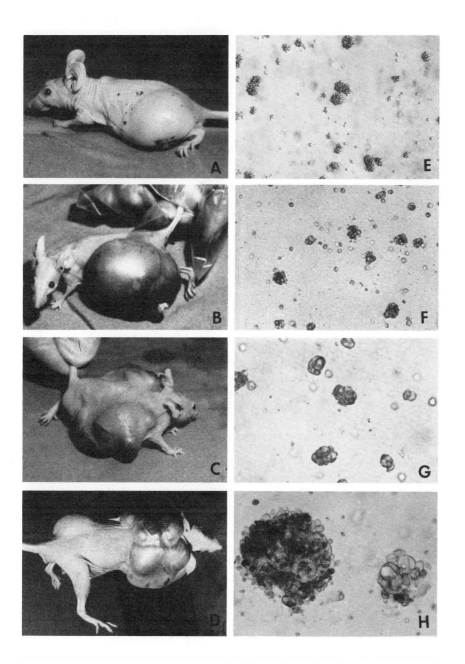

Figure 1. Human Tumor Xenografts, T-Cell Leukemia (A), Sq. Cell Ca. Cervix (B), Melanoma (C), and tumors A, B and C in one mouse (D).

Our experimental chemotherapy studies on xenografts of human solid tumors are based on protocols used in our clinics. Our model systems were xenografts of human melanoma and a variety of human gynecological tumors shown in Figure 1. Drugs were delivered via tail vein infusion or by repeated injections according to the best schedules recommended for a particular protocol. We tested combinations of bleomycin-mitomycin, cytoxan-adriamyin and variations of the high dose methotrexate rescue protocols. Effects on tumor proliferation were monitored by conventional methods of tumor mass measurement, labeling index, and laser flow cytometry. Our data on experimental chemotherapy of these xenografts has been far from encouraging. With the best of protocols available, we have not seen any major lasting effects on the proliferation of the xenograft. Short-term growth inhibition and reduction in tumor mass of between 10-30% was followed by rapid resumption of growth on cessation of therapy.

Needless to say, this data is far from encouraging and indicates the express need for better drug sensitivity and monitoring procedures. We must have tools for monitoring of 1) relative sensitivity of a tumor cell population to chemotherapeutic agents; 2) intracellular uptake and retention of the drugs by the tumor cells in vivo, and 3) the effects of these drugs on tumor cell proliferation and clonogenecity. Fortunately, technical developments within the last few years have provided means to partially answer some of these questions. Our first approach is based on the recent demonstration by Dr. Salmon and his colleagues that human solid tumor colonies can be grown in a soft agar assay. Data in Chart 1 shows the selective drug sensitivity of four different xenografts used in one of our studies.

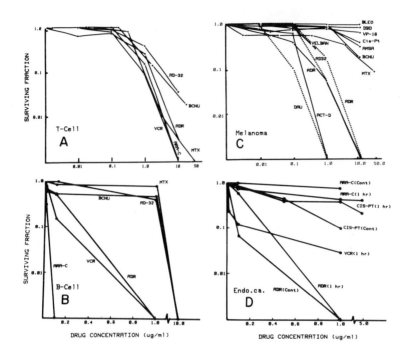

Chart 1. Colony forming assay of human tumors, T-cell (A), B-cell (B), melanoma (C) and endometrial carcinoma (D) in soft agar. Single cell suspensions were treated with various drug concentration for 1 hour, washed and plated. Colonies greater than 25 cells were counted on Day 7 (A and B), Day 10 (C) and Day 14 (D) and the surviving fraction determined.

In the T cell leukemia (A), clinically achievable plasma levels of vincristine, ara-C and adriamycin could have a significant (> 1 log) effect on tumor cell clonogenecity. In contrast, the B cell lymphoblasts (B) were extremely sensitive to ara-C, partially sensitive to vincristine and adriamycin and relatively insensitive to BCNU, methotrexate and AD-32. The human melanoma xenograft (C), showed sensitivity to daunomycin, actinomycin-D, and adriamycin but was resistant to bleomycin, cis-platinum, methotrexate and a number of other agents. The endometrial carcinoma shown in D, was

only sensitive to adriamycin and to vincristine but highly
resistant to ara-C and cis-plantinum.

The soft agar clonogenic assay is an important
technique for the screening of a human solid tumor for its
drug sensitivity in vitro. However, for a number of
pharmacokinetic and pharmacological reasons, it is
important to know whether the drug when given in vivo, is
transported and retained by the target cells. Similarly,
it is important to monitor the effect of the drug on tumor
cell cycle and clonogenecity. We have used the recently
introduced methodology of laser flow cytometry(16) for
monitoring the drug induced perturbations in the tumor
cell cycle and to detect and quantitate the intracellular
transport and retention of some of the important chemotherapeutic agents. In laser flow cytometry, a
monodisperse cell suspension is excited with a laser beam
and data (e.g. cellular DNA content for cell cycle
analysis or drug fluorescence) collected at the rate of
10^5 cells/second. Details of our instrumentation have
been recently published.(14) Drug induced perturbations
in cell cycle traverse of the tumor cells (e.g.
accumulation of cells in G_1, S or G_2/M) can thus be
rapidly determined. Similarly this methodology can be
used to monitor differential response of normal vs tumor
cells or of two sub-population in a solid tumor to a
chemotherapeutic regimen.

We have also recently demonstrated the use of laser
flow cytometry for monitoring the uptake and retention of
anthracycline antibiotics (e.g. adriamycin, daunomycin) in
tumor cells both in vitro and in vivo.(10,11,13) We have
developed two different methods for the detection and
quantitation of the intracellular drug content. Our
indirect method is based on the observation that
anthracyclines including adriamycin and daunomycin compete
with the binding of a DNA intercalating fluorochrome like
propidium iodide.(13) By measuring the quenching of the
propidium iodide fluorescence in drug exposed cells, we
can detect the presence of bound anthracyclines in tumor
cells. Our direct method is based on the observation that
anthracyclines can be excited with the 488 nm laser line
and the emitted fluorescence can be rapidly quantitated
both in vitro and in vivo.(10,11) We have used this
method to correlate drug resistance of adriamycin
resistant P388 cells both in vitro and in vivo.(5) An
example of the kind of data obtained by this methodology
is shown in Chart 2.

LASER EXCIT.OF INTRACELLULAR DAUNOMYCIN IN VIVO

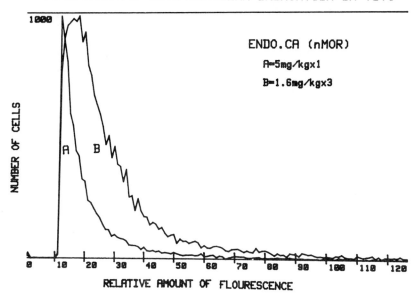

Chart 2. Laser excitation and quantitation of intracellular daunomycin in an adenocarcinoma of endometrium
xenograft treated in vivo. Mice treated i.p. with a bolus
dose (5 mg/kg, A) or multiple doses (1.6 mg/kg/injection x
3 every hour, B) of daunomycin, were sacrificed after 4
hours, and single cell suspensions analyzed. Abscissa
records intracellular fluorescence and the ordinate
represents the number of cells. Note two fold higher drug
fluorescence in tumor treated with multiple doses of drug
(B) compared to bolus injection (A).

In this experiment, nude mice bearing xenografts of an
endometrial carcinoma were administered daunomycin (total
dose 5 mg/kg) either as a single IP injection (curve A) or
as 3 hourly injections of 1.6 mg/kg (curve B). Single
cell suspensions prepared from the tumor biopsies were
analyzed. It is clear that in the tumor from the animal
given the three hourly injections, both the total amount
of intracellular drug fluorescence and the number of
fluorescent cells as significantly greater than that of

tumor cells from the amimal injected with the single dose. These observations are important in view of the recent studies indicating that adriamycin infusion lead to the amelioration of gastrointestinal toxicity with a possible decrease in cardiotoxicity without loss of antitumor activity.(15,19)

In conclusion, we feel that nude mice xenografts provide a unique source of heterotransplanted human solid tumors where questions related to drug induced cytokinetic perturbations (synchronization or recruitment of tumor cells), drug resistance (transport or biochemical) and effect of drugs on tumor cell clonogenecity can be answered.

REFERENCES

1. Bogden AE, Kelton DE, Cobb WR, et al: A rapid screeening method for testing chemotherapeutic agents against human tumor xenografts, in Houchens DP, Ovejera AA (ed): Proc. of the Symposium on the Use of Athymic (Nude) Mice in Cancer Research. New York, Gustav Fisher, 1978, pp 231-250.
2. Cobb LM, Mitchley BCV: The growth of human tumors in immune deprived mice. Eur J Cancer 10:473-476, 1974.
3. Flanagan SP: "Nude", a new hairless gene with pleiotropic effects in the mouse. Genet Res (Camb) 8:295-309, 1966.
4. Fogh J, Giovanella BC: The nude mouse in experimental and clinical research (ed 1). New York, Academic Press, 1978.
5. Ganapathi R, Reiter W, Krishan A, et al: Cytokinetics studies on adriamycin sensitive and resistant P388 cells. Proc Am Assoc Cancer Res 21:267, 1980.
6. Giovanella BC, Fogh J: Present and future trends in investigations with the nude mouse as a recipient of human tumor transplants, in Fogh J, Giovanella BC (ed): The Nude Mouse in Experimental and Clinical Research. New York, Academic Press, 1978, pp 281-312.
7. Giovanella BC, Stehlin JS, Fogh J, et al: Serial transplantation of human malignant tumors in nude mice and their use in experimental chemotherapy, in Houchens HP, Ovejera AA (ed): Proceedings of the Symposium on the Use of Athymic (Nude) Mice in Cancer Research. New York, Gustav Fischer, 1978, pp 163-179.

8. Handler AH, Davis S, Sommers SC: Heterotransplanta-
    tion experiments with human cancers. Cancer Res
    16:32-36, 1956.
9. Houchens DP, Ovejera AA: Proceedings of the
    symposium on the use of athymic (nude) mice in cancer
    research. New York, Gustav Fischer, 1978.
10. Krishan A, Ganapathi, R: Laser flow cytometry and
    cancer chemotherapy: Detection of intracellular
    anthracyclines by flow cytometry. J Histochem
    Cytochem 27:1655-1656, 1979.
11. Krishan A, Ganapathi R: Laser flow cytometric
    studies on the intracellular fluorescence of anthra-
    cyclines. Cancer Res, 1980 (in press).
12. Krishan A, Ganapathi R, Haines H, et al: Gynecologi-
    cal oncology studies in athymic nude mice, in Fogh J,
    Giovanella BC (ed 2): The Nude Mouse in Experimental
    and Clinical Research. New York, Academic Press,
    1980 (in press).
13. Krishan A, Ganapathi R, Israel M: The effect of
    adriamycin and analogs on the nuclear fluorescence of
    propidium iodide stained cells. Cancer Res 38:3656-
    3662, 1978.
14. Krishan A, Pitman SW, Tattersall MHN, et al: Micro-
    fluorometric patterns of human bone marrow and tumor
    cells in response to cancer chemotherapy. Cancer Res
    36:3813-3820, 1976.
15. Legha SS, Benjamin RS, Yap HY, et al: Augmentation
    of adriamycin therapeutic index by prolonged
    continuous I.V. infusion for advanced breast cancer.
    Proc Am Assoc Cancer Res 20:261, 1979.
16. Melamed MR, Mullaney PF, Mendelsohn ML: Flow
    cytometry and sorting, New York, Wiley, 1979.
17. Nomura T, Ohsawa N, Tamaoki N, et al: Proceedings of
    the second international workshop on nude mice. New
    York, Gustav Fischer Verlag, 1977.
18. Osieka R, Houchens DP, Goldin A, et al: Chemotherapy
    of human colon cancer xenografts in athymic nude
    mice. Cancer 40:2640-2650, 1977.
19. Pacciarini MA, Barbieri B, Colombo T, et al: Distri-
    bution and antitumor activity of adriamycin given in
    a high-dose and a repeated low-dose schedule to mice.
    Cancer Treat Rep 62:791-800, 1978.
20. Pantelouris EM: Absence of a thymus in a mouse
    mutant. Nature 217:370-371, 1968.
21. Patterson WB: Transplantation of human cancers to
    hamsters cheek pouches. Cancer Res 28:1637-1651,
    1968.

22.   Povlsen CO: Status of chemotherapy, radiotherapy
      endocrine therapy and immunotherapy studies of human
      cancer in the nude mouse, in Fogh J, Giovanella BC
      (ed):   The Nude Mouse in Experimental and Clinical
      Research.   New York, Academic Press, 1978, pp 437-
      456.
23.   Reed ND, Manning DD: Present status of xenotrans-
      plantation of non-malignant tissue to the nude mouse,
      in Fogh J, Giovanella BC (ed):   The Nude Mice in
      Experimental and Clinical Research.   New York,
      Academic Press, 1978, pp 167-185.
24.   Rostom AY, Thomas JM, Peckham JH, et al: Human
      Tumours in mice and rats. The Lancet Aug 19, 1978.
25.   Rygaard J: The nude mouse - mouse or test tube, in
      Houchens HP, Ovejera AA (ed):   Proceedings of the
      symposium on the Use of Athymic (Nude) Mice in Cancer
      Research. New York, Gustav Fischer, 1978, pp 1-7.
26.   Sharkey FE, Fogh JM, Hajdu SI, et al: Experience in
      surgical pathology with human tumor growth in the
      nude mouse, in Fogh J and Giovanella BC (ed):   The
      Nude Mouse in Experimental and Clinical Research. New
      York, Academic Press, 1978, pp 187-214.
27.   Sordat B, Merenda C, Carrel S: Invasive growth and
      dissemination of human solid tumors and malignant
      cell lines grafted subcutaneously to newborn nude
      mice.   Proc 2nd International Workshop on Nude Mice,
      Univ of Tokyo Press, Tokyo 1977.
28.   Stiles CD, Kawahara AA: The growth behavior of
      virus - transformed cells in nude mice, in Fogh J,
      Giovanella BC (ed):   The Nude Mouse in Experimental
      and Clinical Research.   New York, Academic Press,
      1978 pp 385-409.
29.   Toolan HW: Growth of human tumors in cortisone-
      treated laboratory animals: The possibility of
      obtaining permanently transplantable human tumors.
      Cancer Res 13:389-394, 1953.

Resistance to Therapeutic Agents

R. W. BROCKMAN

Head
Biological Chemistry Division
Southern Research Institute
Birmingham, Alabama 35255

INTRODUCTION

Drug resistance is as old as chemotherapy and has accompanied its development like a shadow.[29]   That this shadow is cast on cancer chemotherapy was established by Burchenal et al.[8] and by Law and Boyle[18] in early studies of resistance to antimetabolites. Resistance to cancer chemotherapeutic agents occurs in populations of tumor cells initially responsive that become resistant under treatment. Overgrowth of drug-resistant cells is, of course, not the only reason for failure of therapy. The kinetics of growth of tumors are an important factor; those tumors in which a large proportion of tumor cells are not in cycle and progressing to cell division are unresponsive to many anticancer agents. Metastasis of tumor cells to so-called sanctuary sites to which some chemotherapeutic agents do not readily gain access is another cause of failure of chemotherapy. Treatment, whether by means of surgery, radiation, or chemotherapy, will be unsuccessful if residual neoplastic cells, sensitive or resistant to therapy, remain viable and escape host defenses. We are concerned here with initial responses to treatment, i.e.   complete or partial remissions, followed by relapse during continued treatment.

It is well established that stable drug-resistant phenotypes of somatic cells in culture arise by mutation.[9,19,30] Selection of resistant phenotypes from a population of cells can then occur under selective pressure of a drug. The full impact of such occurrences in a population of cancer cells can be appreciated when it is realized that the survival of a single cancer cell can

Work from Southern Research Institute reported here was supported by Grant CA-23155 and Grant CA-20070 from the National Large Bowel Cancer Project, and by contract NO1-CM-97309 from the Division of Cancer Treatment, National Cancer Institute, National Institutes of Health, Department of Health and Human Services, U.S.A.

prove fatal.[13]   This has been demonstrated experimentally by implantation of a single viable tumor cell sensitive or resistant to chemotherapeutic agents.[23,36] Although the rate of appearance of mutants resistant to an anticancer agent in a population of tumor cells may be relatively low, the size of that population may be sufficiently large to make it probable that a resistant tumor cell is present.   Schabel et al[25]   demonstrated that the population doubling times for a number of drug-resistant sublines of murine leukemias were similar to those of the parent drug-sensitive lines. The drug-resistant tumor cell population, originating from one variant cell, increases at a faster rate than does the sensitive cell population because the resistant cell population can increase in two ways: (a) by division of resistant cells and (b) by additional mutations to resistance within the much larger sensitive cell population.   The size of the resistant cell population is influenced by the time at which the variant appeared in the sensitive population.   That is, the earlier the appearance of a resistant variant in a population of sensitive cells the larger will be the population of resistant cells at the time of sampling or at the time of treatment.   This is, in fact, the basis of the "fluctuation test" devised by Luria and Delbrück[20] to demonstrate that mutations in bacteria from virus sensitivity to virus resistance occurs by random mutation.   Law[17] applied this concept to mice bearing transplantable leukemia and provided evidence that mutation and selection is a mechanism by which resistant leukemia cells develop.   Study of much experimental data led Skipper[31,32,35] to re-emphasize that "selection and overgrowth of drug-resistant neoplastic cells is a major cause of chemotherapeutic failure."

SELECTION OF DRUG-RESISTANT NEOPLASMS

This was clearly shown in L1210 leukemia undergoing treatment with arabinosylcytosine.[5]   Overgrowth of resistant tumor cells during initially effective drug treatment resulted in failure of therapy and selection of a drug-resistant neoplasm.   In other experiments mice implanted with L1210 leukemia cells were treated with a single dose of palmo-Ara-C, a depot form of Ara-C, and then leukemia cells were harvested from five different treated animals and re-implanted in groups of mice. Sets of animals were treated with palmo-Ara-C and response to therapy was determined; tumor cells in other sets were allowed to grow untreated and then leukemia cells were harvested for enzyme analysis.   The results, summarized in Table 1, clearly show that leukemia cells so treated were completely resistant to Ara-C and that each of the five passage lines was deficient in enzyme capacity for phosphorylation of deoxycytidine and Ara-C.   Uridine-cytidine kinase activity, which served as an internal control, did not differ significantly in sensitive and resistant lines.   Loss of deoxycytidine kinase accompanying resistance to Ara-C is well known and has been described by several groups of investigators (see ref. 4).   This experiment

TABLE 1

Consistent Selection of Leukemia Cells Resistant to Ara-C and
Deficient in Deoxycytidine Kinase

Group	Inocula		Response		Pyrimidine Nucleoside Kinase Activity (nmoles nucleotide/mg protein/min)			
	Cell Source	Size	% ILS	30-day Surv. (%)	Urd	Cyd	dCyd	ara-C
A. Control	Ascites	10^5	212	5/10	2.5	0.58	0.28	0.27
	Spleen	10 mg	257	3/10	1.9	0.51	0.28	0.21
B. AraC-treated	Ascites	10^5	0	0/10	2.0	0.72	0.001	0.0007
	Ascites	10^5	0	0/10	2.6	0.61	0.001	0.0005
	Ascites	10^5	0	0/10	2.8	0.69	0.002	0.0005
	Spleen	10 mg	0	0/10	1.8	0.72	0.002	0.0007
	Spleen	10 mg	0	0/10	2.0	0.50	0.009	0.002

Inocula were obtained from animals implanted with 10^7 L1210 leukemia cells and treated on day 2 with a single dose of palmo-Ara-C (150 mg/kg). The 15th day after implant tumor cells were harvested from five treated mice (group B) and 10^5 cells or 10 mg of leukemic spleen were implanted in recipient mice. One set of animals was treated with palmo-Ara-C (150 mg/kg); ascites tumor cells from the other set, untreated with AraC, were harvested 6 days after cell implant for analysis of pyrimidine nucleoside kinase activity.

serves to emphasize the consistency of this mechanism of resistance in experimental leukemia.

That such events occur in solid tumors is illustrated by the data of Dr. T. H. Corbett in which mice bearing colon adenocarcinoma 36 tumors were treated with palmo-Ara-C. [25] Complete regression of all tumors was observed but two tumors recurred and grew during treatment (Fig. 1). Passage lines of these recurrent tumors were established and examined for sensitivity to palmo-Ara-C; both tumors showed marked resistance to this agent. Results of an analysis of deoxycytidine kinase activity and of capacity to phosphorylate Ara-C by enzyme preparations from sensitive and partially resistant colon tumor 36 showed a 50% decrease in kinase activity relative to that in the parent tumor. Uridine kinase activity was unchanged in the drug-resistant tumor. This result suggests the presence of a mixed population consisting of sensitive cells and of resistant cells deficient in deoxycytidine kinase. Thus, resistance to cancer chemotherapeutic drugs associated with biochemical changes can be demonstrated in murine leukemias and solid tumors in vivo.

New Ways of Looking at Drug Resistance

Goldie and Coldman [14] have presented a mathematical analysis relating the drug sensitivity of tumors to their spontaneous mutation rate to drug resistance. The reader is referred to the original

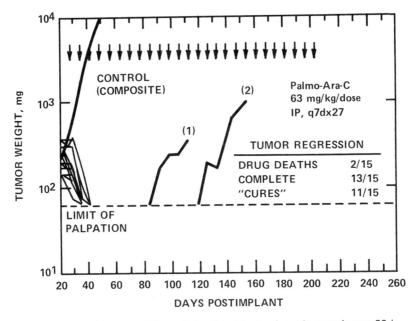

Figure 1.   *Development of lines of Ara-C-resistant colon adenocarcinoma 36 in
mice bearing 0.2-0.3 gram subcutaneous tumors and treated with
palmo-Ara-C once each week for 27 weeks. Median life span of ten
untreated control animals (composite curve) was 54 days. The two
tumors that recurred under treatment were transplanted and shown
to be unresponsive to palmo-Ara-C.*

paper for the derivation of the term that expresses the probability
(P) of finding zero resistant cells in a tumor in relation to the
mutation rate per cell per generation and the number of tumor
cells (N).

$$P = \exp\{-\alpha(N-1)\}$$

As tumor size increases the probability of the presence of resistant
clones increases or, as the graphical expression of the equation
indicates (Fig. 2), the probability of the existence of zero resistant
phenotypes in the population of cells approaches zero.   If it is
assumed that mutation results in complete resistance to treatment,
and if the treatment given is sufficient to eliminate the larger
drug-sensitive population, then P represents the probability of cure
for a tumor of size N.   This mathematical model predicts that as
tumor burden increases the probability of resistant clones increases
and the response to treatment decreases. This is, of course, widely
recognized in experimental and clinical cancer chemotherapy and
finds expression in the dictum that early detection and treatment
increases the likelihood of cure. Dr. H. E. Skipper has tested this
mathematical model by means of experimental results obtained
with groups of mice implanted with increasing numbers of L1210
cells that were treated with Ara-C (Table 2). When these data are
superimposed on the plot of the equation derived by Goldie and
Coldman, good agreement is observed if a mutation rate from

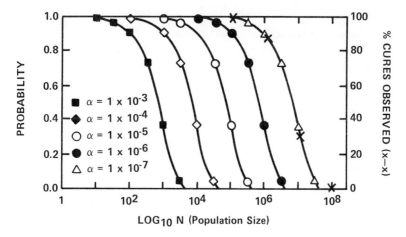

Figure 2. *Relationship of the probability of the existence of no resistant phenotypes to the mutation rate (α) and the number of cells (N) (14). Superimposed on this curve are observed cures (x—x) of mice implanted with increasing numbers of L1210 cells and treated with Ara-C (see Table 2).*

L1210/0 to L1210/Ara-C is assumed to be about 1×10^{-7} (Fig. 2). The development of a resistant clone in any population of tumor cells is a random event and the time of its occurrence is a function of the growth curve of the tumor and the mutation rate. The likelihood of there being at least one resistant cell present in a tumor population can change from a condition of low to high probability over a relatively short interval of growth, and the higher the mutation rate the earlier in the growth of the tumor this transition is likely to occur. The implications of these statements are evident when one considers the development of a clinical cancer in which a single cancer cell and its progeny may go through 27-30 doublings, reaching a size of 10^8 to 10^9 cells, before becoming detectable by means of x-rays or palpation.[11]

CIRCUMVENTION OF RESISTANCE

Combination Chemotherapy

Discussion has thus far emphasized the seemingly inevitable development and selection of drug-resistant tumor cells in a population of sensitive cells. However, chemotherapy alone or in conjunction with other modes of treatment is successful in the treatment of some experimental and clinical cancers. The obstacle to achieving remission and cure that is posed by the emergence of drug-resistant tumor cells can be circumvented by means of judicious combination chemotherapy and appropriate scheduling of treatment. There are, of course, other factors that contribute to the success of combination chemotherapy. Increased cell kill and

TABLE 2

Observed Relationship Between the Cell Burden and Curability
of L1210 Leukemia with Arabinosylcytosine

Treatment Schedule	Courses of Treatment	% Cures in Relation to Leukemia Cell Burden at Initiation of Therapy				
		10^8	10^7	10^6	10^5	10^4
Every	1	--	0	10	50	80
3 Hours	2	0	8	58	--	--
for 8 Doses	3	--	16	65	94	--
	4	0	35	87	100	--

L1210 leukemia cells (10^4 to 10^8 cells) were implanted intraperitoneally in recipient mice and Ara-C was administered i.p. at the maximum tolerated dose (10 mg/kg/dose) every 3 hours for 8 doses with courses of treatment on days 1, 5, 9, and 13 after leukemia cell implants.

access of one or more components of a combination to sites of metastases, e.g. brain, also are compelling reasons for the use of combination chemotherapy. Knowledge of (a) biochemical mechanisms by which drugs act, (b) mechanisms by which tumor cells acquire resistance to active agents, (c) patterns of cross-resistance and sensitivity among chemotherapeutic agents, (d) kinetics of tumor cell growth, and (e) information on pharmacologic and toxic effects of drugs all contribute to the design of drug combinations.[1,3-5,12,22,25,34] In the context of this symposium, it is appropriate to consider some successful clinical examples of combination chemotherapy and to suggest some possibilities for future development based on results of experimental chemotherapy.

Successful combination chemotherapy is well illustrated by the development of regimens for treatment of acute lymphocytic leukemia (ALL) of childhood.[1] Drugs available for therapy twenty years ago were the antimetabolites methotrexate (MTX) and 6-mercaptopurine (6-MP) which, when used alone, gave remission rates of about 25% and which, when used in combination, induced remission in about 45% of patients treated. Combined use of four agents, prednisone, oncovin (vincristine), MTX and purinethiol (6-MP), the so-called POMP regimen, resulted in marked improvement in response of this disease to chemotherapy. Success is achieved in treating ALL in children with sequential combinations of these drugs, i.e., vincristine plus prednisone followed by MTX plus 6-MP. This pattern of treatment - induction of remission with one agent or combination of agents followed by treatment with another agent or combination - is one that would decrease the probability of overgrowth of drug-resistant tumor cells. This is so, provided there is lack of cross-resistance between the two treatments and the population of cells resistant to the first treatment is low.

The development of drug combinations for successful chemotherapy of Hodgkin's disease also is a high point in chemotherapy. DeVita et al [10] developed the combination of mechlorethamine, oncovin (vincristine), procarbazine and prednisone, designated MOPP and Bonadonna et al [2] introduced the combination of adriamycin, bleomycin, vinblastine and dacarbazine (DTIC), designated ABVD. Both of these treatments are effective against Hodgkin's disease with observed absence of cross-resistance between MOPP and ABVD treatment.

Scheduling

The advantage of alternating cycles of treatment has been examined by Skipper [33] and considered on theoretical grounds by Goldie and his associates.* Their analysis considers the problem of the origin of doubly-resistant mutants in a population of tumor cells. Phenotypes resistant to each of two treatments, T_1 or T_2, can arise by mutation-selection, as considered earlier. Lack of cross-resistance would allow successful combination treatment since sensitive cells and cells resistant to T_1 would respond to T_2, and sensitive cells and cells resistant to T_2 would respond to T_1. Failure would result in the event that the population of cells resistant to T_1 or T_2 become large enough for mutation and selection of a doubly-resistant mutant to occur. According to the mathematical analysis by Goldie and his associates, an alternating cycle of treatment (T_1, T_2, T_1, T_2, etc.) increases the likelihood of eradicating the tumor. This assumes that both treatments are equally effective against the sensitive line and that there is no cross resistance. The results of Santoro et al [21] provide an example of improved response by means of alternating treatment with MOPP and ABVD over MOPP alone. If the tumor burden and the mutation rates are low, a single treatment regimen might suffice or, under such favorable circumstances, the sequence of therapy with other regimens might not be so critical. The alternating cycle of treatment increases the probability of success in some circumstances and thus merits further consideration in planning treatment strategies.

Cross-Resistance and Collateral Sensitivity

It has been emphasized that lack of cross-resistance between agents used in combination or in sequence is critical for successful chemotherapy. Much useful information can be obtained from chemotherapy studies with resistant sublines of experimental

---

*The author is indebted to Dr. James H. Goldie and his associates, Cancer Control Agency of British Columbia, Vancouver, for the privilege of referring to their manuscript entitled "A rationale for the use of alternating non-cross resistant chemotherapy," Goldie JH, Coldman AJ, Gudauskas GA.

neoplasms.[25]   For example, it is now recognized that alkylating
agents may differ in modes of transport into cells, in activation by
cellular enzymes, and in reactive alkylating moieties. The observations of Schabel et al[27] on patterns of resistance and therapeutic synergism among alkylating agents in L1210 leukemias
resistant to cyclophosphamide (CPA), BCNU, and L-phenylalanine
mustard (L-PAM) are revealing.   Cyclophosphamide-resistant
L1210 was fully sensitive to BCNU and the other nitrosoureas.
L1210/BCNU, although not completely resistant to BCNU, showed
a marked decrease in sensitivity to other nitrosoureas but was as
responsive to cyclophosphamide and to L-PAM as was the parent
line.   L1210/L-PAM was not completely resistant to L-PAM,
retained sensitivity to cyclophosphamide, and was fully sensitive to
the nitrosoureas.   A piperazinedione derivative with alkylating
activity[7] was active against L1210/BCNU and L1210/L-PAM but
showed decreased activity against L1210/CPA.[26] It is particularly
interesting that certain combinations of alkylating agents show
therapeutic synergism in a number of experimental tumors.[25,27]
For example, cyclophosphamide in combination with nitrosoureas
(BCNU, CCNU, MeCCNU) or with L-PAM exhibited therapeutic
synergism while less than additive toxicity for host animals was
observed. These observations suggest that combinations of certain
alkylating agents merit inclusion in drug combination regimens.

On the other hand it was observed that a line of P388 leukemia
selected for resistance to adriamycin was cross-resistant to actinomycin D, to vincristine, to VP-16 and to an acridine derivative that
was effective against the sensitive line.[25,27]   It has been
suggested that displays of cross-resistance to apparently unrelated
compounds may be a consequence of alterations in cell membrane
and altered transport.[19]   Such unexpected patterns of cross-
resistance pose problems for the design of drug combinations and
sequences of therapy.

The development of resistance to one drug sometimes results in
increased sensitivity to another drug which acts by a different
mechanism.   This phenomenon has been designated collateral
sensitivity and has been studied and reviewed by Dr. Doris
Hutchison and her colleagues.[15,16]   In some experimental
neoplasms the development of resistance to MTX was accompanied
by increased sensitivity to 6-MP and vice versa. [15] Table 3 presents
examples of collateral sensitivity in murine leukemias resistant to
6-MP or to Ara-C.[24,25] Resistance to 6-MP resulted in increased
sensitivity to MTX and resistance to Ara-C resulted in increased
sensitivity to 3-deazauridine, dihydro-5-azacytidine, PALA (N-
phosphonacetyl-L-aspartate), and pyrazofurin. It should be noted,
however, that none of the latter compounds were particularly
active against the parent sensitive line, indicating that they would
not be useful for initial treatment. The combination of MTX and
6-MP used in treatment of ALL may owe some of its efficacy to
collateral sensitivity. Further study of this phenomenon in relation

TABLE 3

Some Examples of Collateral Sensitivity in Murine Leukemia Cells[1]

Agent	Log_{10} Change in Leukemia Cell Population[2,3]		
	L1210/O	L1210/MP	L1210/AraC
Methotrexate	0	−5	
Dichloromethotrexate	−1	−5	
3-Deazauridine	+2		−6

	P388/O	P388/AraC
Dihydro-5-azacytidine	−1	−6
PALA	+2	−3
Pyrazofurin	+3	−2

1. Development of resistance to one agent can result in increased sensitivity to another agent.
2. Based on leukemia cell population at the end of optimal drug treatment.
3. BDF_1 or CDF_1 mice were implanted i.p. with 10^5 L1210 cells or 10^6 P388 cells and treated i.p. q.d. 1-9.

to chemotherapy and drug resistance is warranted as a means of circumventing drug resistance.

CONCLUSIONS

The development of drug-resistant cells in a population of tumor cells is recognized as a major obstacle to successful cancer chemotherapy. A population of drug-resistant tumor cells arises as a consequence of mutation followed by selection in the presence of an effective drug. The rate of mutation to resistance and the size of the population of tumor cells are determining factors, but the occurrence of a resistant clone in a population of tumor cells is a random event. Mutations occurring early in the history of a tumor result in relatively large populations of resistant cells at the time of detection or time of initiation of treatment. Variation in the response of tumors to chemotherapy is in part attributable to this fact.

Combination chemotherapy, appropriately scheduled, offers the best hope of minimizing failure of chemotherapy as a consequence of overgrowth of drug-resistant tumor cells. The development of better agents for use against cancers that are thus far refractory to chemotherapy is essential for further progress. Through understanding of mechanisms of action of drugs, of mechanisms of resistance, and of the process by which sub-populations of resistant cells arise the chemotherapist is better able to "design with nature" in the treatment of cancer.

ACKNOWLEDGMENTS

The author is indebted to Dr. Frank Schabel, Dr. Howard Skipper and Dr. James Goldie for valuable discussions and for permission to use their data to illustrate aspects of this discussion.

REFERENCES

1. Blum RH, Frei E III: Combination chemotherapy, in DeVita VT Jr, Busch H (eds): Cancer Drug Development, Part B. Methods in Cancer Research, Vol. 17. New York, Academic Press, Inc., 1979, pp 215-257.
2. Bonadonna G, Zucali R, Monfardina S, et al.: Combination chemotherapy of Hodgkin's disease with adriamycin, bleomycin, vinblastine, and imidazole-carboxamide versus MOPP. Cancer 36: 252-259, 1975.
3. Brockman RW: Biochemical aspects of drug combinations. Cancer Treat Rep 4 (Pt 2):115-129, 1974.
4. Brockman RW: Mechanisms of resistance, in Sartorelli AC, Johns DG (eds): Antineoplastic and Immunosuppressive Agents, Part I. Handbook of Experimental Pharmacology, Vol. 38. Berlin, Springer-Verlag, 1974, pp 352-410
5. Brockman RW: Circumvention of resistance, in Pharmacological Basis of Cancer Chemotherapy (27th Annual Symposium on Fundamental Cancer Research, 1974, The University of Texas M. D. Anderson Hospital and Tumor Institute). Baltimore, Williams and Wilkins Co. 1975, pp 691-711
6. Brockman RW, Yagisawa Y, Ling V, et al.: Modes of acquiring resistance to chemotherapeutic agents, in Siegenthaler W, Lüthy R (eds): Current Chemotherapy (Proceedings of the 10th International Congress of Chemotherapy, Vol. 1. Washington, American Society for Microbiology, 1978, pp. 97-106
7. Brockman RW, Shaddix SC, Williams M, Struck RF: Studies with 2,5-piperazinedione, 3,6-bis(5-chloro-2-piperidyl)-dihydrochloride. II. Effects on macromolecular synthesis in cell culture and evidence for alkylating activity. Cancer Treat Rep 60:1317-1324, 1976.
8. Burchenal JH, Robinson E, Johnston SF, et al.: The induction of resistance to N^{10}-methylpteroylglutamic acid in a strain of transmitted mouse leukemia. Science 111:116-117, 1950.
9. Clements GB: Selection of biochemically variant, in some cases mutant, mammalial cells in culture, in Klein G, Weinhouse S, Haddow A (eds): Advances in Cancer Research, Vol. 21. New York, Academic Press, 1975, pp 273-390
10. DeVita VT, Serpick AA, Carbone PP: Combination chemotherapy in the treatment of advanced Hodgkin's disease. Ann Intern Med 73:881-895, 1970.

11. DeVita VT, Young RC, Canellos GP: Combination versus single agent chemotherapy: A review of the basis for selection of drug treatment of cancer. Cancer 35:98-110, 1975.
12. Dorr RT, Fritz WL: Cancer Chemotherapy Handbook. New York, Elsevier North Holland, Inc., 1980, pp 50-74
13. Furth J, Kahn MC: The transmission of leukemia of mice with a single cell. Amer J Cancer 31:276-282, 1937.
14. Goldie JH, Coldman AJ: A mathematic model for relating the drug sensitivity of tumors to their spontaneous mutation rate. Cancer Treat Rep 63:1727-1733, 1979.
15. Hutchison DJ: Cross resistance and collateral sensitivity studies in cancer chemotherapy, in Haddow A, Weinhouse S (eds): Advances in Cancer Research, Vol. 7. New York, Academic Press, Inc., 1963, pp 235-350
16. Hutchison DJ, Schmid FA: Cross-resistance and collateral sensitivity, in Mihich (ed): Drug Resistance and Selectivity, Biochemical and Cellular Basis New York, Academic Press, Inc., 1973, pp 73-126
17. Law LW: Origin of the resistance of leukaemic cells to folic acid antagonists. Nature 169: 628-629, 1952.
18. Law PJ, Boyle PJ: Development of resistance to folic acid antagonists in a transplantable lymphoid leukemia. Proc Soc Exp Biol Med 74:599-602, 1950.
19. Ling V: Genetic aspects of drug resistance in somatic cells, in Schabel FM Jr (vol ed): Fundamentals in Cancer Chemotherapy. Antibiotics and Chemotherapy, Vol. 23. Basel, Karger, 1978, pp 191-199
20. Luria SE, Delbrück M: Mutations of bacteria from virus sensivity to virus resistance. Genetics 28:491-511, 1943.
21. Santoro A, Bonadonna G, Bonfante V, Valagussa P: Non cross resistant regimens (MOPP and ABVD) vs MOPP alone in stage IV Hodgkin disease. Proc Am Assoc Clin Oncol 21:470, 1980.
22. Schabel FM Jr: In vivo leukemic cell kill kinetics and "curability" in experimental systems, in The Proliferation and Spread of Neoplastic Cells (21st Annual Symposium on Fundamental Cancer Research, 1967. The University of Texas M. D. Anderson Hospital and Tumor Institute). Baltimore, Williams and Wilkins Co., 1968, pp 397-408.
23. Schabel, FM Jr.: Concepts for treatment of micrometastases developed in murine systems. Am J Roentgenol Radium Ther Nucl Med 126:500-511, 1976.
24. Schabel FM Jr: Test systems for evaluating the antitumor activity of nucleoside analogues, in Walker RT, DeClercq E, Eckstein F (eds): Nucleoside Analogues, Chemistry, Biology and Medical Applications, Vol. 26. NATO Advanced Study Series A: Life Sciences. New York, Plenum Publishing Corp. 1979, pp 363-394

25. Schabel FM Jr, Skipper HE, Trader MW, et al.: Concepts for controlling drug-resistant tumor cells, in Mouridsen HT, Palshof T (eds): Breast Cancer, Experimental and Clinical Aspects. Oxford, Pergamon Press, Ltd, 1980, pp 199-212

26. Schabel FM Jr, Trader MW, Laster WR, et al.: Studies with 2,5-piperazinedione,3,6-bis(5-chloro-2-piperidyl)-dihydrochloride. III. Biochemical and therapeutic effects in L1210 leukemias sensitive and resistant to alkylating agents: Comparison with melphalan, cyclophosphamide, and BCNU. Cancer Treat Rep 60:1325-1333, 1976.

27. Schabel FM Jr, Trader MW, Laster WR, Wheeler GP: Patterns of resistance and therapeutic synergism among alkylating agents, in Schabel FM Jr (vol ed): Fundamentals in Cancer Chemotherapy. Antibiotics and Chemotherapy, Vol. 24. Basel, Karger, 1978, pp 200-215

28. Schmid FA, Hutchison DJ, Otter GM, Stock CC: Development of resistance to combinations of six antimetabolites in mice with L1210 leukemia. Cancer Treat Rep 60:23-27, 1976.

29. Schnitzer RJ, Grunberg E: Drug resistance of microorganisms. New York, Academic Press, 1957.

30. Siminovitch L: On the nature of heritable variation in cultured somatic cells. Cell 7:1-11, 1976.

31. Skipper HE: Reasons for success and failure in treatment of murine leukemias with the drugs now employed in treating human leukemias. Cancer Chemotherapy, Vol. 1. Ann Arbor, MI, University Microfilms International, 1978.

32. Skipper HE: Idealized hypothetical illustrations of the effects of specifically drug-resistant leukemia cells on end-results achievable with single drugs and combinations. Cancer Chemotherapy, Vol. 3. Ann Arbor, MI, University Microfilms International, 1979.

33. Skipper HE: Concurrent comparisons of some 2-,3-, and 4-drug combinations delivered simultaneously and sequentially (L1210 and P388 leukemia systems). Cancer Chemotherapy, Vol. 9: Ann Arbor, MI, University Microfilms International, 1980.

34. Skipper HE, Hutchison DJ, Schabel FM Jr, et al.: A quick reference chart on cross resistance between anticancer agents. Cancer Treat Rep 56:493-498, 1972.

35. Skipper HE, Schabel FM Jr, Lloyd HH: Experimental therapeutics and kinetics: selection and overgrowth of specifically and permanently drug-resistant tumor cells. Semin Hematol 15:207-219, 1978.

36. Skipper HE, Schabel FM Jr, Wilcox WS: Experimental evaluation of potential anticancer agents. XIII. On the criteria and kinetics associated with "curability" of experimental leukemias. Cancer Chemother Rep 35:1-111, 1964.

Rationales for Congener Synthesis

JOHN A. MONTGOMERY

Vice President
Southern Research Institute
Birmingham, Alabama 35255

Although there is admittedly much still to be learned about the optimal utilization of the anticancer agents now in human use, it seems clear that new and better drugs are needed if continuing advances are to be made in cancer treatment. There are at least two reasons for this: a number of important types of human cancer appear to respond poorly to the agents we now have and many cancers that do respond to therapy initially are not cured and eventually develop biochemical resistance to the drug or drugs used. In recent years, new types of agents that are discovered frequently show activity against human cancers unresponsive to all the established drugs. Witness the activity of the nitrosoureas against brain tumors, of DTIC against melanomas, and of cis-platinum against testicular cancers. In addition, they are often effective against neoplasms that have acquired resistance to other agents. It seems likely that this trend will continue, but the development of new leads is difficult because of our inability to identify and define an exploitable biochemical difference between normal mammalian host cells and invading cancer cells such as exists between mammalian cells and bacterial cells and on which the selective toxicity of the highly effective antibacterial agents depends. At the same time, few clinically useful agents have resulted from random screening of synthetically prepared compounds (this remark obviously does not apply to the isolation of useful drugs from complex natural mixtures such as antibiotic beers or plants).

Work referred to herein by the author and his associates was supported by the Division of Cancer Treatment of the National Cancer Institute by Contract NO1-CP-43762 and Grant CA24975.

The development of a congener that is more useful in the treatment of human cancer than the original lead obviously requires that it have greater selectivity in its toxicity to neoplastic cells, that it be better transported to and into the target cancer cells wherever they are in the host, or that it have some special value such as the ability to circumvent acquired drug resistance. To meet any of these requirements, reasonable and specific goals must be defined in terms that can be translated into responses in animal test systems, methods for attaining the goals must be conceived, and progress toward these goals must be accurately measured.

First, how can progress toward these goals be measured? Obviously, in the end, by evaluation in humans. But, despite the real problems that exist in relating animal and human data, it seems unreasonable to suggest that congener comparisons can only be meaningfully made in humans, although more studies of this type should be carried out. Cytotoxicity data can be very important, but not the final basis of selection of a drug for clinical evaluation, since host toxicity cannot be related to activity. So, like it or not, the answer to the question is that appropriate experimental animal models must be used for congener comparisons. This conclusion emphasizes the importance of selecting proper test systems.

If, then, animal models are accepted, what specific goals should be pursued in these models? The discussion that follows sets forth a number of clearly defined goals, the attainment of which could lead to new useful clinical agents. How these goals can be achieved is somewhat more nebulous, but examples of approaches that have been taken with varying degrees of success in the animal models and in clinical applications are given. Often success has been achieved simply by systematic structural alterations of the lead compound guided by feedback from the appropriate animal test system or systems, be they a leukemia, a metastatic solid tumor, a drug-resistant neoplasm, a battery of tumors, or an animal toxicity test.

First, it would be desirable to obtain a significantly better cancer cell kill in a specific test system at host-tolerated doses. This test system should be sensitive to the class of agents in question but not too sensitive; otherwise, meaningful differences in activity cannot be measured. In such a system, or preferably systems, a minimum of a one-log difference in cell kill at the LD_{10}, either alone or in combination with another agent (or agents), should indicate a new congener with potentially recognizably superior clinical activity. That is to say, if a one-log greater cell kill in the animal system is predictive of a one-log greater cell kill at a tolerated dose in man - and there appears to be no data to indicate to the contrary - then the congener should have observably better clinical activity than the parent now in clinical use. Preferably, this log greater cell kill should be demonstrated against solid tumors, and specifically against micrometastases from a solid tumor rather than the primary solid tumor itself, since such activity would indicate its potential utility in surgical adjuvant therapy.

Another measure of improved activity is a better therapeutic index. A congener with a significantly greater difference in its LD_{10} and minimum effective dose, defined here as a dose that will kill a minimum of two or three logs of cells, than the parent should be advantageous, particularly in combination chemotherapy. Drugs do differ in their dose-response curves and in their activity at low fractions of the LD_{10}.

A broader spectrum of activity is a clear indication of increased efficacy. If a congener shows real activity against one or more animal tumors that do not respond to the parent, it should become potentially interesting for clinical investigation, since this simply increases the likelihood that it will be active against some form of the human disease.

A different factor to be considered is the lack of cross resistance (or, in an optimistic vein, collateral sensitivity). If an animal tumor that has become resistant to the parent drug responds to the congener, it should be of interest because of the ease with which neoplasms become resistant to most agents. The evidence today is overwhelming that human cancers that initially respond to drug therapy, but later fail to, have become drug-resistant as a result of the overgrowth of mutant resistant cells selected by the treatment employed. In fact, for obvious reasons, the more effective the treatment (short of cure), the faster resistance develops, if the cancer cell population is about 10^6 or greater, which it almost always is by the time of diagnosis. It is tempting to think that the proper use of new agents effective against cells that are biochemically resistant to clinically useful drugs will at least permit much longer extension of remissions and at best contribute to curative chemotherapy.

Another goal might be to develop a congener with a different limiting toxicity to the host, particularly if the new limiting toxicity is to neither the bone marrow nor the intestinal epithelium, or to eliminate a peculiar toxicity that may be unrelated to the drug's ability to kill neoplastic cells.

The identification of congeners that are metabolized differently is an attractive and, we now know, an attainable goal. Such a difference underlies the activity of certain antimetabolites against neoplasms that have become resistant to closely related compounds. Differential metabolism could be the basis of the selective cytotoxicity of some anticancer agents. Not only do we have some guidelines for successful drug modification based on metabolism, we also understand why certain seemingly logical structural modifications of known drugs did not lead to more active agents.

The development of congeners with more desirable physico-chemical properties but with the same or better activity is a further goal. For example, better stability (either on the shelf or in solution), better solubility in physiologic media, and a more favorable water-lipid solubility ratio (defined by partition coefficient), that might affect drug distribution such as penetration of the blood-brain barrier or of solid tumors are properties that can be designed into certain kinds of agents.

Some of the goals that are important in the development of congeners with better activity have been set forth, as well as at least one suggestion for measuring progress toward these goals. Examples which illustrate how these goals were achieved in specific cases are given below. In general, the strategy for the development of a superior congener depends quite a bit on the type of agent and on the specific agent under the general type. For example, the approach to developing better chemically reactive agents such as the nitrogen mustards or the nitrosoureas is quite different from the approach to developing better antimetabolites, be they analogs of ara-C, 6-mercaptopurine, 5-fluorouracil, or methotrexate. The several ways in which the activity of a lead compound has been modified or improved is discussed below under the headings of some of the types of anticancer agents that have been studied. This is not intended to be a comprehensive review. Rather the choice of agents for discussion is largely based on the research experiences of the author and his associates.

CHEMICALLY REACTIVE COMPOUNDS

The Nitrogen Mustards

From early work on the aliphatic nitrogen mustards, developed during World War II as toxic chemical warfare agents, mechlorethamine (HN2) became the agent of choice for cancer chemotherapy. The synthesis of melphalan (L-PAM) was inspired by the possibility that a nitrogen mustard derivative of a natural amino acid might be directed to a metabolic site critical to neoplastic cells. No compelling evidence has been presented to verify an improvement in the selective action of such agents by facilitated transport, but data generally support the superiority of melphalan over mechlorethamine both in animal systems and in man, although this advantage may be primarily due to the decreased basicity of the nitrogen of the bis(2-chloroethyl)amino group, with the accompanying decrease in chemical reactivity, that results from replacement of the methyl group by a substituted phenyl group.

Although the original premise for the synthesis of phosphorylated nitrogen mustard derivatives is now largely discounted, it led to the development of cyclophosphamide (CPA), one of the most widely used clinical agents today. Proposed as a potentially latent form of bis(2-chloroethyl)amine (nor-HN2), cyclophosphamide (CPA) emerged from the synthesis of more than 500 phosphoramides as the most effective congener in evaluation against the Yoshida ascitic sarcoma in rats. Definitely superior to nor-HN2 and other nitrogen mustards, CPA, which is itself nontoxic to tumor cells in culture, is hydroxylated, primarily in the liver, to 4-hydroxycyclophosphamide, which spontaneously decomposes to the phosphoramide mustard (PM), in all probability the active form of the drug. Ifosfamide (IFA), an isomer of CPA, is superior to it in animal test systems and is, therefore, receiving clinical attention. The phosphoramide mustard (IPM) derivable from IFA is quite active against leukemia L1210 and a subline resistant to CPA, does not require metabolic activation, and does not release acrolein, the metabolite of CPA and IFA that is responsible for their urotoxic effects.

The Nitrosoureas

Interest in the synthesis and evaluation of N-nitroso compounds as potential anticancer agents grew from the observation made in the random screening program of the National Cancer Institute that N-methyl-N'-nitro-N-nitrosoguanidine (MNNG) increased the life span of mice inoculated intraperitoneally with leukemia L1210 cells. The recognition that MNNG is a precursor of diazomethane led to the evaluation of 1-methyl-1-nitrosourea (MNU) in this test system. The nitrosourea proved not only to be much more active than the guanidine against this form of the disease, but also to be effective against this leukemia when cells were implanted intracerebrally in mice, in contrast to the inactivity of well-known anticancer agents such as methotrexate, 6-mercaptopurine, 5-fluorouracil, and cyclophosphamide in a parallel comparison. This unique activity prompted the synthesis and evaluation of a large number of nitrosoureas. Early work led to N,N'-bis(2-chloroethyl)-N-nitrosourea (BCNU), one of the first compounds to effect a high percentage of cures of mice with leukemia L1210 and the first to undergo clinical trials, and to the understanding that the 2-chloro- or fluoroethylnitrosoureido function is essential for a high level of activity. The search for compounds more effective against meningeal leukemia led to the identification of CCNU [N-(2-chloroethyl)-N'-cyclohexyl-N-nitrosourea] and PCNU [N-(2-chloroethyl)-N'-(2,6-dioxo-3-piperidyl)-N-nitrosourea] as two of the most active structures against intracerebrally implanted leukemia L1210; CCNU is now being used clinically for tumors in the brain as well as other forms of cancer.

After the development of CCNU, attention turned to improving the activity of the nitrosoureas against solid tumors using the Lewis lung carcinoma as an animal model for screening. This work resulted in the development of MeCCNU [N-(2-chloroethyl)-N'-(trans-4-methylcyclohexyl)-N-nitrosourea], one of the most active compounds yet tested against the advanced Lewis lung and most other solid tumors in rodents. The sodium salts of cyclohexane-4-carboxylic acid and cyclohexane-4-acetic acid analogs, designed as water-soluble congeners of MeCCNU because of the difficulties in formulating this highly lipid-soluble compound for intravenous injection, are equivalent to it in their activity against solid tumors.

Chlorozotocin tetraacetate was synthesized in a successful attempt to improve the weak anticancer activity of the broad-spectrum antibiotic, streptozotocin, which had shown diabetogenic activity in animals and clinical activity in the treatment of insulinomas in man. The finding that the tetraacetate was less toxic to the bone marrow in mice than BCNU and CCNU (reportedly the limiting toxicity in their clinical use) inspired the synthesis of chlorozotocin itself, which proved to be more active against leukemia L1210 as well as water-soluble, but which retained the low bone marrow toxicity. This work demonstrated the feasibility of altering nitrosourea toxicity while retaining anticancer activity -- at least in experimental animals.

The Imidazole Triazenes

Investigation of the diazotization of AIC with aqueous nitrous acid led to the identification of 5-diazoimidazole-4-carboxamide (diazo-IC), an internally compensated diazonium salt which on standing in aqueous media rearranged to 2-azahypoxanthine. The striking similarity of the structure of diazo-IC to that of the anticancer antibiotics azaserine and DON, compounds known to inhibit an early step in the de novo purine nucleotide biosynthetic pathway, raised the hope that diazo-IC might block a later step in the path and led to the determination of its cytotoxicity to cells in culture. It was quite cytotoxic and showed slight activity in animal tumor systems. Since the diazo-IC did show biologic activity, albeit not enough to warrant consideration for the treatment of human cancer, ways were sought to convert it into derivatives that might have greater selectivity for cancer cells and, therefore, greater potential clinical utility. Among those derivatives were the reaction products of diazo- IC with dialkylamines -- the 5-triazenoimidazole-4-carboxamides. One of the early compounds of this type prepared was the dimethylamine derivative, DTIC [5-(3,3-dimethyl-1-triazeno)imidazole-4-carboxamide], a light-sensitive, but otherwise fairly stable, compound found to be active against all three tumors used at that time as the primary screen of the National Cancer Institute.

DTIC is oxidatively demethylated in vivo and in vitro by liver microsomes to give, presumably, the monomethyl compound, MIC, which then tautomerizes and releases AIC and a methyldiazonium ion. The resulting methylation of DNA is probably ultimately responsible for the activity of DTIC, and not interference with the de novo pathway to purine nucleotides as originally proposed.

Of the many analogs of DTIC that have been prepared, one — BIC   [5-[3,3-bis(2-chloroethyl)-1-triazeno] imidazole-4-carboxamide] -- has shown curative activity in the leukemia L1210 system, but unfortunately has proven to be inferior to DTIC in humans. One reason for the lack of activity in humans may be the ease of cyclization of BIC to a biologically inert derivative. Microsomal oxidases can oxidize a 2-chloroethyl group of BIC as readily as a methyl group of DTIC to give 5-[3-(2-chloroethyl)-1-triazeno] imidazole-4-carboxamide (MCIC), a compound as active against L1210 as BIC, but at one-tenth the dose. Thus, activation would appear to play a vital role in the antileukemic activity of this analog also.

ANTIMETABOLITES

Dihydrofolic Reductase Inhibitors

Aminopterin was the first inhibitor of dihydrofolic reductase shown to have activity in humans; with it temporary remissions could be induced in children with acute leukemia. Because experimental studies suggesting a greater range of therapeutic effectiveness for methotrexate (Mtx) were supported by early clinical experiences, it was eventually chosen over aminopterin for the treatment of human cancer and has been used almost exclusively until recently. Comparative studies in mice on the active transport of aminopterin, methotrexate, and related compounds into gut epithelial cells and into tumor cells have shown that whereas both Mtx and aminopterin are taken up rapidly by the cancer cells, Mtx is not taken up as well by gut cells, but aminopterin is. Thus, aminopterin is more toxic to mice and the clinical results described above are probably attributable to this same differential. Recently 10-deazaaminopterin, although no better than Mtx as an inhibitor of dihydrofolic reductase, was found to be more active in several rodent ascites tumor systems, a result attributed to greater uptake by active transport, by tumor cells, of this analog relative to Mtx.

Purine and Pyrimidine Antimetabolites

The large amount of work on the 6-thiopurines that followed the establishment of 6-mercaptopurine (MP) as a clinically useful agent has led to meager clinical gains, although the impact on biochemical pharmacology has been great. 6-Thioguanine (TG) has been identified as another clinically useful agent, although its clear superiority over MP has never really been demonstrated; both of the compounds may owe their activity to incorporation into DNA as 2'-deoxythioguanylic acid, which requires fewer metabolic steps for TG, a fact that may well explain its greater efficacy on a molar basis (the therapeutic index of these two thiopurines is about the same). 6-(Methylthio)purine ribonucleoside (MeMPR) and MP are therapeutically synergistic against leukemia L1210 and against acute myelogenous leukemia in man, probably because of the lack of cross-resistance between the two agents resulting from the difference in their metabolism and, therefore, their mechanism of resistance.

The 6-thiopurines are the only purines that have earned a place in the treatment of human cancer. A number of nucleosides of adenine -- both synthetic and isolates from antibiotic beers -- have shown activity in animal systems and have produced a number of interesting studies on purine metabolism and enzyme substrate specificities, but have not yet found clinical application. The recent observation of the clinical activity of 9-β-D-arabinofuranosyladenine (Ara-A) coupled with studies demonstrating its enhanced activity in animal tumor systems in the presence of the potent adenosine deaminase inhibitor, 2'-deoxycoformycin (DCF) and the activity of this combination against leukemia P388 resistant to 1-β-D̲-arabinofuranosylcytosine (Ara-C) has led to studies of the effects of DCF on the activity of other adenosine analogs that are extensively deaminated in vivo, and should soon lead to clinical studies with this combination. The 2-fluoro analog of ara-A was synthesized in the hope that this change would prevent deamination but not phosphorylation. This has proved to be the case: F-ara-A is about as active in the L1210 system as ara-A given in combination with DCF. Conversion of F-ara-A to its 5'-phosphate then gave a water-soluble drug resistant to catabolism, lacking rigid schedule dependency, and highly active in the L1210 system.

1-β-D̲-Arabinofuranosylcytosine, useful in the treatment of human cancer particularly acute myelogenous leukemia, is a cell cycle phase specific agent that must be given on a continuous infusion type of schedule to maintain a cytotoxic level of drug in the blood as the proliferating cell population progresses through the S-phase. To overcome the problem of rapid deamination by 2'-deoxycytidine deaminase in serum, a number of O̲-acyl derivatives of the drug have been prepared as depot forms that act by slow release of ara-C. This is a special type of latentiation that alters drastically the water-lipid solubility of the parent.

SUMMARY

The validity of congener synthesis is well established, and there are some guidelines to the types of alteration of a drug that can be made in hopes of effecting improvement in anticancer activity. One of the biggest stumbling blocks so far has been a lack of mutual understanding between the clinicians and the chemists as to worthy goals and as to whether or not these goals have been achieved as measured by the best means we have available -- animal models. This problem is complicated by the lack of appreciation of the magnitude of the difference that must be observed in the tightly staged model to reasonably expect it to be detectable in a much more heterogenous human trial.

GENERAL REFERENCES

Cox, P. J., Lamur, P. B., and Jarmon, M. Proceedings of the Symposium on the Metabolism and Mechanism of Action of Cyclophosphamide. Cancer Treat. Rep., 1976, 60, 299-525.

Hill, D. L. A Review of Cyclophosphamide. Illinois:Thomas, 1975.

Livingston, R. B. and Carter, S. K. Single Agents in Chemotheapy. New York: IFI/Plenum, 1970.

Montgomery, J. A. Experimental Studies at Southern Research Institute with DTIC (NSC 45388). Cancer Treat. Rep., 176, 60, 125-134.

Montgomery, J. A. Chemistry and Structure-Activity Studies of the Nitrosourea. Cancer Treat. Rep., 1976, 60, 651-664.

Montgomery, J. A. Synthetic Chemicals. In V. T. DeVita, Jr. and H. Busch (Eds.), Methods in Cancer Research, XVI, Part A. New York: Academic Press, Inc., 1979, 3-41.

Montgomery, J. A. Nitrosoureas. In M. A. Simkins (Ed.), Medicinal Chemistry VI, Proc. 6th Internat. Sym. Med. Chemistry, Brighton, U.K., 1978. Oxford, U.K.: Cotswold Press, Ltd., 1979, 313-321.

Montgomery, J. A. and Struck, R. F. The Relationship of the Metabolism of Anticancer Agents to their Activity. Fortschr. Arzneimittelforsch, 1973, 17, 320-409.

Montgomery, J. A., Johnston, T. P., and Shealy, Y. F. Drugs for Neoplastic Diseases. In M. Wolfe (Ed.), Medicinal Chemistry, 4th Ed., Part II. New York: Wiley (Interscience), 1979, 595-670.

Sartorelli, A. C. and Johns, D. G. (Eds.), Antineoplastic and Immunosuppressive Agents. Part I and II. Berlin and New York: Springer Verlag, 1975, 484-511.

Schabel, F. M., Jr. Nitrosoureas: A Review of Experimental Antitumor Activity. Cancer Treat. Rep., 1976, 60, 665-693.

Schabel, F. M., Jr. Test Systems for Evaluating the Antitumor Activity of Nucleoside Analogs. In R. T. Walker, E. DeClercq, and F. Eckstein (Eds.), Nucleoside Analogs. New York and London: Plenum Press, 1979, 363-394.

Schabel, F. M., Jr., Griswold, D. P., Jr., Laster, W. R., Jr., et al. Quantitative Evaluation of Anticancer Agent Activity in Experimental Animals. Pharmac. Ther. A, 1977, 1, 411-435.

Sirotnak, F. M., Chello, P. L., and Brockman, R. W. Potential for Exploitation of Transport Systems in Anticancer Drug Design. In V. T. DeVita, Jr. and H. Busch (Eds.), Methods in Cancer Research, XVI, Cancer Drug Development, Part A, New York: Academic Press, 1979, 382-448.

Skipper, H. E. Cancer Chemotherapy I: Reasons for Success and Failure in Treatment of Murine Leukemias with Drugs Now Employed in Treating Human Leukemias, University Microfilms International, Ann Arbor, Michigan, 1978.

Suhadolnik, R. J. Nucleoside Antibiotics. New York: Wiley (Interscience), 1970.

Treatment of Spontaneous Murine
Metastases by the Systemic
Administration of Liposomes Containing
Macrophage-activating Agents

ISAIAH J. FIDLER

Director
Cancer Metastasis and Treatment Laboratory
NCI-Frederick Cancer Research Center
Frederick, Maryland 21701

GEORGE POSTE

Principal Cancer Research Scientist
Department of Experimental Pathology
Roswell Park Memorial Institute
Buffalo, New York 14263

INTRODUCTION

Many primary cancers can be treated successfully with
modern surgical techniques and aggressive chemo- and/or radiotherapy but formation of secondary tumor foci at distant sites
(metastasis) is still responsible for most failures in cancer
treatment.[7,11,31] There are many reasons for this. Metastases may be too small to be detected at the time of surgery,
are often widely disseminated throughout the body, and their
anatomic location(s) may be inaccessible for surgical removal.
The most serious problem, however, is the emergence of metastases that are resistant to conventional therapy. Recent
studies suggesting that metastases may result from the
proliferation of a minor subpopulation of cells within the

This research was supported by the National Cancer Institute
under Contract No. NO1-CO-75380 with Litton Bionetics, Inc.
and USPHS Grants CA13393, CA17609 and CA18260.

77

primary tumor and that tumors are heterogeneous with regard to many phenotypic characteristics, including metastatic potential,[12,25] provide a conceptual basis for explaining the emergence of such relentless tumor deposits. Phenotypic heterogeneity of this kind may also account for reports of differences in the response of primary and metastatic lesions to cytotoxic agents or host effector cells.[19,20,39] Collectively, these studies imply that the only successful approach to the therapy of metastases will be one that circumvents tumor cell heterogeneity and also against which resistance is unlikely to develop.

Although tumor cell populations are heterogeneous with regard to many characteristics, they are susceptible to destruction by activated (tumoricidal) macrophages.[8,21] Macrophages can be rendered tumoricidal by a variety of agents, including lymphokines such as macrophage-activating factor (MAF) released by antigen- and/or mitogen-sensitized lymphocytes.[6,8] Activated macrophages acquire the ability to destroy (in vitro) tumorigenic cells while not harming nontumorigenic cells, even in co-cultivation conditions. Tumoricidal macrophages induce destruction of a variety of target tumor cells from a variety of species by a nonimmunologic mechanism that requires cell-to-cell contact.[6,8,10,21,29,34] How tumoricidal macrophages discriminate between tumorigenic and nontumorigenic cells is not clear. Although tumor cell variants that are resistant to various cytotoxic agents, cytotoxic lymphocytes and natural killer cells have been selected in vitro and in vivo, similar attempts to select tumor cells resistant to macrophage-mediated lysis have been unsuccessful to date.[8,21]

Tumoricidal macrophages have been shown to be effective in controlling cancer metastasis in vivo. Activated syngeneic mouse macrophages injected i.v. reduced the development of B16 melanoma lung tumor colonies,[5] and injection of nonspecifically activated macrophages has been shown to eradicate metastasis in two separate murine tumor systems.[4,10,26] Activated macrophages can also inhibit tumor growth at primary sites.[4] Collectively, these studies suggested that metastases produced by cells originating from heterogeneous neoplasms can be treated successfully by the i.v. injection of activated macrophages, although the degree of success is dependent on tumor burden and number of treatments. For clinical use, however, this approach has several serious limitations. Foremost is the need to transfuse a large number of autologous or histocompatible macrophages. Thus, it would be preferable that autologous macrophages be activated in situ to be rendered tumoricidal. Although macrophages obtained from mice bearing progressively growing neoplasms are not tumoricidal and may also have a reduced ability to respond to host stimuli,[6,24] they are able to respond to exogenous activating stimuli.[6,24,29,32]

The increasing evidence that macrophages are important in host defense against neoplasia has stimulated interest in the potential value of macrophage-activating agents as therapeutic modalities for enhancing macrophage-mediated destruction of tumor cells in vivo. The major pathway for macrophage activation in vivo is thought to be through interaction with the lymphokine, MAF. Recent studies from our laboratories have demonstrated that the phagocytic uptake of liposomes, concentric phospholipid vesicles separated by aqueous compartments[2,15,22,35] containing encapsulated MAF, produces highly efficient activation of rodent macrophages in vitro[32,34,38] and in vivo.[9,14,18] Unlike activation by free MAF, which requires initial binding of MAF to a specific receptor on the macrophage surface,[33] liposome-encapsulated MAF can activate macrophages lacking functional receptors for soluble MAF.[32] Moreover, MAF-encapsulated within liposomes can activate certain types of tissue macrophages (histiocytes) that are refractory to activation by free MAF.[29]

A second major pathway for activation of macrophages in vivo involves their interaction with microorganisms and/or their product(s). However, the use of whole viable microorganisms and/or their products to activate macrophages in vivo often has undesirable side effects, such as granuloma formation and allergic reactions.[1,2] The use of synthetic compounds that are relatively nontoxic, yet possess immune-potentiating activity would thus be preferable. N-acetyl-muramyl-L-alanyl-D-isoglutamine (muramyl dipeptide, MDP; mol. wt. 492) is the minimal structural unit with immune-potentiating activity that can replace Mycobacteria in Freund's complete adjuvant.[3,27,28,37] MDP is known to influence many macrophage functions such as production of prostaglandins and collagenase, inhibition of macrophage migration, enhancement of O_2-generating capacity, enhancement of lymphokine-induced macrophage proliferation and augmentation of macrophage cytolytic activity.[3,27,28,37] We have recently shown that macrophages incubated in vitro with water-soluble MDP can be rendered tumoricidal against syngeneic and allogeneic targets. Moreover, like MAF, MDP encapsulated within liposomes rendered mouse and rat alveolar macrophages tumoricidal in vitro at concentrations at least 1000 times lower than unencapsulated (free) MDP added to the alveolar macrophage culture medium.[37]

Because MAF or MDP encapsulated within liposomes is far more efficient than unencapsulated materials in activating macrophages in vitro[37], we investigated whether liposome-encapsulated agents might be equally efficient in activating mouse macrophages in vivo and thus provide a potential modality for destruction of lymph node and visceral metastases. This report provides a brief review of such in vivo experiments.

THERAPY EXPERIMENTS

The Bl6-BL6 melanoma cell line syngeneic to C57BL/6 mice and the K-1735 melanoma syngeneic to C3H mice were used. Following implantation into the footpad, both tumors metastasized to lymph nodes and the lungs in over 80-90% of the mice. C57BL/6 mice (Bl6-BL6 tumor)[17,30] or C3H mice (K-1735)[23] were given s.c. injections of either 25×10^6 or 50×10^4 viable cells in a volume of 0.05 ml physiological basic saline solution (PBS). Four to five weeks later, when tumors reached the size of 10-15 mm, the leg bearing the tumor and the popliteal lymph node were amputated. Intravenous injections with liposome preparations began 3 days after the surgery. Each treatment consisted of an i.v. injection into the tail vein of 5 μmoles phospholipids of multilamellar liposomes (MLV) suspended in 0.2 ml PBS. MLV were prepared from a 7:3 mole ratio of chromatographically pure egg phosphatidylcholine (PC) and beef brain phosphatidylserine (PS) (purchased from Avanti Biochemicals, Birmingham, Alabama) by mechanically shaking the mixture on a Vortex mixer, as described elsewhere.[34] Encapsulation of MDP, MAF or PBS within liposomes was achieved using methods similar to those described previously.[34,38] We have used PS/PC-MLV as carriers because they are not toxic at the dose used here,[17] and are arrested efficiently in the lungs as well as organs of the reticuloendothelial system following i.v. injections.[13] The internal volume of the MLV has been determined to be 2.4 ± 0.3 μl per μmole phospholipid.[34,38] Thus, for the in vivo studies reported here, mice injected i.v. with 5 umole phospholipid MLV received 12 μl of entrapped suspension.

In experiments designed to evaluate the efficacy of liposome-encapsulated MAF for eradication of spontaneous metastases, control groups of animals were injected i.v. with either PBS, free MAF (200 μl) or with liposomes that contained PBS but were suspended in 200 μl of free MAF. The lymphokine MAF was obtained from cultures of rat lymphocytes sensitized in vitro to concanavalin-A as described previously.[8,34]

In experiments to evaluate the efficacy of liposome-encapsulated MDP in eradicating spontaneous metastases, mice were injected with MLV containing 2.5 μg MDP. Control groups were injected i.v. with either PBS, free MDP (100 μg/mouse) or with liposomes containing PBS and suspended in PBS containing 2-5 μg MDP/mouse. In all experiments, treatments were carried out twice weekly for either 3 or 4 weeks (6 or 8 treatments) as indicated below.

Two major types of experiments are reported here. In the first set of experiments, mice were killed 2 weeks following the final treatment and necropsied; the presence of metastases was determined by the use of a dissecting microscope. All suspected pulmonary and extrapulmonary metastases were confirmed by microscopic examination of fixed histological sections. In a second set of experiments, C57BL/6 mice bearing B16-BL6 metastases were not killed at a predetermined time, but were allowed to survive. The animals were monitored daily, and dead or moribund mice were necropsied. Animals surviving at least 120 days after the last treatment were considered disease-free.[16,36] The in vivo data were analyzed by the Mann-Whitney U-test and Chi square analysis.

Regression of Spontaneous Metastases Following the I.V. Injection of Liposome-encapsulated MAF

Spontaneous pulmonary and lymph node metastases were well established in the C57BL/6 mice at the time liposome treatment began, and many individual metastases could be seen macroscopically.[9] Without therapy, these metastases developed into nodules 1-3 mm in diameter, and the growth or lack of growth of lung metastases could be readily determined by the end of the experiment (Fig. 1). The majority of mice treated with liposome-encapsulated MAF had no macroscopically or microscopically detectable metastases. The results of 2 similar experiments using the B16-BL6 tumor are shown in Table 1. Metastases were present in 17 of 20 PBS-treated control mice and i.v. injection of free MAF or liposomes containing PBS suspended in free MAF failed to alter the incidence of metastasis. However, multiple i.v. injections of liposome-encapsulated MAF significantly reduced the incidence of spontaneous metastases (P < 0.001, Chi square analysis), and metastases were found in only 5 of 20 mice. Moreover, the median number of metastases in the 5 positive mice in this group was significantly reduced relative to the other treatment groups.

Similar data were obtained in C3H mice injected into the footpad with the syngeneic K-1735 melanoma (Table 1). Liposome-encapsulated MAF produced a significant reduction in the incidence of metastasis compared to control mice or animals injected with liposomes containing PBS. Pulmonary metastases in 9 of 10 mice injected with liposomes containing control supernates were both numerous and large. In contrast, only 3 of 10 mice injected with liposome-encapsulated MAF had metastases, which were limited to a few small foci (Fig. 2).

In the next set of experiments with the B16-BL6 tumor, mice were not killed at a predetermined time but were allowed to survive. As shown in Figure 2, virtually all of the mice

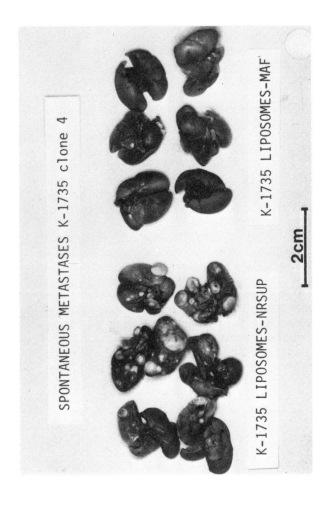

Fig. 1. Spontaneous pulmonary metastases from cells of K-1735 clone 4 melanoma in syngeneic C3H mice at end of experiments. Lungs of control mice treated with liposome-encapsulated NRSUP are laden with large metastases. In contrast, lungs of mice injected with liposome-encapsulated MAF are virtually tumor-free.

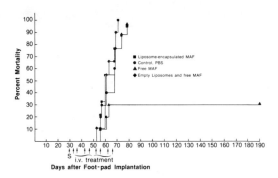

Fig. 2. Survival of C57BL/6 mice bearing spontaneous metastases after multiple i.v. treatments with liposomes containing
MAF.

TABLE 1
Treatment of Spontaneous Metastases in Mice by the I.V.
Injection of Liposome-encapsulated MAF

Treatment Group	Pulmonary Metastasis			
	Positive Mice/ Total Mice	Median	Range	P
K-1735 melanoma in C3H mice				
PBS, control mice	9/10	3	0-10	
Liposomes containing HBSS	9/10	9	0-31	
Liposome-encapsulated MAF	3/10	0	0-5	<0.01
B16-BL6 melanoma in C57BL/6 mice				
PBS, control mice	17/20	10	0-41	
Liposomes containing HBSS suspended in free MAF	16/18	12	0-65	
Free MAF	8/10	13	0-38	
Liposome-encapsulated MAF	5/20	0	0-10	<0.001

injected i.v. with saline solution, free MAF or liposomes
containing PBS suspended in free MAF solution were dead by day
70 of the experiment, i.e. 40 days after the amputation of the
tumor-bearing leg. In marked contrast, 7 of 10 mice injected
i.v. with liposome-encapsulated MAF were alive when the
experiment was terminated at 190 days. The median life span
of mice following implantation of the minimum tumorigenic dose
of 10 cells is 40-50 days.[16,36] Animals surviving at least
120 days longer than any other treated mouse can, therefore,
be considered to be disease free.

Regression of Spontaneous Metastases Following the I.V. Injection of Liposomes Containing MDP

C57BL/6 mice bearing spontaneous B16-BL6 melanoma metastases were injected i.v. with free MDP (100 μg/mouse), liposomes (5 μmoles phospholipids) containing 2.5 μg MDP,
or liposomes containing PBS and suspended in 2.5 μg free
MDP. Mice were injected twice weekly for 4 weeks. Here, as
in the previous experiments, spontaneous lymph node and
pulmonary metastases were well established at the time treatment commenced, i.e., 4-6 weeks after implantation of tumor
cells in the footpad and 3 days after leg amputation. Metastases in the superficial iliac nodes and surface pulmonary
metastases were visible with a dissecting microscope. Many of
these metastases contained hundreds of tumor cells.

As in the previous protocol, mice in the initial set of
experiments were killed 2 weeks after the final (8th) i.v.
treatment. Metastases were found in the majority of control
mice injected with PBS and also those treated i.v. with free
MDP or liposomes containing PBS (Table 2). In contrast, the
incidence of metastasis was reduced significantly in mice
injected i.v. with liposomes containing MDP. Twenty of 27
mice were free of macroscopic tumor foci. Moreover, there was
a significant reduction in the median number of pulmonary
metastases in positive mice in the group treated with liposome-
MDP as compared with all other treatment groups.

In the next set of experiments, mice bearing spontaneous
B16-BL6 metastases were treated as described above and allowed
to survive. The data are shown in Table 3. Each group of
mice consisted of 15 animals. By day 80 of the experiment,
nearly all mice injected with PBS, free MDP or liposomes containing PBS and suspended in PBS containing free MDP had died.
In contrast, 9 of 16 mice (60%) injected i.v. with MLV liposomes containing 2.5 μg MDP/dose survived 120 days after the
last treatment. As stated above, this period greatly exceeded
the time necessary for as few as 10 surviving tumor cells to
kill their hosts.[16,36] On day 190 of the experiment, all
surviving mice, as well as naive control recipients, were

TABLE 2
Treatment of Spontaneous B16-BL6 Metastases in C57BL/6 Mice by the I.V. Injection of Liposome-encapsulated MDP

| Treatment Group | Pulmonary Metastasis | | |
	Positive Mice/ Total Mice	Median	Range
PBS, control mice	24/28	49	0-107
Free MDP (100 µg)	8/10	55	0-94
Liposomes containing PBS suspended in 2.5 µg free MDP	23/26	68	0-308
Liposomes containing 2.5 µg MDP	7/27	0	0-7

The incidence of metastasis in mice treated with liposome-encapsulated MDP was significantly decreased ($P < 0.001$ Chi square analysis). The data are a summary of 2 separate experiments.

TABLE 3
Eradication of Metastases by the I.V. Injection of Liposomes Containing MDP: Survival Studies

| Treatment Group | Survival on Day: | | | |
	40	60	80	190
PBS, control mice	14/14	8/14	0/14	0/14
Free MDP (100 µg)	15/15	9/15	1/15	1/15
Liposomes containing PBS suspended in 0.2 µg MDP	15/15	7/15	1/15	1/15
Liposomes containing 0.2 µg MDP	15/15	9/15	9/15	9/15

Survival: number of live mice/total number of mice. The differences in median life span are highly significant ($P < 0.001$).

challenged s.c. with 2.5×10^4 B16–BL6 cells. All mice developed s.c. tumors by 2 weeks after injection. At this time all
mice were killed and necropsied. No evidence of metastatic
disease was found in the long-term surviving mice.

DISCUSSION AND CONCLUSIONS

Our results indicate that the multiple i.v. injections of
MLV liposomes containing macrophage–activating agents such as
MAF or MDP, but not free agents, eradicated spontaneous
pulmonary and lymph node metastases (arising from B16–BL6
melanoma or K-1735 melanoma primary tumors resected before
therapy) in mice. In mice bearing the B16–BL6 tumor, the
tumor burden in lung and lymph node metastases at the start of
therapy was great (perhaps in excess of 10^7 cells). It is
thus important to note that 70% of mice treated with liposome-
encapsulated MAF and 60% of mice treated with liposome-
encapsulated MDP survived for 190 days after tumors were
implanted into the footpad. In this tumor system, the median
life span of mice inoculated with as few as 10 viable cells
has been shown to be 40–50 days.[16,36] The tumor burden in
surviving mice must have been reduced to below 10 viable
cells, because they survived longer than required to be
classified as disease free.

The ability to activate AM in situ with MAF or MDP-encap-
sulated within liposomes is attractive for several reasons.
Liposomes in general are nonimmunogenic, and their repeated
administration is unlikely to lead to the formation of granulomas or elicit the allergic reactions associated with
systemic administration of certain immune adjuvants.[1,2,16]
MLV liposomes are cleared from the circulation by cells of the
reticuloendothelial system. This can be taken advantage of to
deliver materials encapsulated within liposomes to cells of
the macrophage–histiocyte series. We have shown[34,37] that
the concentration of MDP or MAF encapsulated within MLV
liposomes required to render mouse or rat AM tumoricidal in
vitro is at least 1000 times lower than the amount of the free
agent needed to accomplish this task. Moreover, water-soluble
MDP is cleared from the body in less than 1 hr after parenteral administration.[29] This is too short a time to evoke
the activated state, and free MDP injected i.v. even at high
doses does not render macrophages tumoricidal. The encapsulation of MDP within liposomes leads to retention of MDP within
the macrophage where it is released over 2–3 days and maintains the tumoricidal state. In none of our experiments did
injection of liposomes containing PBS suspended in free MDP
solution lead to any reduction in metastasis. Only liposome-
encapsulated MDP is effective in eradication of established
metastases.

In conclusion, the present experiments demonstrate that multiple i.v. injections of liposome-encapsulated MAF or MDP can induce regression of established spontaneous metastases originating from an s.c. murine melanoma. The optimal conditions for liposome therapy have yet to be defined. Future studies should determine whether increasing the number of treatments or the dose of MDP in each treatment, or both, could be more effective against increased tumor burden. The lack of toxic effects of this therapy on normal cells, as well as the susceptibility of all tumorigenic cells to destruction by tumoricidal macrophages (at least in vitro), suggests that this new approach may be a valuable addition to the regimens now being used for the treatment of cancer metastases.

REFERENCES

1. Allison AC: Mode of action of immunological adjuvants. J Reticuloendothel Soc 26:619-630, 1979.
2. Allison AC, Gregoriadis G: Liposomes as immunological adjuvants. Nature 252:252-254, 1974.
3. Chedid L, Carelli L, Audibert F: Recent developments concerning muramyl dipeptide, a synthetic immunoregulating molecule. J Reticuloendothel Soc 26:631-641, 1979.
4. Den Otter E, Dullens Hub FJ, Van Lovern H, Pels E: Anti-tumor effects of macrophages injected into animals: A review, in James K, McBride B, Stuart A (eds.): The Macrophage and Cancer. Edinburgh, Econoprint, 1977, pp 119-140.
5. Fidler IJ: Inhibition of pulmonary metastasis by intravenous injection of specifically activated macrophages. Cancer Res 34:1074-1078, 1974.
6. Fidler IJ: Activation in vitro of mouse macrophages by syngeneic, allogeneic or xenogeneic lymphocyte supernatants. J Natl Cancer Inst 55:1159-1163, 1975.
7. Fidler IJ: Tumor heterogeneity and the biology of cancer invasion and metastasis. Cancer Res 38:2651-2660, 1978.
8. Fidler IJ: Recognition and destruction of target cells by tumoricidal macrophages. Isr J Med Sci 14:177-191, 1978.
9. Fidler IJ: Therapy of spontaneous metastases by intravenous injection of liposomes containing lymphokines. Science 208:1469-1471, 1980.
10. Fidler IJ, Fogler WE, Connor J: The rationale for the treatment of established experimental micrometastases with the injection of tumoricidal macrophages, in Terry W, Yamamura T (eds.): Immunobiology and Immunotherapy of Cancer. Amsterdam, Elsevier, 1979, pp 361-372.
11. Fidler IJ, Gersten DM, Hart IR: The biology of cancer invasion and metastasis. Adv Cancer Res 28:149-250, 1978.

12. Fidler IJ, Kripke ML: Metastasis results from
     preexisting variant cells within a malignant tumor.
     Science 197:893-895, 1977.
13. Fidler IJ, Raz A, Fogler WE, Kirsh R, Bugelski P, Poste
     G: The design of liposomes to improve delivery of
     macrophage-augmenting agents to alveolar macrophages.
     Cancer Res, in press, 1980.
14. Fogler WE, Raz A, Fidler IJ: In situ activation of
     murine macrophages by liposomes containing lymphokines.
     Cell Immunol, in press, 1980.
15. Gregoriadis G: Tailoring liposome structure. Nature
     283:814-815, 1980.
16. Griswold, DP Jr: Consideration of the subcutaneously
     implanted B16 melanoma as a screening model for potential
     anticancer agents. Cancer Chemother Rep 3:315-323, 1972.
17. Hart IR: Selection and characterization of an invasive
     variant of the B16 melanoma. Am J Pathol 97:587-600.
18. Hart IR, Fogler WE, Poste G, Fidler IJ: Toxicity studies
     of liposome-encapsulated immunomodulators administered
     intravenously into dogs and mice. Cancer Immunol Immuno-
     ther, in press, 1980.
19. Hakansson L, Trope C: On the presence within tumors of
     clones that differ in sensitivity to cytostatic drugs.
     Acta Path Microbiol Scand 82:35-40, 1974.
20. Heppner GH, Dexter DL, De Nucci T, Miller FR, Calabresi
     P: Heterogeneity in drug sensitivity among tumor cell
     subpopulations of a single mammary tumor. Cancer Res
     38:3758-3763, 1978.
21. Hibbs JB Jr: Discrimination between neoplastic and
     non-neoplastic cells in vitro by activated macrophages.
     J Natl Cancer Inst 53:1487-1492, 1974.
22. Kimelberg HK, Mayhew EG: Properties and biological
     effects of liposomes and their uses in pharmacology and
     toxicology. CRC Crit Rev Toxicol 9:25-44, 1978.
23. Kripke ML: Speculations on the role of ultraviolet
     radiation in the development of malignant melanoma.   J
     Natl Cancer Inst 63:541-544, 1979.
24. Kripke ML, Budmen MB, Fidler IJ: Production of specific
     macrophage-activating factor by lymphocytes from tumor-
     bearing mice. Cell Immunol 30:341-350, 1977.
25. Kripke ML, Gruys E, Fidler IJ: Metastatic heterogeneity
     of cells from an ultraviolet light-induced murine fibro-
     sarcoma of recent origin. Cancer Res 38:2962-2967, 1978.
26. Liotta LA, Gattozzi C, Kleinerman J, Saidel G: Reduction
     of tumor cell entry into vessels by BCG-activated macro-
     phages. Br J Cancer 36: 639-641, 1977.

27. Matter A: The effects of muramyldipeptide (MDP) in cell-mediated immunity. A comparison between in vitro and in vivo systems. Cancer Immunol Immunother 6:201-210, 1979.

28. Parant M, Parant F, Chedid L, Yapo A, Petit JF, Lederer E: Fate of the synthetic immunoadjuvant, muramyl dipeptide (^{14}C-labelled) in the mouse. Int J Immunopharmacol 1:35-41, 1979.

29. Poste G: The tumoricidal properties of inflammatory tissue macrophages and multinucleate giant cells. Am J Pathol 96:595-608, 1979.

30. Poste G, Doll J, Hart IR, Fidler IJ: In vitro selection of murine B16 melanoma variants with enhanced tissue-invasive properties. Cancer Res 40:1636-1644, 1980.

31. Poste G, Fidler IJ: The pathogenesis of cancer metastasis. Nature 283:139-146, 1979.

32. Poste G, Kirsh R: Rapid decay of tumoricidal activity and loss of responsiveness to lymphokines in inflammatory macrophages. Cancer Res 39:2582-2590, 1979.

33. Poste G, Kirsh R, Fidler IJ: Cell surface receptors for lymphokines. Cell Immunol 44:71-88, 1979.

34. Poste G, Kirsh R, Fogler WE, Fidler IJ: Activation of tumoricidal properties in mouse macrophages by lymphokines encapsulated in liposomes. Cancer Res 39:881-892, 1979.

35. Poste G, Papahadjopoulos D: Lipid vesicles as a carrier for introducing materials into culture cells: Influence of vesicle lipid composition on mechanism(s) of vesicle incorporation into cells. Proc Natl Acad Sci USA 73:1603-1607, 1976.

36. Schabel FM Jr, Griswold DP Jr, Laster WR Jr, Corbett TH, Lloyd HH: Quantitative evaluation of anticancer agent activity in experimental animals. Pharmacol Ther [A] 1: 411-435, 1977.

37. Sone S, Fidler IJ: In vitro activation of tumoricidal properties in rat alveolar macrophages by synthetic muramyl dipeptide encapsulated in liposomes. Cell Immunol, in press, 1980.

38. Sone S, Poste G, Fidler IJ: Rat alveolar macrophages are susceptible to activation by free and liposome-encapsulated lymphokines. J Immunol 124:2197-2202, 1980.

39. Trope C: Different sensitivity to cytostatic drugs of primary tumor and metastasis of the Lewis carcinoma. Neoplasma 22:171-180, 1975.

Pharmacology

PHARMACOLOGY

EMIL FREI III, M.D.

Director and Physician-in-Chief
Sidney Farber Cancer Institute
Boston, Massachusetts

One of the major sciences underpinning cancer chemotherapy is pharmacology. The science of pharmacology as it
relates to anticancer drug development includes 1) the identification of new antitumor agents through drug synthesis and
the isolation of natural products, 2) the study of the
structure-activity relationships of given drug classes with
congener synthesis, 3) studies of the mechanism of action and
drug resistance at a molecular level, 4) preclinical toxicology, and 5) preclinical and clinical pharmacology. Since
some of these topics have been covered elsewhere in this symposium, I will focus my remarks on clinical pharmacology and
the identification of biochemical targets for chemotherapeutic attack.

THE STEEP DOSE-RESPONSE CURVE

The dose-response curve for chemotherapeutic agents
against both the tumor and normal host tissues is steep, and
the therapeutic dose range is correspondingly narrow. Initial evidence for this derived from animal tumor studies. In
Figure 1 survival of mice bearing L1210 leukemia is plotted
as a function of dose. The dose producing the maximal antitumor effect is 1 mg/kg/day. If one decreases the dose by 25
or 50 percent, the therapeutic effect is largely lost. In
addition, if one doubles the optimal dose, the improvement in
survival is largely lost, as a result of drug toxicity. Indeed, for most cancer chemotherapeutic agents, twice the dose
that will kill 10 percent of rodents will kill 90 percent of
such animals. That this relationship also applies to the
clinic has been demonstrated in randomized comparative
studies for lymphoma (Table 1). Here a two-fold difference in
response on the one hand, and a similar difference in toxicity. Finally, and more recently, it has been demonstrated

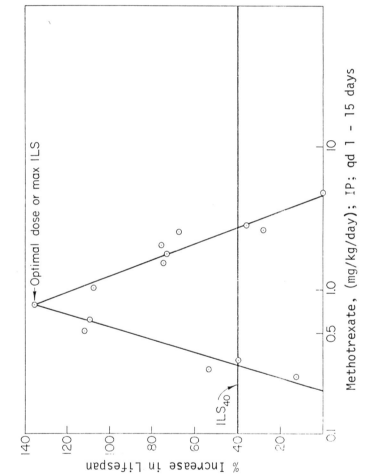

Figure 1. Effect of Dose on Response of Mouse Leukemia L1210 to Methotrexate

TABLE 1
Dose Effect of Chemotherapy in Lymphoma

Dose	Number of patients	Objective response		Significant toxicity*	
		No.	%	No.	%
Thiotepa					
0.2	9	1	11	2	22
0.4	22	13	59	12	55
Folic acid antagonists+					
Low dose	16	3	19	3	19
High dose	30	15	50	17	68

*Decrease in white blood cells to less than 3000 cells per cu. mm. and decrease in platelets to less than 75,000 per cu. mm.
Dose in mg/kg/day x 4, then weekly, all intravenously.
+Low dose: MTX 0.075 or DCM (dichloromethotrexate) 0.375 mg/kg/day for 42 days; high dose: MTX 0.15 or DCM 0.75 mg/kg/day for 42 days. All folic acid antagonists given by mouth.

that long-term disease-free survival in the adjuvant treatment of breast cancer with CMF is markedly dose-related
(Table 2). In this study by Bonadonna of premenopausal patients with breast cancer, the patients were divided into
those who received over 85 percent of the protocol-prescribed
dose, 65 to 85 percent, and less than 65 percent. This relatively slight difference in dose makes a substantial and significant difference in disease-free survival. The same has
been demonstrated for CMF in patients with postmenopausal
breast cancer and for adriamycin in osteogenic sarcoma.
These adjuvant situations represent curative-intent treatment
and are consistent with the position that not only palliation
but cure as well for chemotherapeutic agents is influenced by
relatively slight differences in dose rate.[4] Thus the clinical cancer chemotherapist in order to optimize treatment usually tries to deliver the maximum safe dose and must recognize that a change by 25 or 50 percent in drug concentration
delivered to host target tissues on the one hand, and tumor
on the other, may result in either excess toxicity or inadequate therapeutic effect. Anything that modifies the body's
manipulation of the drug after it is administered becomes important in this context, and this of course is clinical pharmacology.

GENERAL PHARMACOLOGIC CONSIDERATIONS

General pharmacologic considerations are presented in
Figure 2. The various aspects of clinical pharmacology will
be reviewed in sequence, indicating examples where such may
impact on the pharmacology of cancer chemotherapeutic agents.
Absorption into the bloodstream is assured by intravenous administration. Giving drugs by mouth represents a practical
advantage. However, again in view of this steep dose-response
curve, it must be demonstrated by pharmacologic studies that
significant biotransformation in the gastrointestinal tract
does not occur and that absorption is reproducibly complete.
Fluorouracil was commonly given by mouth in clinical protocols
several years ago. However, it was demonstrated that, in contrast to intravenous administration, blood levels following
oral administration were highly variable, indicating incomplete and variable absorption, not only between patients but
within the same patient. With that study, the oral use of FU
was essentially terminated.

Once in the plasma many drugs bind with variable avidity
to plasma albumin. For example, methotrexate is approximately 60 percent bound to plasma albumin and can be displaced
by weak organic acids such as aspirin and probenacid, increasing thereby its bioavailability.

TABLE 2
Breast Cancer: CMF Dose-Response†

PERCENT OPTIMAL DOSE	ADVANCED DISEASE CR + PR (%) ALL PATIENTS	ADJUVANT THERAPY			
		DISEASE-FREE SURVIVAL*			SURVIVAL*
		ALL PTS.	PRE-MENO. PTS.	POST-MENO. PTS.	ALL PTS.
≥ 85%	66.7	75.5	75.6	74.2	82.1
85-65%	52.6	56.4	57.5	55.6	76.0
≤ 65%	35.3	46.3	48.2	45.9	66.5
ALL DOSES CMF	52.6	62.8	64.9	59.8	76.6
NO CHEMOTHERAPY	-	48.2	44.3	51.5	64.4

*All node-positive patients, 5-year follow-up.

† Milan, 1980

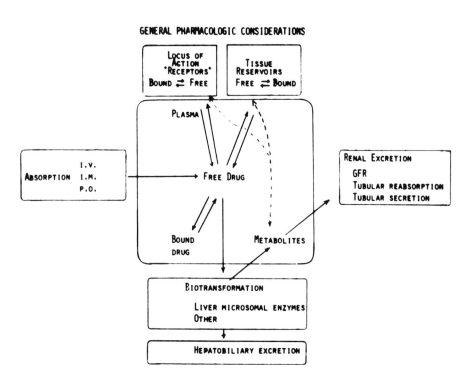

Figure 2. Clinical Pharmacology -- Schematic Diagram

A major site of biotransformation of drugs is the liver. Here microsomal enzymes biotransform and/or conjugate drugs in the direction of a marked decrease in biological activity and an increase in water solubility, such that the metabolites are more readily excreted by the kidney. There are several important antitumor agents which are so biotransformed and wherein this biotransformation may be substantially influenced by liver disease and particularly by other drugs. The second major mechanism for drug elimination relates to the kidney (see below). As we will see in a moment, drug-drug interaction at this level which influences glomerular infiltration or tubular function can have a major impact on the pharmacology of antitumor agents. Tissue reservoirs may be important, particularly for lipid-soluble drugs such as ortho-p-DDD (Mitotane).

The balance of these and other factors determines the concentration and half-time of free drug in the plasma and the amount of drug available for binding to the receptor site, that is the site that mediates the biologic effect. Since many patients with metastatic cancer are elderly and have varying degrees of compromise in, for example, liver and renal function, knowledge as to their pharmacology is essential to the optimal use of the agent in the individual patient.

An increasingly important aspect of clinical chemotherapeutics relates to drug-drug interaction. In a survey of forty inpatients during one day at the Farber hospital, it was found that these patients received 82 different drugs; and the average number of drugs per patient on that day was 5.6. In Table 3 the classes of drugs employed in these 40 patients are indicated in descending order of usage. As few as 2 and as many as 15 drugs were employed within the individual categories. Thus, in addition to combinations of cancer chemotherapeutic agents, it is important to appreciate that most patients with cancer, and particularly inpatients with cancer, are receiving a variety of other agents as well. What is not as widely appreciated is the fact that 60 percent of drugs which are not cancer chemotherapeutic agents are capable of perturbing the pharmacology and/or toxicology of one or more cancer chemotherapeutic agents. Only a few examples are listed in Table 4. Thus methotrexate is quantitatively excreted by the kidney. Changes in GFR induced by diuretics and competition for renal secretion of methotrexate by weak organic acids such as aspirin and probenecid may decrease the renal excretion of methotrexate and thereby increase its toxicity. Tubular damage may be induced by the use of aminoglycoside antibiotics, which are commonly

TABLE 3

A DAY AT THE FARBER HOSPITAL

DRUG USE IN 40 INPATIENTS IN ONE DAY

CLASS	NO. OF DIFFERENT AGENTS	PATIENTS RECEIVING (%)
SEDATIVES, TRANQUILIZERS HYPNOTICS	5	78
ANALGESICS	7	68
ANTITUMOR AGENTS	13	63
ANTIBIOTICS	15	60
CONSTIPATION-DIARRHEA	6	42
ANTIEMETICS	6	40
CORTICOSTEROID-ENDOCRINE	4	22
ANTACIDS	2	16
ANTIDURITICS	3	10
ANTISEIZURE	2	7
OTHER	8	--

SFCI DATA

TABLE 4

DRUG - CHEMOTHERAPEUTIC AGENT INTERACTION

60% of drugs used in cancer patients may perturb
Pharmacology - Toxicology of one or more cancer
chemotherapeutic agents.

Examples

Renal Elimination		Modify toxicity of
GFR	↓ by diuretics	MTX
Tubular function	↓ by aminoglysides	Platinum
Tubular secretion	↓ by ASA, proben.	MTX

Liver

Microsomal enzyme

Induction	Barb, antidepressants, anticoagulants	⎧ Cyclophosphamide
Inhibition	Allopurinal, darvon, phenylbutazone	⎨ Adriamycin
		⎩ DTIC

Binding Site Displacement	ASA, probenecid	MTX

| Ototoxicity | Aminoglycosides, etha-crynic acid | Platinum |

employed in patients with cancer, which may result in additive toxicity with platinum, a nephrotoxic cancer chemotherapeutic agent.

A number of commonly employed pharmaceuticals, such as, for example, the barbiturates, antidepressants and anticoagulants, cause induction of microsomal drug metabolizing enzymes of the liver. This will modify the pharmacology of cyclophosphamide, adriamycin, and DTIC and in general should tend to decrease their toxicity. On the other hand, the liver microsomal enzymes may be inhibited by allopurinal, darvon, and phenylbutazone, which would have the opposite effect. Finally, ototoxicity may occur with commonly employed antibiotics and diuretics, such as aminoglycosides and ethacrynic acid, which, if given concurrently with platinum, will increase the risk of eighth nerve damage and hearing loss.

The above represent only a few of the multiple interactions between, not only antitumor agents, but between antitumor agents and other commonly employed pharmaceuticals. Thus plus modifications of organ function, particularly with respect to the liver, the kidney, and the bone marrow, which commonly are present in patients with cancer, provides the basis for very substantial variability in the pharmacology of antitumor agents. Increasingly, monitoring of plasma curves of individual agents is being employed to guide the clinician in this setting. Certainly a thorough knowledge of these potential pharmacologic perturbations on the part of the medical and pediatric oncologist are essential. It is reflex on the part of all of us in many such complex clinical situations to reduce the dose of chemotherapeutic agents and err on the side of safety. It is important, however, to remember that the dose-response curve for our agents is steep, and thus that such downward modification may have significant adverse impact on the antitumor effect. The skillful clinician with a good knowledge of clinical pharmacology is best capable of selecting the proper agents and safe doses and schedules on the one hand, and of treating sufficiently vigorously to maximize the therapeutic effect on the other.

COMPARATIVE PHARMACOLOGY

Another important aspect of pharmacology which has been insufficiently emphasized is what I refer to as comparative pharmacology. There have been a number of circumstances where it has been found that a given drug has substantial activity against a number of experimental *in vivo* tumors. On the other hand, when that drug is tested in the clinic it is found to be negative. We should pursue these negative correlations more vigorously than we have in the past. There is an explanation for everything, and one possible explanation for this discordance may be a difference in pharmacology; for example a difference in the biotransformation of a given drug in the experimental animal and in man. Such differences provide the basic pharmacologist an opportunity to identify the active biotransformation products and particularly the opportunity to synthesize congeners of the drug in question, which might provide active biotransformation products in patients as well as in experimental animals. Up to the present time, we have tended to get involved in extensive clinical pharmacologic studies only for agents which show some evidence for clinical activity. This is important. On the other hand, in many ways it is more important to conduct comparative laboratory, animal, and clinical pharmacologic studies on all agents which show high promise on the basis of their activity in experimental tumors and have been inactive in man. We need new and active agents, and the possibility that exploitable therapeutic approaches might derive from such comparative pharmacology studies is real.

REGIONAL CHEMOTHERAPY

The use of chemotherapeutic agents by isolation perfusion, or by regional arterial infusion, began over twenty years ago. However, the primary science underlying this approach is pharmacology, and the application of pharmacology to such studies has occurred only in the last several years. Again, the primary rationale for this approach is the steep dose- or concentration-response curve. If by regional administration one can achieve a substantially higher drug concentration into the tumor bed, as compared to normal dose-limiting organs such as the bone marrow, an improved therapeutic effect might be anticipated.

Liver tumors commonly dominate the clinical situation, in patients with metastatic colorectal cancer for example, and hepatic artery infusion has commonly been employed in this setting (Figure 3). The potential advantage of this approach can be outlined from this figure. Thus the hepatic artery, while it supplies only one-third of the blood to the liver, as a whole commonly supplies ninety percent of the blood to the tumor. Secondly, if the drug is extensively metabolized by the normal liver, which is true for many drugs, a decrease in concentration gradient across the liver could

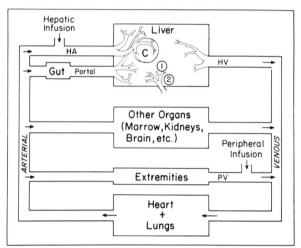

Scheme for hepatic infusion study showing sites of infusion in hepatic artery (*HA*) or peripheral vein and sites for blood sampling. This diagram also indicates preferential tumor (C) blood supply from the hepatic artery, and two mechanims for hepatic extraction: (*1*) catabolism by hepatocytes and (*2*) hepatobiliary excretion. With peripheral infusion of drug, hepatic arterial, PV, and HV samples are taken.

Figure 3. Hepatic Artery Infusion -- Schematic Diagram

be expected, so that the ratio of drug delivered to the tumor as compared to that which is seen by the normal organs, which are responsible for dose-limiting toxicity, could be high. This contrasts, of course, to peripheral blood infusions, where such a distributional advantage would not be expected. Recently pharmacologic studies addressed to intrahepatic artery infusion have been performed.[3] For fluorodesoxyuridine, for example, it has been found that 80% is extracted in a single pass through the liver. In part because of this, and because of the aforementioned factors, the concentration of drug in the hepatic artery at equilibrium when given at the same dose rate is one hundred-fold higher when given by intrahepatic artery infusion, as compared to peripheral vein infusion (Table 5). Because of extraction of drug by the liver, a four-fold higher dose rate of FUDR can be delivered into the hepatic artery as compared to the peripheral vein per equitoxic effect. Hence, at equitoxic doses it should be possible to achieve a four hundred-fold greater concentration of FUDR in hepatic tumors when the drug is given by hepatic artery infusion.

However, concentration in the hepatic artery obviously does not equate directly the concentration within the tumor. Since approximately 40 percent of patients do not respond to hepatic artery FUDR infusions, the question was asked as to whether this might not be a function of poor vascular perfusion of the tumor.[8] With bolus contrast angiography, some 80 to 90 percent of tumors filled adequately. However, by using radionuclide scans and varying the flow rate, it was found that with high flow rates the tumors filled in the majority of patients; but at the relatively slow rates commonly employed for FUDR infusion, only 50 percent of patients had tumors that were well visualized. When this was analyzed as a function of response to FUDR, it was found that patients with good perfusion at low flow rates, that is FUDR flow rates, had in excess of an 80 percent response rate, that is tumor regression rate; whereas the response rate was less than 20 percent for patients with poor perfusion, that is circumstances where the FUDR presumably did not distribute into the tumor. By using altered flow rates, by attempting to modify the vascularity by the use of vasoactive drugs, and by the use of chemotherapeutic agents which might have different perfusion characteristics, we are attempting to improve the response rates with this technique. At the very least, pharmacologic and hemodynamic studies have provided an important background for the selection of agents for use in this system, have explained the effectiveness or lack of in certain circumstances, and thus have provided a much more

TABLE 5

REGIONAL CHEMOTHERAPY - HEPATIC ARTERY INFUSION

FUdR given by continuous infusion into:

	Peripheral vein Total body	Hepatic artery 80% extracted in 1st pass thru liver
Distribution		
Concentration in hepatic artery at equilibrium (same dose rate)	$2-4 \times 10^{-6}M$	$3 \times 10^{-4}M$ (100 x greater)
Four-fold higher dose rate can be given by intra- hepatic artery		(x 4)
Final relative concentration of FUdR in tumor bed	1	400

rational and scientific basis for proceeding with this approach in the future.

Another common clinical problem, for example in ovarian carcinoma, is multiple superficial seeding of the peritoneal surface with metastasis. The group at NCI have performed experimental and clinical pharmacologic studies of several cancer chemotherapeutic agents, employing peritoneal dialysis-like techniques.[13] In the example presented in Figure 4 two liters of dialysate with a 4 millimolar concentration of fluorouracil were instilled into the peritoneal cavity. The peritoneal fluid concentration of fluorouracil was in all instances one hundred-fold or more greater than those in the plasma. The comparative concentrations in the plasma following single dose intravenous (IV) or continuous administration of standard doses are presented for purposes of comparison. The critical question, of course, is the concentration of drug achieved in small tumors on or immediately under the peritoneal surface. Nevertheless, from the toxicological point of view, this approach is feasible; and from the pharmacological point of view, much higher concentrations are provided within the peritoneal fluid, as compared to the plasma.

A third approach, which really represents a systemic approach to regional chemotherapy of the central nervous system, is as follows. Carboxypeptidase is an enzyme that cleaves glutamic acid from both folic acid and methotrexate, with resultant products which are essentially inactive. If methotrexate is given in high concentration for, for example, thirty-six hours, as in the study in figure 5, very high concentrations are achieved in the serum; and substantially lower but therapeutic concentrations are achieved in the spinal fluid (Figure 5). This difference is a result of the blood-brain barrier, which largely excludes methotrexate. This dose of methotrexate would be highly toxic in the absence of leucovorin rescue. Unfortunately, leucovorin, for example, rescues not only the systemic effect of methotrexate but also, since it enters the central nervous system, precludes any further therapeutic effect of methotrexate against brain parenchymal or meningeal tumors. On the other hand, carboxypeptidase is a macromolecular enzyme which does not penetrate the central nervous system. It eliminates methotrexate from the serum very promptly with a half-time of a few minutes; but since it does not enter the central nervous system, unopposed methotrexate at relatively high and therapeutic concentrations will persist in the central nervous system for relatively long periods -- again, a systemic approach to regional therapy.[1]

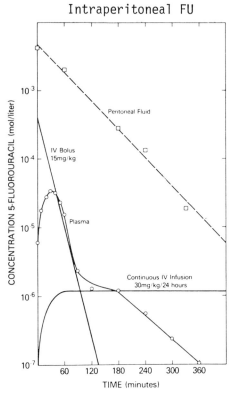

Intraperitoneal FU

Chart 2. 5-FU concentrations in a patient after 2 liters of dialysate with a 4 mM concentration was instilled. □, peritoneal fluid; ○, plasma. Values for i.v. bolus derived from the literature (2–6, 10, 12, 14, 22, 26); values for continuous i.v. infusion from the literature (4, 14, 15).

Speyer et al.

Figure 4. Peritoneal Dialysis with Fluorouracil --
Pharmacology

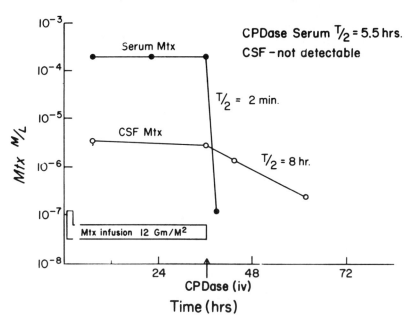

Figure 5. The Pharmacology of High-Dose Methotrexate with Carboxypeptidase Rescue

METABOLIC MODULATION

One pharmacologic approach to improving the effectiveness of established chemotherapeutic agents is to modulate
such agents in the direction of an improved therapeutic index. The antimetabolite fluorouracil has been a subject of
this approach. In Figure 6 a schematic diagram of the biochemical pharmacology of fluorouracil is presented, along
with two areas wherein modulation might be accomplished.
Fluorouracil is converted to FUMP by an enzyme that requires
PRPP. Increasing the availability of PRPP, which can be accomplished with methotrexate or the adenosine analog MMPR,
should increase the conversion of FU to FUMP. This should
increase the biological activity of FU, since FUMP, as a result of incorporation into RNA or as a result of a conversion
to the analog which inhibits DNA synthesis, is responsible
for the biological activity of FU. Another qualitatively different approach involves inhibition of pyrimidine biosynthesis with the antimetabolite PALA. This would decrease
UMP pools, which by decreasing competition for the related
fluorourinated substrate, in terms of incorporation into RNA
on the one hand, or inhibition of DNA synthesis on the other
should increase the biological effect. That this in fact can
be accomplished *in vitro* is evident in Table 6. In this *in
vitro* study of breast cancer cells, tritiated fluorouracil
was added to the medium, and its incorporation into RNA was
measured as a function of modulating materials. With tritiated FU only, incorporation into RNA was set at 1. The addition of PALA increased this some 3-fold, as did MMPR. With
the use of various combinations, such as PALA plus methotrexate, or PALA plus MMPR, approaches that involve both inhibition of pyrimidine biosynthesis and increasing the availability of PRPP, a 7- to 10-fold increase in FU incorporation
into RNA was achieved. Clearly *in vitro* one can modulate FU
in the direction of increasing the biological effect.
Whether this can be translated to an improved therapeutic effect *in vivo*, and particularly in the clinic, remains to be
determined.[2,9,10]

CHEMOTHERAPEUTIC TARGETS

While improving the use of established antitumor agents
through modulation or other means is important, it is at
least equally important to develop new cancer chemotherapeutic agents, either as structural analogs of known agents
or, still better, as new structures. The empirical and

INTRACELLULAR MODULATION OF 5-FU METABOLISM

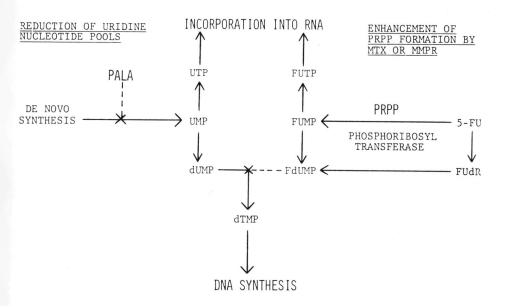

Figure 6. Biochemical Pathways Related to Fluorouracil:
Metabolic Modulation

TABLE 6
Metabolic Modulation of Fluorouracil

EFFECT OF VARIOUS DRUG COMBINATIONS
ON INCORPORATION OF [^{3}H]FU INTO MCF-7 RNA
AND ON INTRACELLULAR PRPP LEVELS

DRUG COMBINATION	PRPP (mean + S.D.)	RATIO [^{3}H]FU/^{32}P
Control	1.0 + .24	1.0
PALA	2.9 + .19	3.4 + 1.5
MTX	3.2 + .34	1.7 + 0.1
MMPR	4.3 + .65	2.5 + 0.5
MTX/MMPR	1.7 + .15	2.6 + 0.2
PALA/MTX	3.8 + .60	7.2 + 1.0
PALA/MMPR	7.4 + .23	9.0 + 1.9
PALA/MTX/MMPR	2.6 + .96	9.6 + 2.8

rational screening employing a wide net for antitumor activity represents an importnat approach, which is being increasingly supplemented by basic and pharmacologic science directed at defining therapeutic targets. The ideal chemotherapeutic target is one wherein the target is present in the tumor cells and where the drug in question interacting with the target will kill these tumor cells. Finally, and critically important for specificity, is the fact that the target must be minimally present or absent in normal cells. The target may represent a critical enzyme, other receptors, incorporation into macromolecules, etc. Some targets of current major interest are presented in Table 7. Dihydrofolate reductase, and to some extent thymidylate synthetase, is the target for a number of folic acid antagonists and will be discussed elsewhere in this symposium. Some tumors, such as melanoma, have metabolic pathways, such as the tyrosinase-melanin pathway that is prominently represented within the tumor but otherwise present only in noncritical G-O normal cells. A number of experimental approaches to the treatment of melanoma are based upon this rationale.

Enzyme deletion which may occur at the level of gene regulation, and thus amino acid dependence in, for example, the case of asparagine and cysteine, have been described. I will present cysteine in more detail shortly. In contrast, enzyme elevation, such as adenosine deaminase in T-cell lymphocytic neoplasms, has been a target for the antimetabolite deoxycoformycin.

Cell surface targets, such as tumor-associated antigens, are of substantial current interest. Such antigens have great specificity for the tumor, a specificity that far exceeds that of the classical chemotherapeutic agents. The complexing of such agents with highly cytotoxic materials represents an opportunity to exploit the specificity of antibodies with the potency of certain chemotherapeutic agents. More about this shortly.

Chemotherapeutic targets may be inferred empirically from evidence that a given agent has substantial specificity for tumors. This obtains, for example, for the anthracyclines. The basis for this specificity is under study.

I would like to enlarge upon several of these areas. First, cysteine dependence. Cysteine is a nonessential amino acid for normal tissues. It was demonstrated eight years ago that many leukemia cells and some nonleukemia tumor cells in culture required cystine, that is were cysteine-dependent (Table 8). An investigation at a pharmacologic level of this phenomenon led to the following explanation: It was found by analyzing the biochemical pathway involved in the

TABLE 7

CHEMOTHERAPEUTIC TARGETS

-- Dihydrofolate reductase, thymidylate synthetase.

-- Tyrosinase-melanin system in melanoma cells

-- Enzyme deletion, aminoacid dependence;
   e.g. asparagine, cystine.

   Enzyme elevation; e.g. adenosine deaminase

-- Cell surface targets. Receptors, tumor-associated
   antigens.

-- Anthracycline targets.

TABLE 8

CYSTEINE DEPENDENCE

Observation

1) Cysteine not required for normal cells.

2) Cysteine required for culture of human leukemia
   cell lines.

Explanation

Cystathionase (C'ase)
Methionine → homocysteine + serine → cystathionine → cysteine

10- to 50-fold decrease in C'ase as measured by:

   1) radiosubstrate enzyme activity.

   2) immunoprecipitation of enzyme protein.

30-fold decrease in mRNA for C'ase as measured by
poly A RNA C'ase generation system.

synthesis of cysteine that the final enzyme in the pathway, cystathionase, which is responsible for the conversion of cystathionine to cysteine, was markedly decreased in leukemic cells. This was determined by activity assays using radiosubstrates and by direct enzyme protein titration by immunologic means. Using the poly A RNA cystathionase generating system, it was found that these cells had a comparable decrease occurred at a translational level. That this decrease obtains not only for cells in culture but *in vitro* in man is demonstrated in Figure 7, wherein there is 10-fold less enzyme activity in human leukemic cells taken from the marrow, as compared to mononuclear cells from the normal marrow. These observations strongly support a therapeutic approach involving reduction of cysteine in extracellular fluid *in vivo*. After examining several cysteine-degrading enzymes, the most promising is beta-cystathionase. In order to get sufficient material for *in vivo* work, recombinant DNA techniques are being employed.[15,6]

A second approach to specificity that I would like to illustrate briefly is that of the combined antibody drug approach (Figure 8). One such approach that is being pursued at an experimental level involves the highly cytotoxic natural product known as ricin. This compound is cytotoxic at 10^{-9} molar. The F(ab) fragment of an antibody specific for human IGG is employed. This antibody will react with B lymphocytes, which have surface IGG, but not with T-lymphocytes or other cells which do not bear surface immunoglobulin. The F(ab)$_2$ fragment is split at the disulfide bond by reduction and activated by Ellmen's reagent. Ricin is similarly split by reduction between the alpha moiety, which is cytotoxic, and the beta moiety, which is receptor-oriented. By chromatography the cytotoxic alpha moiety can be separated. This is then reacted with the activated F(ab)$_1$ fragment, and a complex is produced including the antibody and the alpha fragment united by disulfide bonds. The specificity of the F(ab)$_1$-alpha complex is demonstrated in Table 9. The cells along increase in culture at the times indicated. If the F(ab)$_1$-alpha chain is added, there is a marked reduction. Such a reduction does not occur with T-cells or other cells that do not bear surface immunoglobulin. The alpha chain and the F(ab)$_1$ fragment alone are not active, nor are they active together. Human gamma globulin added to the F(ab)$_1$-alpha chain inhibits its activity by competing for antigenic sites. This specificity is confirmed by demonstrating that bovine gamma globulin which does not react with the human IGG receptor site does not interfere with the cytotoxicity of the F(ab)$_1$-alpha chain *in vitro*. This immunopharmacologic

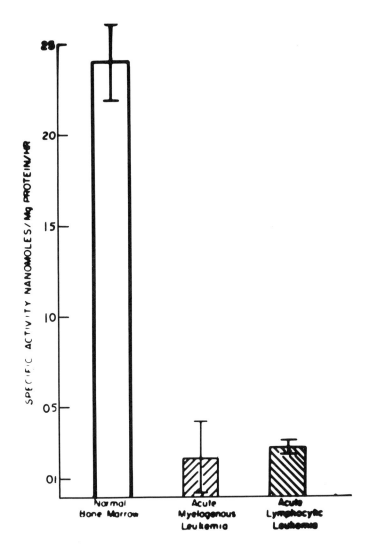

Figure 7. Cystathionase Levels in the Normal Marrow and Acute Leukemic Cells

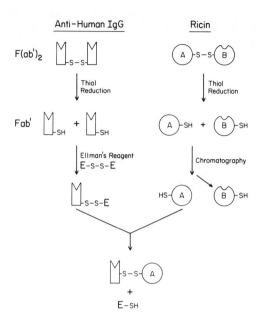

Figure 8. The Complexing of Monoclonal Antibodies with Ricin

TABLE 9

Specificity of the Toxicity of F(ab)$_1$-alpha Chain for Ig on Daudi Cells

Addition	Cells/ml x 10^{-4}			
	0 hrs	72 hrs	96 hrs	120 hrs
Cells Alone	38	162	165	141
+ Fab'-A Chain	38	52	24	4
+ A Chain	38	166	152	150
+ Fab'-E	38	120	144	143
+ A Chain + Fab'-E	38	179	145	145
+ Fab'-A Chain + HGG	38	183	180	167
+ Fab'-A Chain + BGG	38	45	27	6

approach to systemic cancer therapy is just beginning. There
are an increasing number of monoclonal antibody systems with
substantial tumor specificity. Similarly, we have a number
of exceedingly toxic chemical materials. Whether these can
in fact effectively be combined and produce antitumor activity *in vivo* remains to be determined.[12]

A final example relates to the anthracyclines (Figure
9). Adriamycin is an important antitumor agent, and attempts
have been made to improve upon its activity by modifying its
structure. Adriamycin is superior to a related analog,
daunorubicin, as a result of slight differences in the molecule at the fourteen carbon. More important is the fact that
the amino grlup of the amino sugar is important to the water
solubility of adriamycin, and particularly to its binding to
DNA. Accordingly, a number of modifications of these sites
were rendered, of which AD 32 has the greatest biological
activity. AD 32 is more lipid-soluble than adriamycin and
hence may more readily enter cells, and its binding to DNA
as compared to adriamycin has been substantially altered. In
terms of antileukemic activity in experimental *in vivo*
systems, it is substantially superior to adriamycin (Tables
10 and 11). Similarly, it has superior activity in breast,
colon, and melanoma cancer models. A major limitation in
the use of anthracyclines in man is the production of delayed
cardiac toxicity, which is questionably reversible. Accordingly, adriamycin and AD 32 were compared in terms of their
ability to produce cardiac toxicity in the rabbit (Table 12).
At equimyelotoxic doses AD 32 has little or no cardiac
toxicity, in circumstances where adriamycin produced death
from cardiotoxicity in the majority of animals. Thus in addition to metabolic modulation one can take an established
antitumor agent and by appropriate structural modification,
guided by biological and biochemical feedback, develop an
improved analog. AD 32 is currently the subject of a clinical trial.[7,11]

I have tried to look a bit into the future in terms of
cancer pharmacology. It remains to deal with more basic
science and a more long-range look at the potential for tumor
specificity. Only two of many possible examples will be
cited (Table 13). There is substantial evidence for abnormality in regulation of gene expression by most and perhaps
all tumors. Most, and perhaps all, human tumors demonstrate
an increase in production of ectopic hormones and/or oncofetal proteins. Also, as I have already indicated, there is
a reduction in enzyme production by certain tumors, which at
least in some circumstances occurs at the level of transcription. There is recent evidence for great heterogeneity of

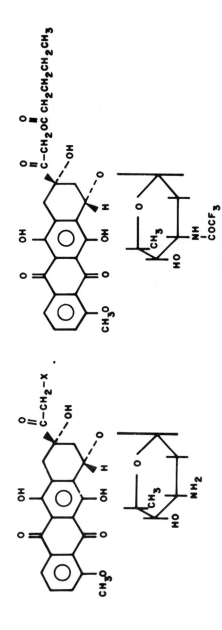

Daunorubicin: X = H
Adriamycin: X = OH

AD 32

Figure 9. Structural Formula of Adriamycin and AD 32

117

TABLE 10
Effect of AD 32 on Mouse Leukemias

Mouse Leukemia	Drug	Optimal Dose mg/kg/day, ip days 1-4	Increase in Median Life Span (%)	"Cure"
L1210	Adriamycin	4	45	0/5
	AD 32	60	445+	4/5
P388	Adriamycin	4	132	0/6
	AD 32	40	429	4/5'

*"Cure" = 30 day tumor-free survivors, expressed as a fraction of surviving/treated leukemic mice

TABLE 11
Effect of AD 32 on Solid Tumors in Mice

COMPARATIVE ACTIVITY OF AD 32 AND ADRIAMYCIN AGAINST SOME MURINE SOLID TUMORS

DATA OF SOUTHERN RESEARCH INSTITUTE (DR. D. P. GRISWOLD)

TUMOR (ROUTE)	AGENT	DOSE,* MG/KG, IP	SCHEDULE	% ILS	MEDIAN DELAY, DAYS[+] (T-C VALUE)
COLON TUMOR No. 38 (SC-IMPLANTED)	ADRIAMYCIN	7.5	DAYS 3, 10, 17	12	4.0
	AD 32	105.0	DAYS 3, 10, 17	26	17.1
C3H MAMMARY TUMOR No. 13/C (SC-IMPLANTED)	ADRIAMYCIN	7.5	DAYS 20, 27, 34	28	9.3
	AD 32	79.0	DAYS 20, 27, 34	100	19.9
B16 MELANOMA (SC-IMPLANTED)	ADRIAMYCIN	1.5	QD X 8 (DAYS 2-9)	0	1.0
	AD 32	30.0	QD X 8 (DAYS 3-10)	28	5.0

*HIGHEST NONTOXIC DOSE LEVEL.

[+]ANALOGOUS TO DURATION OF REMISSION.

APRIL 1976

TABLE 12
Adriamycin and AD 32 - Studies of Cardiac Toxicity in the Rabbit

HISTOLOGIC SCORES FOR CARDIOTOXICITY
IN RABBITS TREATED WITH ADRIAMYCIN OR AD 32

TREATMENT GROUP	NUMBER RABBITS EVALUABLE	NUMBER OF RABBITS WITH HISTOLOGIC SCORE			
		0	1+	2+	3+
CONTROL	4	4	-	-	-
ADRIAMYCIN	14	1 (7%)	-	1	12 (86%)
AD 32	9	4 (44%)	2	1	2 (22%)

TABLE 13
Potential Molecular Biological Targets for Chemotherapy

Regulation of Gene Expression in Tumors.

Abnormal in that:

1) ↑ in ectopic hormones and oncofetal proteins.

2) Enzyme deletion as above.

3) Other.

Regulation of Transcription.

Role of non-histone chromosomal proteins.

Major differences in structural and functional properties of non-histone chromosomal proteins have been observed between normal and tumor tissues. May be basis of alkylating agent specificity (Stein, CR, 1978).

Regulation of Translation.

Base methylation of tRNA.

tRNA methylases markedly increased in tumors with alteration of tRNA profiles.

S-adenosyl homocysteine is a competitive inhibitor of selected tRNA methylase. Such analogs may regulate translational events and have the potential for therapeutic specificity.

119

non-histone chromosomal proteins, and most particularly for
major structural and functional differences among non-histone
chromosomal proteins between normal and tumor tissues.[14]
These observations as they are extended might be expected to
form a basis for chemotherapeutic attack, and there is preliminary evidence that specificity of alkylating agents may
in part depend upon these chromosomal proteins. At the level
of regulation of translation, there is widely confirmed evidence for both quantitative and qualitative alteration in
base methylation of transfer RNA (tRNA) in tumors. Thus
transfer RNA methylases are markedly increased in tumors,
with resultant alteration in tRNA profiles. These tRNA
methylases may be quite specific for amino acids. S-adenosyl
homocysteine is a competitive inhibitor for selected tRNA
methylases. Such analogs may regulate translational events
and have the potential for therapeutic specificity.[5]

The above represent only a few principles and examples
as to why clinical and basic cancer pharmacology is important,
indeed essential, to progress in cancer treatment. Further
examples will be given in the symposia later on today.

References

1.   Abelson HT, Ensminger W, Kufe D, et al.: High-dose methotrexate-carboxypeptidase - A selective approach to therapy of the central nervous system tumors, in Kisliuk, R and Brown, G (eds): Chemistry and Biology of Pteridines. New York, Elsevier North Holland, 1979, pp 629-633.

2.   Cadman E, Heimer R, Davis L: Enhanced 5-fluorouracil nucleotide formation after methotrexate administration: Explanation for drug synergism. Science 205:1135-1137, 1979.

3.   Ensminger WD, Rosowsky A, Raso V, et al.: A clinical pharmacological evaluation of hepatic artery infusion of FU and FUDR. Cancer Res 37:3784-3792, 1978.

4.   Frei E III, Canellos GP: Dose - A critical variable in cancer chemotherapy. Amer J. Med, in press.

5.   Glick JM, Ross S, Leboy PS: S-adenosylhomocysteine inhibition in 3 purified RNA methyltransferases from rat liver. Nucleic Acid Res 2: 1639-1651, 1975.

6.   Glode M, Green H, Bickel I: Cystathionase in normal and leukemic cells. Cancer Treat Rep 63:1081-1088, 1979.

7.   Israel M, Modest EJ, Frei E III: AD 32, an analog with greater experimental antitumor activity and less toxicity than adriamycin. Cancer Res 35:1365-1368, 1975.

8.   Kaplan WD, Ensminger WD, Come S et al. Radionuclide angiography prediction of response to hepatic artery chemotherapy. Cancer Treat Rep, in press.

9.   Kufe DW, Egan ME: Enhancement of fluorouracil incorporation into human lymphoblast RNA. Biochem Pharmacol, in press.

10. Martin D, Stolfi R, Spiegelman S: Striking augmentation of the *in vivo* cancer activity of 5-fluorouracil (FU) by combination with pyrimidine nucleosides: An RNA effect. Proc Amer Assoc Cancer Res 19:221, 1978.

11. Parker L, Hirst M, and Israel M: AD 32 - Additional mouse antitumor and toxicity studies. Cancer Treat Rep 62: 119-127, 1978.

12. Raso V, Griffin T: Specific cytotoxicity of a human immunoglobulin directed F(ab)-ricin A chain conjugate. J. Immunol, in press.

13. Speyer JL, Collins JM, Dedrick RL, et al.: Phase I and pharmacological studies of 5-fluorouracil administered intraperitoneally. Cancer Res 40:567-572, 1980.
14. Stein GS, Stein JL, Thomson JA: Chromosomal proteins in transformed and neoplastic cells: A review. Cancer Res 38: 1181-1201, 1978.
15. Uren J, Lazarus H: Cysteine requirements of malignant cells and progress towards depletion therapy. Cancer Treat Rep 63:1073-1079, 1979.

MODULATION OF CHEMOTHERAPY WITH CYTOSINE ARABINOSIDE

PETER H. ELLIMS
ROSS C. DONEHOWER
BRUCE A. CHABNER

Clinical Pharmacology Branch
Division of Cancer Treatment
National Cancer Institute, NIH
Bethesda, Maryland 20205

Cytosine arabinoside (ara-C; 1-β-D-arabinofuranosylcytosine), used in combination with an anthracycline (either doxorubicin or daunomycin), is a standard agent for primary treatment of acute myeloblastic leukemia. These combinations now yield complete remissions in the majority of patients treated, and a small but finite (approximately 10%) fraction of long-term disease-free survivors. An important objective of pharmacologic research concerning ara-C is to increase its effectiveness by modulation of its metabolism within tumor cells. In order to understand these new approaches to cancer treatment, it is necessary to briefly review the mechanism of action of ara-C and the basic steps in its conversion to active and inactive products.

The cytotoxic activity of ara-C is believed to result from inhibition of DNA polymerase by the metabolite ara-CTP; a second action is the incorporation of ara-C into DNA. Ara-C incorporation into DNA has been shown to cause defective ligation of DNA subunits, failure of elongation of growing strands of DNA, and reiterative synthesis of fragments of DNA. The active mediator of each of these effects is ara-CTP, and the ability of leukemic cells to form and retain ara-CTP has been correlated with the duration of clinical response (1).

Ara-CTP is synthesized by a series of phosphorylation reactions catalyzed in sequence by deoxycytidine kinase, pyrimidine nucleoside monophosphate kinase (also known as dCMP kinase), and nucleoside diphosphate kinase. These steps are shown in Figure 1. Ara-C is inactivated to ara-uracil (ara-U)

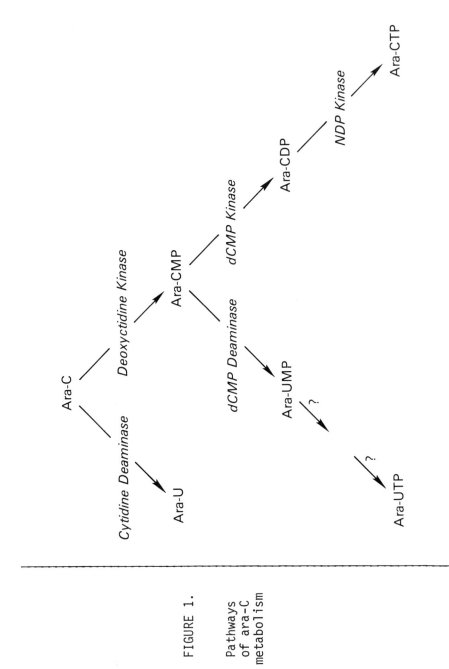

FIGURE 1.

Pathways
of ara-C
metabolism

124

by cytidine deaminase, and ara-CMP is deaminated and inactivated to ara-UMP by a second degradative enzyme, deoxycytidylate (dCMP) deaminase.

Each of the potential cytotoxic effects of ara-CTP is opposed by the naturally occurring pyrimidine dCTP. Thus, the
intracellular pool of dCTP is a crucial determinant of ara-C
sensitivity in experimental studies, and probably in clinical
therapy. dCTP pool size is regulated by multiple enzymes, but
two appear to be of particular importance (Fig. 2). Ribonucleotide reductase, which catalyzes the reduction of diphosphate ribonucleotides to deoxyribonucleotides, is the first of
these critical junctions. Conversion of CDP to dCDP by this
enzyme is inhibited by dCTP, dTTP, and dGTP, and is stimulated
by ATP.

FIGURE 2.   Ara-C:TdR Interaction

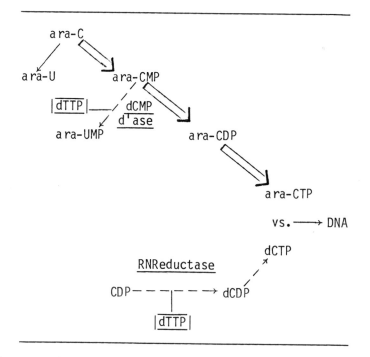

The second important regulatory step is dCMP deaminase,
which catalyzes the irreversible hydrolytic deamination of
dCMP to dUMP. The enzyme has been isolated from a number of
sources and the mammalian activity has been purified and characterized from donkey spleen (2) and recently from human
spleen (3) and cultured human leukemic cells (4). Despite

extensive investigation of the properties of this enzyme, the physiological importance of dCMP deamination in determining the intracellular dCTP and dTTP content has only recently been appreciated. Two recent reports (5,6) suggest that dCMP deamination is the primary pathway of cellular dUMP synthesis and the primary regulator of dTTP content of the mammalian cell. Like the activity from other sources, mammalian dCMP deaminase is an allosteric enzyme. The major control over enzyme activity is exerted by the positive allosteric effector dCTP with a K_m of activation 0.3 μM and the negative allosteric effector dTTP which produces a 50% inhibition of enzyme activity at a concentration of 2 μM (3). Substrates for the human enzyme are dCMP, CMP, and ara-CMP, with dCMP being approximately 20-fold more effective than CMP and 10-fold more than ara-CMP. Experimental studies have pointed out the importance of this enzyme in regulating the dCTP pool.

In studies of ara-C resistant Hamster fibroblasts, deSaint Vincent et al. (6) identified several lines deficient in dCMP deaminase; this deficiency was associated with an expanded intracellular pool of dCTP and a reduced pool of dTTP. These findings suggest that the primary influence of this enzyme on ara-C response is mediated through its control of intracellular dCTP. In other cell lines, the same workers found resistant mutants with high dCTP pools but normal dCMP deaminase activity. In the latter cells, the high concentrations of dCTP would be expected to activate dCMP deaminase, reduce its K_m for ara-CMP from 10 mM to 1 mM, and convert the drug to the inactive ara-UMP. High dCTP levels would also inhibit the phosphorylation of ara-C by deoxycytidine kinase and would compete with ara-CTP for catalytic sites on DNA polymerase. In this second group of cells (with high dCTP pools and normal dCMP deaminase activity) the explanation for increased nucleotide pools was unclear.

Other mechanisms of resistance to ara-C have been documented in cell culture experiments and in murine leukemias treated with the drug in vivo. The most common mechanism in murine lymphoblastic leukemias appears to be deletion of deoxycytidine kinase (7). An increase in cytidine deaminase has been implicated in one study of resistant human leukemic cells (8), but has never been observed in animal tumor models or in tissue culture variants selected for ara-C resistance.

In an effort to alter ara-C metabolism and to favorably modulate the ratio of ara-CTP to dCTP, several naturally occurring nucleosides and antimetabolites have been used in combination with ara-C. A few of these combinations have entered clinical trial, while for the remainder the biochemical interactions are being studied in cultured tumor cells and in animal tumor models in order to clarify the potential clinical value of each combination.

In the succeeding discussion, we describe the influence of these potentially valuable modulators on the metabolism and antitumor effect of ara-C.

ARA-C AND THYMIDINE

The inhibitory effects of the pyrimidine deoxyribonucleoside thymidine (TdR) on the growth of cultured mammalian cell lines are well known and have been used to synchronize proliferating cell populations (9). The major biochemical mechanism of this inhibition is thought to be the negative allosteric regulation exerted by the metabolite dTTP on ribonucleotide reductase activity (10). Accumulation of dTTP inhibits reduction of CDP to dCDP and stimulates the reduction of GDP to dGDP, resulting in a fall of dCTP and a rise in dGTP intracellular content. The low level of intracellular dCTP is insufficient to support DNA synthesis and cell proliferation. Inhibitory feedback control is also exerted by high dTTP concentrations on other enzymes regulating pyrimidine nucleotide biosynthesis and interconversions, including TdR kinase, dTMP synthetase, and dCMP deaminase, but the role played by each of these activities in the thymidine block of DNA synthesis is unclear, and probably less important than the effects on dCTP pools.

Cultured tumor cell lines differ in their sensitivity to TdR inhibition. Some types of cultured mouse tumor cells and human T- and null-leukemia cells are sensitive to μM concentrations of TdR (11,12) while growth inhibition of other cell lines requires TdR in mM concentrations (12). Inhibition of cell proliferation at either "low" or "high" TdR concentrations correlates with a depletion of intracellular dCTP content. The biochemical basis of differential sensitivity to TdR has been elucidated in some cell lines with sensitivity to "low" concentrations and has been attributed to reduced activity of the catabolic enzyme thymidine phosphorylase (11).

These data have formed the basis of several investigations that have examined the effect of TdR depletion of intracellular dCTP content on the antitumor activity of ara-C. Plagemann et al. (13) found that 100 μM TdR increased the incorporation of ara-C into the DNA of cultured Novikoff rat hepatoma cells but did not significantly alter total cellular ara-CTP content. In cultured mouse tumor cells, Harris et al. (14) observed that the sensitivity of several cell lines to ara-C was enhanced by thymidine concentrations as low as 10 μM. Enhanced antitumor effect correlated with a fall in dCTP levels, while,

conversely, the intracellular dCTP content of those cell lines
which did not show TdR augmentation of ara-C cytotoxicity did
not fall despite a rise in the dTTP pool. The reason(s) for
this differential effect of exogenous TdR on the dCTP pools
of various mouse tumor cell lines was not apparent from this
work. Two possible mechanisms for this phenomenon are an
alteration in the regulation of ribonucleotide reductase, or a
deletion of deoxycytidylate deaminase, metabolic defects known
to be associated with raised intracellular dCTP levels (6) and
thymidine resistance.

Thymidine has also been found to enhance the antitumor effect of ara-C against the L1210 mouse leukemia cell line (15).
Maximum cytotoxicity was observed when cells were pretreated
with 100 μMTdR for 5 hours prior to ara-C exposure and these
findings correlated with increased ara-CTP levels and decreased dCTP content compared to cells exposed to ara-C only. Pre-
treatment with higher concentrations of TdR or for less than
5 hours caused less enhancement of ara-C cytotoxicity. In an
in vivo study of the combination of TdR and ara-C in rats
bearing a transplanted colonic carcinoma, Danhauser and Rustum
(16) found maximal advantage for antitumor activity when the
thymidine infusion was given for 24 hours prior to ara-C administration, as compared to alternative schedules or ara-C
alone. Pretreatment with TdR caused increased tumor ara-CTP
levels but without tissue specificity as those host tissues
examined exhibited the same phenomenon.

In summary, these investigations indicate that ara-C and
thymidine are synergistic in selected situations, but in clinical trials careful attention will need to be given to both
the schedule and dosage of administration if maximum effects
are to be realized. For example, most mammalian cells in culture are unaffected by μM concentrations of thymidine. Higher
concentrations, above 1 mM, are required to decrease intracellular dCTP and produce cytotoxic effects in most cell lines.
Sensitivity to thymidine may be determined by the cellular
content of thymidine phosphorylase, which cleaves TdR to an
inactive product. Sublines of cultured human lymphoblasts
which lack this enzyme have greatly increased sensitivity to
TdR, suggesting that this enzyme might be useful as a marker
for TdR responsiveness in man.

A serious drawback to the combination of TdR and ara-C may
be the coincident development of resistance to both modalities, as observed by deSaint Vincent and Buttin (6). As mentioned previously, cell lines exposed to ara-C alone were
found to develop resistance associated with increased dCTP
pools, and were simultaneously resistant to TdR. This observation suggests that human cells resistant to ara-C will show

little additional response to ara-C plus TdR, if resistance is due to dCTP pool expansion.

ARA-C AND DEOXYGUAUOSINE

The purine deoxyribonucleoside GdR is a more potent inhibitor of the human myeloblastic leukemia cell line HL-60 than TdR (17) and an approximately equal inhibitor of cultured T- and null-leukemia cells (18). Akman et al. (17) have examined the effect of deoxyguauosine on the inhibition of HL-60 cell lines by ara-C. The addition of 10 µM ara-C or 100 µM GdR alone did not affect HL-60 cloning but 5 µM ara-C with 100 µM GdR reduced cloning efficiency to 40%, indicating synergism. GdR toxicity to T- and null-leukemia cells is mediated by high intracellular dGTP levels which inhibit ribonucleotide reductase, leading to a fall in dCTP content (18). The decrease in intracellular dCTP content could explain the synergism between ara-C and CdR; however, Akman et al. (17) have found additional GdR effects on ara-C metabolism. GdR in high concentration (500 µM) inhibits ara-C uptake but enhances ara-C incorporation into nucleic acid, the latter probably due to decreased dCTP pools competing with ara-CTP. At all GdR concentrations examined, total cellular ara-CTP content fell by 30%. These data indicate that deoxyguauosine can influence ara-C metabolism by two mechanisms, one being a negative effect on ara-C uptake and the other an enhancement of ara-CTP incorporation into DNA polymerase. Further investigation of this potentially interesting combination is warranted.

ARA-C AND TETRAHYDROURIDINE

The reduced uridine analogue tetrahydrouridine (THU) is a tight-binding competitive inhibitor of cytidine deaminase (K_i 4 x 10^{-8}M) (19) which catalyzes the deamination of ara-C to the inactive metabolite ara-U. Interest in the combination of ara-C and THU has arisen because of the high levels of cytidine deaminase activity found in human tissues, including liver, spleen, and leukemic blast cells (19), and the work of Steuart and Burke (8) who showed a correlation between high leukemic blast cell enzyme activity and resistant disease.

In clinical trials, THU has enhanced ara-C potency but the combination has not demonstrated superior therapeutic effect as compared to ara-C alone (20). When used against various animal tumors, the combination has generally shown no clear advantage over ara-C alone, although most of the tumor systems tested did not contain high concentrations of cytidine deaminase, as found in human acute myeloblastic leukemia. It should

be emphasized that in using this, as well as other combinations, tumors resistant to ara-C by virtue of deletion of
deoxycytidine kinase or because of expanded dCTP pools would
not be expected to have an enhanced response, since neither
of these resistance mechanisms would be overcome by cytidine
deaminase inhibition. Indeed, inhibition of cytidine deaminase might lead to expansion of intracellular dCTP pools and
decreased dTTP content, both being the biochemical characteristics of ara-C resistant cells.

ARA-C AND HYDROXYUREA

Ara-C cytotoxicity is specific for the S-phase of the cell
cycle, and its combination with a cell cycle synchronizing
agent such as hydroxyurea could potentially enhance the antitumor effect of ara-C. Hydroxyurea inhibits mammalian cell
DNA synthesis by interference with ribonucleotide reductase
activity. The effect of hydroxyurea on ara-C activity has
been examined in cultured tumor cell lines. Plagemann et al.
(13) found that 1 mM hydroxyurea markedly increased the intracellular ara-CTP content of Norikoff hepatoma cells but actually reduced ara-C incorporation into DNA. In cultured L1210
mouse leukemia cells, Walsh et al. (21) observed that preincubation of cells with hydroxyurea in concentrations from 0.1 to
10 mM prior to ara-C (1 μM) significantly increased ara-CTP
content. A similar hydroxyurea effect on ara-C metabolism was
found in vivo, with a 2-fold increase in the ara-CTP content
of L1210 leukemia cells when the animals were treated with hydroxyurea and ara-C together as compared to ara-C alone (21).
Hydroxyurea enhancement of ara-CTP concentrations appeared to
be tumor cell specific as the effect was not found in the
normal host tissues examined. The biochemical mechanism of
the hydroxyurea effect on ara-C metabolism was examined by
these investigators and a role for decreased dCTP levels was
suggested, but the exact mode of interaction between hydroxyurea and ara-C metabolism remains unclear.

ARA-C AND 3-DEAZAURIDINE

Paterson and colleagues have described an enhancement of
ara-CTP formation in some murine and human cell lines by 3-
deazauridine (22,23). The latter is an inhibitor of CTP synthetase, and thus decreases both CTP and dCTP pools. It also
inhibits, albeit with modest potency, cytidine deaminase and
dCMP deaminase (24). The basis for enhanced formation of ara-
CTP is not clear, but is likely mediated by the reduction in
dCTP pools; this reduction would tend to release inhibition of

deoxycytidine kinase and would decrease the activity of dCMP deaminase. In preliminary work, Donehower et al. have found that ara-CMP deamination is probably an unimportant component of ara-C metabolism, and that the more important action is enhanced deoxycytidine kinase activity (25) secondary to a fall in dCTP pools. The potency of ara-C:3-deazacytidine synergism is not striking in cell culture systems. However, both drugs are active against human myeloblastic leukemia, and a clinical trial of the combination is warranted.

A second poorly understood interaction is observed between methotrexate and ara-C. Pretreatment of cells with the antifolate leads to increased formation of ara-C derived nucleotides, and synergistic cytotoxicity versus the L1210 cell line in tissue culture (26). These findings are surprising and unexplained, since methotrexate would tend to lower TTP pools and expand dCTP pools; both these effects are associated with ara-C resistance.

In conclusion, a number of possible ways exist for manipulating the metabolism of ara-C and the formation of its competitor dCTP. The effect of various nucleosides and antimetabolites on ara-C metabolism will depend on the activity of critical enzymes in the leukemic cell. Clinical trials of these combinations should include pretreatment measurement of these activities so that a rational interpretation of results can be accomplished. Further advances in biochemical technique, particularly in the accurate measurement of dCTP concentrations in clinical leukemia cell samples, are needed to allow an interpretation of functional enzyme activity in the patient, as opposed to the artificial setting of a cell-supernatant, where assays do not reflect the regulatory influence of nucleotides.

REFERENCES

1. Rustum YM, Preisler HD: Correlation between leukemic cell retention of 1-β-D-arabinofuraosylcytosine 5'-triphosphate and response to therapy. Cancer Res 39:42-49, 1979.
2. Geraci G, Rossi M, Scarano E: Deoxycytidylate aminohydrolase. I. Purification and properties of the homogenous enzyme. Biochemistry 6:182-191, 1967.
3. Ellims PH, Chabner BA: Unpublished observations.
4. Ellims PH, Chabner BA: Unpublished observations.
5. Jackson RC: The regulation of thymidylate biosynthesis in Novikoff hepatoma cells and the effects of amethopterin,

5-fluorodeoxyuridine, and 3-deazauridine. J Biol Chem 253:7440-7446, 1978.

6. deSaint Vincent BR, Dechamps M, Buttin G: The modulation of the thymidine triphosphate pool of Chinese hamster cells by dCMP deaminase and UDP reductase. J Biol Chem 255:162-167, 1980.

7. Schrecker AW, Urshel MJ: Metabolism of 1-β-D-arabinofuranosylcytosine in leukemia L1210 cells: Studies with intact cells. Cancer Res 28:793-801, 1968.

8. Steuart CD, Burke PJ: Cytidine deaminase and the development of resistance to arabinosylcytosine. Nature (New Biol) 233:109-110, 1971.

9. Xeros N: Deoxyriboside control and synchronization of mitoses. Nature (Lond) 194:682-683, 1962.

10. Eriksson S, Thelander L, Akerman M: Allosteric regulation of calf thymus ribonucleoside diphosphate reductase. Biochemistry 18:2948-2952, 1979.

11. Fox RM, Tripp EH, Piddington SK, et al: Thymidine sensitivity of cultured leukemic lymphocytes. Lancet 391-393, 1979.

12. Reynolds EC, Harris AW, Finch LR: Deoxyribonucleoside triphosphate pools and differential thymidine sensitivities of cultured mouse lymphoma and myeloma cells. Biochim Biophys Acta 561:110-123, 1979.

13. Plagemann PG, Marz R, Wohlheuter RM: Transport and metabolism of 1-β-D-arabinofuranosyl-cytosine into cultured Novikoff rat hepatoma cells. Relationship to phosphorylation, and regulation of triphosphate synthesis. Cancer Res 38:978-989, 1978.

14. Harris AW, Reynolds EC, Finch LR: Effect of thymidine on the sensitivity of cultured mouse tumor cells to 1-β-D-arabinofuranosylcytosine. Cancer Res 39:538-541, 1979.

15. Grant S, Lehman C, Cadman E: Enhancement of 1-β-D-arabinofuranosyl-cytosine accumulation within L1210 cells and increased cytotoxicity following thymidine exposure. Cancer Res 40:1525-1531, 1980.

16. Danhauser LL, Rustum YM: Effect of thymidine on the toxicity, antitumor activity, and metabolism of 1-β-D-arabinofuranosylcytosine in rats bearing a chemically induced colonic carcinoma. Cancer Res 40:1274-1280, 1980.

17. Akman S, Ross D, Salinger C, et al: Augmentation of effect of cytosine arabinoside (ara-C) on human myeloblastic leukemia cell line HL-60 by deoxyguanosine (GdR). Proc Amer Assoc Cancer Res 1130:282, 1980.

18. Fox RM, Tripp EH, Piddington SK, et al: Sensitivity of leukemic human null lymphocytes to deoxynucleosides. Cancer Res 40:3383-3386, 1980.

19. Stoller RG, Myers CE, Chabner BA: Analysis of cytidine deaminase and tetrahydrouridine interaction by use of ligand techniques. Biochem Pharmacol 27:53-59, 1977.
20. Kreis W, Woodcock TM, Gordon CS, et al: Tetrahydrouridine: Physiologic disposition and effect upon deamination of cytosine arabinoside in man. Cancer Treat Rep 61:1347-1353, 1977.
21. Walsh CT, Craig RW, Agarwal RP: Increased activation of 1-β-D-arabinofuranosylcytosine by hydroxyurea in L1210 cells. Cancer Res 40:3286-3292, 1980.
22. Lauzon GJ, Paran JH, Paterson ARP: Formation of 1-β-D-arabinofuranosylcytosine diphosphate choline in cultured human leukemic RPMI 6410 cells. Cancer Res 38:1723-1729, 1978.
23. Lauzon GJ, Paterson ARP, Belch AW: Formation of 1-β-D-arabinofuranosylcytosine diphosphate choline in neoplastic and normal cells. Cancer Res 38:1730-1734, 1978.
24. Drake JC, Hande KR, Fuller RW, et al: Cytidine and deoxycytidylate deaminase inhibition by uridine analogs. Biochem Pharmacol 29:807-811, 1980.
25. Donehower RC, Drake JC, Chabner BA: Unpublished observation.
26. Cadman E, Eiferman F: Mechanism of synergistic cell killing when methotrexate precedes cytosine arabinoside. J Clin Invest 64:788-797, 1979.

Biological Response Modifiers in Cancer Therapeutics

E. MIHICH, M.D.

Director, Grace Cancer Drug Center and Dept.
of Experimental Therapeutics
Roswell Park Memorial Institute
New York State Dept. of Health
Buffalo, New York

During the past 20 years, evidence has been accumulated suggesting that tumor-host interactions may be altered therapeutically. Recently, the biological response modifiers (BRM) have been defined as agents or approaches which may alter the interactions between tumor and host through a modification of the biological responses of the host to tumor*. Modifications of biological responses may be effected in different ways, such as: (a) to increase host anti-tumor responses through augmentation or restoration of effector mechanisms or mediators of host defense, or decrease of undesirable components of the host reaction, (b) to increase host defenses by the administration of natural or synthetic mediators, or effector cells, (c) to increase the efficacy of host responses through changes in tumor cells which might stimulate a greater host response or increase tumor cell sensitivity to a response, (d) to decrease the development (transformation) of, and/or increase the differentiation (maturation) of, tumor cells, (e) to increase the ability of the host to tolerate

*Interim Report on BRM, dated September 30, 1979, by the Ad Hoc Subcommittee of the Board of Scientific Counselors of the Division of Cancer Treatment (DCT) of the National Cancer Institute (USA). This Subcommittee was instituted by Dr. V.T. DeVita Jr., to formulate programmatic recommendations for DCT and it includes: E. Mihich (Chairman), A. Fefer (Vice-chairman), J. Bertram, A. Goldstein, E. Hersh, M. Krim, M. Mastrangelo, M. Mitchell, H. Oettgen, J. Whisnant, A. Goldin (Special NCI Advisor) and M. Chirigos (NCI liason).

damage by cytotoxic modalities of cancer treatment.

In this presentation only some aspects of the potential
role of BRM in cancer therapeutics and of the requirements
for their optimal utilization can be briefly considered.
Thus, this discussion is focussed on immunostimulating and
immunomodulating agents and on thymic hormones. Although the
clinical studies of interferons are outlined elsewhere in
this Symposium, a few comments on the development of these
agents are also included because of current interest in this
area. The utilization of tumor immunity in developing new
strategies with tumor vaccines, immune cells or antibodies,
the implementation of chemopreventive treatments with retinoids or other agents, the development of therapeutic approaches based on the induction of differentiation of cancer
cells are not included herein.

Immunostimulating and Immunomodulating Agents. Many substances have been found to modify host responses to tumor and
other immunogens and are usually defined as immunosuppressive, immunostimulating, immunorestorative or immunomodulating. It is becoming increasingly apparent that most of them
are capable of causing suppression or stimulation of the
overall response depending on experimental conditions and,
most likely, on the status of the host defense systems at the
time these systems are exposed to the agent. By definition
immunomodulating agents act on the regulatory mechanisms of
different host defense systems. Although for most substances
proof for this is lacking, the term is used to define operationally agents which alter the balance among various components of a host defense system and/or are capable of causing
opposite effects under different conditions.

The diversity of host defense systems and their controls
provide numerous opportunities for selective intervention by
immunomodulating agents. Based on experimental data, only in
part verified in humans, the effector cells capable of at-
tacking a tumor cell encompass T cells, macrophages (Mϕ),
killer (null) cells and natural killer cells (NK); plasma
cells are also involved as they produce complement-dependent
cytotoxic antibodies as well as the cytophilic antibodies.
The development of these effectors is modulated through complex interplays such as those involving helper, accessory and
suppressor functions. Most of these functions, as well as
the effector development they modify, are regulated through
lymphokines.

An awareness of the complexities of the host defense systems is important for an appreciation of the potentiality for
success of immunointervention. Indeed the capacity to develop effective clinical immunotherapy with immunostimulat-

ing/immunomodulating agents is likely to be dependent on
knowledge in three basic areas, namely; 1) the mechanisms
involved in the regulation of antitumor host defenses in humans, including the central role of tumor antigens, 2) the
methodologies required to assess the status of antitumor defense systems in individual patients at the onset of treatment and thereafter, and 3) the mechanisms involved in the
action of immunotherapeutic agents under different conditions. The lack of sufficient knowledge in each of these
areas has imposed major elements of empiricism on the design
of the early immunotherapy trials and this has no doubt contributed to the relatively modest successes achieved through
this approach in the past.

Progress is, however, being achieved in defining the
antigenicity of human tumors and the complexities of host
defenses[14,15]. Moreover, during the past 5-10 years many
techniques have been developed to measure in patients T cell
subset functions, other suppressor and accessory functions,
and other indicators of host defenses. Thus it is now reasonable to expect that the new immunostimulating/immunomodu-
lating agents may provide a useful modality of cancer treatment. These agents essentially fall into three main groups,
namely, natural products, synthetic products and biologicals
from mammalian sources.

The natural products are represented by cells and cell
fractionation products[13] such as BCG, MER, C. Parvum, OK
432, Nocardia rubra skeleton and by extraction products[13,4]
such as muramyl dipeptides, polysaccharides, glucans, endo-
toxins, Bestatin, Lentinan and cyclomunine. Although each
substance or group of substances has individual characteristics and determines different profiles of altered immune
parameters, a few generalizations can be made: 1) most of
these products stimulate the development and/or the function
of Mϕ ; 2) several of these products induce the production of
interferons (IF) and/or stimulate the function of NK; 3) most
of these products appear responsible for tumor regression
when given in conjunction with different chemotherapeutic
agents in a variety of experimental tumor models. Although
several of these products have been or are being tested in
humans, the majority of the clinical trials during the last
10 years have been carried out with BCG, C. Parvum and related fractions. Only BCG is discussed herein as an example
(see Ref 10 for early reports).

Attempts to stimulate the defenses of the host non-speci-
fically in order to augment their reactivity against tumor
were encouraged by the pioneering work of Mathe's group suggesting prolongation of survival in children with acute lym-

phoblastic leukemia treated with cytoreductive chemotherapy
followed by BCG. Shortly afterwards Morton's group reported
that intratumor inoculation of BCG caused regression of neoplastic skin nodules in malignant melanoma. Following other
early promising reports, numerous trials have indicated that
in most disease types BCG does not alter substantially survival rate, that it provides clear therapeutic advantages only
in patients with dermal metastasis from malignant melanoma[9]
and that it prolongs survival of patients with acute myeloblastic leukemia[16]. Suggestive evidence in other tumor
types such as ovarian carcinoma[1], lymphoma[6], stage I
non-oat cell carcinoma of the lung[8] and superficial bladder cancer[12] must await validation.

     Certain conclusions have emerged from the studies of BCG
which may have relevance also to other immunostimulating
agents. 1) Many of the earlier studies in humans were limited by slow patient accrual within each disease type, excessive diversification of study goals, variability of potency among preparations used, lack of adequate comparability of
prospective variables in treatment and control groups, and
premature reporting. 2) Studies suggesting an effect of immunostimulants must be carefully repeated in randomized
trials, especially when the suggestions are consistent with
what is known about the agent considered. For instance the
study of BCG given by local instillation to patients with
recurrent superficial bladder cancer[12], or as a single
intrapleural injection after surgery to patients with stage I
non-oat cell lung carcinoma[8] are both consistent with the
notion acquired in animal studies and confirmed in patients
with malignant melanoma that BCG has the greatest chance to
exert antitumor effects when placed in close association with
the tumor. 3) Unexpectedly, a group of patients receiving
both BCG and Levamisole in a recent lung tumor study[17] are
doing worse than the controls. An observation of possible
analogous significance has been made in patients with AML
immunized with neuraminidase-treated allogeneic myeloblasts,
in which the additional treatment with MER reduced the advantages of immunization[5]. Therefore combining two presumably different types of immunostimulating treatments need not
provide greater therapeutic advantages but may reduce them.
4) In some of the few well controlled randomized studies with
BCG in combination with chemotherapy completed to date, a
prolongation of median survival time without increase of survival rate, has been observed in the BCG treated group as
compared to the group given chemotherapy alone. The reason
for the ultimate convergence of the control and treated survival curves has not yet been elucidated nor has this clinic-

al observation been correlated with changes in relevant parameters of host response throughout the period of survival.
5) Based on information accrued in animals and in humans, it
is unlikely that immunostimulation may be therapeutically
effective against large tumor masses[3].

The experience gained during the past 10 years indicates
the need to evaluate extraction products which would allow
more precise dosing and might eventually lend themselves to
chemical synthesis or modifications. Many such substances
are being developed at present[13,4].

Synthetic compounds with immunostimulating and immunomodulating activity[13,4] include derivatives such as peptido-
glycans, polynucleotides, pyran copolymers, phospholipid
derivatives, Levamisole, isoprinosine, NTP 15392, and benzi-
midazole derivatives. Certain anticancer agents, such as,
6-mercaptopurine (6 MP), cyclophosphamide (Cy) and Adriamycin
(AM) also have shown immunomodulating activity. The immunomodulating effects of AM are outlined herein to stress the
fact that chemotherapeutic agents originally developed for
their anti-proliferative action may also have BRM activity[11].

The effects of AM on the immune system have been studied
primarily in this laboratory and at the Negri Institute in
Milan using various in vivo and in vitro mouse systems and,
to the knowledge of this reviewer, have not yet been validated in humans. In various mouse systems AM has sparing effects on monocytic-macrophage cells and augments the development of phagocytic cells from non-phagocytic precursors.
Also, AM and C. Parvum, a Mϕ stimulator, had synergistic
anti-tumor effects. In mice AM inhibits the development of
humoral responses against allogeneic lymphoma cells under
conditions of optimal response whereas it augments both this
and the T cytolytic cells responses under conditions of suboptimal response; such opposite effects are also seen in primary CML cultures against the same target cells. Effects on
T suppressor (Ts) function have been noted in at least six
different systems. The reduction of suppressor function and
the increase of Mϕ function may be instrumental, at least in
part, in the augmentation of immune responses induced by AM.
In addition, it was found by others[4] that AM augments NK
activity in peritoneal cell populations but not in the spleen
where there is actually some depression.

Some of the effects of AM are comparable to those of
other anticancer drugs. For instance, depending on conditions, Cy may depress or augment T cell lytic responses or
may selectively inhibit Ts development. In 1966 6 MP was
reported by Chanmougan and Schwartz (see ref 11) to augment

or inhibit antibody responses to bovine γ globulins in rabbits depending on dose of drug, dose of antigen and time between drug and antigen administration. The possibility that immunomodulating effects may be exerted by anticancer drugs in humans under conditons of anticancer treatment deserves investigation.

Thymic Factors. Thymosin was the first extract from thymic tissue found to replace the thymus in the development of T cell dependent immune functions in neonatally thymectomized or athymic nude mice and in restoring these functions in adult mice rendered immunodeficient[3]. A large number of factors have since been isolated from thymic tissues and blood which have shown at least some "thymic-like" activity. Thymosin itself has been purified to Fraction 5 (Fr-5) which contains several active polypeptides with molecular weights ranging from 1000 to 15,000; of these polypeptides, thymosin α_1 is the most studied. The other known thymic-like factors are Thymic humoral factor (THF), Thymopoietin (TP) and its active pentapeptide TP5, Thymic factor (TFX), Facteur thymique serique (FTS), homeostatic thymic factor, lymphocytopoietic factors, hypocalcemic and lymphocytopoietic substances TP_1 and TP_2, thymic epithelial supernatant, thymosterin, human serum prealbumin factor and thymus-dependent human serum factor. It is not yet known to what extent these preparations are biologically different and whether some of them have the same active moiety[3]. To date, the best characterized substances include Fr-5 and its polypeptide components, THF, TP, TP5, TFX and FTS; of these, thymosin α_1, TP5 and FTS have been chemically synthesized.

Based on functional assays, cell surface markers and terminal nucleotidyl transferase activity, it has been proposed[3] that the various polypeptides contained in Fr-5 affect predominantly distinct stages of T cell maturation. Because of such selectivities and the chemical differences established between thymosin α_1, TP and FTS, it seems important that all the preparations with thymic-like activities found in different laboratories be thoroughly characterized and compared, both structurally and functionally in attempts to define the regulation of the thymus dependent immune systems. The knowledge thus acquired might be utilized towards the development of BRM treatments.

The rationale for the clinical use of Fr-5 and of other preparations with thymic-like activity, lies in the ability of these substances to stimulate the maturation of T cells from precursor cells in individuals with immunodeficiencies related to thymic hypoplasia or dysfunction. In cancer patients the rationale is to reverse the immunosuppressive effects of the tumor itself or of chemotherapy and other treatment modalities through a similar stimulation of T cells maturation.

Fr-5 proved to be of benefit in primary immunodeficiency diseases such as DiGeorge Syndrome, chronic mucocutaneous candidiasis and Wiskott-Aldrich Syndrome[3]. Correlations were found between pre-treatment increase of MLC reactivity by Fr-5 _in vitro_ and post-treatment increase in MLC reactivity. The effects of thymic factors in immunodeficiency diseases cannot yet be definitely evaluated as in most instances the treated patients were not randomized against placebo and the number of cases with any given syndrome was small. Nevertheless, there is little doubt that thymic hormone replacement may be effective in children with thymic aplasia or dysplasia. After current limitations in supply of thymosin preparations are overcome through the availability of products obtained by chemical synthesis or genetic engineering, it should become feasible to carry out definitive clinical trials to validate the positive indications derived from past studies.

After several preliminary trials of Fr-5 in patients with cancer, the first randomized Phase II trial was carried out in 55 patients with non-resectable small cell carcinoma of the lung[2]. Patients received intensive combination chemotherapy for remission induction and were randomized to placebo, 20 mg/m^2 Fr-5 or 60 mg/m^2 Fr-5 given twice a week for the 6 weeks of chemotherapy. Remission rate was comparable in the three groups. The patients given 60 mg Fr-5 had significantly prolonged remission duration, with median survival increased to 450 days from 240 days in the placebo group, and about 30% of them were alive at 500 days, with 28% free of detectable tumor. Prolongation of survival by Fr-5 was correlated with initial low levels of α2HS glycoprotein and T cell numbers in blood. Although randomized, this study has limitations related to the small number of patients and shorter survival of the chemotherapy-placebo group as compared to that reported by others using the same chemotherapy. Should these results be validated in a large number of patients, they would indicate a role of thymic factors in the treatment of certain neoplastic diseases.

Interferons. The results obtained to date by the use of IF in cancer patients have been outlined in another part of this Symposium. Type I IF are secretory glycoproteins produced by eukaryotic cells in response to viral infection or other agents, which are capable of inducing a state of cellular resistance to viral infection[7]. Type II, or "immune", IF is produced by lymphocytes stimulated by antigen or mito-

gens. These glycoproteins are essentially species-specific.
In addition to their broad spectrum of antiviral effects, IF
affect immune responses specifically and in opposite directions depending on timing of administration, antigen and response studied. One of the most consistent effects is the
stimulation of NK cells, an index that may be used to monitor
the BRM action of IF in humans. The antitumor effects of IF
have been demonstrated in a variety of mouse models and appear to be more marked when tumor burden is small and IF is
given repeatedly[7]. Close contact of IF with target cells
seems required for activity and consequently prophylactic
treatments are ineffective. Although the mechanisms of the
antitumor effects are not yet known, they may be related to
both immunomodulation and direct antiproliferative action.
That alterations in cell surface characteristics or other
cellular effects of IF may contribute to the antitumor effects cannot be excluded at this time. It is important to
note that antiviral and antitumor activity seem to co-purify
in preparation of both mouse and human IF.

Three types of IF have been used in humans, namely, leuc-
ocyte IF (HuLe IF) which is obtained from induced human buffy
coat cells in short-term cultures, lymphoblast IF (HuLy-IF)
which is obtained from induced lymphoblast culture and fibro-
blast IF (HuFi-IF) which is obtained from induced fore-skin
fibroblasts in culture. Each of these IF is structurally
different although similarities exist between HuLe-IF and
HuLy-IF. There is uncertainty as to which type of IF may
provide greater therapeutic potential, and it has been recently suggested that each may find optimal use in different
types of cancer when given by different routes and schedules.

As a whole, the data available suggest that HuLe-IF has
objectively measurable antitumor effects in some patients
with some types of cancer (see Chapter). These effects are
generally not marked and not always reproducible using different batches of HuLe-IF. The number of patients is too
small to reach any conclusion at this time. The HuLe-IF preparations used are only about 0.1% pure, a standard that
would be unacceptable in trials using a chemical agent.
Moreover, the clinical results have been obtained with possibly suboptimal regimens designed without the support of
information from Phase I trials, to which IF has not yet been
subjected. Therefore, it is reasonable to expect that future
trials with purified IF given according to the results of
Phase I trials and pharmacological studies of BRM activity
may show activity against certain forms of cancer.

Studies are currently underway using HuLy-IF and HuFi-IF,
respectively, by systemic administration. The preparation of

HuLy-IF used in the United Kingdom is 10-100 fold more pure
than HuLe-IF and yet its toxicity occurs at IF-equivalent
doses comparable to those of HuLe-IF causing similar toxicity[13]; this suggests that the activity resides in the IF
molecule or is co-purified with IF. In initial comparative
and cross-over trials, HuFi-IF showed a spectrum of antitumor
action which did not totally coincide with that of HuLe-
IF[13]. The toxicity of the three types of IF tested in humans has been generally similar, usually mild and somewhat
transient.

Finally, it should be noted that HuLe-IF has been shown
to exert encouraging antiviral effects. This activity may
provide advantages in cancer therapeutics not only in possibly affording protection against viral infection in immunosuppressed or immunodeficient patients, but also in improving
the opportunities for survival of patients with leukemia
given bone marrow transplantation who have a high incidence
of CMV-induced pneumonia.

<u>Concluding Remarks</u>. Some of the pharmacological require-
ments for the optimal clinical study of BRM are similar to
those which have been identified in cancer chemotherapy.
Thus, for instance, it is important that the purity of a BRM
be assured or, if the active moiety is not structurally defined, that consistent and reproducible preparations be used. This requirement has not yet been strictly met for such
bacterial products as BCG or for IF. Some of the discrepanc-
ies and frustrations which have characterized the development
of BRM in the past are in part attributable to deficiencies
in this respect. Limitations in supply of BRM preparation
have also represented a major obstacle. Chemically defined
derivatives of bacterial preparations and active moieties of
thymic factors and interferons are being currently identified
and this should provide improved opportunities for the production of reliable preparations either through chemical synthesis or genetic engineering.

It is as essential that Phase I studies be carried out
for BRM as it is in classical chemotherapy approaches. However, in the case of BRM, these Phase I trials should not be
restricted to measurements of possible dose-limiting toxicities and of the pharmacokinetics and disposition of the substance, but should also include measurements of the biological response(s) expected to be modified. Indeed in the case
of the BRM, optimal regimens are likely to be rather different from regimens based on maximum tolerated doses (MTD).
Moreover, it is important that Phase II trials be designed

using regimens known to cause the expected modification of
biological response: only then would it be possible to ascertain the relationship of antitumor to BRM activity and to
identify likely reasons for success or failure. The search
for relevant assays of BRM activity is therefore an important
component of therapeutic development in this area.

It appears likely that the activity of certain classes of
BRM is dependent on the status of host defenses at the time
of treatment. With the advent of monoclonal antibodies, the
rapidly increasing knowledge of cell markers defining cell
subsets with specific functions in the systems of host defense and the improved methodologies to measure the functional specificities of those cell subsets, it should eventually
become possible to estimate more precisely the status of
antitumor defenses in patients. These measurements should be
applied, as relevant, to the Phase II studies of BRM.

Although the value of most BRM in cancer therapeutics has
not yet been unequivocally proven, it should be anticipated
that agents capable of increasing the efficacy of host responses to tumor would ultimately provide essential tools in
the definitive treatment of certain forms of cancer. Because
BRM are likely to be effective primarily against a small tumor load, this type of agent may be most effective against
tumors which are clinically undetectable but are destined to
recur. Consequently, in most cases, BRM may be useful after
reduction of tumor burden by other modalities of treatment.
These agents need not be restricted to treatment of minimal
residual disease, however, because they may also reduce some
of the toxicities of cytoreductive treatments. Because at
least some of the BRM are unlikely to exert antitumor effects
measurable according to customary criteria, prolongation of
disease-free interval and of survival and modifications of
functional parameters of host response may provide the only
realistic assessment of their activity. Because BRM are expected to act through physiological mechanisms, it is possible that they have relatively moderate toxicities and it is
probable that these toxicities are not directly related to
the desired therapeutic action.

In conclusion, it seems reasonable to continue vigorously
the development of known classes and approaches of BRM towards potential utilization in cancer therapeutics while also
exploring new leads in tumor specific immunity, chemopreven-
tion and the control of cell differentiation. It should be
reiterated, however, that the acquisition of basic information on the mode of action of BRM and on the prerequisites

for BRM action is essential for a profitable development of this area of therapeutics.

REFERENCES

1. Alberts, D.S., Moon, T., O'Toole, R., et al.: BCG as an adjuvant to Adriamycin-Cytoxan for advanced ovarian cancer: a SWOG study, in Jones, S. and Salmon, S.E. (eds.) Second International Conference on Adjuvant Therapy of Cancer II. New York, Grune and Stratton, 1979, pp. 483-494.
2. Cohen, M.H., Chretien, P.B., Ihde, D.C., et al.: Thymosin fraction V and intensive combination chemotherapy. J. Am. Med. Assoc. 241:1813-1815, 1979.
3. Goldstein, A.L., Low, T.L.K., Thurman, G.B., et al.: Thymosins and other hormonal-like factors of the thymus gland, in Mihich, E. (ed.) Immunological Aspects of Cancer Therapeutics, New York, J. Wiley and Sons, 1981, in press.
4. Hersh, E.M., Chirigos, M., Mastrangelo, M.J. (eds): Proceedings of Workshop on Augmenting Agents in Cancer Therapy: Progress in Cancer Research and Therapy, New York, Raven Press, 1980, in press.
5. Holland, J.F. and Bekesi, J.G.: Comparison of chemotherapy with chemotherapy plus VCN-treated cells in acute myelocytic leukemia. Prog. Cancer. Res. Ther. 6:347-353, 1978.
6. Jones, S.E., Salmon, S.E., Fisher, R.: Adjuvant immunotherapy with BCG in non-Hodgkin's lymphoma: a SWOG controlled clinical trial, in Jones, S. and Salmon, S.E. (eds) Adjuvant Therapy of Cancer II. New York, Grune and Stratton, 1979, pp. 163- 172.
7. Krim, M.: Towards tumor therapy with interferons. Blood 55:711-721 and 875-883, 1980.
8. McKneally, M.F., Maver, C. and Kausel, H.W.: Regional immunotherapy of lung cancer with intrapleural BCG. Lancet 1:377-379, 1976.
9. Mastrangelo, M.J., Berd, D., Bellet, R.E.: Critical review of previous reported clinical trials of cancer immunotherapy with non-specific immunostimulants. Ann. N.Y. Acad. Sci. 277:94-123, 1976.
10. Mihich, E.: Chemotherapy and immunotherapy as a combined modality of cancer treatment. Proc. 7th Intl. Symposium on Biological Characterization of Human Tumors, Budapest, in Excerpta Medica Intl. Congress Series No. 420. Advances in Tumor Prevention, Detection and Char-

acterization, Vol. 4, Amsterdam, 1978, pp. 113-121.

11. Mihich, E.: Cancer chemotherapy and immunity, in Mihich, E. (ed.) Immunological Aspects of Cancer Therapeutics, New York, J. Wiley and Sons, 1981, in press.

12. Morales, A., Eidinger, D., Bruce, A.W.: Adjuvant BCG immunotherapy in recurrent superficial bladder cancer, in Terry, W.D. and Windhurst, D. (eds.) Immunotherapy of Cancer: Overall Status of Trials in Man. New York, Raven Press, 1978, pp. 225-230.

13. Mullen, P.W., Hadden, J.W.: Abstracts of the First International Conference on Immunopharmacology, Int. J. Immunolpharm. 2:153-267, 1980.

14. Old, L.J.: Cancer Immunology: The search for specificity. GHA Clowes Memorial Lecture 1980. Cancer Research, 1981, in press.

15. Ozer, H.: Tumor immunity and escape mechanisms in man, in Mihich, E. (ed.) Immunological Aspects of Cancer Therapeutics, New York, J. Wiley and Sons, 1981, in press.

16. Powles, R.L., Russell, J., Lister, T.A., et al.: Immunotherapy for acute myelogenous leukaemia: A controlled clinical study 2½ years after entry of the last patient. Br. J. Cancer 35:265-272, 1977.

17. Wright, P.W., Hill, L.D., Peterson, A.V., et al.: Levamisole (L) results in immunosuppression and lacks antitumor activity when combined with intrapleural BCG (Ip-BCG) in patients with resected non-small cell lung cancer. Proc. Am. Soc. Clin. Oncol. 21:452, 1980.

Pharmacology of New Cancer Chemotherapy Agents

TI LI LOO

Professor of Therapeutics
Chief, Pharmacology Branch
Department of Developmental Therapeutics
M.D. Anderson Hospital and Tumor Institute
Houston, Texas 77030

This review summarizes for you our recent pharmacologic studies of 3 relatively new anticancer agents, namely TCN (NSC-154020, 3-amino-1,5-dihydro-5-methyl-1-β-D-ribofuranosyl-1,4,5,6,8-pentaazaacenaphthylene), DHAQ (NSC-301739,1,4-dihydroxy-5,8-bis[2-[(2-hydroxyethyl)-amino]ethylamino]-9,10-anthracenedione dihydrochloride), and 5-MTHHF (NSC-139490, 5-methyl-tetrahydrohomofolate). The definition of "new" is arbitrary, since it often takes more than 5 years for a promising agent to advance from the laboratory to the clinic; by then the agent may no longer be new to those credited with its discovery and development. We are currently involved in pharmacologic studies of a variety of new agents. However, our discussion shall be confined to the three mentioned above, each chosen for a specific reason. To illustrate our systematic approach to delineate the disposition, metabolism, and mechanisms of action of an antitumor agent, we should like to summarize for you our studies of TCN: in this work, we have brought some of the most powerful sophisticated analytical methodologies to bear on the problem. DHAQ, a synthetic compound somewhat related to the anthracycline antibiotics, is now in clinical trial at several centers on account of its impressive activities in experimental tumor systems; consequently the results of our research with this agent may be of some general interest. Although 5-MTHHF is not yet in clinical trial, we are nevertheless able to conduct limited clinical pharmacological studies with tracer doses of this agent. Potentially our findings could significantly contribute to the design and conduct of future clinical trials with this agent.

TCN

     Methodical structural modifications by Townsend and
collaborators (1) of the naturally occurring antineoplastic
antibiotics toyocamycin and sangivamycin with the purpose
of improving their therapeutic efficacies against transplantable animal tumor culminated in the synthesis of TCN (Fig. 1).
The significant activity of TCN in experimental systems coupled with novel structure made it an attractive candidate
for clinical trial. We therefore investigated the pharmacologic fate of TCN in preparation for its possible phase 1
studies.
     Radioactive [5-^{14}CH$_3$]TCN was administered as an intra-
venous (i.v.) bolus in 10 min to 8 beagle dogs at 5-25 mg/kg
(ca. 100-500 mg/m^2), 100 μCi per animal. Blood and urine
specimens were collected in the usual fashion. In 5 dogs,
bile samples were also obtained by catheterization of the
common bile duct. Plasma clearance of total radioactivity
was fast, with an average terminal $t_{\frac{1}{2}}$ of 3.6 hr (Fig. 2).
The apparent volume of distribution of TCN and metabolites
(see later) exceeds the total body water content of the dog,
suggesting localization of the drug in certain body compartments. This received support from the finding that the
radioactivity in red blood cells (RBC) was 20 times as high
as that in the plasma. Additionally, although less than 5%
of the administered dose was excreted in the urine in 5 hr,
the average total plasma clearance was 65 ml/kg/min, more
than 16-fold higher than the creatinine clearance in the dog.
The high clearance was accounted for by the rapid concentrative excretion of TCN in the bile, 55% in 5 hr (Fig. 3). In
fact, in the dose range of 5-25 mg/kg, the drug often crys-
tallized in the bile. An unfortunate consequence of this
finding was that the clinical trial of TCN was postponed
indefinitely. Another unusual property of TCN resides in its
extensive binding to plasma which averaged 65% in the concentration range of 0.1-100 μg/ml in human plasma; higher
than any other ribonucleoside that we have come across.
     In the bile of the beagle dog TCN was excreted unchanged.
But in the urine, several metabolites were detected by radiochemical and chromatographic techniques; however, unchanged
TCN remained the major component. The concentrative uptake
of TCN by human and dog RBC as well as by Chinese hamster
ovary (CHO) cells was followed by the intracellular formation of TCN 5'-monophosphate (TCN-MP), but unaccompanied
by formation of the di- or triphosphate. The identity of

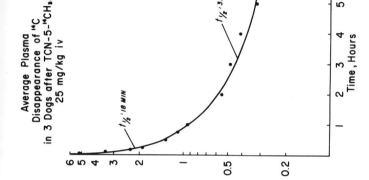

TCN

Figure 1

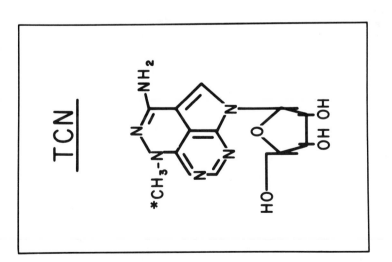

Average Plasma
Disappearance of ^{14}C
in 3 Dogs after TCN-5-^{14}CH$_3$,
25 mg/kg iv

$t_{1/2}$: 18 MIN

$t_{1/2}$: 3.5 HR

Conc, µg/ml, in Drug Equivalent

Time, Hours

Figure 2

149

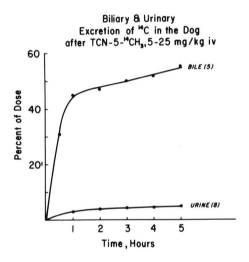

Figure 3

TCN-MP was established chemically and physicochemically
by comparison with an authentic synthetic specimen provided by Professor LeRoy Townsend. We shall discuss
the in vitro metabolism of TCN by RBC in more detail later.
It suffices to point out that none of the TCN metabolites
were formed through simple N-demethylation, deamination, or
loss of the ribofuranosyl group. Similiar to tubercidin
(7-deazaadenosine) to which TCN is structually closely related, the conversion of TCN to TCN-MP was mediated by
adenosine kinase (EC 2.7.1.20). A subline of CHO cells
deleted of adenosine kinase failed to effect this conversion.
For this reason, the intracellular transformation of TCN to
its 5'-monophosphate by RBC obeyed Michaelis-Menten Kinetics,
(Fig. 5) and exhibited saturation at high TCN concentrations.
    Analysis of RBC lysate by high pressure liquid chromato-
graphy (HPLC) showed the presence of 3 other metabolites (I,
II, and III) in addition to TCN and TCN-MP. Incubation of
TCN with 30% H_2O_2 at 37° led to the formation of metabolites
II and III; but instead of metabolite I, a new metabolite, IV,
was detected. Incubation of II but not III with RBC's
afforded I. Conversely, incubation of I with either alkaline
phosphatase (EC 3.1.3.1) or 5'-nucleotidase (EC 3.1.3.5) produced II exclusively, not III. Both II and III had identical
mass spectra. These results suggested that II and III were
anomeric, II being the natural β-anomer, and that I was the
5'-monophosphate of II. Also, mass spectrometric studies
showed that IV differed from II and III in the absence of the
ribofuranosyl moiety. Since the molecular weight of II was
4 units more than that of TCN, it was likely that TCN gave
rise to II by losing a carbon and gaining an oxygen. Based
on mass spectrometric and other physicochemical evidence we
assigned to II the structure 1-methyl-3-amino-5-β-D-ribo-
furanosylamino-pyrimidino[4,5-c]pyridazin-4-one, and postulated that it was formed by the sequence of transformations
shown in Fig. 5.
    The uptake and intracellular conversion of TCN to TCN-
MP by RBC's is reminiscent of another antimetabolite, 6-
methylmercaptopurine riboside (MMPR,9-β-D-ribofuranosyl
6-methylthiopurine) which behaves similarly in this regard.
It is therefore reasonable to compare their mechanisms of
antitumor action. MMPR 5'-monophosphate blocks the de novo
biosynthesis of purine ribonucleotides by inhibiting the
formation of 5-phospho-β-D-ribofuranosylamine. This reaction
is mediated by amidophosphoribosyltransferase (EC 2.4.2.14).
MMPR cytotoxicity can accordingly be reversed by hypoxanthine,

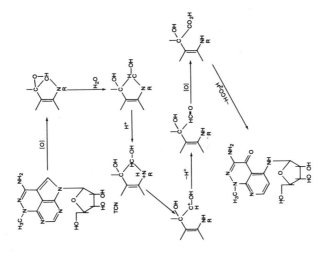

Figure 5

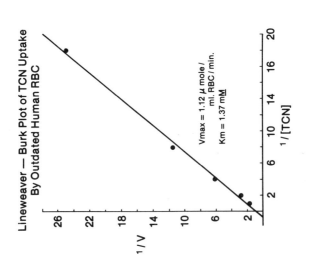

Lineweaver – Burk Plot of TCN Uptake
By Outdated Human RBC

Vmax = 1.12 μ mole /
ml. RBC / min.

Km = 1.37 m$\underline{M}$

Figure 4

152

adenine plus guanine, or 5-amino-imidazole-4-carboxamide
(AIC). Independent of Plagemann (2) and Bennett (3), we
noted that TCN cytotoxicity was not reversed by these compounds in CHO cells. In agreement with Bennett and Plageman,
we likewise concluded that TCN and MMPR could not have identical loci of action. Incubation of CHO cells with 50 μM of
either agent at 37° for 4 hr resulted in noticeably different
effects on ATP and GTP biosynthesis. The 2 agents were similar in that none affected pyrimidine nucleotide synthesis
significantly and both inhibited formate incorporation into
ATP and GTP to less than 2% of control. But they differed
in 2 major aspects. First, TCN inhibited hypoxanthine incorporation into GTP at least 5 times more than into ATP, while
MMPR inhibited this incorporation to the extent of about 30%.
Second, and most strikingly, although MMPR reduced ATP and
GTP concentrations to about 40% of control, in contrast, TCN
only lowered ATP concentration to 80%. This was actually
accompanied by an elevation of GTP concentration to over 130%
of control. These results are summarized in Table I.

Table 1. Effects of 50 μM TCN or MMPR on Purine
Nucleotide Biosynthesis in CHO cells. Incubation
at 37⁰ for 4 hr. Average results of 6-8 experiments
expressed as % of control

	TCN		MMPR	
	ATP	GTP	ATP	GTP
Concentration	79	131	38	35
Formate Incorp.	1.9	0.5	0.5	0.3
Hx Incorp.	55	10	33	26

In other words, if TCN reduced hypoxanthine incorporation into
GTP moderately and formate incorporation markedly, why then
did GTP concentration become elevated instead of lowered as
was with MMPR? We felt that, despite TCN inhibition of GMP
and consequently GTP biosynthesis, GTP nevertheless accumulated because its utilization was diminished, possibly in
protein synthesis. Accordingly, we examined the effects of
TCN on macromolecular syntheses, particularly protein synthesis, using cycloheximide (CHX) as a reference compound.

In 6 hr both TCN and MMPR decreased thymidine incorpora-

tion into perchlorate-insoluble materials of CHO cells to
about 40% of control as compared with 10% after CHX incubation.   The effects of these 3 agents on L-leucine incorporation were dramatically different.   TCN reduced leucine incorporation to about 35% of control; however, MMPR virtually
had no effect, while CHX almost completely inhibited this incorporation within 1 hr.   The TCN inhibition of amino acid
incorporation into proteins was not confined to leucine;
similar effects were observed with histidine, phenylalanine,
proline, tryptophan, and tyrosine.   We are unclear why the incorporation of these amino acids was inhibited to nearly the
same extent, 30% of control and no further; possibly the rate
limiting step is the availability of TCN-MP or some other
metabolite.   Evidently further work needs to be done.   To define more precisely the specificity of TCN inhibition of macromolecular syntheses, CHO cells were pulse treated for 45
min. with 50 nM to 50 μM of either TCN or CHX together with
leucine, thymidine, or uridine.   The general inhibition
pattern was similar with both agents.   Further, they both
inhibited leucine and thymidine more than uridine incorporation.   However, TCN exerted the same effect on leucine and
thymidine incorporation, but CHX was clearly a more potent
and selective inhibitor of leucine incorporation.   Since CHX
is far more cytotoxic than TCN and requires no activation to
be toxic, it is a more powerful inhibitor of precursor incorporation than TCN.

DHAQ

In an effort to reduce the toxicity of the antitumor anthracycline antibiotics without adversely affecting their
activity, a number of aminoanthracenedione derivatives were
synthesized.   Among these DHAQ exhibited the highest activity
against a broad spectrum of experimental tumors (4).   For
this reason it was selected for clinical trial and concurrent
clinical pharmacological investigations.   We now briefly
describe our results.

DHAQ labeled with ^{14}C in all 4 carbons of the bis(2-hy-
droxyethyl) moiety {generously supplied by the NCI} was administered as an i.v. bolus in 15 min. at 1-4 mg/m^2, 100-200
μCi per patient, to 10 patients participating in the phase I
trial.   None of these participants showed markedly abnormal
hepatic or renal function tests.   However, as noted in Table
2, there was ascites in one patient, and leg edema in another.
Pharmacologic studies were performed on day 1 of the first
course, except 3 patients in whom the studies were carried
out on day 1 of the second course instead.   A course of treat-

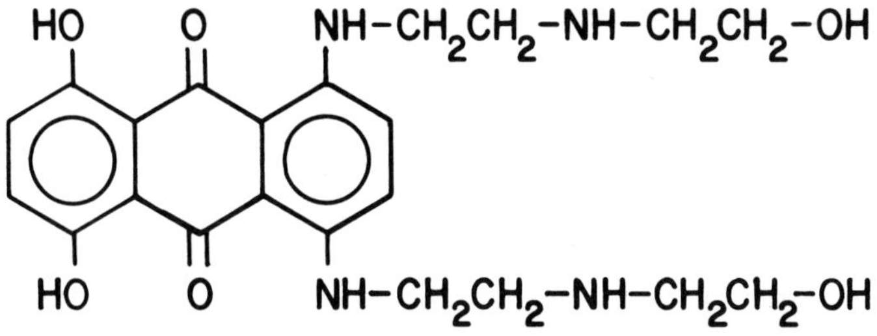

DHAQ

Figure 6

Table 2. Clinical Pharmacokinetic Parameters of DHAQ

Dose mg/m²	Plasma t½ Initial min	Plasma t½ Terminal hr	Vd ml/kg	Clearance ml/kg/hr	Urinary Excretion,% 24 hr	Urinary Excretion,% 96 hr
1	58	58	1160	142	9	11
2	32	61	346	106	13	ND[a]
3	20	53	811	159	4	5
3	27	50	1263	363	6	8
3	58	52	1542	285	8	11
3[b]	31	80	620	155	3	4
4[c]	52	73	878	80	7	8
2[d]	61	187	1723	35	6	9
3[d]	29	128	713	76	4	5
3[d]	68	182	3224	155	4	6

a ND: Not done. c This patient had leg edema.
b This patient had ascites. d Determined on day 1 of 2nd course instead of 1st course.

ment consisted of 5 daily administrations at the dose indicated, followed by a 2-day rest. Blood and urine specimens
were collected at intervals in the customary way. Drug
analysis was by HPLC, using unlabeled DHAQ as a marker. The
absorbance of the eluent was monitored at 254 nm, and the
DHAQ peak was collected and counted.

In all patients plasma DHAQ disappearance followed
biexponential kinetics (Table 2). In the 5 patients studied
on day 1 of the first course, the average terminal $t_{\frac{1}{2}}$ of
DHAQ was very long, about 55 hr. In the 2 patients with an
abnormal "third space", it was still longer, about 77 hr.
The longest terminal $t_{\frac{1}{2}}$ was in the 3 patients studies on
day 1 of the second course; it was nearly 7 days. The
apparent volume of distribution and total clearance of
DHAQ showed large variations. The average clearance was
slightly higher than creatinine clearance (90-110 ml/kg/hr);
consequently some tubular excretion of DHAQ was possible.
The cumulative urinary excretion of DHAQ, was low, averaging
about 7% in 24 hr and less than 9% in 96 hr. In 1 patient
bile was available for analysis. The biliary excretion was
also low, less than 3% in 96 hr. All these results strongly
suggest persistence of DHAQ in the body, and therefore
caution against frequent intermittent administration of this
agent. In the urine, 1 major and 1 minor unidentified DHAQ
metabolites were detected.

One of the mechanisms of cytotoxicity of DHAQ seems to
rest on its intercalation with cellular DNA, similar to
doxorubicin or adriamycin. We have confirmed this in mouse
L1210 leukemia cells [V.I. Avramis, S. Feldman, G.A. Alianell,
and Ti Li Loo, to be published]. We have also found that
the experimental therapeutic activities of the aminoanthra-
cenediones correlated well with their in vitro genetic toxicity as revealed by cytogenetic assays. DHAQ was most active
in induction of chromosomal damage. In cytogenetic assays,
the activities of these agents were reduced in the presence
of microsomal enzymes (the so-called S9 system) (5).

5-MTHHF

Homofolate, a synthetic folate analogue, possesses an
extra methylene group between the $9-CH_2$-and 10-NH-of folate.
Its reduced 5,6,7,8-tetrahydro derivative (THHF) proves to
be active against mouse L1210 leukemia resistant to folate
antagonists. However, MTHHF excels THHF in being not only
more stable but also less toxic. Moreover, cellular transport mechanism for MTHHF is distinctly different from that

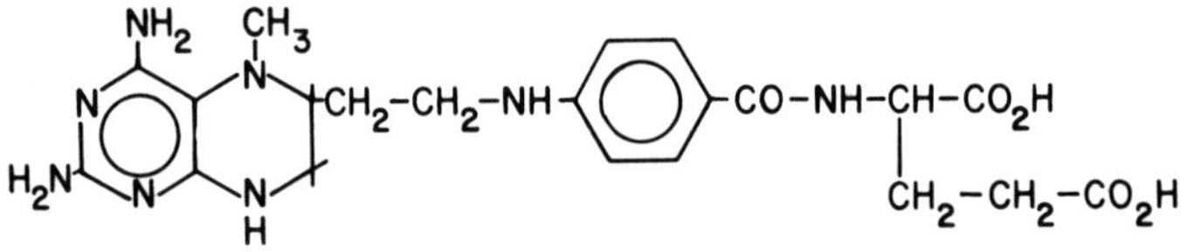

5-Methyl-tetrahydrohomofolate

Figure 7

for both reduced folates and folate antagonists. Therapeutically this different transport mechanism is an advantage that is potentially explorable to circumvent resistance to folate antagonists. These reasons constituted the basis for the scheduled phase 1 studies of MTHHF.

We therefore undertook a series of investigations of MTHHF in patients with a view to learning certain pertinent pharmacokinetic properties of this agent so as to facilitate the design and execution of its scheculed clinical trial. Our work derived considerable benefits from published information on the disposition of MTHHF in experimental animals (6).

Radioactive MTHHF labeled with ^{14}C in the 5-CH$_3$ moiety provided by the NCI was administered as a single i.v. bolus in 15 min to 4 patients selected for the study with their informed consent. The dose was about 14 mg/m^2 (Table 3), 100-200 μCi per patient, and calculated not to produce any therapeutic or toxic effects based on animal studies. Blood and urine specimens were analyzed by HPLC and radiochemical methodologies similar to our research with DHAQ. Table 3 lists the pharmacokinetic parameters.

There was no evidence that MTHHF was metabolized in man, similar to published findings in animals (6). The plasma clearance of MTHHF followed triphasic patterns; the average longest $t_{\frac{1}{2}}$ was over 3 days. The apparent volume of distribution of this agent suggests that it was distributed mostly in extracellular water. Very little of the drug was found in the CSF. Its long plasma $t_{\frac{1}{2}}$ and low total clearance in man may be contrasted with its much shorter $t_{\frac{1}{2}}$ and higher clearance rate in animals. The possibility of drug persistence in the body must be seriously considered. The low urinary excretion suggests possible high biliary excretion.

In future clinical trials with MTHHF, it would be prudent to avoid repeated dosing, and to reduce its dosage judiciously in patients with hepatic malfunction.

SUMMARY

1. TCN is an agent with an interesting mechanism of action. Its metabolism in vitro is unique. Sophisticated instrumentation has greatly advanced our research.
2. Both DHAQ and MTHHF may accumulate in the body. Repeated dosing with these agents must not proceed except with extreme caution.

Table 3.   Pharmacokinetic Parameters of MTHHF in 4 Patients.

Dose	Plasma $t_{\frac{1}{2}}$			Vd	Clearance	Urinary Excretion
	α	β	γ			
mg/m²	min	hr	hr	ml/kg	ml/kg/min	%, 96 hr
14	13.2	3.4	58	117	0.2	62
16	54.2	14.4	58	140	0.3	59
16	34.5	4.4	116	119	0.2	88
13	11.1	3.3	116	80	0.3	59
	28.3±10[a]	6.4±2.7[a]	87±17[a]	114±12[a]	0.23±0.1[a]	67±7[a]

[a] Mean ± S.E.

3. Clinical pharmacological investigations of anticancer
    agents in conjunction with, and occasionally even
    before, the therapeutic evaluations of these agents
    in man, often provide invaluable information to aid
    in the design and execution of Phase I and Phase II
    clinical trials.

ACKNOWLEDGEMENT

This brief review summarizes the work done in collaboration with the following colleagues.
    William Au, Robert S. Benjamin, Jie-Shi Liu,
    Katherine Lu, Niramol Savaraj, Paul Schweinsberg,
    Manuel Valdivieso, Boh Seng Yap.
    I am grateful for their generosity in making their
results available to me.

REFERENCES

1. L.B. Townsend and G.H. Milne. Synthesis, chemical
    reactivity, and chemotherapeutic activity of certain
    selenonucleosides and nucleosides related to the
    pyrrolo[2,3-d]pyrimidine nucleoside antibiotics.
    Ann. N.Y. Acad. Sci., 255: 91-103, 1975.
2. P.G.W. Plagemann. Transport, phosphorylation, and toxi-
    city of a tricyclic nucleoside in cultured Novikoff rat
    hepatoma cells and other cell lines and release of its
    monophosphate by the cells. J.N.C.I., 57: 1283-1295,
    1976.
3. L.L. Bennett, Jr., D. Smithers, D.L. Hill, L.M. Rose,
    and Jo Ann Alexander. Biochemical properties of the
    nucleoside of 3-amino-1,5-dihydro-5-methyl-1,4,5,6,8-
    pentaazaacenaphthylene. Biochem. Pharmac., 27: 233-
    241, 1978.
4. R.K. Johnson, R.K.Y. Zee-Cheng, W.W. Lee, E.M. Acton,
    D.W. Henry and C.C. Cheng. Experimental antitumor
    activity of aminoanthraquinones. Cancer Treat. Rep.,
    63: 425-439, 1979.
5. W.W. Au, M.A. Butler, T.S. Matney, and Ti Li Loo. A
    comparative structure-genotoxic study of three amino-
    anthracenedione drugs and doxorubicin. Cancer Res.,
    (in press).
6. S.M. El Dareer, K.F. Tillery, and D.L. Hill. Disposition
    of 5-methyltetrahydrohomofolate in mice, dogs, and monkeys.
    Cancer Treat. Rep., 63: 201-207, 1979.

Recent Trends In Preclinical
Toxicologic And Phase I-II Study of
New Anti-Cancer Drugs

CHARLES W. YOUNG, M.D.[1]

Chief, Developmental
Chemotherapy Service
Department Of Medicine
Memorial Sloan-Kettering Cancer Center
New York, New York

INTRODUCTION

The purpose and design of preclinical toxicologic studies on
candidate anticancer drugs is being influenced both by the
economic realities of research in the 1980s and the growing
clinical success of cancer chemotherapy that has been produced by new drugs with disparate toxic effects. Our approach
to pharmacologic and toxicologic study of new agents during
Phase I and II of their clinical development is also becoming
increasingly involved with sophisticated technology. This
communication will discuss these changes in some detail.

Over the past 15 years increasingly successful regimens
have been developed in the treatment of acute leukemia,
malignant lymphoma, germ cell neoplasms and breast cancer. In
the past 5 years modest but encouraging advances have been
made in the treatment of ovarian, colorectal, head and neck
and lung cancers. These favorable clinical results have produced a climate of "rising expectations" within the oncologic
research community with regard to the therapeutic and commercial potential of new drug research. Because of this impetus
the number of novel candidate drugs and of analogues of established drugs being considered for clinical trial continues to
burgeon. However, continuing inflation has made the financial
cost of developing a drug for clinical trial uncomfortably
large, occasioning counter pressure both to reduce the number
of drugs actually chosen for clinical development and to re-

1. Reprint Requests:
Charles W. Young, M.D.
1275 York Avenue
New York, New York 10021

evaluate the basic preclinical studies required to initiate a
Phase I trial both from the points of view of inherent merit
and cost-effectiveness.

Although a reduction in the scope of routine preclinical
evaluation of candidate antineoplastics is being considered,
an expansion of study in animal models seems desirable in
specific areas of analogue development. Important new drug
varieties that have contributed to the aforementioned clinical
success produce major or dose-limiting toxicity in tissues
other than the gut and bone marrow. These include anthracyclines and cardiomyopathy, organoplatinum complexes and nephrotoxicity, bleomycins and pulmonary toxicity.

Whether or not these organ toxicities were detected in the
orginal toxicologic screen prior to their clinical introduction, rational selection of a specific analogue for clinical
development should be based not only upon testing for antitumor efficacy but for efficacy in relation to the specific
organ toxicity that proved troublesome in clinical use. This
consideration makes desirable the development of quantitative
animal models for organ toxicity to the heart, lung and kidney
In a like manner further development of candidate vinca alkaloids has included testing in model systems for neurotoxicity.
Since many anticancer drugs have strong emetic properties,
further quantitative development of animal models for emetics
is desirable.

REASSESSMENT OF PRECLINICAL
TOXICOLOGY REQUIREMENTS FOR PHASE I
AND II EVALUATION OF CANDIDATE
ANTICANCER DRUGS

Although in any individual patient chemotherapy is administered with therapeutic intent, the pruposes of a Phase I
study are: a) to develop a drug dose and schedule that reliably produce a visible biologic effect and is appropriate for
use in disease-oriented Phase II studies; b) to characterize
and quantitate acute toxic effects of the drug at escalating
dosages up to that which produces dose-limiting toxicity.
Phase I studies enlist patients with advanced cancer non-re-
sponsive to conventional therapy; these patients usually have
limited life-expectency. Although responding patients will be
continued on the test drug, chronic administration of the a-
gent in this study phase is uncommon. Unless unpredictable,
irreversible and unacceptible toxic effects occur during Phase
I, all candidate agents are advanced to Phase II trial where
the primary test of clinical anticancer activity is to be
made.

Phase II studies are organized to enlist patients with

specific diseases; although they have measurable cancer not responsive to conventional therapy they are in relatively good physical condition. Stable and responding patients are maintained on the test drug until clear evidence of disease progression has developed; exposure to the drug repeatedly over a period of months will commonly occur.

Both Phase I and Phase II studies are carried out in cancer centers by oncologists with extensive experience in such studies. The patients are closely monitored clinically and with laboratory studies that can detect subtle indications of drug injury to the bone marrow, kidney, liver, red cell mass, blood coagulation system and somewhat less successfully to the brain, pancreas, lung, heart and peripheral nerves. Although the clinical investigators value animal study indications that toxicity will manifest in specific organ systems they rely on the animal studies primarily to provide a safe initial dose; they look to the clinical studies to provide the basic information regarding organ toxicity in humans.

Quantitative Considerations

Phase I trials begin with a low dose that is judged to be below the maximally tolerated dose (MTD) in humans based upon projections from animal studies. This dose is progressively escalated in a predetermined manner, usually according to a modified Fibonacci progression. Preclinical toxicology studies in animals have traditionally provided a safe starting dose and an indication of the likely pattern of organ toxicity. The traditional pattern of extensive testing in multiple species was codified by the Laboratory of Toxicology of the National Cancer Institute for use by its contractors.[17] Approved as a model by the Food and Drug Administration this rigorous protocol has subsequently been criticized as a roadblock to the entry of promising drugs into clinical trial by reason of its cost, $100,000/compound in 1977, and the time required to complete it, from 8 to 12 months.

Multiple workers now have urged that the starting clinical dose can be adequately developed through studies in mice. Examining data on 18 anticancer drugs Freireich et al concluded that, expressing dose on a mg/m^2 of body surface area basis, the MTD of a given drug in mouse, rat, dog, monkey and human was quite similar.[4] The concept has been refined and extended by Homan[8], Goldsmith et al[6] comparing the accuracy of human dose prediction based upon one-third the toxic dose low (TDL) in monkeys or dogs and one-third the LD_{10} in mice.

Noting the developing opinion in favor os using mouse toxicity data as a major factor in determining the clinical dose

Guarino et al[7] pointed out sources of variability in the retrospectively gathered murine toxicity data, urging that this
could be reduced in prospective LD_{10}, LD_{50}, LD_{90} studies. In
the report by Penta et al[15] on 12 drugs entering clinical trial between 1972 and 1978 one-third the murine LD_{10} yielded a
safe starting dose in 9 of 11 drugs; one-tenth the LD_{10} would
have been safe for the remaining two drugs.

As a result of these analyses a revised preclinical toxicology protocol is being urged wherein, on a single i.v. dose
and a daily x 5 basis, the LD_{10}, LD_{50} and LD_{90} will be derived
in mice then a toxic and non-toxic dose be obtained in dogs by
testing one-tenth the murine LD_{10} and the LD_{10} (or further
fractions or multiples thereof as needed). Detailed clinical
chemistry and clinical hematology studies will be made in both
species. Animals will be sacrificed early and late to examine
acute and delayed histopathalogic findings but the sections
will usually not be examined until the Phase I clinical trial
is in progress.

The delay in interpreting the histologic sections until the
clinical trial has actually been initiated is perhaps the most
widely argued aspect of the proposed revisions. Schein and
colleagues[18,19] have published a detailed review of the dog
and monkey toxicologic predition of human organ toxicity. The
data in dogs in particular proved rather adequate predictors
of hematopoietic effects; the dog was similarly superior for
predicting gastrointestinal effects. As the studies were performed the dog and monkey data over-predicted hepatic and renal toxicity compared with that observed in clinical drug use.
In the latter circumstance, drug administration is usually adjusted to the dose that produces dose-limiting toxicity most
commonly either gut or bone marrow injury.

In view of these analyses and upon reflection on the basis
for decision making during Phase I studies, it has been urged
that while the histopathologic toxicity results are desirable
at any time, they are not mandatory to guide the clinician in
this initial phase. The concept is that clinical observation,
plus the clinical chemistries and hematologic laboratory observations obtained as the study is occurring provides the basic information on which the oncologist makes treatment decisions regardless of what the histopathology had shown. If this
is the case and if the histopathologic assessment presents a
serious point of delay in making a potentially useful drug
clinically available why not do the histopathology during the
Phase I trial. It remains the intent to perform an extensive
evaluation including chronic toxicity studies for those clinically active drugs that will receive large scale patient usage.

ANIMAL MODELS FOR DRUG INJURY TO
ORGANS THAT LACK PROLIFERATING
CELL POPULATIONS

The anthracycline antibiotics daunomycin and adriamycin are
valuable additions to cancer therapy; analogues are being
sought that will provide an enhanced therapeutic index. Particular emphasis is being given to seeking analogues that
have a diminished cardiomyopathic liability. After the cardiotoxic properties of this drug group were discovered in clinical use animal models were developed in the rabbit[9], rat[12,14]
and mouse[1]. Although the relevance of the rabbit model is the
most generally accepted, the murine model reported by Bertazzoli et al[1] offers the potential advantages of requiring smaller quantities of a test drug and being inherently less expensive. It appears quantitative and reliable at least in the
laboratory that developed it and is using it to assist in selection of new anthracyclines for clinical development.

The vinca alkaloids vinblastine and vincristine are widely
used in the treatment of leukemia, lymphoma, germ cell tumors
and breast cancer. In analogue development a less neurotoxic
derivative was sought. Although dogs and rodents proved un-
suitable for assessing the neurotoxicity of these agents Todd
et al[21] found that the chicken, cat and monkey could provide
clinically predictive information. Although the methodology
is still in development it may be that the unsheathed cat
sciatic nerve may also provide a useful model for the study
of the neurotoxic effects of these agents[13]. The prediction
of these models that vindesine would be less neurotoxic than
vincristine has been borne out clinically.

DETECTION OF SUBCLINICAL DRUG
INJURY TO THE HEART, LUNG AND KIDNEY

Billingham and colleagues[2] have established endomyocardial
biopsy as the standard for detection and quantitation of an-
thracycline-induced cardiotoxic effects. Measurable changes
commonly preceed clinical evidence of cardiac decompensation.
Subsequently, gated radionuclide cardiac blood pool scans
with and without exercise are being widely explored as a non-
invasive technique for detecting and quantitating the drug-
induced functional impairment[11,21]. It seems likely that both
of these procedures will be used to provide the basis for comparison of analogues and of proposed protective substances.

The lung injury produced by bleomycin is routinely followed by detailed pulmonary function studies. The usual con-
vention has been to continue treatment in responding patients

until over all function had deteriorated to a clinically
meaningful degree. Recently the single breath carbon monoxide-diffusing capacity has been advocated as the most useful of the pulmonary function studies examined[3].

Jones et al[10] have pointed out that patients who receive
cisplatin almost universally experience reversible enzymuria
and β_2 microglobulinuria. The most sensitive of the tests
was the appearance in urine of the brush border tubular enzyme leucine aminopeptidase. The tubular lysosomal enzyme
N-acetyl-β-glucosaminidase appeared in the urine in comparable
numbers of patients. The low molecular weight protein β_2
microglobulin, that is normally all but totally reabsorbed
from the glomerular filtrate in the proximal convoluted tubule
appears in the urine of a smaller number of patients. Its
appearance and continued presence suggests a degree of lasting structural injury. These urinary proteins appear to provide the necessary sensitivity to permit comparison of analogues for nephrotoxic effects at drug dosages that do not
threaten irreversible clinical renal damage.

REFERENCES

1. Bertazzoli C, Bellini D, Magrini V, et al: Quantitative
   experimental evaluation of adriamycin cardiotoxicity in
   the mouse. Cancer Treat Rep 63:1877-1883, 1979.
2. Billingham ME, Mason JW, Bristow MR, Daniels JR: Anthracycline cardiomyopathy monitored by morphologic
   changes. Cancer Treat Rep 62:865-872, 1978.
3. Comis RL, Kuppinger MS, Ginsberg SJ, et al: Role of single
   breath carbon monoxide-diffusing capacity in monitoring
   the pulmonary effects of bleomycin in germ cell tumor
   patients. Cancer Res 39:5076-5080, 1979.
4. Freireich EJ, Geham EA, Rall DP, et al: Quantitative comparison of toxicity of anticancer agents in mouse, rat,
   hamster, dog, monkey and man. Cancer Chemother Rep 50:
   219-244, 1966.
5. Glylys JA, Doran KM, Buyniski: Antagonism of cisplatinum
   induced emesis in the dog. Res Comm Chem Pathol Pharmacol
   238:61-68, 1979.
7. Guarino AM, Rozencweig M, Kline I, et al: Adequacies and
   inadequacies in assessing murine toxicity data with antineoplastic agents. Cancer Res 39:2204-2210, 1979.
8. Homan ER: Quantitative relationships between toxic doses
   of antitumor chemotherapeutic agents in animals and man.
   Cancer Chemother Rep 3(Part 3):13-19, 1972.
9. Jaenke RS: Delayed and progressive mycoardial lesions

after adriamycin administration in the rabbit. Cancer Res 36:2958-2966, 1976.

10. Jones BR, Bhalla RB, Mladlek J, et al: Comparison of methods of evaluating nephrotoxicity of cis-platinum. Clin Pharmacol Therap 27:557-562, 1980.

11. Kennedy JW, Sorenson SG, Ritchie JL, et al: Radionuclide angiography for the evaluation of anthracycline therapy. Cancer Treat Rep 62:941-943, 1978.

12. Mettler FP, Young DM, Ward JM: Adriamycin-induced cardio-toxicity (cardio-myopathy and congestive heart failure) in rats. Cancer Res 37:2705-2713, 1977.

13. Ochs S, Worth RM, Chan SY: Calcium requirement for axo-plasmic transport in mammalian nerve. Nature 270:748-750, 1977.

14. Olson HM, Capen CC: Chronic cardiotoxicity of doxorubicin (adriamycin) in the rat: morphologic and biochemical in-vestigations. Toxicol Appl Pharmacol 44:605-616, 1978.

15. Penta JS, Rozencweig M, Guarino AM, Muggia FM: Mouse and large animal toxicology studies of twelve antitumor agents: relevance for starting dose Phase I clinical trials. Cancer Chemother Pharmacol 3:97-101, 1979.

16. Prestayko AW, Bradner WT, Huftalen JB, et al: Anti-leukemic (L1210) activity and toxicity of cis-dichlor-diammineplatinum (II) analogs. Cancer Treat Rep 63:1503-1508, 1979.

17. Prieur DJ, Young DM, Davis RD, et al: Procedures for pre-clinical toxicologic evaluation of cancer chemotherapeutic agents: protocols of the laboratory of toxicology. Cancer Chemother Rep 4(Part 3):1-30, 1973.

18. Schein PS: Preclinical toxicology of anticancer agents. Cancer Res 37:1934-1937, 1977.

19. Schein PS, Davis RO, Carter SK, et al: The evaluation of anticancer drugs in man. Clin Pharmacol Therap 14:3-40, 1970.

20. Singer JW, Narahara KA, Ritchie JL, et al: Time- and dose-dependent changes in ejection fraction determined by radionuclide angiography after anthracycline therapy. Cancer Treat Rep 62:945-948, 1978.

21. Todd GC, Griffing WJ, Gibson WR, Morton DM: Animal models for comparative assessment of neurotoxicity following re-peated aministration of vinca alkaloids. Cancer Treat Rep 63:35-41, 1979.

22. Ward JM, Fauvie KA: The nephrotoxic effects of cis-diam-mine-dichloroplatinum (II) (NSC-119875) in male F344 rats. Toxical Appl Pharmacol 38:535-547, 1976.

Pediatric Tumors

Progress in the Study, Treatment and Cure of

The Cancers of Children

DENMAN HAMMOND, M.D.

Director
Kenneth Norris, Jr., Cancer Research Institute
Comprehensive Cancer Center
University of Southern California
and
Chairman
Childrens Cancer Study Group
Los Angeles, California

The progress of the last two decades in the treatment and cure of the cancers of infants and children is, perhaps, the most gratifying achievement in the entire field of cancer therapy. Cancer remains the leading medical cause of death from one year through adolescence; however, the cancer mortality of this age group has decreased forty-three percent since 1950. Pediatric oncologists, surgeons and radiation therapists have begun to direct their concerns to the increasing numbers of young adult patients who were cured of cancer during childhood and who exhibit various adverse effects of successful therapies administered years ago.

It is an appropriate time to review the accomplishments of the last two decades to identify the important milestones of progress and the lessons that should be learned from them, and to identify the new challenges of the next decade.

DIFFERENCES BETWEEN CANCERS OF ADULTS AND CHILDREN

The principal cancers of children differ from those of adults with respect to site, histopathology, clinical stage at diagnosis and other prognostic factors which are associated closely with outcome. The

Supported in part by grant no. CA13539 to the Childrens Cancer Study Group from the National Cancer Institute, NIH, USPHS. CCSG Operations Office, 1721 Griffin Avenue, Los Angeles, CA 90031

common cancers of adults, such as lung, breast, gastrointestinal and genito-urinary tract, are rarely seen in children. Other than hematologic neoplasias, the organs most frequently involved in children are the nervous system, muscles, bones and kidneys. Histologically, glandular tumors are rare in children, so the typical solid tumor is a sarcoma rather than a carcinoma. The majority of children with cancer are diagnosed at a late stage of clinical involvement, often after there is spread to sites remote from the primary. Since superficial cancers are rare in childhood, opportunities for early detection by such techniques as exfoliative cytology, mammography, or abnormal intestinal blood loss do not occur among pediatric cancer patients. There is no practical cancer screening procedure that is cost effective when applied to apparently healthy asymptomatic children.

There are additional therapeutic and management differences between the cancers of adults and children. In this country, most children with cancer are referred to major pediatric medical centers and are managed by teams of physicians specializing in diagnosis and treatment of childhood cancers. Most adult cancer patients are managed in community hospitals, and most commonly are treated by one specialist after another, often with long intervals between.

The principles and objectives of surgery and techniques of radiation therapy have undergone major changes as applied to children. Many of the chemotherapeutic agents useful in the treatment of cancers of adults, appear to have no place in pediatric cancer . The cancers of children, fortunately, are generally responsive to treatment and, therefore, the clinical outcomes to treatment of children's cancers are much more favorable at present than for cancers of adults.

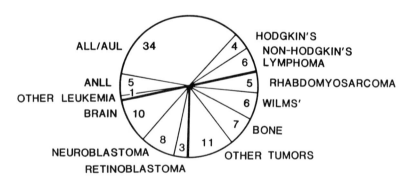

Figure 1. Percent Distribution of the principal cancers of infants and children among 13,601 patients registered by institutions participating in the Childrens Cancer Study Group, 1974-1980.

Figure 1 shows the frequency of the principal cancers among children registered by the 28 institutions participating in the Childrens Cancer Study Group. Leukemia accounted for 40% of the cancer diagnoses in this large group, and the lymphomas constituted another 10%. Cancers of the nervous system, including the brain, neuroblastoma and retinoblastoma, accounted for over 20% of the total. The remaining 30% are primarily cancers of the musculo-skeletal system and the kidney. Many cancers of children are so uncommon that no single institution can accumulate a significant body of clinical information over a reasonably brief span of years.

ACUTE LYMPHOCYTIC LEUKEMIA

A major event in the treatment of cancer of children occurred with the first demonstration that a clinical remission of acute lymphocytic leukemia could be induced by chemotherapy. This occurred in the late 1940's, and by 1955 there were several agents, each of which was known to be capable of inducing clinical remission. The National Cancer Institute sponsored a coordinated national effort to exploit the chemotherapy of acute leukemia by organizing and funding groups of multiple institutions for cooperative clinical investigation of the chemotherapy of leukemia.

There has been progressive improvement in the survival of children with acute lymphocytic and undifferentiated leukemia who were treated on the therapeutic trials of multi-institution cancer clinical investigation groups since 1956.

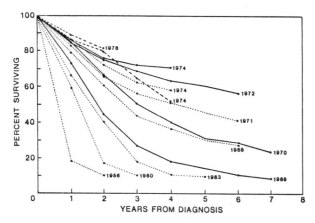

Figure 2. The improving survival of children with Acute Lymphocytic and Undifferentiated Leukemia diagnosed between 1956 and 1976. Composite experience of Cancer and Acute Leukemia Group B, the Childrens Cancer Study Group and the Southwest Oncology Group.

Median survival has increased from approximately 6 months in 1956, to longer than 6 years for trials begun in 1972. A group of studies begun in 1974 show up to 70% survival at 4 years and studies begun in 1976 show 2 year survival between 80 and 90%.

Figure 3 illustrates the duration of the initial complete remission of over 2,000 patients treated on four successive protocols of the Childrens Cancer Study Group, begun between 1972 and 1977. Study CCG-101, begun in 1972, shows continuous complete remission for 5 years of over 50% of all patients entered. Furthermore, the curve appears to have been horizontal for the past three and one half years. Subsequent studies may achieve even better outcome.

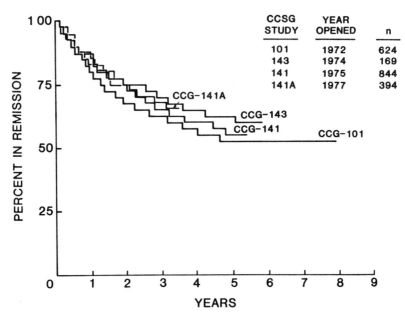

Figure 3. Curves of the Duration of the Initial Complete Remission of 2,031 children with Acute Lymphocytic Leukemia treated according to recent studies of the Childrens Cancer Study Group. All patients who achieved Complete Remission were included in the analysis.

While the general prognosis for acute lymphocytic leukemia in children has improved dramatically during the last decade, the heterogeneity of patients with this diagnosis has become increasingly apparent. At the time of diagnosis, subgroups can be identified which have excellent prognosis for survival and cure, while others have extremely poor outcome. Consequently, the accurate identification and understanding of prognostic variables has become essential for the development of improved treatment strategies and for appropriate design and analysis of clinical studies.

The large population of patients included in the studies illustrated in Figure 3 have been analyzed to determine the association with outcome of a large number of clinical, biologic and laboratory evaluations. Some of these emerge consistently as being important predictors of the achievement of complete remission, the duration of the initial complete remission, the duration of survival, or all of these outcomes. When prognostic variables are analyzed in detail it becomes apparent that many are strongly interrelated and a somewhat smaller set of variables appears to have prognostic significance as independent variables.

Table I lists a number of prognostic variables ranked according to their importance and usefulness in predicting outcome to treatment, as determined by multivariate analysis. Such a technique assists in the identification of those factors which have major associations with outcome, those which have moderate or minor association and others which may be useful indicators of prognosis when analyzed individually, but which because of their close association with other variates of greater significance appear to have little or no additional value as predictors of outcome.

TABLE I
Acute Lymphocytic Leukemia

Prognostic Variables Ranked According to
Relative Importance in Predicting Outcome

Major

- o   WBC at Diagnosis
- o   Blast Cell Morphology
- o   Cell Surface Antigens
- o   Immunoglobulin Levels

Minor

- o   Node Enlargement
- o   Spleen Enlargement
- o   Race

Moderate

- o   Age
- o   Sex
- o   Marrow Response (Day 14)
- o   CNS Leukemia at Diagnosis
- o   Hemoglobin

Little or None

- o   Platelet Count
- o   Mediastinal Mass
- o   Liver Enlargement

A variety of subgroups of patients with acute lymphocytic leukemia can be selected according to known prognostic variables. For example, a group with a highly favorable prognosis might include patients with WBC at diagnosis of 10,000/mm^3 or less, age between 1 and 10 years, with no T or B cell surface receptor antigens on lymphoblasts, marrow lymphoblasts with L1 or L1/L2 morphology (French/American/British classification), no significant decrease in the levels of immunoglobulin A, G or M, minimal evidence of extramedullary involvement by leukemia, (CNS, liver, spleen, peripheral lymph nodes or mediastinum) and whose response to initial therapy is rapid when evaluated by examination of the bone marrow after the first two weeks of therapy. Experience to date with such good prognosis patients indicates that the rate of achieving complete remission would be close to 100%, the proportion remaining in continuous complete remission for 8 years would be over 80% and most of this population would be cured. Current data suggest that this group would not only have a very favorable outcome to treatment but, in addition, could be treated adequately with much less chemotherapy and radiation therapy than has been the standard for many years.

Recognition of the heterogeneity of acute lymphocytic leukemia has led to the concept that there are subsets of this clinical syndrome which result from neoplasia of different varieties of cells of the lymphoid system. These have fundamentally different biologic behavior and respond differently to current treatments. They will doubtless ultimately have different diagnostic names.

Recognition that a large number of clinical and biological measurements have a very strong association with outcome has made it mandatory to determine the characteristics of a population of patients under treatment in order to be able to make valid comparisons among the regimens of a clinical trial and meaningful comparisons between studies done at different times or by different institutions. It is essential to know the proportion of patients of different risk groups which are included or excluded in clinical trials or valid comparisons cannot be made. Furthermore, it is now essential to have large enough populations for clinical trials to permit stratification into more homogeneous subgroups which are then still large enough for valid statistical analysis. Thus, even for the most common cancer of children, therapeutic studies by single institutions are subject to strong limitations.

Finally, the immunologic and biochemical tests currently being studied as potentially valuable cell markers, and those yet to be developed, must be applied to patient groups that are well characterized according to clinical and biological variables already known to have strong association with outcome, in order to evaluate their usefulness.

MILESTONES IN THE SUCCESSFUL TREATMENT OF
THE PRINCIPAL SOLID TUMORS OF CHILDREN

Since the widespread application of the three principal therapeutic modalities in the treatment of the tumors of children, virtually all have shown an increasing proportion of favorable responses, significant prolongation of the duration of response and increased survival. Figure 4 illustrates the progressive improvement in the two year survival experience of the principal solid tumors of children since 1940 when attempt at surgical removal was the only therapy widely employed.

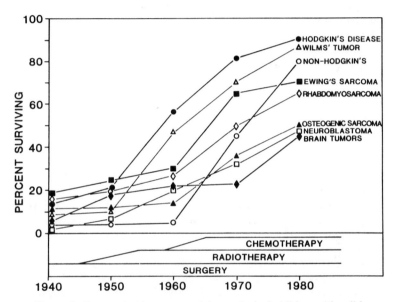

Figure 4. Progressive improvement in survival of children with solid tumors, 1940 to 1980. Proportion surviving two years from diagnosis. Data from multiple sources are shown relative to the chronology of the general application of the three principal therapeutic modalities to the tumors of children.

Radiation therapy began to be widely applied to selected solid tumors of childen in the 1940's, and in the mid 1950's was generally applied to all pediatric tumors felt to be radiosensitive. Initial radiation therapy was with orthovoltage equipment. Since then, megavoltage therapy has become more generally available, and there is an increasing use of simulators, patient molds and more sophisticated dosimetry so tumoricidal therapy can be administered. Chemotherapy was not being used widely in the treatment of tumors of children much before 1960, but, perhaps by 1965, the chemotherapeutic agents then available were being generally applied to a variety of pediatric tumors.

In 1940, the two year survival of the principal cancers of children ranged from nil to about 20%. Following the use of radiation therapy for Hodgkin's disease and Wilms' tumor, there were significant improvements in survival by 1960, and the trend continued with the application of megavoltage therapy and the introduction of chemotherapy. The other principal cancers of children, except for malignant brain tumors, showed significant improvement in survival by 1970. Essentially all tumors showed significant improvement in two year survival rates by 1980, ranging from 40% to 90%. Although the two year survival figure is not synonymous with long-term survival or cure, it is a significantly sensitive index of the progress that has been realized through the introduction of combined modality therapy.

It is unique that the great majority of children with cancer are managed in this country by teams of diagnostic and therapeutic specialists working in collaboration. This is not yet the pattern of care for the majority of adult patients with cancer; however, for an increasing variety of cancers of adults, coordinated multidisciplinary teamwork offers the greatest hope for favorable outcome.

It is instructive to review the events that have provided important milestones in the increasingly successful management of the cancers of children. Table 2 lists many of these in rough chronological order. Historically, cancer therapy involved only attempts at surgical removal. When radiation therapy was introduced it was used primarily postoperatively, particularly in patients whose surgery was believed to be unsuccessful. Subsequently, there was demonstration that chemotherapeutic agents given alone could cause regression of some solid tumors. There ensued a succession of studies identifying additional active chemotherapeutic agents, and their use in combinations led to increasing success. When it was demonstrated that chemotherapy was beneficial when given to patients whose tumors were thought to have been completely resected surgically, the role of chemotherapy was firmly established. It became of great importance to introduce chemotherapy as a principal therapeutic modality for early disease. Chemotherapists became involved in multi-modality cancer treatment programs in conjunction with radiation therapy and the era of combined modality therapy was a reality.

TABLE 2
Milestones in the Successful Treatment of Solid Tumors of Children

1. Extirpative Surgery
2. Post Operative Radiation Therapy
3. Activity of Single Chemotherapeutic Agents
4. Effective Combinations of Active Agents
5. Effectiveness of Chemotherapy for Surgically "Resected" Tumors
6. Combined Modality Therapy
7. Development of Multidiscipline Therapy Teams
   at Principal Pediatric Institutions
8. Development and Refinement of Systems of Staging
9. New Principles of Surgical Management
10. New Principles of Radiation Therapy
11. Identification of Additional Factors Influencing Outcome
12. Design of Therapy for Subgroups Stratified
    According to Factors Influencing Prognosis
13. Less Aggressive Therapy for Subgroups with Good Prognosis
14. Different Therapeutic Strategies for Subgroups with Poor Prognosis
15. Widespread Application of New Technologies
    by Various Cancer Control Interventions
    o   Development of Networks for Professional Education
    o   Increasing Availability of Pediatric Oncology Consultants
    o   Increasing Referral of Patients to Principal Pediatric Centers
         for Multidisciplinary Evaluation and Management

For the cancers of children this trend began to emerge significantly by the mid-1960's, and by the early 1970's principal pediatric
institutions throughout the nation responsible for treating significant
numbers of children with cancer had developed, or were developing, a
coordinated multidisciplinary approach involving preoperative diagnosis, staging and treatment planning for children with cancer. This
led to refinements in all therapeutic modalities and to the development and refinement of new systems for the clinical, surgical and
histologic staging of the principal cancers of children.

The involvement of pediatric surgeons, radiation therapists and
pathologists in large scale multi-institutional cooperative clinical
trials was begun in 1968. Their increasing participation and acceptance of responsibility for the design, conduct and analysis of
controlled clinical trials led to the development of new principles of
surgical management and radiation therapy and the identification of
many clinical, biologic and laboratory evaluations that were strongly
associated with outcome to therapy. During the past decade,
numerous clinical trials have been designed for subgroups of patients

stratified according to such factors in order to have more homogeneous groups of patients for study, to permit more refined analysis of outcomes and to stimulate the development of therapies tailored to the prognosis of the population under therapy. Repeated studies have now demonstrated that less aggressive therapy is quite adequate for patients with an inherently good prognosis. Those groups known to have unfavorable prognostic characteristics have provided the challenge of developing different therapeutic strategies than the traditional therapies known not to be effective.

Another significant milestone has been the development of systems for the widespread application of the new techniques for managing pediatric cancers. Networks for continuing professional education have been developed in the regions surrounding the nation's major pediatric medical centers. Such institutions make expert consultation in various aspects of pediatric oncology increasingly available to pediatric patients with cancer in their region. Due to the infrequency of pediatric cancers, only major referral institutions can acquire a significant level of expertise in their management. Only in such institutions can there be developed successfully an adequate staff of the needed diagnostic and therapeutic specialists who are appropriately experienced in pediatric cancer management.

The successful model of cancer control for the cancers of infants and children has been to create the essential personnel, facilities and resources for sophisticated management of pediatric cancers in the nation's major pediatric referral centers. Systems of easy communication with experts and easy availability of referral centers to physicians and hospitals throughout the surrounding region is making more widely available the multidisciplinary evaluation, treatment planning and management that is required for cure of the cancers of children.

Whereas 20 years ago it mattered little where, or by whom, a child with cancer was managed, it has come to matter enormously. Institutions that accept children with cancer for management should recognize their obligation to develop multidisciplinary cancer management teams supported by the appropriate resources. Those that do not have such teams or resources should develop referral arrangement with institutions that do.

STAGING AND OTHER FACTORS INFLUENCING PROGNOSIS

Clinical staging of cancer based upon the size and extent of the tumor at the time of diagnosis has been useful in stratifying patient groups according to appropriate therapeutic management, and expected outcome.

A typical staging system for tumors of children is outlined in Table 3. This illustrates the general scheme of a staging system, based upon the extent of the cancer at the time of diagnosis, the nature of its surgical management, and the histologic evaluation and subclassification of the specimen. In addition to these, staging to identify groups of similar prognostic outcome may include the site of involvement for those tumors of children that occur in a variety of locations, some of which have been found to have much more favorable outcome than others.

TABLE 3
Tumors of Children
Typical Staging System

Clinical
    Stage I   Localized
    Stage II   Regional Adjacent
    Stage III   Regional Distant
    Stage IV   Metastatic

Surgical
    a.   Complete Removal
    b.   Microscopic Residual Tumor
    c.   Gross Residual Tumor

Histologic
    Cellular or Tissue Patterns
    Associated with Good or Poor Outcome

Preoperative clinical staging has been done for many years. Further staging has been based upon the surgical management which was accomplished at operation.

For decades, tumor pathologists have recognized variations in cellular or tissue patterns within certain classes of cancers of children. Only in recent years, however, have large scale multi-institutional, cooperative studies enabled pathologists to examine large numbers of specimens with the same general diagnosis. This has permitted them to recognize different histopathologic classifications, and to study their correlation with clinical course and outcome. During the last decade, several new variants of pediatric cancer diagnoses have been identified, which have important associations with either favorable or unfavorable outcome.

In addition to clinical stage, surgical management, histopathology and site of tumor, two additional evaluations may have an important influence on prognosis, including the age of the patient at diagnosis and the rapidity and completeness of the patient's response to therapy.

CHANGES IN SURGICAL MANAGEMENT

The principles of surgical management of the tumors of children, and even the objectives of surgery, have undergone significant change. A list of some of the important changes in surgical objectives, or the specifics of surgical management that have evolved primarily during the last decade, is presented in Table 4.

TABLE 4
Tumors of Children
Changes in Surgical Management

1. Debulking of Unresectable Tumors
2. Assessment of Chemotherapy Effect on Tumor
3. Fewer Radical Extirpative Procedures
4. Limb Salvage and Prostheses
5. Second Look Surgery Following Chemotherapy and RT
6. Resection of Metastases
7. Regional Node Dissections
8. Bench Surgery of Removed Organ
9. Interstitial Endocurie Therapy
10. Two Team Approach For Dumbbell Lesions
11. Preoperative Multidiscipline Treatment Planning
12. Supportive Procedures:
    o   Marking Tumor Bed for Follow-Up
    o   Surgical Staging Systems
    o   Ostomies for Nutrition
    o   Catheterization for Parenteral Feeding
    o   Catheterization for Dialysis
    o   Open Lung Biopsy
    o   Relocation of Abdominal Organs from RT Field
    o   Pneumothorax Prior to RT of Chest Wall

Since radiation therapy and chemotherapy are much more effective in the treatment of minimal residual tumor than gross tumor, the tumors that cannot be completely removed are nonetheless no longer considered "inoperable". Pediatric oncologic surgeons now remove as much tumor tissue as is technically feasible, but rely upon radiation therapy and chemotherapy for treatment of residual tumor and seldom do radical extirpative procedures. New techniques of limb salvage have developed around the use of prostheses to replace removed bone segments. An entirely new objective of surgery, in some cases, is the assessment of preoperative chemotherapeutic effect on the tumor tissue to guide postoperative chemotherapy.

Second look surgical explorations of the primary operative site are being done in some patients who are believed to be tumor free following postoperative chemotherapy and radiation therapy. This has been done both to assess the completeness of response to therapy and also to accomplish additional extirpative surgery, which could not be done at the primary operation.

It is considered appropriate at present to surgically remove distant metastases, even when multiple, following apparently successful treatment of a primary tumor. Metastases which were undetectable at the time of initial surgery, or during the initial courses of therapy, may become apparent later in patients whose primary cancer appears to have been treated successfully. The opportunity to follow large numbers of patients having cancers of specific sites has disclosed that there are patterns of recurrences in regional groups of lymph nodes which were not immediately associated with the tumor. Such new information about patterns of tumor spread and recurrence has modified the objectives of surgery for tumors at specific sites such as, for example, paratesticular rhabdomyosarcoma.

The surgical approach to Wilms' tumor, particularly when bilateral, may require meticulous removal of tumor tissue from the kidney in order to preserve maximum renal function. A technique has been developed which involves removal of an affected kidney from the patient so delicate surgery can be accomplished, following which the organ is re-implanted. There has been renewed interest in interstitial endocurie therapy procedures, which involve close teamwork between the surgeon and the radiation oncologist applying radionuclide sources within inoperable tumor tissue, employing after-loading techniques and templates for the placement of needles, which will provide the desired dose distributioin. Some tumors extend contiguously from one body compartment to another, but are technically completely resectable. Abdominal tumors, which extend above the diaphragm into the chest or into the spinal canal, have led to a two surgical team approach to accomplish complete removal.

One of the most significant changes in surgical management of cancers in children is that it has become widespread established practice to involve all appropriate members of the diagnostic and therapeutic disciplines in complete pretreatment diagnosis, staging, study and evaluation of the child with cancer, and in the development of a plan for management that involves each therapeutic modality as appropriate. The tumor board approach to the management of the child with cancer is an accepted way of life in the principal institutions treating children with cancer throughout the United States. This is an evolution that has taken place primarily within the past decade, and has undoubtedly been responsible for some of the major successes in pediatric cancer management.

Finally, pediatric surgeons have become much more frequently involved in the performance of procedures designed to support and facilitate the treatment plan, in addition to primary surgical procedures.

One is inescapably left with the impression that the surgical management of the cancers of children has undergone very pronounced change during the past decade or so.

Since pediatric surgeons became full participants in multidisciplinary team management of the cancers of children, and have become significantly involved in clinical investigation, not only have new surgical techniques evolved, but the concepts of surgical management, and even the objectives for which surgery is performed, have undergone significant change.

TABLE 5
Tumors of Children
Changes in Radiation Therapy

1.	Transition from Orthovoltage to Megavoltage
2.	Increased Use of RT Simulators
3.	Increased Use of Patient Molds
4.	Improved Tumor Imaging Techniques
5.	Precision of Tumor Geometry and Dosimetry
6.	Tumoricidal Therapy to Tumor
7.	Maximum Sparing of Normal Tissues
8.	Refinements in Total Body and Hemibody Irradiation
9.	Determination of Minimal Effective Dose
10.	Appropriate Sequencing with Other Therapies
11.	Coordination with Chemotherapy
12.	Quality Control Procedures
13.	Radiation Enhancers

CHANGES IN RADIATION THERAPY

Table 5 summarizes some of the significant changes in the radiation therapy management of the cancers of children, which have led to more effective and potentially curative radiation therapy, and to its coordination and appropriate sequencing with surgery and chemotherapy.

During the past decade, there has been a progressive transition from use of orthovoltage therapy to megavoltage equipment, a more widespread use of radiation therapy simulators and patient molds to permit greater precision in dosimetry. Improved tumor imaging techniques, such as computerized tomographic scanning, also have permitted much greater precision in determining the geometry of tumors. This enables the therapist to deliver tumoricidal therapy to a larger proportion of tumors treated, and with maximal sparing of adjacent normal tissues. There have been major refinements in techniques for delivering total body and hemibody irradiation, using different radiation sources. Radiation oncologists have participated in the design, conduct and analysis of numerous controlled clinical trials for evaluation of reduced doses of radiation therapy for specific cancers of various stages. This has led to reduction in dose of radiation therapy to the central nervous system for prevention of CNS leukemia, the elimination of radiation therapy for Stage I Wilms' tumor, and reduced volume and dose for the treatment of numerous manifestations of rhabdomyosarcoma.

These are important advances, particularly in reducing the likelihood of adverse late effects of therapy among long-term survivors. The role of radiation therapy is variable, depending upon the tumor, the site and the stage. In some circumstances, radiation therapy has become the standard of primary therapy, rather than surgery or systemic therapy. Close collaboration between radiation oncologists and chemotherapists has become essential since toxic effects, late adverse effects and acute radiation effects may be additive when given concurrently with chemotherapy. Radiation therapists and chemotherapists are continuing to learn how to modify their dose and course to enable the patient to achieve optimum therapy with each modality at the appropriate time during the course of treatment.

Another important change in radiation therapy which is of particular importance for infants and children, is the increasing variety of quality control procedures, designed to insure maximum information about tumor volume and geometry, precise dose distribution, reproduceability of treatment portals, avoidance of inappropriate overlap and of therapy gaps and adequate documentation of the specific therapy administered. Such procedures are continuing to evolve at the principal institutions providing radiation therapy for pediatric patients. The current emphasis is the result of more sophisticated and scientifically based concepts of radiation therapy, new equipment and an increasing cadre of persons trained specifically in radiation oncology as applied to infants and children.

The full impact of this variety of improvements in the precision and quality of radiation therapy for the cancers of children is yet to be fully realized, but will certainly emerge in future years as patients who have had the advantage of better quality and more effective therapy demonstrate their improved survival experience.

One area of current research specifically involving radiation oncology is the use of techniques which may enhance radiation therapy effects, including hyperoxygenation, agents which simulate hyperoxygenation and hyperthermia.

TABLE 6
Tumors of Children
Progress in Chemotherapy

1.	Demonstration of Activity of Many New Agents
2.	Increased Effectiveness of Multiple Agent Chemotherapy
3.	Combining Drugs for Synergistic Effects
4.	Combining Drugs to Avoid Additive Toxicity
5.	Effectiveness of Chemotherapy for "Resected" Tumors
6.	Sequencing of Chemotherapy with Surgery and RT
7.	The Role of Pre-Operative Chemotherapy
8.	Evaluation of Chemotherapy Effect on Tumor Specimen
9.	Refinements of Dose
10.	Supralethal Pulse Dose With "Rescue"
11.	Refinements of Schedule, Course and Duration
12.	Determination of Minimal Effective Therapy

PROGRESS IN CHEMOTHERAPY

There are numerous examples of advances in the chemotherapy of the cancers of children, particularly those that have been largely realized within the last decade. Table 6 lists some of the notable areas of progress, including the discovery of many new agents active against the cancers of children, the repeated documentation of the increased effectiveness of chemotherapy employing multiple agents used concurrently or in cycles, the combination of agents for their synergistic effects and combining agents that have different manifestations of toxicity to avoid incurring additive toxicity.

The demonstration of the benefits of chemotherapy for patients with tumors thought to have been completely resected by surgery was perhaps the most important single milestone that enabled the widespread application of chemotherapy early in the course of disease. Over a decade ago, chemotherapy was primarily employed in pediatric patients with metastatic or recurrent cancer, or following unsuccessful surgery and one or more courses of radiation therapy. It is expected practice now to determine the appropriate sequencing of chemotherapy, surgery and radiation therapy by multidisciplinary pretreatment patient evaluation and treatment planning. In an increasing number of cases, chemotherapy is selected as the treatment of first choice, and may enable successful removal of an otherwise inoperable tumor. Clinical trials are now underway to determine the feasibility and usefulness of histopathologic examination of a surgically removed tumor specimen following chemotherapy. Experience is evolving which may provide information of value in planning postoperative chemotherapy.

During the chemotherapy era, there have been almost continual refinements of dose, route, schedule, appropriate course interval and the duration of chemotherapy as may be appropriate for various cancers of children. In some circumstances, significant improvements in therapy appear to have been achieved by the use of supralethal doses of chemotherapy, followed by the administration of agents which will prevent the development of life threatening toxicity which would otherwise occur. Thus, the maximum therapeutic effect of the chemotherapeutic agent may be realized by techniques which will "rescue" the patient from the possible deleterious effects of such large doses. On the other hand, there are now several examples of clinical trials which demonstrate that, for certain stages of cancer, traditional chemotherapies do not contribute to improved response or survival and that less aggressive chemotherapy should be used.

MULTIDISCIPLINARY MANAGEMENT AND PEDIATRIC CANCER CONTROL

Numerous advances which have resulted from collaboration among the medical disciplines involved in the diagnosis and treatment of cancers of children have been enumerated above. It is significant that the majority of children with cancer diagnosed in the United States are managed not by one specialist after another, but by teams that have been developed in the nation's major pediatric referral institutions. The examples cited have stressed the important contributions made by pediatric oncologists, surgeons, radiation therapists, and pathologists. Groups of these specialists were formally organized in 1968 for participation in multimodality, cooperative, clinical therapeutic investigations of childhood cancers. They have been responsible for developing an increasing level of sophistication in the application, quality control, and evaluation of each diagnostic and therapeutic modality as protocol requirements became more precise, more demanding, more quantitative and more evaluable.

The variety of disciplines required for sophisticated management of infants and children with cancer include many more than have been mentioned. Table 7 presents a more extensive multidisciplinary management team for diagnosis, staging, treatment plannning, treatment and rehabilitation of infants and children with cancer.

TABLE 7
Multidisciplinary Management Team

Primary Physician	Nurse
Radiologist	Pharmacologist
Pathologist	Clinical Pharmacist
Biochemist	Microbiologist
Immunologist	Nutritionist
Surgeon	Rehabilitationist
Chemotherapist	Psychologist
Radiation Therapist	Social Worker

Persons skilled in these disciplines are represented at the nation's principal referral centers for the diagnosis and treatment of the cancers of children. All of these constitute the pediatric oncology team. Many of the nation's pediatric medical centers, having developed such teams, are devoting significant effort to professional education of the pediatricians, surgeons, radiation therapists, and others in the institutions in their metropolitan area, state and region.

The trained personnel, facilities, equipment and other resources needed to provide the best available treatment for the cancers of children cannot be developed in most of the nation's community hospitals. It is a mission more appropriate for a pediatric medical center providing tertiary care. However, centers capable of providing state of the art pediatric cancer management are having a significant nationwide impact on the management of the cancers of infants and children through cancer control programs which make pediatric oncologic specialists, their expertise and their institutional facilities more widely known and available to the professionals involved in the medical care of children in their region.

The National Cancer Institute has provided funds to enable several of the cooperative clinical cancer investigation groups to develop cancer control programs designed to provide easy access to expert consultation, to equipment and other resources that may be needed to provide state of the art cancer care to infants and children on a more wide scale basis. The expertise of pediatric oncologic specialists is being more widely applied to the nation's pediatric cancer population. Surely the impact of this will be discernable in time as it is translated to improved national statistics on the survival and cure of children with cancer.

References

Baehner, R., Bernstein, I., Sather, H., et al: Improved remission induction rate with D-Zapo but unimproved remission duration with addition of immunotherapy to chemotherapy in previously untreated children with ANLL. Med. and Ped. Oncology 7:127-139, 1979.

Beckwith, J., & Palmer, N.: Histopathology and prognosis of Wilms' tumor: Results from the first Wilms' Tumor Study. Cancer 41: 1937-1948, 1978.

Breslow, N., Palmer, N., Hill, L., et al: Wilms' tumor: Prognostic factors for patients without metastases at diagnosis. Cancer 41: 1577-1589, 1978.

D'Angio, G. J., Beckwith, J. B., Breslow, N., et al: Results of the National Wilms' Tumor Study II. Proceedings of ASCO, 20:309, 1979.

Evans, A., Albo, V., D'Angio, et al: Factors influencing survival of children with nonmetastatic neuroblastoma. Cancer 38:661-666, 1976.

Evans, A., D'Angio, G., & Randolph, J.: Proposed staging for children with neuroblastoma: Childrens Cancer Study Group A. Year Book of Cancer, p. 374, 1972.

Finklestein, J. Z., Klemperer, M. R., Evans, A., et al: Multiagent Chemotherapy for Children with Metastatic Neuroblastoma: A Report from Childrens Cancer Study Group. Med. and Ped. Oncology 6:179-188, 1979.

Ghavimi, F., Exelby, P. R., D'Angio, G. J., et al: Multidisciplinary treatment of embryonal rhabdomyosarcoma in children. Cancer 35:677-686, 1975.

Hammond, D.: Pediatric malignancies, Chapter I of Cancer Research: Impact of the Cooperative Groups. B. Hoogstraten (Ed.) Masson Publishing USA, Inc., NY, NY, 1980.

Heyn, R., Holland, R., Joo, P., et al: Treatment of rhabdomyosarcoma in children with surgery, radiotherapy and chemotherapy. Med. and Ped. Oncology 3:21-32, 1977.

Jenkin, R. D. T., Anderson, J., Chilcote, R., et al: Grossly Localized Childhood Non-Hodgkin's Lymphoma (NHL), Response to Irradiation and Elective 4 or 10 Drug Combination Chemotherapy. Proc. Amer. Assoc. Cancer Res., 1979.

Jenkin, R. D. T., & Berry, M. P.: Hodgkin's disease in children. Seminars in Onc. 7:202-211, 1980.

Leikin, S., Evans, A., Heyn, R., et al: The impact of chemotherapy on advanced neuroblastoma. Survival of patients diagnosed in 1956, 1962, and 1966-68 in Childrens Cancer Study Group. Am J Pediat. 84:131-134, 1973.

Miller, D., Leikin, S., Albo, V., et al: The use of prognostic factors in improving the design and efficiency of clinical trials in childhood cancer. Cancer Chemother. Rep., 1980.

Nesbit, M., Robison, L., Ortega, J., et al: Testicular relapse in childhood acute lymphoblastic leukemia: Association with pretreatment patient characteristics and treatment. Cancer, 45:2009-2016, 1980.

Raney, B., Hays, D., Lawrence, W., et al: Paratesticular rhabdomyosarcoma in childhood. Cancer 42:729-736, 1978.

Razek, A., Perez, P. A., Tefft, M., et al: Intergroup Ewing's Sarcoma study: Local control related to radiation, dose, volume, and site of primary lesion in Ewing's Sarcoma. Cancer 46:516-521, 1980.

Tefft, M., & D'Angio, G. J.: Patterns of intra-abdominal relapse in patients with Wilms' Tumor who received radiation therapy: Analysis by histology favorable vs. unfavorable. A report of National Wilms' Tumor Study I & II. Proceedings of AACR, 20:480, 1979.

Tefft, M., Razek, A., Perez, P. A., et al: Local control and survival related to radiation dose and volume and to chemotherapy in nonmetastatic Ewing's Sarcoma of pelvic bone. Int J of Rad. Onc. 4:367-372, 1978.

Wara, W., Jenkin, R., Evans, A., et al: Tumors of the pineal and suprasellar region: Childrens Cancer Study Group treatment results 1960-1975. Cancer 43:698-701, 1979.

Wilms' Tumor

D'ANGIO, G.J. and BELASCO, J.B.

The Departments of Radiation Therapy and Pediatrics,
The University of Pennsylvania;
and The Children's Cancer Research Center,
Children's Hospital of Philadelphia,
Philadelphia, PA 19104

A review of the progress made in the management of children with Wilms' tumor provides at the same time a review of the progress made in pediatric oncology, the Wilms' tumor serving as the solid tumor counterpart for acute leukemia.
The goals of those caring for children with cancer have been: (a) to cure the disease, (b) with the least associated morbidity, and (c) to gain a better understanding of pediatric malignant processes, thus furthering the first two goals, while striving to achieve the ultimate aim: prevention.(1) Death was the dispirited watch-word in the early years of this century.(2) (Table I) Virtually no children with Wilms' tumor survived, the highest percentage of them receiving no treatment and being left to die. Then came the era of the pioneering pediatric surgeons, notably at the Boston Children's Hospital, and survival became the

The authors thank the many surgeons, radiation therapists, pediatricians and pathologists and the past and present members of the NWTS Committee, and the Study Centers, all of whom have contributed so much to the study of Wilms' tumor.
Supported in part by U.S.P.H.S. Grants Nos. CA-11722 and CA-14489.

TABLE I

Wilms' Tumor Survival

Year	% Alive at 2 Years*
1920	8
1930	15
1940	32
1950	47
1965	81
1975	90

*Survival for years 1920-1960 based on data published by the Boston Children's Hospital. The 1975 figure is estimated from the survival rates obtained using the most successful regimens of the National Wilms' Tumor Study.(2)

key-word. Yet, more than one out of five children died as a result of surgery at that institution, and fewer than 10% were alive two years later. The subsequent history at the Boston Children's Hospital allows us to trace what happened, with the fewest confounding influences entering the story. Improvements in anesthesia and pre- and post-operative care accounted for the first major advances. The operative mortality dropped to less than 5% in the 1930's and early 1940's, and the overall survival rose to the 40% range. The first two goals were implicitly being observed: attempts at cure were being made, while lessening the morbidity which in this case all-too-often proved to be lethal. It then was found that the Wilms' tumor was responsive to irradiation. Gross and his colleagues gave post-operative irradiation routinely to the flank, and attributed the rise in survival to almost 50% to the use of the combined modalities.(3) This was the embryo of the modern multi-modal team, the surgeon and radiation therapist working in concert in every case. It is of interest that even in these early years, both the acute and long-term morbidity associated with radiation was being studied. Neuhauser, Wittenborg and their colleagues wrote land-mark articles pointing out the need to include the whole epiphyseal plate in the irradiation beams so that the inevitable growth disturbance produced would be symmetrical, and not lead to an obligatory structural scoliosis.(3,4) They also made seminal observations with respect to the interplay of dose and age, and correctly pointed out that the bone changes were inversely proportional to age, and directly proportional to the dose delivered. Thus, thirty or more years ago the elements of the modern team approach, and the stress on cure with the fewest possible side effects were already established tenets among specialists devoted to the care of children. Then came the revolutionary discovery that simple chemicals could effect a remission in patients with neoplastic diseases. The first major observation was in leukemia with the antifols by Farber and his colleagues at the Boston institution; and that team among others shortly described the efficiency of actinomycin-D against the Wilms' tumor.(5) Others were busy, too, of course.(6) Memorial Sloan-Kettering Cancer Center investigators explored the actinomycins in a series of clinical and laboratory investigations, while Sutow, Sullivan and their co-workers at the M.D. Anderson Hospital made similar observations with respect to vincristine.(7,8) In this same era, refinements of therapy already were being sought. Was it necessary to deliver routine post operative irradiation to all children with Wilms' tumor? Noting that babies with Wilms' tumor had had an excellent prognosis even before irradiation or the chemotherapeutic agents were

introduced into routine management, Boston Children's
Hospital investigators initiated a pilot study where no
post operative radiation was given to infants with localized tumors that were totally excised, and found that the
babies so managed fared well.

It can be seen that individuals and groups of individuals in single institutions were making provocative and
stimulating discoveries with respect to neoplastic diseases
in general, and the Wilms' tumor in particular. It also can
be seen that one of the land-mark advances was the appearance of the multi-modal team.(1)   Surely, much of the success in pediatric oncology can be ascribed to the appearance
of these groups in specialized centers, thus permitting
each child to obtain the benefit of expert consultations
and care from the moment of diagnosis. But no single
institution, no matter how large, could amass enough
patients sufficiently rapidly to address some of the questions that were being asked. The cooperative group came
into being as a result. This was the only means whereby
large numbers of patients could be accumulated to answer
pressing clinical questions within a reasonable period of
time.   These studies were carefully designed, and--it must
be said--with ethical considerations constantly in mind.
Cancer and Acute Leukemia Group B confirmed that actinomycin-D used as a surgical adjuvant improved survival.(9)
Children's Cancer Study Group (CCSG) showed that children
who received actinomycin-D systematically over a period of
15 months had a better relapse-free survival experience than
their counterparts who were given a single para-operative
course.(10,11)   Southwest Oncology Group demonstrated the
value of vincristine in Wilms' tumor patients, including
those resistant to actinomycin D.(12,13)   Now it was time
to seek answers to more precise questions, and even more
patients were needed in order to sub-divide the patient
population appropriately. The first intergroup organization
was formed for this purpose, and the National Wilms' Tumor
Study (NWTS) group came into being. It has since conducted
two clinical trials, stratifying patients according to a
clinical-pathologic grouping system.(14,15)   (Table II)

TABLE II

Abbreviated National Wilms' Tumor Study Grouping System*

Group I   -   Tumor limited to the kidney and completely
               excised
Group II   -   Tumor extends beyond the kidney but is
               completely excised
Group III -   Residual nonhematotgenous tumor confined
               to abdomen
Group IV   -   Hematogenous metastases

*See Ref. 14 for more detailed exposition.

The NWTS has so far shown the following, adriamycin meanwhile having been identified as an active agent.(16,17) (Table III):

   1.   Routine post operative radiation therapy need not be given Group I children who receive both actinomycin-D (AMD) and vincristine (VCR) for a period of at least six months.

   2.   Vincristine added to actinomycin appears to substitute for postoperative irradiation.

   3.   The combination of actinomycin plus vincristine is superior to either of the two agents alone.

   4.   Adriamycin (ADR) added to actinomycin and vincristine gives a better result than actinomycin plus vincristine.

   5.   Pre-operative vincristine simplifies surgery in patients with metastatic disease at diagnosis, but does not improve survival.

There are some points to be made from these data. The over-all two-year survival rate for the first NWTS is 80%. Thus, the results at the Boston Children's Hospital years ago that promised 80% survival if modern, multi-modal therapy were used has been achieved in a multiple institution study using such regimens. This is a practical result that goes beyond the figures cited. It means that relatively straight-forward but well-defined surgical, radiotherapeutic and chemotherapeutic techniques can be used successfully by any team of well-trained specialists.

In turn, the result of constant building is apparent in the second NWTS. The best regimens of NWTS-1 predicted a two-year survival rate in the 90% range; this has been realized in NWTS-2, where the rate is 87%. The second study, of course, not only used the best regimens of NWTS-1, but sought to improve on them.

Table III
Two Year Results of the
National Wilms' Tumor Study*

Study	Group/Regimen**	RFS(%)***	Survival(%)
NWTS-1	I/A+RT	83	97
NWTS-2	I/A+V	85	95
NWTS-1	II+III/A	57	67
	/V	55	72
	/A+V	81	86
NWTS-2	II+III+IV/A+V	67	79
	/A+V+Ad	80	86

*Actuarial estimates
**A = actinomycin D; V = vincristine; Ad = adriamycin
***RFS = relapse-free survival

Other cooperative groups were not idle. The International Society of Pediatric Oncology conducted the first Wilms' tumor trial, and showed that pre-operative irradiation lessened the frequency of intra-operative rupture.(18) Patients so treated needed whole abdominal irradiation less often than their non-irradiated counterparts. This has clear implications regarding the gonads, especially in girls. SIOP also showed that the relapse-free survival experience and survival rate for patients given multiple courses of actinomycin-D (as it was used in the CCSG and NWTS studies) were not better than the children given a single course of AMD. This result is different from that reported by the CCSG investigators, of course, and there is no immediate explanation for the discrepancy. Meanwhile, the Medical Research Council Study showed that vincristine given more intensively than in the NWTS seemed superior to actinomycin-D.(19) Indeed, the relapse-free survival results using VCR alone in that fashion more than matched the NWTS data for the two agents in combination. The MRC patient numbers are small, but about 85% of 23 Group II and III patients given VCR were disease-free at two years. This is to be compared with 81% for 59 NWTS Group II and III children given both AMD and VCR.

Cooperative group studies have been designed to do more than compare therapeutic options, however. Data concerning the surgical, radiologic, radiotherapeutic, pathologic, and epidemiologic aspects of Wilms' tumor are being collected--and more recently, information regarding the status of long-term survivors.(2) The result has been a torrent of information with respect to Wilms' tumor. Not only have histologic subtypes of prognostic import been described, but new entities have been identified. These have been described by Beckwith and Palmer, who divided Wilms' tumor into two broad categories according to histopathologic criteria.(20) These are aggregated under the terms Favorable Histology (FH) and Unfavorable Histology (UH), which have profound implications with respect to survival. UH tumors made up but 11% of the 427 cases reviewed in NWTS-1, yet accounted for 43% of the deaths among those patients. The two year survival rates for FH and UH children respectively were 89% and 39%. The UH group is actually composed of four sub-types: focal anaplasia, diffuse anaplasia, and the rhabdoid and clear cell sarcoma types. Indeed, the latter two categories may not be Wilms' tumors at all, but rather sarcomas that tend to occur in the kidney but are not restricted to that site. In any case, the rhabdoid tumor is associated not only with cerebral metastases, but the appearance of independent, second brain

tumors arising in the posterior fossa. The clear cell sarcoma
on the other hand tends to metastasize to bone, an association
described independently by Marsden and his colleagues.(21)
These observations are of importance in defining the entity
or entities that previously were clustered under a single
term, and thus provide opportunity for study not only for the
morphologist, but also for the etiologist and the embryologist
in manners that will be obvious. They have their practical
aspects, too. There is little need to obtain base-line brain
scans or skeletal surveys in every child with Wilms' tumor;
rather, they ought to be reserved for the types that tend to
involve those organs. The result is lessened exposure to
radiation, and lower medical costs in financial terms.

Factors of importance to the surgeon, the diagnostic
radiologist, and the radiation therapist also have been reported in detail in multiple publications pertaining to those
specialties. For example, the importance of lymph node involvement, already noted by Jereb, et al.(22) has been
strongly confirmed by the more extensive and homogeneous data
accummulated in both the NWTS and the SIOP studies.(23,24)
This has obvious importance not only for surgeons and radiation therapists, but to chemotherapists who now can know that
patients with lymph nodal involvement are at increased risk.

The NWTS required of its investigators that all patients
with a preoperative diagnosis of Wilms' tumor be registered.
This has given the NWTS Group an opportunity to review such
ancillary but important questions as the management of
children with bilateral Wilms' tumors, mesoblastic nephromas,
or renal cell carcinomas, as well as several subsidiary
questions that are still undergoing analysis.(2)

Cooperative group data can and should be used for a
variety of other purposes as well. These can go beyond the
relatively narrow issues of the therapeutic trial; indeed,
beyond the disease itself.(25,26)

It should be noted that these several observations concerning Wilms' tumor over the years constitute a kaleidoscope.
The basic elements may be the same, but they are made to
change in relation to each other, and thus the pattern
changes. Some of the prognostic factors found to be
important in the first National Wilms' Tumor Study are no
longer of significance in the second because treatments have
improved. An example is the age factor. Group I children
over two years of age had a worse outcome than those under
that age in the first study. The difference disappeared in
the second trial. Moreover, children of whatever age had
superior relapse-free survival experience, even though none
of the children were irradiated, because two-agent chemotherapy was used. As Beckwith also has pointed out, prog-

nostic factors will shift with time as better treatments are
devised.(27) One result is that high-risk patients who require more intensive treatment, will become increasingly
obvious. Another result, however, is that those at low risk
will be obscured. It is important to identify them if refinement of therapy remains one of the goals of the pediatric
oncologist. It is important, of course, because low-risk
children are eligible for even less treatment. Ancient records
must be reviewed for this purpose--and once again, the fruitful interplay between individual institutions and the cooperative group becomes apparent. Only single institutions
going carefully over Wilms' tumor records that antedate the
chemotherapy era and--if possible--before routine post operative radiation therapy was given can derive the necessary
information. The patterns of relapse in patients who had
only radical nephrectomy performed provides the necessary
basic information. Thus, reports such as those from the
Toronto and Boston groups which analyze patterns of relapse
provide important information in this regard.(28,29)

There thus is ample room for individual institutions to
continue to conduct careful analyses of specific points.
These kinds of observations are the basic ingredients on
which cooperative group trials can and should be built.
Single institutions, when it is feasible to do so, should--
of course--conduct their own clinical trials and reach their
own conclusions. That is seldom possible given the subdi-
visions of each tumor type according to sex, age, location,
histologic type, and other important variables which are becoming recognized with increasing frequency. Nonetheless,
pilot investigations made in single institutions often provide the bases on which cooperative trials can be built. At
the same time, there is no reason why cooperative groups
cannot mount their own innovative, forward-looking studies--
and the record just reviewed shows that this has been done
by investigators of many nationalities in several parts of
the world.

This rich legacy of information gathered over the years
from single institutions and from cooperative groups have
been used to construct the third National Wilms' Tumor Study
which was launched in 1979.(2) It divides patients between
those with favorable histology and those with unfavorable
histology so that further reductions of therapy can be made
on the one hand, and more aggressive treatments on the other.
The three goals of pediatric oncology are implicit in the
design; for example, concern for the potential late cardiac
damage of adriamycin has led to a trial of a more intensive
AMD and VCR regimen rather than merely accepting the superiority of the three-drug regimen.

The questions being posed in NWTS-3, thus, are:
    1.   <u>Favorable Histology</u>.
        A.   Are the results in Stage I patients given AMD plus VCR for ten weeks different from those in children who get both agents for six months?
        B.   Is more intensive use of AMD plus VCR as good as the three drugs AMD plus VCR plus ADR?
        C.   Is routine post operative radiation therapy of the flank necessary in Stage II patients who get effective chemotherapy as well?
        D.   Is the result better in Stage III patients, given effective chemotherapy, who receive 2000 vs. 1000 rad?
    2.   <u>Unfavorable Histology, any Stage and Stage IV, any Histology</u>
        A.   Are better results provided when cyclophosphamide is added to AMD plus VCR plus ADR in these patients who are at high risk?
        B.   Are there any differences when radiation doses ranging from 1200 to more than 4000 rad are used?

NWTS-3 also is accumulating information regarding the health and well-being of long-term survivors of the first two trials. In addition, the NWTS has since its inception been supplying epidemiologic information to epidemiologists and others who study etiologic factors in attempts to understand the disease better. It is to be hoped that this collaboration will provide clues that will lead eventually to a reduction in the incidence of the disease through genetic counselling and through identification of possible pre-natal causative factors such as parental occupational and environmental exposures.

Thus, the goals of pediatric oncology are exemplified by the progress made in Wilms' tumor. They are being fulfilled through the untiring work of individual investigators, whether working in single institutions or banded together in cooperative groups. The result has been that survival has climbed steadily over the years from less than 10% to more than 85%--a proud achievement for modern medicine.

REFERENCES

1.   D'Angio, G.J.: Perspectives of pediatric oncology-- battlegrounds, old and new. <u>Care of the Child with Cancer</u> (American Cancer Society) 1979.
2.   D'Angio, G.J., Beckwith, J.B., Breslow, N.E.: Wilms' tumor: an update. Cancer <u>45</u>:1791-1798, 1980.

3. Gross, R.E., and Neuhauser, E.B.D.: Treatment of mixed
    tumors of the kidney in childhood. Pediatrics
    6:843-852, 1950.
4. Neuhauser, E.B.D., Wittenborg, M.H., Berman, C.Z. and
    Cohen, J.: Irradiation effects of roentgen therapy on
    the growing spine. Radiology 59:637650, 1952.
5. Farber, S.: Chemotherapy in the treatment of leukemia
    and Wilms' tumor. J. Am. Med. Assoc. 198 826-838, 1966.
6. The actinomycins and their importance in the treatment
    of tumors in animals and man. Ed.: S.A. Waksman. Ann.
    N.Y. Acad. Sciences 89:283-486, 1960.
7. Sutow, W. and Sullivan, M.P.: Vincristine in primary
    treatment of Wilms' tumor. Texas State J. Med. 61:
    794-799, 1965.
8. Sullivan, M.P.: Vincristine (NSC-67574) therapy for
    Wilms' tumor. Cancer Chemotherapy Reports 52:481-484,
    1968.
9. Burgert, E.O., Jr., and Glidewell, O.: Dactinomycin
    in Wilms' tumor. J. Am. Med. Assoc. 199:464-468, 1967.
10. Wolff, J.A., Krivit, W., Newton, W.A., Jr., et al.:
    Single versus multiple dose dactinomycin therapy of
    Wilms' tumor. N. Engl. J. Med. 279:290-294, 1968.
11. Wolff, J.A., D'Angio, G.J., Hartmann, J., et al.:
    Long-term evaluation of single versus multiple course
    of actinomycin D therapy of Wilms' tumor. N. Engl.
    J. Med. 290:84-86, 1974.
12. Vietti, T.J., Sullivan, M.P., Haggard, M.E., et al.:
    Vincristine sulfate and radiation therapy in metastatic
    Wilms' tumor. Cancer 25:12-20, 1970.
13. Sutow, W.W., Thurman, W.C., and Windmiller, J.:
    Vincristine (leurocristine) sulfate in the treatment
    of children with metastatic Wilms' tumor. Pediatrics
    32:880-887, 1963.
14. D'Angio, G.J., Evans, A.E., Breslow, N., et al.: The
    treatment of Wilms' tumor--Results of the National
    Wilms' Tumor Study. Cancer 38:633-646, 1976.
15. D'Angio, G.J., Evans, A.E., Breslow, N., et al.: The
    treatment of Wilms' tumor--Results of the National
    Wilms' Tumor Study. Cancer (In press)
16. Bonadonna, G., Monfardini, S., Delena, M., et al.:
    Phase I and preliminary phase II evaluation of adriamycin.
    Cancer Res. 30:2572-2582, 1970.
17. Tan, C., Etcubanas, E., Wollner, N., et al.: Adriamycin--
    an antitumor antibiotic in the treatment of neoplastic
    disease. Cancer 32:9-17, 1973.

18. Lemerle, J., Voute, P.A., Tournade, M.F., et al.:
    Preoperative versus post-operative radiotherapy,single
    versus multiple courses of actinomycin D, in the treatment
    of Wilms' tumor. Cancer 38:647-654, 1976.
19. MorrisJones, P.H.: Med. Res. Council's Working Party
    on Embryonal Tumors in Childhood: Management of nephro-
    blastoma in childhood. Arch. Dis. Child. 53:112119,1978.
20. Beckwith, J.B., and Palmer, N.F.: Histopathology and
    prognosis of Wilms' tumor--Results from the First
    National Wilms' Tumor Study. Cancer 41:1937-1948, 1978.
21. Marsden, H.B., Lawler, W., and Kumar, P.M.: Bone
    metastasizing renal tumor of childhood: Morphologic
    and clinical features and differences from Wilms' tumor
    Cancer 24:1922-1928, 1978.
22. Jereb, B., and Eklund, G.: Factors influencing the
    cure rate in nephroblastoma. Acta. Radiol. Ther.
    12:84-106, 1973.
23. Breslow, N.E., Palmer, N.F., Hill, L.R., et al.:
    Wilms' tumor: Prognostic factors for patients without
    metastases at diagnosis--Results of the National Wilms'
    Tumor Study. Cancer 4:1577-1589, 1978.
24. Jereb, B., Tournade, M.F., Lemerle, J.: Lymph node
    invasion and prognosis in nephroblastoma. Cancer
    45:1632-1636, 1980.
25. Farewell, V.T., and D'Angio, G.J.: A simulated study
    of historical controls using real data. Biometrics
    (In press)
26. Farewell, V.T., D'Angio, G.J., Breslow, N., and
    Norkool, P.: Retrospective validation of a new
    staging system for Wilms' tumor. Cancer Clinical
    Trials (In press)
27. Beckwith, J.B.: Grading of pediatric tumors. Care
    of the Child with Cancer (American Cancer Society)
    1979 (pp. 39-44).
28. Jeal, P.N., and Jenkin, R.D.: Abdominal irradiation
    in the treatment of Wilms' tumor. Int. J. Radiation
    Oncology Biol. Phys. 6:655-661, 1980.
29. Cassady, J.R., Jaffe, N., and Filler, R.M.: The
    increasing importance of radiation therapy in the
    improved prognosis of children with Wilms' tumor.
    Cancer 39:825828, 1977.

RHABDOMYOSARCOMA

Harold M. Maurer, M.D.*

Professor and Chairman
Department of Pediatrics
Medical College of Virginia
Virginia Commonwealth University
Richmond, Virginia

*For the Intergroup Rhabdomyosarcoma Study Committee of
Children's Cancer Study Group and Southwest Oncology Group:
W.M. Crist, M.D., M. Donaldson, M.D., E.A. Gehan, Ph.D.,
D.Hammond, M.D., D.M. Hays, M.D., R. Heyn, M.D., W. Lawrence,
M.D., R. Lindberg, M.D., W. Newton, M.D., A. Ragab, M.D.,
R.B. Raney, M.D., F. Ruymann, M.D., E.H. Soule, M.D., W.W.
Sutow, M.D., M. Tefft, M.D.
    Supported by U.S. PHS Grant Numbers: CA24507, CA04646,
CA12014, CA16943, CA13539, CA16118

Rhabdomyosarcoma (RMS), the most common soft tissue sarcoma occurring in patients under age 21, poses a considerable
challenge to the clinician-investigator. Because the cancer
arises from embryonic mesenchyme, unlike most other childhood
tumors it can develop virtually anywhere in the body, and
each site of origin has its own set of special problems.
Adding to the complexity of study and management of RMS are
the variety of histologic subtypes which appear to have differing patterns of behavior.
    Despite this complexity, significant progress has been
made recently in improving the survival rate of patients with
this disease. Survival rates have increased dramatically,
from less than 20% 15 years ago to approximately 70% at the
present time in patients without metastasis, as a result of
a better understanding of the biologic characteristics of the
cancer, improved histologic classification, careful staging,
new techniques for accurately defining disease extent, effective chemotherapy coordinated with improved radiation
therapy and surgery and, finally, vigorous use of improved
supportive therapy.
    The purpose of this report is to review the recent accom-
plishments in the treatment of RMS, to identify the challeng-

es ahead and to assess the future prospects for cure.

ACCOMPLISHMENTS

   Important conceptual advances have resulted from the Intergroup Rhabdomyosarcoma Studies (IRS) conducted since 1972
collaboratively by multidisciplinary members of Children's
Cancer Study Group, Southwest Oncology Group, and Cancer and
Leukemia Group B. The significance of the results of the
major aspects of the study are summarized as follows:

1. The clinical grouping classification designed to assess
    extent of disease in patients appears to be valid in
    defining prognosis and, as such, is an effective frame-
    work for treatment planning and study (Tables 1,2). (5,6)
2. In the treatment of Group I patients, no postoperative
    radiotherapy to the tumor bed appears necessary when VAC
    chemotherapy is given. The 3-year survival rate is 92%
    in this group without radiation therapy and with the
    omission of radiation therapy the risk of late effects
    from the treatment itself is decreased. In IRS-II,
    attempts to refine treatment in this group of patients
    continues and, therefore, cyclophosphamide has been de-
    leted from the chemotherapy regimen.
3. In the treatment of Group II patients, it has been possi-
    ble to omit cyclophosphamide from the chemotherapy regi-
    men, although all patients do receive postoperative radi-
    ation to the the tumor bed. The omission of the drug
    will obviate the risk of cyclophosphamide-related late
    effects, especially hemorrhagic cystitis, cardiomyopathy,
    bone marrow suppression and gonadal dysfunction. The
    3-year survival rate for these patients is 74%.
4. In patients with gross residual (Group III) or metastatic
    disease (Group IV) at diagnosis, the use of pulse-VAC
    chemotherapy with or without the addition of adriamycin,
    plus radiation therapy, produced a complete response rate
    of 66% in Group III and 46% in Group IV, with the CR +
    PR rates being 85% to 76%, respectively. The disease-
    free survival rates at 3 years were 57% in Group III and
    29% in Group IV. In IRS-II, high doses of cyclophospha-
    mide are given intermittently in association with repeti-
    tive courses of pulse VAC for two years and radiation to
    the primary tumor and sites of metastases. Treatment is
    further intensified by incorporating adriamycin into the
    program. This additional therapy was considered necessary
    for patients with advanced disease.
5. Patients with primary lesions of the genitourinary tract

TABLE 1
CLINICAL GROUPING CLASSIFICATION - IRS

Group I   Localized disease, completely resected
     II   Microscopic residual or nodal involvement
     III Incomplete resection or biopsy with gross residual
          disease
     IV   Metastasis present at diagnosis

TABLE 2
3-YEAR SURVIVAL RATES BY GROUP - IRS-I

Group	No.	Disease-Free Survival	Survival (%)
I	79	83	90
II	143	66	72
III	165	57	*58
IV	53	29	**18

*251 patients; **115 patients

(bladder, prostate, vagina, uterus) had exceedingly good
survival rates (Group I 96%, II 77%, III 72%) at three
years, including those with lesions of the prostate, a
classically unfavorable site prognostically, but at a cost
of radical surgery (Table 3). IRS-II is testing the possibility that, in these patients, preoperative chemotherapy and, if necessary, radiation therapy may permit less
extensive surgery and achieve a similarly high cure rate
with retention of organ function. Thus far, of 16 evaluable patients (8 prostate, 6 bladder, 2 vagina) on study
only 2 have required exenterative surgery, and all are a-
live and in remission from 8-58 weeks. In this study surgery is scheduled at week 16; however, clinical assessment
of response at week 8 permits identification of the cases
in which earlier surgical intervention is indicated.
6. Survival rates in patients with primary lesions of the
orbit were also exceedingly good, with over 85% of patients alive at 3 years in Groups I-III. (10)
7. Special problems have been identified in IRS-I which led
to special approaches to treatment for certain lesions in
IRS-II.
   a. It was noted that 40% (57/141) of patients with primary tumors of the head and neck area had involvement
of parameningeal sites (nasopharynx, nasal cavity,
paranasal sinuses or middle ear-mastoid area) and of
these patients, 35% (20/57) showed evidence of direct
meningeal extension and all but 1 (19/20) died in 1
year. (11) In IRS-II, patients with parameningeal

TABLE 3
3-YEAR SURVIVAL RATES BY PRIMARY SITE - IRS-I

	Site	Group I No.	%	II No.	%	III No.	%	IV No.	%
Disease-Free Survival*	H&N	5	80	32	70	101	42	22	13
	Orbit	1	100	17	94	35	72	2	0
	GU	37	93	32	76	28	66	25	30
	Extremity	23	71	35	57	25	18	29	3
Survival	H&N		100		78		53		14
	Orbit		100		94		87		0
	GU		96		77		72		37
	Extremity		83		69		34		3

*Time on study in Groups III & IV

lesions are considered to be at high risk of meningeal involvement if they show cranial nerve dysfunction or evidence of bone erosion at the base of the
skull. Such patients and those with evidence of direct meningeal involvement documented by tumor cells
in the CSF, CT scan and/or arteriography demonstrating intracranial tumor, or evidence of spinal cord
involvement, receive craniospinal radiation and intrathecal courses of hydrocortisone, methotrexate and
cytosine arabinoside in combination, in addition to
systemic chemotherapy and radiation to the primary
tumor. Thus far, of 32 evaluable patients with either
cranial nerve palsy (23) bone erosion at the base of
the skull (21) or documented intracranial tumor (11),
16 (50%) achieved a complete response and another 10
(31%) a partial response. (8) Fourteen patients are
relapse-free for a median of 10+ months; only 2 patients with intracranial tumor have developed progressive disease. Toxicity (neutropenia, mucositis) has
been moderate to severe in most patients, but is reversible. Although these results must be considered
very preliminary, already the duration and rate of
survival has improved significantly for these patients.
b. In IRS-I, it was noted that patients with primary
tumors of the extremity had the highest relapse rate
and lowest survival rate, compared to patients with
tumors in other sites. (2) The relapse rate at 3
years in patients treated by primary extremity amputation was 5/6, in Group I 29%, Group II 43%, Group III
82%, and Group IV 97%. The percentage of patients in
this series of extremity lesions with the alveolar

histologic subtype was 44% versus 18 in the total series. The poor prognosis of extremity lesions relative
to other sites can be largely explained on the basis
of the relative frequency of the alveolar histologic
subtype. The survival rates of patients with non-
alveolar histologic subtypes of extremity tumors is
not significantly lower than in patients with tumors
of the head and neck area, and genitourinary tract.
A greater degree of local tumor control may be
achieved by more aggressive surgery (short of amputation). However, the major problem in this site is
the high incidence of dissemination in patients with
alveolar histology. In IRS-II, this problem has been
approached by treating all patients with alveolar
extremity lesions in Group I and II and all patients
in which primary extremity amputation is performed,
i.e., those with the poorest prognosis, with intensive chemotherapy regimens ordinarily reserved for
patients in Groups III and IV. The results thus far
are two preliminary to report at this time.

c. Initial data on the frequency of lymph node involvement by RMS have become available through review of
patients in the IRS. (3) Although biopsy of regional nodes was not a routine practice early in the
study, the information available showed that lesions
of the genitourinary tract and extremity had a higher incidence of lymphatic spread then was previously
realized (17%-19%). Retroperitoneal lymph node involvement in primary tumors of the paratesticular
region was 40% (6/15). (7) It is probable that this
important piece of biological information, critical
in disease staging and treatment planning, was largely responsible for the 89% survival rate in patients
with primary paratesticular lesions. Regional node
dissection or biopsy is now advisable in all patients
with pelvic, paratesticular and extremity tumors.
A positive regional node in an extremity tumor should
lead to a consideration of exploration for biopsy of
more proximal node groups to fully evaluate the extent of the disease.

6. Earlier reports have indicated the need to deliver doses
of radiation in the order of 5000 to 6000 rad to achieve
local tumor control of RMS. Enhancement of radiation effects against soft tissues occurs with concomittent
multi-agent chemotherapy and leads to severe contractures
of soft tissue and necrosis of underlying bone in patients who receive high levels of radiation. This effect

is more pronounced in young children. Secondary onco-
genesis may also occur later in life. Therefore, refinement in local treatment is desirable as long as control
of local tumor and ultimate survival are not compromised.
The results of IRS-I indicate that lowering radiation
doses to between 4000 and 5000 rad and volume of tissue
treated, yield satisfactory rates of local tumor control
and survival when patients receive maintenance systemic
chemotherapy. (12) Local control was achieved in 91% of
children 6 years of age or less whether doses were less
or greater than 4000 rad. However, children over 6 years
achieved a lower local control rate (68%) at the lowest
doses, as compared to doses between 4000-5000 rad (88%).
The data also suggest an increased risk of local failure
when tumors are more than 5 cm in diameter. As a result
of these findings, in IRS-II all patients in Group II
receive between 4000-5000 rad. Patients in Group II who
are 6 years of age or less with tumors of less than 5 cm
receive the same dose. However, those over 6 years or
with tumors equal to or greater than 5 cm receive between
4500 and 5000 rad. The results of this study should provide better guidelines for radiation therapy for RMS.

9. Evaluation of the tumor histology in over 800 patients,
    and study of the post-mortem material of patients placed
    on the IRS have revealed several important clinically
    relevant facts: (1)

    a. The alveolar histologic pattern, which accounts for
        18% of the cases, is associated with a significantly
        shorter survival rate at 3 years when compared to all
        other histologic types (Table 4).

    b. A new histologic variant of RMS has been identified in
        7% of cases. This histologic subtype, which has been
        called extraskeletal Ewing's tumor, is somewhat more
        common in an extremity lesion and has a good response
        rate to treatment. (9)

TABLE 4

3-YEAR SURVIVAL RATES BY CELL TYPE - IRS-I

		Group I		II		III		IV	
	Cell Type	No.	%	No.	%	No.	%	No.	%
Disease-Free	Alveolar	14	53	32	43	33	34	33	0
Survival*	Embryonal	40	88	75	73	150	44	60	20
	All other	23	90	30	68	57	40	20	17

*Time on study in Groups III & IV

c. There is involvement of the CNS in a high proportion
    of tumors of the head and neck area and extremity. On
    post-mortem examination the CNS was involved in 28 of
    46 patients (61%) with head and neck tumors and in 15
    of 38 patients (39%) with primary extremity tumors.
    Seventeen of the 28 patients with the primary site in
    the head and neck died with CNS tumor without spread
    elsewhere, while patients with an extremity primary
    site always showed spread to multiple sites, often
    including the CNS.
d. There is involvement of the regional lymph nodes in a
    high proportion tumors of the genitourinary tract
    (62%) and lower extremity (57%) on post-mortem examin-
    ation, as compared to the upper extremity (25%) and
    other primary sites (28%).

At the present time a very detailed histologic analysis of
the over 800 specimens of tissue is being correlated with
clinical data in an attempt to identify a pathologic staging
classification for RMS. A similar approach was highly successful in the case of Wilms' tumor.

CHALLENGES

The challenges ahead are apparent. It is essential that
the biologic characteristics of rhabdomyosarcoma be fully
identified, including any special features related to histology, tumor size and location so that disease patterns and
prognosis can be anticipated and treatment maximized. Further
work is needed in tissue culture, electron microscopy, and
biochemical and cell surface antigenic markers of rhabdomyosarcoma to delineate the histogenesis of the various subtypes
and to study methods for detecting subclinical residual disease.

The etiology of rhabdomyosarcoma remains to be explained.
It is hoped that the special epidemiologic studies which are
being designed in the IRS will shed light on this area and
provide important leads for future study.

A number of important management questions remain to be
answered. We need to know why extremity lesions convey such
a poor prognosis even when seemingly "localized" at the time
of diagnosis.

With the recognition of the clinical importance of CNS disease in patients with parameningeal lesions of the head and
neck area, we need prophylactic CNS treatment which will prevent meningeal disease, be well tolerated and be free of late
side effects.

Which lesions can be approached by primary chemotherapy and radiation therapy rather then primary surgery is another challenging question. IRS-II may shed light on this question for lesions of the genitourinary tract.

Reduction in radiation dose and volume is a desirable goal when good local control and survival rates are achieved. The late effects of radiation therapy in patients with RMS of the orbit, a prognostically favorable site, would justify the study of lower doses and volumes of radiation for these patients.

The need for better treatment for patients in Clinical Groups III and IV is obvious. The use of cis-platinum as a front-line drug for RMS should be studied, but more new active drugs are needed. In patients with Group IV disease, a trial of hemi-body irradiation combined with intensive chemotherapy and marrow preservation and restoration would seem to be justified.

Data on the late effects of presumably "well-tolerated" chemotherapy radiotherapy regimens are still incomplete. Therefore, reduction in therapy is a desirable goal. In patients with Group I disease further reduction in therapy may be possible without jeopardizing disease control and survival.

FUTURE PROSPECTS

The prospects for further improvement in the survival and cure rates of patients with RMS are good, even with the treatments available today. As we unravel the complex nature of RMS and design treatment strategies more knowledgeably, survival rates will improve. The optimal regimen employing surgery, radiation therapy and chemotherapy has yet to be designed. With the development of new agents and the better use of existing agents and treatment modalities, employed in conjunction with a better understanding of the disease itself, RMS should be curable in the vast majority, if not all of the patients.

REFERENCES

1. Gaiger AM, Soule EH, Newton WA: Pathology of rhabdomyo-
    sarcoma. Experience of the IRS (1972-1978), J Nat'l Can-
    cer Inst (In Press).
2. Hays D, Lawrence W, Sutow W, et al: Primary extremity
    lesions in the Intergroup Rhabdomyosarcoma Study (1972-
    1977). Progress report, Proc Am Soc Clin Oncol, 21:389,
    1980.

3. Lawrence W, Hays D, Moon T: Lymphatic metastasis with childhood rhabdomyosarcoma, Cancer 39:556, 1977.
4. Maurer HM: The Intergroup Rhabdomyosarcoma Study II: Objectives and study design, J Pediatr Surg 15:371, 1980.
5. Maurer HM, Donaldson M, Gehan EA et al: The Intergroup Rhabdomyosarcoma Study - Update 1978, J Nat'l Cancer Inst (In Press).
6. Maurer HM, Moon T, Donaldson M et al: The Intergroup Rhabdomyosarcoma Study: A preliminary report, Cancer 40:2015, 1977.
7. Raney RB, Hays D, Lawrence W et al: Paratesticular rhabdomyosarcoma in childhood, Cancer 42:729, 1978.
8. Raney RB, Tefft M, Maurer HM: Treatment of cranial parameningeal sarcoma with meningeal radiotherapy and chemotherapy: Preliminary results of the IRS-II, Proc Am Soc Clin Oncol 21:386, 1980.
9. Soule EH, Newton W, Moon T, Tefft M: Extraskeletal Ewing's Sarcoma: A preliminary review of 26 cases encountered in the IRS, Cancer 42:259, 1978.
10. Sutow WW, Lindberg R, Gehan E et al: Rhabdomyosarcoma of the head and neck, including the orbits in children. Results of the IRS, Proc Am Soc Clin Oncol 20:343, 1979.
11. Tefft M, Fernandez C, Donaldson M et al: Incidence of meningeal involvement by rhabdomyosarcoma of the head and neck in children: A report of the IRS, Cancer 42:253, 1978.
12. Tefft M, Lindberg R, Gehan E: Radiation of rhabdomyosarcoma in children combined with systemic chemotherapy: Local control in patients enrolled in the Intergroup Rhabdomyosarcoma Study, J Nat'l Cancer Inst (In Press).

Current Management of Malignant
Bone Sarcomas

GERALD ROSEN

Attending Physician
Departments of Pediatrics & Medicine
Memorial Sloan-Kettering Cancer Center
New York, New York

OSTEOGENIC SARCOMA

Introduction

The definition of the activity of high dose methotrexate
with citrovorum factor rescue[1] and the dose of high dose
methotrexate necessary to obtain a response in evaluable osteogenic sarcoma during the past eight years at Memorial
Sloan-Kettering Cancer Center[8] has enabled us to utilize this
agent along with adriamycin and the combination of bleomycin,
cyclophosphamide and dactinomycin (BCD)[3] for the treatment of
patients with primary osteogenic sarcoma.

In a protocol (T-7) initiated in 1976 and utilized through
1978, 61 patients were treated with high dose methotrexate
given at the dose of $8gm/M^2$ for adolescents and adults, and
$12gm/M^2$ for pre-pubescent children. All patients received
doses of methotrexate between 12 and 20 grams. The protocol
also contained adriamycin at the dose of $90mg/M^2$ per course,
and the combination of BCD. Sixty-one patients with fully
malignant primary osteogenic sarcoma of the extremity were
entered into the treatment protocol. At a median follow-up
time of three years (2-4 years) 51 (84%) of the 61 patients
treated with this chemotherapy protocol in addition to surgery are surviving free of disease.[8] The majority of patients
treated on that protocol received chemotherapy prior to surgical resection of extremity lesions or endoprosthetic replacement of the femur and knee.[9] In addition, patients with

lesions of the humerus received preoperative chemotherapy followed by modified Tikhoff-Linberg resection of the proximal
humerus and shoulder joint.[2] Most patients received between
four and sixteen weeks of chemotherapy prior to surgical resection of the primary tumor.

Histologic review of multiple sections taken from the
specimens resected following preoperative chemotherapy revealed varying degrees of tumor necrosis attributable to preoperative chemotherapy. Patients were divided into two groups
based on the effect of preoperative chemotherapy on the primary tumor. The majority of patients had greater than 90%
tumor necrosis within the entire resected specimen (grade III
and IV effect of preoperative chemotherapy on the primary
tumor). All of the patients demonstrating the latter effect
of preoperative chemotherapy on the primary tumor have remained disease-free survivors. The ten patients who relapsed
with metastatic disease all had either no effect of preoperative chemotherapy on the primary tumor (grade I) or only a
partial effect (grade II).[8]

This positive corelation between a good histologic effect
of preoperative chemotherapy on the primary tumor and disease-
free survival has enabled us to identify patients who will be
cured if kept on the same chemotherapy postoperatively, and a
sub-group of patients who are at a high risk (60%) of developing metastases if continued on the same chemotherapy protocol. Although the latter patients are in the minority it
would be desirable to identify those high risk patients being
given this particular chemotherapy protocol and take steps to
further increase their chance for disease-free survival. It
is assumed in this group of poor responders that the tumor is
not as totally responsive to high dose methotrexate with
citrovorum factor rescue as in patients who have a histologic
grade III or IV effect of preoperative chemotherapy on the
primary tumor.[10]

Methods

Our current chemotherapy protocol for osteogenic sarcoma
calls for preoperative weekly high dose methotrexate with
citrovorum factor rescue. The effect of this single agent on
the primary tumor is carefully determined. Patients undergoing amputation or resection of the proximal humerus have
surgery following four weekly high dose methotrexate treatments. However, patients awaiting the custom-production of an
endoprosthesis for lesions of the distal femur have sixteen
weeks of preoperative chemotherapy as indicated in Figure 1.

Following surgical resection of the primary tumor the entire
specimen is examined by a single pathologist (A.G. Huvos) and

Induction Chemotherapy for Osteogenic Sarcoma
(T - 10)

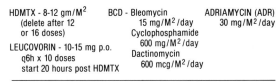

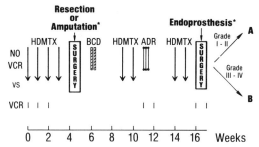

*Patients who are to undergo resection or amputation will have surgery at approximately four weeks; patients who are to undergo endoprosthetic replacement will have surgery at approximately 16 weeks.

Figure 1.T-10 induction chemotherapy for osteogenic sarcoma.

the effect of preoperative chemotherapy on the primary tumor is determined. Patients not having a complete effect of preoperative chemotherapy on the primary tumor (grades I and II) are assigned to an alternate postoperative chemotherapy regimen containing the agent cis-platinum, given in a single dose of 120mg/M^2 with mannitol diuresis,[11] in combination with adriamycin at a dose of 30mg/M^2 daily for two consecutive days. The combination of BCD chemotherapy is also utilized in these patients (Figure 2, regimen A). However, the patients who have a complete or near complete effect of preoperative chemotherapy on the primary tumor (grades III and IV) continue on the same chemotherapy, including high dose methotrexate with citrovorum factor rescue, postoperatively. In this group of patients we are attempting to reduce the total number of methotrexate doses needed to achieve disease-free survival in all patients (Figure 2, regimen B).

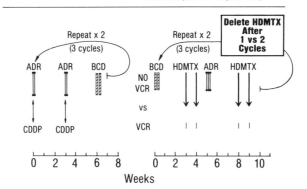

Maintenance Chemotherapy for Osteogenic Sarcoma

Histologic Response of Primary Tumor

GRADE I - II	GRADE III - IV
(T - 10A)	(T - 10B)

ADR 30 mg/M^2/day
CDDP 120 mg/M^2 or 3 mg/kg

Bleomycin 15 mg/M^2/day
Cyclophosphamide 600 mg/M^2/day
Dactinomycin 600 mcg/M^2/day

Figure 2.T-10 maintenance chemotherapy for osteogenic sarcoma.

Results

Initial results are quite encouraging. Of the past 87 patients with classic osteogenic sarcoma of an extremity treated
with preoperative chemotherapy, 45 patients had grade III and
IV histologic effects of preoperative chemotherapy on the primary tumor; all 45 (100%) patients have remained free of any
evidence of metastatic disease. Ten of 16 patients having a
grade I or II response to preoperative T-7 chemotherapy have
relapsed; none of these patients received high dose cis-
platinum following surgery. However, on the new T-10 chemotherapy protocol 26 patients were found to have only a partial
effect of preoperative chemotherapy on the primary tumor
(grade I-II) and received high dose cis-platinum (regimen A)
postoperatively; only two patients have relapsed and 24 have
remained free of disease. One of these two patients who relapsed had only a solitary pulmonary nodule and is currently
free of disease following thoracotomy. Thus, 69 of 71 patients (97%) treated with optimal "individualized" therapy
according to the response of the primary tumor to preoperative

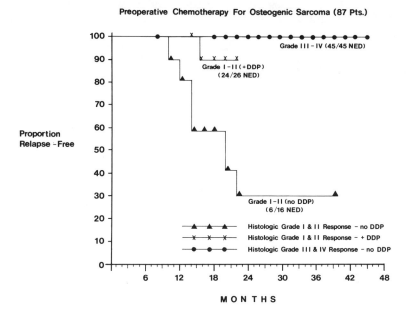

Figure 3.Of 87 patients with primary osteogenic sarcoma to undergo preoperative chemotherapy, 45 of 45 patients having a grade III or IV response to preoperative chemotherapy are surviving free of disease. 24 of 26 patients having a grade I or II response to preoperative chemotherapy have remained free of disease on the new T-10 chemotherapy protocol. Only 6 of 16 patients having a grade I or II effect of preoperative chemotherapy where high dose cis-platinum was not added to their regimen in the past have remained free of disease (lower line).

chemotherapy have remained free of recurrent disease from 8 to 26 months (median 16 months) from the start of treatment (Figure 3).

Discussion

These extremely encouraging initial results emphasize the importance of preoperative chemotherapy for primary osteogenic sarcoma. With this approach it is hoped that we can individualize therapy by selecting a group of patients that will not be expected to have a high percentage of disease-free survivors if continued on high dose methotrexate therapy postoperatively. This allows us to select the poor risk patient and offer "second-line" therapy before he actually relapses, giving even the poor risk patient a better chance for cure. In addition, this approach allows us to continue with effective chemotherapy in good responders, 100% of whom are expected to survive free of disease, without exposing them to the possible risk of permanent renal and hearing damage associated with high dose cis-platinum therapy.

EWING'S SARCOMA

Introduction

1980 represents the tenth year of the use of adjuvant chemotherapy in the treatment of Ewing's sarcoma at Memorial Sloan-Kettering Cancer Center. Of particular note is the fact that the very effective agent adriamycin has been used in this regimen since 1970.[12,6] Over the past ten years 67 patients with primary Ewing's sarcoma have been treated with chemotherapy and radiation therapy and/or surgery for the primary tumor.

Methods and Results

Current chemotherapy for Ewing's sarcoma consists of very aggressive combination chemotherapy (Figure 4) which, in addition to being able to keep approximately 80% of patients free of metastases, has the ability to rapidly shrink primary tumors, allowing us to delay radiation therapy to the axial skeleton until the patient has completed most of his chemotherapy. This has resulted in a lower incidence of distant metastases in patients with pelvic tumors; in addition, the ability to rapidly shrink primary pelvic tumors with chemotherapy (Figure 5) has enabled us to resect many of these tumors and then employ moderate dose radiation therapy (3,000 rad) to the operative site.[4] With this approach we have not had any incidence of local recurrence in pelvic and extremity tumors.

Our ten-year experience has shown that the local recurrence rate is still approximately 20% for patients who receive high dose radiation therapy alone to the primary tumor in an effort to avoid a major amputation; however, there have been no local recurrences in a comparable size group of patients treated with surgical resection and moderate dose radiation therapy. Therefore, we prefer to employ surgical resection in addition to moderate dose radiation therapy for the local treatment of

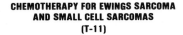

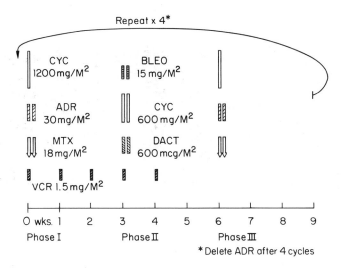

Figure 4.Current combination chemotherapy for small cell sarcomas including Ewing's sarcoma of bone. This chemotherapy is very aggressive and patients must be meticulously followed and return to the hospital for supportive care as necessary.

Ewing's sarcoma. This has resulted in no local recurrences, as well as end results functionally superior to either amputation or radiation therapy alone.[12,6]

The timing of local therapy following intensive chemotherapy is fundamental. It is essential to administer the majority of chemotherapy prior to local therapy so patients can tolerate this intensive chemotherapy prior to having radiation therapy, and without delays in their systemic therapy due to surgical procedures which can permit the establishment of distant metastases. It is also essential to meticulously follow the patient to document unequivocal evidence of local control by combination chemotherapy. This is accomplished by serial bone scans, CTT scans and physical examination.

Intensive combination chemotherapy is dangerous and the majority of patients undergoing T-11 chemotherapy have had to return to the hospital for transfusions (we routinely keep the hemoglobin above 10gm/dl) or for brief hospitalizations during

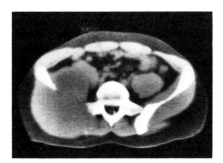 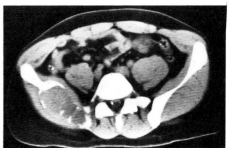

Figure 5.CTT scans before and after T-11 chemotherapy in a patient with Ewing's sarcoma of the pelvis. Note the great reduction in the size of the soft tissue mass following T-11 chemotherapy. This made surgical resection of the primary tumor relatively simple. Following surgical resection chemotherapy was continued and the patient received moderate dose (3,000 rad) radiation therapy.

periods of leukopenia and fever. When the latter occurs appropriate dose reductions are made in further courses of chemotherapy.

Figure 6 shows the disease-free survival of 53/67 patients with Ewing's sarcoma treated with chemotherapy at Memorial Sloan-Kettering Cancer Center since 1970. The T-2 protocol was used from 1970 to 1975.[12] From 1975 to 1978 combination chemotherapy for Ewing's sarcoma was utilized (T-6 protocol).[4,5] Since 1978 only abbreviated combination chemotherapy has been utilized for approximately 9-10 months (T-9 protocol).[7] Figure 4 shows the further modified protocol in use at this time.

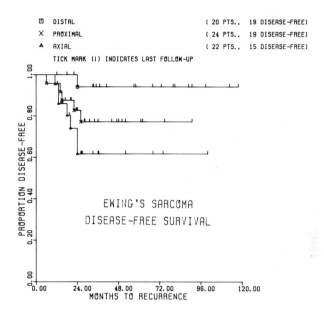

Figure 6. From 1970 to 1979, 67 patients with Ewing's sarcoma were treated with adjuvant chemotherapy. One patient never achieved disease-free status. Of the remaining 66 patients to be rendered free of disease 53 have continuously remained free of disease with all patients followed from 19 to 125 months. No patient has relapsed after six months from the completion of chemotherapy. All of the above patients have been off chemotherapy from 10 to 101 months.

Discussion

In addition to increasing disease-free survival in even the poor risk (axial lesions) patients with Ewing's sarcoma, a further advantage of intensive chemotherapy prior to local therapy for patients with extremity tumors is the ability to have the pathologically eroded bone heal prior to radiation therapy. This results in a lower incidence of late fractures, particularly in weight-bearing bones; we hope it will also result in a lower incidence of local recurrence than that ob-served following radiation therapy alone due to a significant reduction or complete eradication of the primary tumor prior to radiation therapy by the intensive chemotherapy necessary

to prevent systemic metastases. It is expected that preoperative intensive chemotherapy will eventually allow us to
reduce the total dose of radiation therapy needed to control
the primary tumor sparing patients the late morbidity associated with high dose radiation therapy.

SUMMARY

    Thus, in the management of both osteogenic sarcoma and
Ewing's sarcoma the use of early preoperative or pre-local
therapy chemotherapy has the following advantages:

1. The early institution of systemic therapy to prevent meta-
    stases.
2. The ability to insure that patients are responding to the
    given chemotherapy regimen by observing regression and
    histologic evidence of destruction of the primary tumor.
3. The ability to produce better long term function through a
    multidisciplinary approach combining chemotherapy, surgery
    and/or radiation therapy in the treatment of the primary
    tumor. Frequently, the reduction in size of the primary
    tumor by chemotherapy makes surgical resection more feasi-
    ble, and hopefully will allow for lower doses of radiation
    therapy to obtain complete and permanent control in the
    primary tumor area when dealing with Ewing's sarcoma.
4. It is expected with this approach that there will be a
    higher proportion of disease-free survivors and a lower
    incidence of long term complications and debility due to
    the aggressive local therapy that is necessary to control
    malignant bone tumors.

REFERENCES

1. Jaffe N, Frei E, Traggis D, Bishio Y: Adjuvant metho-
    trexate and citrovorum factor treatment of osteogenic
    sarcoma. N Engl J Med 291:994-997, 1974.
2. Kotz R, Salzer M: Resection therapy of malignant tumors
    of the shoulder girdle. Osterreichische Zeitschrift fur
    Onkologie 2:97-109, 1975.
3. Mosende C, Gutierrez M, Caparros B, Rosen G: Combination
    chemotherapy with bleomycin, cyclophosphamide and dac-
    tinomycin for the treatment of osteogenic sarcoma.
    Cancer 40:2779-2786, 1977.

4. Rosen G: Primary Ewing's sarcoma.The multidisciplinary lesion. Int J Radiation Oncology Biol Phys 4:527-532, 1978.
5. Rosen G: Malignant musculoskeletal tumors.The clinical investigative approach to combined therapy, in: Care of the Child with Cancer. Washington, D.C., American Cancer Society, 1979, pp 71-82.
6. Rosen G, Caparros B, Nirenberg A, et al.: Ewing's sarcoma.Ten-year experience with adjuvant chemotherapy. Cancer (in press).
7. Rosen G, Juergens H, Nirenberg A, et al.: Combination chemotherapy in the multidisciplinary treatment of Ewing's sarcoma. J Natl Cancer Inst (in press).
8. Rosen G, Marcove R, Caparros B, et al.: Primary osteogenic sarcoma.The rationale for preoperative chemotherapy and delayed surgery. Cancer 43:2163-2177, 1979.
9. Rosen G, Murphy ML, Huvos AG, et al.: Chemotherapy, en bloc resection, and prosthetic bone replacement in the treatment of osteogenic sarcoma. Cancer 37:1-11, 1976.
10. Rosen G, Nirenberg A, Caparros B: Evaluation of high dose methotrexate (HDMTX) with citrovorum factor rescue (CFR) single agent chemotherapy in osteogenic sarcoma (OSA). Proc Am Assoc Cancer Res 21:177, 1980.
11. Rosen G, Nirenberg A, Caparros B, et al.: Cisplatin in metastatic osteogenic sarcoma, in Prestayko AW, Crooke ST, Carter SK (ed): Cisplatin.Current Status and New Developments. New York, Academic Press, 1980, pp 465-475.
12. Rosen G, Wollner N, Tan C, et al.: Disease-free survival in children with Ewing's sarcoma treated with radiation therapy and adjuvant four-drug sequential chemotherapy. Cancer 33:384-393, 1974.

Long-Term Survival in Childhood Non-Hodgkin's Lymphoma

STUART E. SIEGEL, M.D.[1,2]
DEREK JENKIN, M.D.[2]
JACK WILSON, M.D.[2]
JAMES ANDERSON, M.D.[2] AND
DENMAN HAMMOND, M.D.[2]

[1]Head, Division of Hematology-Oncology,
Childrens Hospital of Los Angeles, and
Associate Professor of Pediatrics
University of Southern California School of Medicine;

[2]Childrens Cancer Study Group
Los Angeles, California

The past decade has seen major advances in the treatment of lymphoid malignancies. The dramatic improvement in the initial response, long-term survival and, even cure, of acute lymphoblastic leukemia (ALL) in childhood have recently been matched for non-Hodgkin's lymphoma (NHL)[1-5]. These developments are not surprising, given the increasing evidence that pathologically and biologically these malignancies of the lymphoid system, whether their origin is in the bone marrow or an extramedullary site, are closely related and response to similar therapeutic approaches.

Together ALL and NHL make up 41% of all new childhood cancers registered with the Childrens Cancer Study Group (CCSG) between 1974 and 1978. NHL accounted for 5% of the total patients seen at the member institutions. The most common age range for NHL in children is 8-10 years, but cases have been recorded as early as the first year of life. All authors have reported a consistent male predominance with ratios of 3-5:1 generally described[6]. The anatomic site of

Address for Reprints: Stuart E. Siegel, M.D.
                          Childrens Hospital of Los Angeles
                          Division of Hematology-Oncology
                          4650 Sunset Boulevard
                          Los Angeles, CA 90027

primary presentation is the abdomen in 35% of cases, the
mediastinum in 25%, peripheral nodal areas in 25%, the head
and neck in 5% and other sites such as the testes, skin or
bone in 10% of cases[1-9].

The clinical staging of NHL in childhood has been the
subject of some controversy, but the schema shown in Table 1
has been accepted by most major centers. In general, approximately 40% of patients will present with localized or Stage
I and II disease, while 60% demonstrate generalized or Stage
III and IV disease at diagnosis[1-4].

TABLE 1

Staging of Childhood Non-Hodgkin's Lymphoma

Stage I   Limited to one single site, excluding
                 mediastinal disease. (Nodal or Extranodal).
Stage II   Limited to two or more sites on the same side
                 of the diaphragm excluding mediastinal
                 disease. (Nodal or Extranodal).
Stage III   Mediastinal disease; or one or more sites on
                 opposite sides of the diaphragm (Nodal or
                 Extranodal) without bone marrow or central
                 nervous system involvement.
Stage IV   Any of the above distributions with bone
                 marrow and/or central nervous system
                 involvement.

Until the mid-1970's the prognosis for NHL in childhood
was poor and Figure 1, depicting almost two decades of experience from 1956 to 1971 by Jenkin and his colleagues in
Toronto is typical[6]. Only 20-25% of children survived two
years from diagnosis at a time when surgery and radiation
therapy were the primary therapeutic modalities, and chemotherapy was generally reserved for patients with advanced or
recurrent disease. When utilized, such chemotherapy usually
consisted of single agents of the type used for ALL. As
late as 1977, one reviewer of the status of NHL in childhood
stated that "although the survival rate for Hodgkin's disease
in the pediatric age group has shown significant improvement
in the past few years, the prognosis for NHL remains very
dismal"[7].

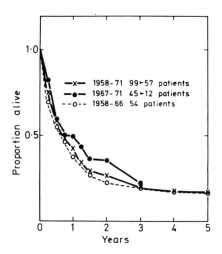

FM: Jenkin, 1974

Figure 1. Survival of non-Hodgkin's lymphoma in children age
16 years or less. From Jenkin, R.D.T. 1973.(Ref.6)

In 1971 Drs. Wollner, Burchenal and their colleagues at
Memorial Sloan Kettering Cancer Center initiated a therapeutic trial for childhood NHL using a multi-drug program called
LSA_2-L_2, derived, in part, from previous experience with the
L_2 leukemia regimen and a regimen employing high-dose cyclophosphamide for NHL - LSA_1[3,4]. The induction and consolidation phases were designed to rapidly decrease bulky disease
by utilizing high-dose cyclophosphamide and local radiation
to mass disease and, at the same time, initiate an intensive
leukemia-type chemotherapy program to prevent marrow and central nervous system (CNS) involvement, the most common causes
of failure in previous treatment programs[6,7].

The maintenance program consisted of 5-day cycles of
chemotherapy repeated in sequence every 2-3 weeks. Intrathecal methotrexate was given at the completion of each cycle and
patients were treated for a total of 18 months. In Figure 2,
the results of the protocol for the first 43 patients are compared to a group of children treated with a variety of chemotherapeutic regimens, usually using single agents with or
without maintenance therapy. Patients on LSA_2-L_2 had a 76%
projected survival compared to 11% for the non-protocol
group[4].

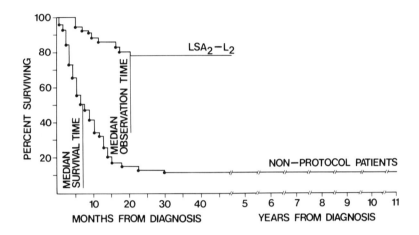

Figure 2. Actuarial survival of 43 patients on LSA$_2$-L$_2$
          compared to survival of 45 non-protocol patients.
          Modified from Wollner, N. et al., 1976, (Ref. 3).

When analyzed by stage of disease at diagnosis, all
Stage I and II patients were alive without disease, while 65-
70% of patients with Stages III and IV disease were surviving
without recurrence. As of 1979, of the 135 patients evaluated on the LSA$_2$-L$_2$ regimen, 76% remained alive with a median
follow-up of 42 months and virtually all are free of disease.
Of the 35 failures, 25 were due to recurrent disease or induction failure and 6 due to infectious deaths. One additional patient was lost to follow-up. (Wollner, personal communication).

Drs. Murphy and Hustu at St. Jude's Childrens Research
Hospital initiated a study for childhood NHL in 1975 utilizing high-dose cyclophosphamide, vincristine and prednisone
for induction and oral 6-MP and methotrexate therapy for
maintenance[1,8]. Sixty-nine patients were entered on that
study, with a complete response rate of 88% and a two year
actual disease-free survival rate of 55% (Figure 3). Once
again the long-term response rate was most favorable for
patients with localized disease.

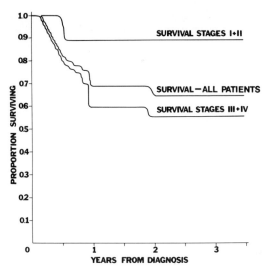

Figure 3. Survival of 69 patients with N.H.L. treated with
          S.J.R.H. protocol. Modified from Murphy, S.B., et
          al., 1980. (Ref. 8).

The questions of radiation in bulk disease in Stages II and IV
and CNS prophylaxis for Stages II-IV disease were also investigated in a prospective randomized fashion. No benefit for
radiation to bulk tumor in patients with disseminated disease
could be demonstrated, but CNS prophylaxis was effective in
virtually eliminating CNS relapse[1,8].

Weinstein and his colleagues at the Sidney Farber Cancer
Institution chose to investigate the patients with lymphoblastic lymphoma involving the mediastinum using a chemotherapy regimen employing adriamycin, vincristine and prednisone, or "APO", combined with 6-MP, L-asparaginase, cranial
radiation and IT methotrexate[2,5]. Radiation to the mediastinum was reserved only for relief of respiratory distress
due to compression by tumor or for patients with incomplete
regression of primary disease after induction therapy. Of
the 12 patients entered on the study, 86% or 10/12 remained
in remission with a median follow-up of 41 months.

In the studies of Wollner and Murphy, disseminated abdominal lymphomas had a particularly poor prognosis[1,3,4,8].
Approximately 25-50% of these are histologically classified as
Burkitt's type[1,7]. Arseneau et al. in 1975 summarized the
results of 30 cases of American Burkitt's lymphoma treated
with chemotherapy, including cyclophosphamide, treated at the

NCI[9]. As before, patients with extensive disease, primarily in the abdomen, had a poor prognosis with only a 30-40% 2-year survival. Similar results were reported by Ziegler et al. at NCI Uganda Lymphoma studies[10]. Patients with widespread abdominal disease in the Uganda series also had a poor outcome, with only 20% surviving 2 years following diagnosis.

In 1977, the CCSG initiated a multidisciplinary trial for all stages and sites of NHL, CCG-551[11]. The design of this study is shown in Figure 4.

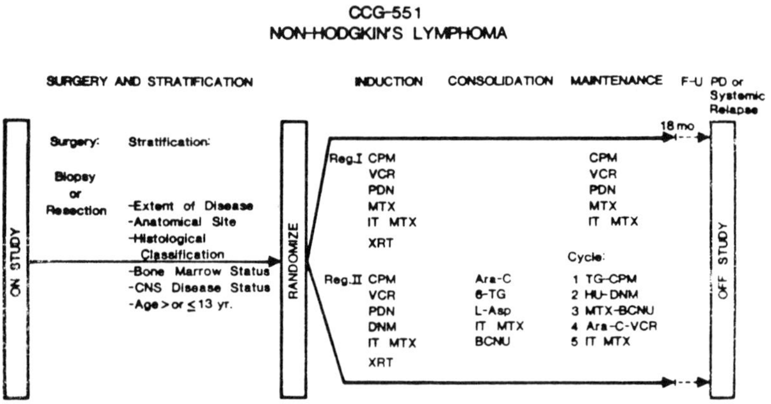

Figure 4. Study design of CCG-551 protocol for childhood non-Hodgkin's lymphoma.

To be eligible, patients must be aged 17 years or less, have no prior treatment with chemotherapy or radiation therapy and have a diagnosis of NHL established by histologic or cytologic techniques. After informed consent is obtained, patients are randomized to receive either a regimen consisting of high-dose cyclophosphamide, in conjunction with vincristine, prednisone and methotrexate induction, followed by maintenance with cyclophosphamide and methotrexate, or a modified LSA_2-L_2 regimen. Both groups receive IT methotrexate for CNS prophylaxis during the initial therapy and in maintenance, and therapy is continued for a total of 18 months. Two hundred and forty-seven patients have been entered on the study as of February 1980. At this time the projected 2-year survival rate is 90%, with 59% of patients disease-free (Figure 5).

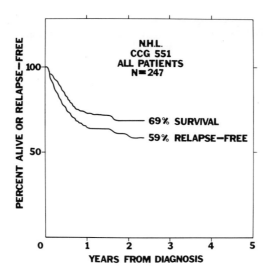

Figure 5. Survival of 247 children with NHL treated on CCG-551

Response was dependent on extent of disease, with 84% of patients with localized disease (Stage I and II) relapse free, while 46% of patients with disseminated disease (Stages III and IV) have remained disease-free. Patients with 25% or more lymphoblasts in their bone marrow were treated on ALL protocols and were not included in this study unless their bone marrow was infiltrated by "Burkitt's" leukemia/lymphoma cells.

Diagnostic tissue from 117 patients has undergone central group pathology review as part of this study, and separated into groups on the basis of the Rappaport histologic classification[12,13]. Seventy-six percent of mediastinal lesions demonstrated lymphoblastic histology, while 88% of abdominal lesions were either of the Burkitt's or pleomorphic undifferentiated histology. Nodal primaries were approximately equally divided between the lymphoblastic and pleomorphic histologies.

Preliminary analysis of the therapeutic outcome of patients on CCG-551 was carried out with relation to the histologic classification of the tumor at diagnosis, determined by the Group pathology review. There was no difference in outcome between the two treatment regimens for patients with localized disease. However, patients with generalized or Stages III and IV disease, demonstrated significant differences in response to the two theapeutic regimens, depending on histology. Patients with lymphoblastic histology had a much better relapse-free survival when treated with regimen 2 or the LSA2-L2 arm, while those with non-

lymphoblastic histologies, that is Burkitt's, pleomorphic and
histiocytic types, responded better to regimen 1, which employed primarily cyclophosphamide and methotrexate. As one
would anticipate, mediastinal primaries responded very favorably to regimen 2, with an 85% relapse-free 2-year survival
noted. The therapeutic advantage of regimen 2 over regimen 1
was demonstrated also for lymphoblastic lesions with primary
sites other than the mediastinum (Figure 6).

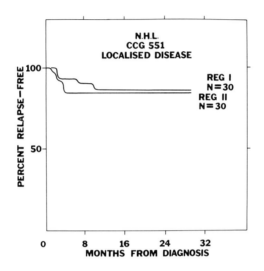

Figure 6.   Disease-free survival on CCG-551 by a) extent of
disease (above), lymphoblastic histology vs. treatment regimen (facing page, top), and c) non-lympho-
blastic histology vs. treatment regimen (facing page,
bottom).

Finally, in considering this increasingly fascinating
group of childhood neoplasms, we must briefly note the emerging importance of the functional characterization of malignant lymphoid cell populations in both NHL and ALL. By virtue
of the identification of specific antigenic determinants on
the surface of the cell and raising of specific monoclonal
antibody reagents to those antigens, several steps in the
maturation of lymphoid cells have now been described and, not
surprisingly, neoplastic disorders of cells at a number of
these stages of maturation have also been recently identified.
[14-17] The identification of E-rosette positive or surface
immunoglobulin positive lymphomas and leukemias has been described for several years.[16,17] However, a large number of
patients with ALL and a smaller number with NHL had malignant

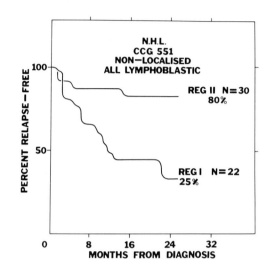

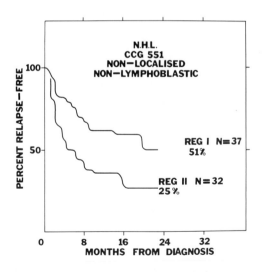

cell populations which had none of these surface markers detectable and were, therefore, designated as "null" cell disorders. With the new techniques now available, some of these cases can now be defined as disorders of "pre-T" or "Pre-B" lymphoid cells.[14,15,17]

A number of authors have reported the importance of these functional characteristics of the malignant population to the prognosis and outcome of treatment. Drs. Coccia and Kersey from the University of Minnesota have divided a group of 73 children with ALL and NHL on the basis of such functional studies.[16,17] Patients were monoclonal IgM on their blast cells, morphologic features of Burkitt's lymphoma, abdominal masses ("B-cell") had a very poor prognosis. A second group of patients had receptors for sheep red blood cells, complement or both ("T-cell") and mediastinal or nodal disease and, again, poor survival. Finally, group III patients had no such surface markers ("null cell"). Those with initial WBC's greater than 100,000/cu.mm. (IIIA) had a poor survival, while patients with initial WBC's of less than 100,000/cu.mm. (IIIB) had a relatively good prognosis.

In the face of very rapid developments in the characterization of NHL, where do we find ourselves in the approach to this tumor in 1980? A number of unsolved problems still face us. How do we attain long-term control for patients with massive disseminated abdominal disease, especially Burkitt's lymphoma? How do we rescue the failures on the current therapeutic regimens? How much and what type of CNS prophylaxis is needed for patients with localized vs. generalized disease? How long do patients require maintenance chemotherapy and what are the late affects of therapy in the disease process? Is radiotherapy to bulk disease required for all primary sites? Is the separation of ALL and NHL on the basis of bone marrow involvement appropriate to design of the therapeutic approach to the patient, or should we instead focus on the functional characterization of these disorders?

The answers to these questions may come from several directions. The work of Schlossman and others defining a number of monoclonal antibodies directed at T-lymphocytes makes possible attempts at serotherapy, especially for patients with abdominal Burkitt's lymphoma and patients failing initial, less intensive chemotherapy regimens.[10,17] We certainly need new agents for those patients failing our current approaches and these could include the biological response modifiers. New techniques of radiotherapy including sequential half-body radiation and radiation sensitizers may also have applicability to NHL.[19,20] The role of radiotherapy to bulk disease, especially in patients with advanced disease seems certain to be settled in the next few years, as will the question of duration of chemotherapy for patients with localized disease. Finally, the current thrust of biological research in NHL emphasizing the characterization of lymphoid malignancies as a whole may provide both new therapeutic leads for the clinical oncologist as well as insight into the pathogenesis of these diseases. If the next 10 years of research into childhood NHL are as productive as the last decade, there will be much to discuss at the time of the next review of this subject.

REFERENCES

1. Murphy, SB: Classification, staging and end results of treatment of childhood non-Hodgkin's lymphomas: Dissimilarities from lymphomas in adults. Semin Oncol 7:332-339, 1980.
2. Weinstein, HJ, Link, MP: Non-Hodgkin's lymphoma in childhood. Clin Hemat 8:699-713, 1979.
3. Wollner, N, Burchenal, JH, Lieberman, PH, et al: Non-Hodgkin's lymphoma in children. A comparative study of two modalities of therapy. Cancer 37:123-134, 1976.
4. Wollner, N, Burchenal, JH, Lieberman, PH, et al: Non-Hodgkin's lymphoma in children. Med and Pediat Oncol 1:235-263, 1975.
5. Weinstein, HJ, Vance, ZB, Jaffe, N, et al: Improved prognosis for patients with mediastinal lymphoblastic lymphoma. Blood 63:687-694, 1979.
6. Jenkin RDT: The management of malignant lymphomas in childhood, in Deelek TJ (ed) Modern Radiotherapy - Malignant Diseases in Children, London, Butterworths, 1973, pp-341-359.
7. Dehner LP: Non-Hodgkin's lymphomas and malignant histiocytosis in children. Semin Oncol 4:273-286, 1977.
8. Murphy JB, and Hustu, HO: A randomized trial of combined modality therapy of childhood non-Hodkin's lymphoma. Cancer 45:630-637, 1980.
9. Arseneau, JC, Canellos, GP, Banks PM, et al: American Burkitt's lymphomas. A clinicopathologic study of 30 cases. Am J Med 58:314-321, 1975.
10. Ziegler, JL, Deisseroth, AB, Applebaum, FR, et al: Burkitt's lymphoma - A model for intensive chemotherapy. Semin Oncol 4:317-323, 1977.
11. Jenkin, RDT, Anderson J, Chilcote R, et al: Grossly localized childhood non-Hodgkin's lymphoma (NHL) Response to irradiation and elective 4 or 10 drug combination chemotherapy. Proc ASCO 20:354, 1979.

12. Sheehan, WW, Rappaport, H: Morphological criteria in
    the classification of the malignant lymphomas. Proc
    Natl Cancer Conf 6:59-71, 1970.
13. Berard, CW, Dorfman, RF: Histopathology of malignant
    lymphomas. Clin Haematol 3:39-76, 1974.
14. Reinherz, EL, Kung, PC, Goldstein, G, et al: Separation
    of functional subsets of human T cells by monoclonal
    antibody. Proc Natl Acad Sci USC 76:4061-4065, 1979.
15. Reinherz, EL, Schlossman, SF: Regulation of the immune-
    response - Inducer and suppressor T-lymphocyte subsets
    in human beings. New Eng J Med 303:370-373, 1980.
16. Coccia, PF, Kersey, JH, Gajl-Peczalska, KH, et al:
    Prognostic significance of surface markers analysis in
    childhood non-Hodgkin's lymphoproliferative malignan-
    cies. Am J Hematol L:405-417, 1976.
17. Kersey, JH, LeBien, TW, Hurwitz, R, et al: Childhood
    leukemia-lymphoma. Heterogeneity of phenotypes and
    prognoses. Amer J Clin Pth 72 (Suppl):746-753, 1979.
18. O'Leary, M., Rabsay, NK, Nesbit, ME, Kriuit, W, Coccia
    PF, Kim, TH, Kersey, JH: Bone marrow transplantation
    for childhood non-Hodgkin's lymphoma. Proc Am Assoc
    Cancer Res 21:173, 1980.
19. Thar, TL, Million RR, Noyes, WD: Total body irradiation
    in non-Hodgkin's lymphoma. Int J Radiation Oncol Biol
    Phys 3:171-176, 1979.
20. Thar, TL, Million, RR: Total body irradiation in non-
    Hodgkin's lymphoma. Cancer 42:926-931, 1978.
21. Johnson, RE: Total body irradiation (TBI) as primary
    therapy for advanced lymphosarcoma. Cancer 35:242-246,
    1975.

Neuroblastoma

ALVIN M. MAUER, M.D.
Director

F. ANN HAYES, M.D.
Hematology/Oncology

ALEXANDER A. GREEN, M.D.
Hematology/Oncology
St. Jude Children's Research Hospital
Memphis, Tennessee

Neuroblastoma is a malignant tumor arising from the primitive neurocrest cells that form the adrenal medulla and
sympathetic nervous system. This tumor occurs at an annual
rate of about 1 per 100,000 children under the age of 15
years. It is a tumor of young children: 30% of patients
have been identified by 1 year of age, 40% by 2 years of age
and 90% before the age of 10 years. In the United States it
is one of the more common solid tumors of childhood.

One of the unfortunate characteristics of this tumor is
that about two-thirds of the patients have disseminated
disease at the time of diagnosis. Treatment for these
patients must be based on regimens of chemotherapy. Leikin
and co-workers (1974) reviewed the results of different
treatment programs and found little improvement in the
median survival rates with the passing of time. The use of
treatment programs found to be of value in other tumors of
childhood had resulted in no apparent benefit to patients
with neuroblastoma.

It will be the purpose of this paper to describe the
development of a treatment regimen for disseminated neuroblastoma at St. Jude Children's Research Hospital. A careful review of the previous treatment results was conducted
to sharply define the clinical problem. Growth characteristics of the neuroblastoma cells were studied to determine
some of the biological features of importance in designing
treatment programs. The clinical and laboratory evaluation
of the treatment regimen has provided new insights into the

management of disseminated cancer. The future directions
for continued study of this tumor and its treatment will be
indicated.

REVIEW OF CLINICAL EXPERIENCE

The first step in the design of a new treatment program
was a careful review of all children with neuroblastoma seen
at this institution from 1962 to 1974. This review was done
to define our previous experience and to identify the objectives for new programs.

One of the important objectives of any retrospective
review is to identify clinical features in the patients
which will help predict outcome and expected clinical
course. Two important prognostic factors for children with
neuroblastoma had already been identified; age of the patient and extent of disease at diagnosis (Wilson and co-
workers, 1974). These prognostic factors were also identified in this retrospective review. Children under the age
of 1 year had about a 60% expectation of survival and there
was lesser influence of disease extent found. Over the age
of 1, survival was related primarily to the extent of
disease at diagnosis.

The system developed to assess extent of disease is shown
in Table 1. It varies little in concept from the proposed
staging system of Evans and co-workers (1971) but is simpler
in application and results in well-defined groups with
respect to clinical outcome regardless of age. All patients
who were classed as stage I or II-A survived. More than 50%
of patients classed as stage II-B were alive and without
evidence of disease. Unfortunately, most patients with
stage III disease died within the first year of diagnosis
and there were few long term survivors. As already indicated, more than two-thirds of patients with neuroblastoma
fall into the stage III category at diagnosis. The decision
was made to focus efforts on improving treatment results for
these patients.

TABLE 1
Clinical Staging

1.   Stage I
Localized tumor completely resected.

2.   Stage II
Localized tumor incompletely resected.

Stage IIA
Resected but histologically proven to have capsule invasion; however, only microscopic residual disease remains.

Stage IIB
Locally unresectable or gross residual tumor following surgery confined to a single radiation area without invasion of adjacent organs, i.e., cervical, thoracic, abdominal with only adrenal or paraspinal involvement.

3.   Stage III
Regional or systemic spread of disease.

Stage IIIA
Regional or systemic spread of disease without bone or bone marrow involvement, i.e., liver, lymph nodes, skin or thoracoabdominal extension.

Stage IIIB
Local bone destruction without evidence of generalized bone or bone marrow involvement.

Stage IIIC
Generalized bone and/or bone marrow involvement by tumor.

Perhaps one of the most important prognostic factors to emerge from this review was the effect of response to therapy. The criteria of response used in this review and in judging the results of proposed treatment programs is shown in Table 2. For patients with stage III neuroblastoma, a significant improvement in survival was experienced only in those patients achieving a complete response to therapy regardless of the nature of the treatment programs. No survival advantage was experienced in those patients who achieved only a partial response or no response. This

relationship of prognosis for survival to response to treatment has also been observed by Leikin and co-workers. The
proportion of patients with stage III neuroblastoma achieving a complete response was small being about 1 in 5.

TABLE 2
Definition of Response

1. Complete Clinical Response (CCR)
Total regression of all apparent tumor including
healing of bone lesions and absence of tumor in at least two
consecutive marrow aspirates. The response must be attained
before and maintained throughout the 4 months of induction
therapy.

2. Partial Response (PR)
Greater than 50% regression of all apparent tumor
plus at least 50% clearing of bone marrow tumor on 2 consecutive marrow aspirates with no progression of disease at
any site. This response must be maintained through the 4
months of induction therapy.

3. No Response (NR)
Less than 50% regression at any site and all
patients, no matter what the degree of response, who have
progressive disease during the 4 months of induction
therapy.

4. Progressive Disease (PD)
Progressive disease at any site, even if regression occurs at other sites, is defined as greater than 25%
increase or appearance of new lesions.

From this review the objectives of the new treatment
program emerged. If the results of treatment for patients
with stage III neuroblastoma were to be improved, the first
step was to increase the proportion of these patients
achieving a complete clinical response.

ANALYSIS OF THERAPEUTIC IMPEDIMENTS AND DESIGN OF THERAPY

Treatment of patients with disseminated cancer depends
primarily on chemotherapy. A survey of the experience in
this institution and that reported in the literature concerning single drug responses in neuroblastoma was conducted
(Carli and co-workers, in press). It was determined that

cyclophosphamide and adriamycin were the two best single agents and were combined in the initial treatment program. Subsequently, two additional drugs, the epipodophyllotoxin VM-26 and cis-diamminedichloroplatinum, have also proven to be effective and have been incorporated into subsequent treatment regimens (Hayes and co-workers, 1979, and Green and co-workers, 1980). The next step in the design of the initial treatment program was to define the doses and scheduling of cyclophosphamide and adriamycin. Preliminary studies of neuroblastoma tumor cell kinetics had indicated that there was a relatively low proliferative activity in neuroblastoma tumor cell populations (Hayes and co-workers, 1977). Thus, one mechanism for drug resistance might be the large proportion of tumor cells in a relatively drug resistant resting phase. It seemed appropriate therefore to design a schedule for these two drugs to increase the proportion of cells actively dividing and thus to enhance their sensitivity to treatment.

Cyclophosphamide is relatively effective in killing both dividing and resting tumor cells. Therefore, treatment was begun with 7 days of this drug at a dose of 150 mg/m^2. The purpose of this phase of the regimen was to kill as many tumor cells as possible, reduce the tumor cell density, and increase the proliferative activity among the surviving cells. On the 8th day, adriamycin in a dose of 35 mg/m^2 was given with the expectation that an increased proportion of residual tumor cells would be susceptible to its drug action which maximally affects cells in DNA synthesis and delays cell cycle progression late in G_1 and during G_2. This treatment was then to be repeated every three weeks for a period of four months. At the end of four months of therapy the clinical response was to be evaluated according to the criteria shown in Table 2.

In order to evaluate the changes induced in tumor cell proliferative activity, studies were done in those patients who had tumor cells in their bone marrow. The proliferative activity of these tumor cells was determined by measuring the tritiated thymidine labeling index autoradiographically and the mitotic index microscopically. Determinations were made before and after the week of cyclophosphamide and serially for 48 hours after the administration of adriamycin. The degree of perturbation of tumor cell proliferative activity was compared to the clinical responses in those patients.

CLINICAL RESULTS

The results achieved with this regimen during the years 1974-1979 are compared to the results in the initial group of patients treated from 1962-1974 and shown in Table 3. The results are shown to indicate the portion of patients achieving a complete response prior to and following the implementation of the new treatment program. The clinical response is also depicted by age of the patient at diagnosis. The result of the treatment program was a significant improvement in the proportion of patients with disseminated neuroblastoma achieving a complete clinical response.

TABLE 3
The Response to Chemotherapy of
Children With Disseminated Neuroblastoma

Age at Diagnosis	1962-1974	1974-1979
< 6 months	*5/10+	5/7
6-12 months	2/6	7/9
> 12 months	10/61	23/52
Total	17/77 (22%)	35/68 (52%)

*No attaining CR
+Total number treated

It had already been noted from the original survey that an improved survival experience was observed only in patients achieving a complete clinical response. It was therefore important to determine if patients achieving a complete clinical response on the new program would have the same survival advantage experienced in the previous studies. The survival curves for patients achieving a complete response were identical for both series. Thus, the realization of one of the objectives of this study, that is to improve the complete response rate, also achieved the objective of improving the survival experience for this group of patients as well.

The survival experience of patients achieving only a partial response or no response at all was also identical for both groups. Thus, with this treatment regimen, no survival advantage was observed in patients achieving partial response to treatment. This observation emphasizes the importance of achieving a complete response in disseminated neuroblastoma. In this respect it is important to realize the similarities emerging between treatment problems for this disseminated solid tumor and the problems posed in the early days of the design of treatment programs for acute leukemia. One of the earliest lessons learned in the study of acute leukemia was the necessity for achieving a complete remission.

ANALYSIS OF RESIDUAL CLINICAL PROBLEMS

It is necessary in the evolution of treatment programs for cancer to continually review results, not only to determine the effectiveness of treatment programs but to identify residual or newly emerging clinical problems. As these problems are identified, then the objectives for new treatment programs can be set and regimens designed to answer these objectives. Analysis of the results of these clinical studies results in the identification of two major problem areas. The first area is the need to improve the initial complete clinical response rate. As indicated in Table 3, almost half of the patients have shown no benefit from the first treatment program and have not realized survival improvement. One approach is to attempt to treat the tumors resistant to the initial combination of agents with other agents which would not be expected to have cross resistance. To this end studies were done with the other two agents showing the best single drug responses, the epipodophyllotoxin VM-26 and the metallic drug cis-diamminedichloroplatinum (Hayes and co-workers, 1979 and Green and co-workers, 1980). Initial studies were done in order to determine the most effective sequence in which to give these two drugs as indicated by the pattern of perturbation of tumor cell proliferative activity. Based on these studies a sequence of cis-diamminedichloroplatinum followed in 48 hours by VM-26 was chosen (Hayes and co-workers, 1979). Initial studies have indicated the effectiveness of these two drugs in combination. They have now been incorporated into the current treatment program for children over 1 year of age with disseminated neuroblastoma. With the use of two effective drug combinations during the initial treatment period it is hoped that an increasing portion of patients can achieve a complete clinical response. The studies at this time are too early in their evaluation to determine if that objective has been achieved.

The other clinical problem that became evident was the problem of maintaining the complete clinical response in patients over 1 year of age. Here again the analogy with the treatment of acute leukemia became evident. Following the achievement of a complete remission it is necessary to have a period of continuation therapy to prevent early relapse. It was found that simply continuing the initially successful regimen of cyclophosphamide and adriamycin would neither avoid relapse in some patients nor did it prolong the period of disease-free status. It is also true that in acute leukemia agents maximally effective in the induction of remission are not necessarily good agents during the continuation phase. Furthermore, the cumulative toxicity of adriamycin precludes its long term use. Thus, it may be necessary to develop a treatment phase to prevent relapse in the initially responding patients similar to the continuation phase in acute leukemia. The drugs for that phase should be different from those used in the induction phase and be capable of being administered over a long period of time without the risk of cumulative toxicity. Our therapeutic armamentarium for disseminated neuroblastoma must be expanded.

CORRELATION OF CLINICAL AND LABORATORY OBSERVATIONS

During the course of the evaluation of the initial studies of the new treatment program an interesting series of observations emerged regarding the correlation of the cell kinetic and clinical response to chemotherapy. These observations have not only been of interest from the standpoint of the biological characteristics of neuroblastoma, but also been of value in designing treatment programs for individual patients.

In the initial series of patients treated according to the new program there were 15 who could be evaluated for changes in their bone marrow tumor cell kinetic patterns. Of these, 10 had increases in labeling and mitotic indices following cyclophosphamide therapy as predicted from the rationale of the treatment design. Five patients, however, had either no change or actual decreases in labeling and mitotic indices. When these patients were then examined for clinical responses, it was found that of the ten patients exhibiting increased tumor cell proliferative activity, 7 attained a complete clinical response and 2 had partial clinical responses. The 1 remaining child had early marrow suppression and infection after the first course of therapy and subsequently had rapidly progressive disease during the time when treatment was not given. Of the 5 children who did not have increased proliferative activity of marrow tumor cells, none achieved even a partial remission.

Of this initial group of 15 patients, 11 had adequate marrow samples for serial evaluation of the labeling and mitotic indices after adriamycin. In 4 children there were no cell kinetic changes attributable to an adriamycin effect. In contrast, in 5 children, the results indicated tumor cell lysis in the phase of DNA synthesis, a block in the G_2 phase and a block at the interphase of G_1 and DNA synthesis. In two other patients some but not all of the expected adriamycin effects were seen.

In these 11 children the results from studies following adriamycin provided an even better correlation between the observed tumor cell kinetic changes and the clinical response to therapy. In the 5 patients demonstrating a complete cyclophosphamide and adriamycin tumor cell effect, all attained a complete clinical response. If the tumor cell response to adriamycin was incomplete or absent, only a partial clinical response was observed even though the full cyclophosphamide tumor cell effect had been demonstrated. Thus, combining the observations of tumor cell effect following cyclophosphamide and adriamycin in this first study, a perfect correlation between cell kinetic and clinical responses were found (Hayes and co-workers, 1977). Since this first set of observations these studies have been continued and the correlation maintained.

These correlations have proved to be of real value in identifying within the first weeks of therapy that important group of patients in whom clinical responses cannot be anticipated to be complete and the ineffective drug regimen can be stopped without a prolonged period of exposure to its toxic side effects. Recently patients showing complete or partial cell kinetic non-responsiveness are immediately switched to the combination of the epipodophyllotoxin VM-26 and the metallic drug cis-diamminedichloroplatinum (Hayes and co-workers, 1979).

The initial degree of tumor cell proliferative activity showed no relationship to the liklihood of a complete or partial clinical response. This observation is similar to those already reported for acute leukemia. The inital tumor cell proliferative activity, however, did demonstrate a relationship with the subsequent duration of clinical response just as has been shown in acute myeloblastic leukemia. Patients with initial labeling indices in bone marrow tumor cells greater than 15% had relatively short periods of

clinical response in comparison with those patients whose
tumor cell labeling indices were less than 15%. Another
important correlation was found between tumor cell proliferative activity at the time of relapse and response to reinduction treatment. Those patients whose tumor cells had
labeling indices greater than 15% were unlikely to respond
to reinduction therapy.

While these correlations of tumor cell biological characteristics and clinical response are important in designing
therapy for the individual patient and anticipating clinical
courses, they have biological implications that are even
greater. The differences of tumor cell populations between
patients and in the same patient at different phases of the
disease must be explained. Much work remains to be done in
order to achieve an understanding of these differences and
their meaning for the design of new treatment programs. In
many respects neuroblastoma can serve as a model disease to
further our understanding of disseminated cancer.

CONSIDERATIONS FOR THE FUTURE

In this paper there has been an attempt to trace the
history of the development of a treatment protocol for a
difficult and resistant childhood tumor. The objective of
the initial protocol study was achieved in that there was an
improvement in the initial complete response rate from
approximately 1 in 5 patients to 1 in 2 patients. While
this result is obviously encouraging, further efforts must
be made to continue to improve this initial complete response rate. Evidence has been presented that achievement
of a complete response rate is the essential initial step to
improvement in survival.

At this time it appears that we are about at the stage we
were with acute lymphocytic leukemia in 1960. Complete remissions were being frequently achieved at that time but
patients were subsequently relapsing. It was during the
1960's that we became aware of some of the components of
treatment such as the continuation phase and the importance
of sanctuary sites. Much of what we have learned in the
treatment of acute lymphoblastic leukemia has been applied
to the development of the treatment protocol for children
with disseminated neuroblastoma. In a similar fashion much
of what we have learned from this series of studies of
neuroblastoma may be useful in treatment programs for other
forms of disseminated cancer as well. Currently, in treating children with disseminated neuroblastoma, studies are

needed to identify useful continuation therapy regimens in order to provide a longer period of disease-free survival and potentially cure. There needs to be continued exploration of new initial treatment regimens to improve the proportion of patients achieving a complete clinical response. It is necessary to learn more about the reasons for treatment failure both initially and during the subsequent relapse. The finding that tumor cell populations with greater proliferative activity at diagnosis are more likely to relapse early provides a possibly important clue to the acquisition of drug resistance in these patients' tumor cells. There must be an assessment of patients with neuroblastoma in order to determine if sanctuary sites for tumor cells might exist as they do within the central nervous system in acute lymphoblastic leukemia. Such sanctuary sites might be residual nests of tumor cells within the primary site which survive chemotherapy to form the focus for subsequent redissemination. In the current series of studies careful evaluation of the primary tumor at the completion of four months of treatment is being done in order to aid our understanding of this tumor's behavior.

It is also clear that one of the limitations for the effective treatment of neuroblastoma is the limited number of agents available for use. At the time the initial treatment program was begun, only cyclophosphamide and adriamycin showed significant clinical response rates as single agents. Since that time, as mentioned above, two additional drugs have been demonstrated to be effective. There must now be a search for other new agents to be tested for singly and then in combination to build up our armamentarium of effective agents for the treatment of this tumor.

Further studies are also in order to define the relationship between the tumor cells characteristics with respect to cell proliferation and the clinical response to chemotherapy. The studies to date have certainly indicated close correlations between the biological and clinical behavior of an individual patient's tumor. Pursuit of these correlations will no doubt lead to a better understanding of the tumor and an opportunity for design of more rational and hopefully effective treatment programs.

These studies have had the gratifying result in improving treatment results for some patients with disseminated neuroblastoma. They have also provided the opportunity for important new insights into the relationships between the biological and clinical characteristics of this kind of cancer. New avenues for research have been developed and the objectives for new clinical studies defined. The work for the next years has been clearly defined.

REFERENCES

Carli, Modesto, Green, Alexander A., Hayes, F. Ann, Rivera,
    Gaston, and Pratt, Charles B.: Therapeutic efficacy of
    single drugs for childhood neuroblastoma: A review.
    Cancer Treat. Rep. (In Press).
Evans, Audrey, E., D'Angio, Giulio J., and Randolph, Judson:
    A proposed staging for children with neuroblastoma.
    Children's Cancer Study Group A. Cancer 27 (2): 374-378,
    1971.
Green, Alexander A., Hayes, F. Ann, Pratt, Charles B.,
    Evans, William E., Howarth, Cathryn B., and Senzer, Neil:
    Phase II evaluation of cisplatinum in children with neuro-
    blastoma and other solid tumors. In, Crooke, S.,
    Prestayko, A., Carter, S. (eds), Current Status and New
    Developments, Chap. 35, pp. 477-484. Academic Press, New
    York, 1980.
Hayes, F.A., Green, A.A., and Evans, W.: Treatment of
    neuroblastoma with cis-Platinum (CDDP) and VM-26: Re-
    sponse and toxicity. Proceedings of the 11th ICC and the
    19th ICAAC, 1979, pp. 1642-1643. Editors J.D. Nelson and
    C. Grassi.
Hayes, Frances Ann, Green, Alexander A., and Mauer, Alvin
    M.: Correlation of cell kinetic and clinical response to
    chemotherapy in disseminated neuroblastoma. Cancer Res.
    37: 3766-3770, 1977.
Leikin, Sanford, M.D., Evans, Audrey, M.D., Heyn, Ruth,
    M.D., and Newton, William, M.D.: The impact of chemo-
    therapy on advanced neuroblastoma. Survival of patients
    diagnosed in 1956, 1962, and 1966-68 in Children's Cancer
    Study Group A. J. Pediatr. 84 (1):131-134, 1974.
Wilson, L.M. Kinnier and Draper, G.J.: Neuroblastoma, Its
    natural history and prognosis: A study of 487 cases. Br.
    Med. J. 507:301-307, 1974.

Leukemias

Leukemia Overview

JOSEPH H. BURCHENAL, M.D.

Director, Clinical Investigation
Memorial Sloan-Kettering Cancer Center
New York, New York

This overview of leukemia will attempt to cover the progress
that has been made in the diagnosis, the understanding, and
the treatment of this group of diseases. Leukemia is, in
essence, a cancer of the blood, usually originating in the
bone marrow, with cells that can spread through the blood
stream to almost all organs. Thus, the symptoms of the disease may be protean in nature. Leukemia was first recognized
in 1845, almost simultaneously by Cragie and Bennett in
Scotland, and by Virchow in Germany. The case described by
Virchow had such a high white count that at postmortem the
blood appeared almost white. He gave it the name "weisses
blut" or leukemia. The next milestone was the description
by Lissauer in 1865 of two cases of leukemia treated with
potassium with apparently some success, that is with diminution in size of spleen and nodes with concomitant benefit to
the patient. The next outstanding advance was the development by the great Paul Ehrlich of methylene blue, followed
later by polychrome staining to differentiate the white cells
of the several different kinds of leukemia. This in turn
gave rise to the great morphologic schools under Naegli, the
discoverer of the myeloblast, and Schilling-Torgau, who first
diagnosed acute monocytic leukemia, both of whom used fixed
cell preparations of the peripheral blood, and Sabin and Doan
who used supravital staining. Schulten did much to advance
bone marrow aspiration as a diagnostic method. Prior to this
time, the leukemias had been classified as acute, with survival times of about one year, and chronic, with survivals of
two or three years and sometimes even longer. These morphologic studies also differentiated the acute from the chronic
leukemias, and then further into the lymphoid, myeloid,
erythroid and monocytic varieties. This differentiation was
of great value prognostically at that time and later for

This work was supported by NCI Grants CA-05826 and CA-18856;
ACS Grant CH-27V; and a Grant from the Hearst Foundation.

determining the appropriate form of therapy. In recent years
studies of other special markers have added a great deal more
precision to the cytological diagnosis and determination of
therapy. These will be discussed in detail later.

ETIOLOGY

As to the etiology of leukemia, it is probably multifactorial. There are a plethora of conjectures and few hard
facts. Radiation certainly increases the incidence of some
types of leukemia as demonstrated by the experience with the
early radiologists and the victims of the atomic bombing at
Hiroshima. However, it is important to note that although in
those maximally exposed in Hiroshima the incidence of leukemia increased 15-25 fold over the normal population, only one
in fifty developed leukemia. Thus, although radiation may
have triggered leukemia, it obviously was not the only factor
in these patients. The same can probably be said of the increased incidence of leukemia among benzene workers as reported by Bernard and among patients on long-term chemotherapy.

Host factors, including immunity and genetics, are also
important. Identical twins of leukemic patients have a 700-
fold increased incidence of leukemia, whereas nonidentical
siblings have only a four-fold increased incidence. It does
not appear that leukemic cells pass through the placenta
since women with overt leukemia at the time of parturition
have had normally-developing children, and women bearing
children with congenital leukemia have shown no evidence of
contracting the disease.

Patients with impaired immunity, as in Bloom's Syndrome
(350-fold) and in severe combined immunodeficiency, ataxia,
telangectasia, and the various other immunologic disorders,
show a much higher incidence of leukemia and non-Hodgkin's
lymphoma than normal individuals or individuals with normal
immune systems. It has also been noted that kidney-trans-
plant patients under continuous immunosuppression have a
higher incidence of leukemia than normal individuals.

Viruses are known to cause leukemia in mice, rats, guinea
pigs, hamsters, cats, cattle, gibbon apes, chickens, and even
pike, and ten years ago it was felt that it was only a matter
of a very short time before viruses would be found to be etiologic in human leukemia as well. To date, however, no virus
has been proven to be etiologic in leukemia. Even the
Epstein-Barr virus (EBV), which has been known for fifteen
years to be present in essentially all cases of African
lymphoma of Burkitt's type, has not been solidly confirmed as

the cause of Burkitt's lymphoma, although it may well be a
necessary factor along with holo-endemic malaria in the development of the disease. On the other hand, it appears to
have been proven that the EB virus in America and Europe is
the causative agent of infectious mononucleosis, a self-
limiting, leukemia-like disease in young adults.[33] The recent studies of Kaplan et al.[34] have demonstrated C-type
particles in certain lymphomas, but, again, the etiological
significance remains obscure.

ACCESSION OF NEW AGENTS

In the treatment of the leukemias, it is natural that the
chronic leukemias with their high counts and slower courses
were the ones that were most studied (Fig. 1). Chronic myelocytic leukemia responded particularly well to potassium
arsenite, as previously mentioned and as demonstrated in
studies repeated in 1934 by Forkner, to benzene, as reported
by Kalapos and Korenyi, and to urethane, as reported by
Haddow in 1945. Some improvement in chronic lymphocytic
leukemia was also noted with these agents, but the primary
effect was in reducing the count and spleen size of patients
with chronic myelocytic leukemia. The development of the

ACCESSION OF AGENTS FOR TREATMENT OF LEUKEMIA

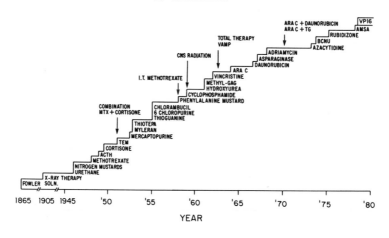

Figure 1

alkylating agents such as the nitrogen mustards in World War
II gave compounds which were shown by Goodman, Wintrobe, et
al.[28] to be highly effective in lowering the counts, decreasing the size of the spleen in chronic myelocytic leukemia,
and of lymph nodes also in chronic lymphocytic leukemia.
The development of the orally available effective derivatives
such as chlorambucil, myleran, and the ethyleneimino compound
TEM, made the treatment of these diseases by a chronic, gradual administration of drug much more effective and pleas-
ant.[25,29,49] These have continued as the mainstays of the
treatment of these two chronic forms of leukemia up to the
present time.

In the treatment of acute leukemia, the nitrogen mustards
were able to reduce the count in most patients with high
counts and perhaps reduce the splenomegaly and lymphadenopathy, but there was no improvement in the levels of platelets
or hemoglobin, or a return of normal leukocyte picture. The
great progress in the treatment of acute leukemia was started
by the discovery by Farber et al.[20] that aminopterin, the
4-amino antagonist of folic acid, would produce temporary,
complete remissions in both the peripheral blood and bone
marrow of children with acute lymphocytic leukemia. Eventually, however, resistance developed and the patients succumbed to the disease. Shortly thereafter, the pituitary
hormone ACTH and the adrenal corticosteroid cortisone (compound E) were both shown to produce very rapid remissions in
acute leukemia, but again these were temporary. The steroids,
however, could produce remissions in children whose disease
had become resistant to the folic acid antagonist. In 1953,
it was demonstrated that children and occasionally adults
with acute leukemia could be induced into remission with a
purine antagonist, 6-mercaptopurine,[12] and shortly thereafter
by the related compounds 6-chloro-purine and thioguanine.[42]
These complete remissions (CR) could be achieved not only in
untreated patients, but in those resistant to folic acid antagonists and steroids.

The years between 1955 and 1965 were a time of regrouping.
New agents were being developed both in industry and in the
tremendous screening program of the Cancer Chemotherapy National Service Center which was now in full-swing. The first
development was cyclophosphamide by Brock in 1958.[8] This new
alkylating agent, which is inactive as an alkylating agent
until the phosphamide linkage in the ring is broken by a
phosphamidase, was supposed to be contained particularly in
the cancer cell. Actually, it now appears that cyclophosphamide is activated by the liver, but, regardless of the rationale, cyclophosphamide seemed to have unique properties in

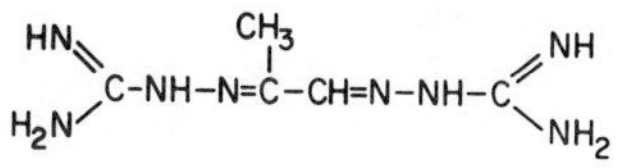

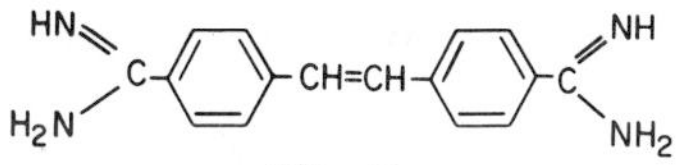

Methylglyoxal bis (guanylhydrazone)

Stilbamidine

Figure 2.   Chemical Structures of Methyl-GAG & Stilbamidine.

that it would produce remission in acute leukemia in children
which other alkylating agents rarely did.   This was followed
in 1960 by a series of alkaloids derived from the shrub Vinca
rosea, discovered by Nobel and Johnson and their groups.
The first of these was vinblastine which was shown by Armstrong et al.[2] to have a marked effect in lymphomas, but did
not appear to be particularly active against other forms of
leukemia.   A derivative of this, vincristine, in 1962, proved
extremely valuable in the treatment of leukemia in that it
would induce remissions without producing leukopenia or
thrombocytopenia, and exerted most of its toxicity on the
peripheral nervous system.[50]   At about that time, methyl-
glyoxal bis (guanylhydrazone) (Methyl GAG) (Fig. 2) was reported by Freireich et al.[23] (1962) to be very active in acute
non-lymphocytic leukemia, producing CR in 9/18 patients.
In a cooperative group study, however, the toxicity was so
great as to make it very difficult to use, and it has not
achieved the prominence it might deserve if it were carefully
studied clinically, particularly in combination with various
anti-cancer agents.   In that regard it is of interest (Fig.3)

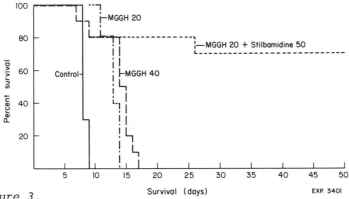

SYNERGISTIC EFFECTS OF METHYLGLYOXAL BIS (GUANYLHYDRAZONE)
(MGGH) AND STILBAMIDINE AGAINST LEUKEMIA L 1210

DOSE IN MG/KG GIVEN DAYS 1-10 ip

Figure 3.

that its activity, even at low doses, against mouse leukemia
L1210 was markedly potentiated by nontoxic doses of stilbamidine and hydroxystilbamidine, drugs with antileishmanial but
no antileukemic activity.[14] Studies presently in progress
suggest some potentiation also with pentamidine, a more
available derivative. In view of the resurgence of interest
in methyl-GAG, new knowledge about its pharmacology in man,
and its proven activity in HD, NHL, lung and esophageal cancer, its antileukemic activity should be again studied clinically, either alone or in combination with one of the diami-
dine compounds such as stilbamidine or pentamidine. Arabinosyl cytosine (ara-C), an analog and antagonist of deoxycytidine, was shown to be active in mouse leukemias in 1964 by
Evans et al.,[19] and later in patients with acute leukemia.
After various changes in scheduling and dosage by Ellison in
1968,[18] this compound turned out to be the mainstay of the
treatment of acute non-lymphocytic leukemia, particularly in
adults. Two compounds which are inhibitors of ribonucleoside
reductase and demonstrate good activity against mouse leukemias are guanazole and hydroxyurea. Guanazole, when tried in
Phase I and II studies in patients, did not appear to have
antileukemic activity, but hydroxyurea has demonstrated activity in chronic myelocytic leukemia,[36] and has been used also
in combination with other agents as maintenance therapy in
ANNL. Azacytidine, an analog of cytidine, was also discovered about this time by Piskala and Sorm (1964), but its use
in leukemia required a great deal of scheduling studies since
its therapeutic index is relatively low.[35] A close derivative,
pseudoisocytidine, which could be called 1-deaza-5-azacyti-
dine, has shown activity in experimental leukemias,[11] and because of its chemical structure was thought to be much more
stable and much less likely to give toxic decomposition
products. In patients, however, hepatic toxicity was seen
before doses were reached which could demonstrate antileukemic activity. It is now being restudied in other combinations which may allow it to be given in lower doses and still
exert its antileukemic effect. The discovery of the clinical
antileukemic and antitumor activity of the anthracycline compounds daunorubicin (1967),[51,3] adriamycin (1970),[6,52] and rubidazone (1975), added another extremely important group of
antileukemic agents. A series of acridine derivatives synthesized by Cain produced the clinically useful 4'-(9-acrid-
inyl-amino)methanesulfon-m-anisidide (AMSA) with which remissions have been achieved in ANNL both alone[37] and as a replacement for daunomycin in combination with ara-C and thioguanine.[1] The chemically modified podophyllotoxin alkaloids
VM26 and VP16 have shown high activity in mouse leukemia both

alone and in combination with other agents. VM26 has been
reported to show some activity in acute monocytic leukemia.
VP16 has been reported of value in combination with azacytidine in the treatment of ara-C-refractory ANNL.[40] Because
of its excellent activity both alone and in combination with
ara-C or cis platinum dichloro diammine (PDD) in mouse leukemia and clinically in oat cell carcinoma of the lung and
other solid tumors, VP16 deserves a more thorough study in
combinations in acute leukemia.

RESULTS OF THERAPY IN THE 1950's

The different types of agents discovered since 1955 with
different mechanisms of action and no cross-resistance laid
the foundation for effective combination chemotherapy, first
in ALL, and more recently and with somewhat less spectacular
results in ANNL. It might be worthwhile to pause a moment
and see what had been actually accomplished by the late
1950's when acute leukemia was generally considered to be
hopelessly incurable. In 1963, a survey was begun under the
aegis of the Acute Leukemia Task Force of all hematologists
in the American Society of Hematology and the International
Society of Hematology to find out how many patients with a
proven acute leukemia had survived five or more years with
or without evidence of disease. By 1965, records had been
received on 108 patients, and by 1968, on 157 with bona fide
acute leukemia who had survived for over five years. Of
these 30 adults and 127 children, 103 were living and well
with no evidence of disease 5-17 years from the diagnosis
and first treatment of their disease.[10] With only one exception, these patients who were free of disease had been
treated only with methotrexate, steroids, or mercaptopurine,
or combinations thereof. With the kind cooperation of physicians all over the world, the follow-up was continued in
1971, 1976, and 1980. Of the 93 patients living and well
with no evidence of disease in 1971, by 1976 one was lost to
follow-up, three had died of leukemia 12, 15, and 19 years
after diagnosis, and three had died of unrelated causes,
leaving 86 living and well with no evidence of disease for
14-26 years. Of these, 24 had been free of disease for over
20 years. Follow-up in 1980 was made difficult by the fact
that the mortality rate was much greater among the doctors
than among the patients, but of the 61 original patients in
the 1968 and 1976 surveys who were traceable, only one was
reported to have died of leukemia and one of unrelated causes
in the intervening four years. Whether the former, who died

at 22 years was a relapse or a new induced leukemia is open
to question. The remainder are now living and well more than
18 years from the start of the disease, the longest being 30
years from diagnosis. This study was designed originally to
determine whether with the methods of chemotherapy then
available any cures of acute leukemia could be achieved.
For the numerator of 80-odd cases, there was no available
denominator, but the cure rate was roughly estimated to be
between 0.1% and 1.0%. The study did demonstrate, however,
that even with these meager tools, bona fide acute leukemia
was occasionally curable.

DEVELOPMENT OF CURATIVE THERAPY

   Building on the base of these occasional and very rare
cures, let us now trace the use of combination therapy in
the gradual progression towards the development of curative
chemotherapy in the acute leukemias. Great discoveries in
science rarely spring full-grown as Athena is said to have
done from the brow of Zeus. Rather, they usually are the
result of many small contributions from many different investigators. It is the scientist with the prepared mind
who believes in the possibility of achieving the goal who
is capable of utilizing these as building blocks.
   Originally, it took the successful chemotherapy of infectious disease to convince investigators that the curative
chemotherapy of leukemia might be possible. As has been
mentioned, testing various compounds against experimental
leukemias and tumors followed. Then, the successful palliation of various forms of clinical lymphomas and leukemias by
alkylating agents, antimetabolites, antibiotics, and plant
alkaloids, followed by the striking cures reported in two
rare diseases, choriocarcinoma by Li, Hertz, et al.,[39] and
Burkitt's tumor by Burkitt, Oettgen, Clifford, et al.,[43,44]
brought home the realization that widespread cancer could be
cured by chemotherapy alone.
   In the great majority of cancers, however, cures could
not be achieved by single-agent chemotherapy. Combination
chemotherapy in many situations had improved the results of
infectious disease chemotherapy, particularly in the septi-
cemias and in tuberculosis. Experimental studies of combination chemotherapy in animal leukemias and tumors by Skipper,
Schabel and their group at Southern Research Institute, Martin and Gelhorn at Columbia, and Goldin et al. at the National Cancer Institute, and the demonstration that many of
the various agents which all had activity against human

cancer had quite different limiting toxicity, laid the groundwork for much of the combination chemotherapy of today. The first small step in clinical combination chemotherapy, however, antedated these animal studies, and was with the combination of cortisone and aminopterin by Bernard et al. in 1951.[4] Although this combination was of value in increasing the percentage of complete remissions, it did not produce cures. The combination of mercaptopurine and azaserine had shown activity in sarcoma 180 and leukemia L1210 in mice and was tried in a selected series of 29 children with acute leukemia. In this series, 20/29 children achieved complete remissions, with an average duration of 5.8 months,[13] but further studies by Heyn et al.[32] of Acute Leukemia Group A could not demonstrate an advantage of the combination over mercaptopurine alone, although with this regimen there were a few long-term survivors. Frei, Freireich, Pinkel, Holland, et al.[21] from Acute Leukemia Group B reported in 1961 that the combination of 6-mercaptopurine and methotrexate gave a higher remission rate than either 6-mercaptopurine or methotrexate alone. The median duration of the complete remissions of the three treatments was not different (4-5 months), however, and there were no differences between the three treatment programs as regards median survival (9 months). Here again, however, long-lasting remissions were more frequent in patients receiving the combination therapy. This last observation was important, however, since this reflects the situation in mice where increased survival time (equivalent to increase in remission rate in man) is then followed occasionally by long-term survivals where the combination of drugs has been able to destroy all the leukemic cells.

With the increasing lifespan of children with acute leukemia, it became obvious to many investigators that chemotherapy which was achieving complete remission in the marrow and blood was not preventing central nervous system involvement, particularly meningeal leukemia. Previous pharmacologic studies had shown that neither methotrexate nor mercaptopurine in standard doses reached significant levels in the spinal fluid and, for that reason, Whiteside et al.[55] studied the intracisternal administration of methotrexate in dogs and then the intrathecal administration in patients. He found that by this method high levels could be achieved and tolerated in the spinal fluid and the significant levels persisted for up to six days. This therapy had a dramatic effect on leukemic meningitis, although it was much less effective in the treatment of deep-seated neurologic lesions. Intrathecal methotrexate was then regularly used by our group and others for the treatment of meningeal leukemia, but the first

randomized study of the prophylactic use in the asymptomatic
patient to prevent clinical disease was reported by Frei et
al.[22] in 1965 for the ALGB. During the first third of the
study aminopterin at 2.5 mg/M^2 was given every 28 days, but
for the remiander, 12 mg/M^2 of methotrexate was given on the
same schedule. No overall increase in duration of remission
was noted on this arm of the protocol, but meningeal leukemia
occurred significantly less frequently in these patients.
In 1959, D'Angio, Evans, and Mitus demonstrated that radiation penetrates uniformly through the tissues of the CNS and
can be expected to destroy leukemic cells in the deep peri-
vascular arachnoids as well as in the superficial arachnoids
adjacent to cerebrospinal fluid channels. This sparked the
careful studies of Pinkel[27] and his group who pioneered the
prophylactic use of cranio-spinal irradiation. He also demonstrated how much easier it was to prevent the occurrence
of meningeal leukemic infiltration in contrast to the difficulty of controlling it once it became clinically manifest.
The radiation dosage of 500 rads was first chosen because it
usually produced responses in clinically diagnosed CNS leukemia. This was later increased to 1200 rads, a dose above
that which cleared CSF pleocytosis, and finally to 2400 rads.
    As near as can be dated from the time of publication, the
dates of submission for publication, and figures on survival
given in the articles, the successful chemotherapy with a
significant percentage of cures of acute childhood leukemia
began simultaneously and independently in November, 1962,
with the work of Freireich, Karon, and Frei[24] with the VAMP
program at the National Cancer Institute, and the work of
Pinkel and collaborators[46] on the concept of "Total Therapy"
at St. Jude's Hospital in Memphis. The VAMP protocol[24] consisted of vincristine, 2 mg/M^2 IV weekly, amethopterin, 20
mg/M^2 IV q4d, 6-mercaptopurine, 60 mg/M^2 orally daily, and
prednisone, 40 mg/M^2 orally daily. This was given in 10-day
courses followed by minimum intermittent intervals of ten
days. Five such courses of therapy were given over three to
six months. Fourteen of sixteen consecutive patients admitted to this protocol between November, 1962, and May, 1963,
achieved complete clinical and hematologic remission, and
seven were still in remission one to seven months after completion of the six-month course of therapy. Here, for the
first time, was intensive intermittent combination chemotherapy using four drugs with different mechanisms of action.
The short, intensive courses were designed to cause massive
leukemic cell kill and prevent the development of resistant
cells, while the intervals between the courses allowed time
for the normal cells to recover. This protocol was followed

by BIKE which called for induction with prednisone and vincristine until remission was achieved, and then sequential maintenance courses with methotrexate, 15 mg/M^2 IV daily for five days, 6-mercaptopurine, 1000 mg/M^2 IV daily for five days, and cyclophosphamide, 1000 mg/M^2 IV in a single dose. Courses one, two and three were then repeated one more time. Thirteen of fifteen patients admitted for this protocol between May, 1963, and December, 1963, achieved complete remission. A new protocol, designated POMP, used five-day courses consisting of prednisolone, 1000 mg/M^2 IV days 1-5, vincristine, 2 mg/M^2 IV day 1, methotrexate, 7.5 mg/M^2 IV days 1-5, and 6-mercaptopurine, 500 mg/M^2 IV days 1-5. Courses were given at 5-10-day intervals until remission was achieved, and then four consolidation courses were given ten days apart followed by 12 monthly maintenance courses. Thirty-one of thirty-four patients admitted to this protocol between January, 1964, and October, 1965, achieved complete remission. Leventhal et al.[38] reviewing these 65 patients in 1975, found 10 still surviving ten-plus years. One patient had had multiple relapses; four were still in their initial remission; and five were in prolonged second remission. Thus, these protocols, between 1962 and 1965, gave 15% ten-year survivors and probably 14% cures.

Pinkel's group[46] also starting in November of 1962, used vincristine and prednisone for induction, followed by 500 rads craniospinal radiation, and maintenance with daily 6-mercaptopurine and weekly methotrexate and cyclophosphamide. A second study starting a few months later used similar induction, intensive consolidation with methotrexate, 10 mg/M^2 IV qdx3, and cyclophosphamide, 600 mg/M^2 x 1, followed by maintenance with 6-mercaptopurine, 50 mg/M^2 PO qd, methotrexate, 20 mg/M^2 IV, cyclophosphamide, 200 mg/M^2 IV, and vincristine, 1.0 mg/M^2 IV, all weekly. Early in maintenance, 1200 rads craniospinal radiation was given. Of the patients treated by Pinkel's group between 1962 and 1965, 7/41 (17%) have been in continuous remission 13-15 years from the start of treatment. Since these patients have received no further therapy for 9-12 years, they can be presumed to be cures.[47] Thus, the curative results of these two series in the period 1962 to 1965 were approximately equal.

Since that time, the development of better combinations and the discovery of new classes of antileukemic agents with differing toxicities and no cross-resistance to conventional agents have improved results enormously. An indication of the progressive improvement in survival and cure rates is shown in Hammond's compilation[31] of the results of major cooperative groups treating childhood leukemia with an increase

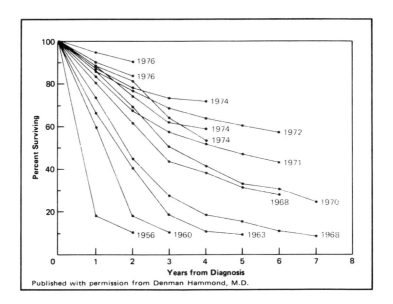

Figure 4. Combined experience of major cooperative groups treating childhood leukemia. Dates indicate when treatment began. Progressive improvement in survival with time is shown.

in four-year survival from 10% to 70% in protocols started from 1963 to 1974 (Fig. 4). The overall data from CALGB on all children treated from 1963 to 1975 shows 500 out of 2,230 children (22%) surviving without evidence of leukemia 5-17 years from the diagnosis.[26] Series confined to later years naturally show better results. Haghbin et al.[30] reported from Memorial Sloan-Kettering Cancer Center (MSKCC) that of 75 children entered on the L-2 protocol from 1969 to 1974, 40 (53%) are free of disease 6-10 years from the start of therapy. The Children's Cancer Study Group data from 1972 to 1974 show 426 out of 736 (58%) patients living with no evidence of disease from 6-8 years from the beginning of treatment.[48] Adults with ALL are generally not thought to do as well as children, but, surprisingly, the three groups of adults treated at MSKCC by Clarkson et al. with the L-2, L-10, and L-10M regimens have had a 79-85% complete remission (CR) rate and show continuous remission rates of 21%, 44%, and 58%, respectively, with median follow-ups of nine, five, and two years, respectively.[41] All these protocols differ considerably from one another, but have three main features in common: 1) induction with relatively non-marrow-suppressive agents such as vincristine, prednisone, asparaginase, and sometimes adriamycin; 2) prophylaxis of CNS leukemia with methotrexate given either intrathecally or by Ommaya reservoir in the high-count leukemias, intermittently throughout the whole course of therapy, or with craniospinal radiation or cranial radiation plus intrathecal methotrexate; and 3) maintenance therapies using mercaptopurine and methotrexate as the backbone. Oftentimes, various other agents are added, and sometimes reinduction courses of vincristine and prednisone are repeated. Most treatment regimens in ALL now last two to three years.

The situation in acute non-lymphocytic leukemia presents quite a different picture. Long-term survivors have increased since the early '60's, but are still in the 4-25% range. The percentage of complete remissions which has been achieved, however, is much higher than before, and this augurs well for a higher long-term remission rate in the future. The figures reported by Ellison for CALGB show 89 out of 2,186 patients (4%) treated before 1975 surviving in CR more than three years, and 68 (3%) surviving without evidence of disease at six years where the actuarial line plateaus.[17] A recent compilation of the SWOG figures show 54 out of 624 (9%) patients treated between 1965 and 1975 living and well without evidence of disease 5-13 years from the beginning of treatment.[16] The L-6 data of the Memorial group show 13 out of 101 (13%) patients surviving without evidence of disease from 7-10 years. Weinstein, Frei, et al., using a protocol of only 14 months duration employing early and late intensification in 83 patients with ANNL under 50 years of age (35 in the 0-17 year group, and 23 in the 18-50 year group), reported a CR of 70% with a median observation time of 12 months. Of those in CR, 40-50% by Kaplan-Meier actuarial analysis would still be expected to be in their original remission out to 4.5 years. No relapses have been seen after 28 months (14 months off therapy). Age had no significant effect on percent of CR or on duration.[54]

All these protocols, again, have something in common: most use ara-C as the backbone of treatment, and the preferred schedule seems to be five to seven days of continuous intravenous dosage at 100-200 mg/M^2. This is supplemented by two to three doses of an anthracycline, either daunorubicin or adriamycin, and often in many protocols with thioguanine given at 100 mg/M^2 twice daily again for five to seven days.

The marked improvement in the complete remission rate in
acute promyelocytic leukemia is due to the addition by Bernard[5] of an anthracycline and an anticoagulant to the regimen
which has caused the remission rate to increase tremendously
in these cases. It now remains to achieve an adequate maintenance therapy for these patients. In most protocols, intrathecal CNS prophylaxis is not given because leukemic meningitis has, so far, not been a particularly striking complication of ANNL. Maintenance, which usually lasts for a period of two to three years, is achieved by repeated courses of
the induction therapy in some cases, or in others by giving
every 3-4 weeks four or five days of a different cycle-spe-
cific agent such as methotrexate, thioguanine, or hydroxyurea
by mouth, or subcutaneous injections of ara-C followed by a
single dose of a cycle-non-specific agent such as an anthracycline, vincristine, cyclophosphamide or BCNU. Although the
results so far as long-term survivors are concerned are not
nearly as good as in childhood ALL, the gradual increase in
the percentage of complete remissions that are achieved with
therapy suggest that it is only a matter of time before the
long-term survivors and potential cures will markedly increase.

     In the meantime, however, some investigators are offering
any patient with ANNL in whom a CR is induced and who has an
HLA-matched sibling donor the choice of bone marrow transplant with no more chemotherapy instead of three more years
of fairly intensive chemotherapy. The results of the transplant program in ANNL and ALL will be discussed in detail
later in the program, but it appears that there are several
general considerations. For marrow transplants in leukemia
probably an allogeneic, HLA-matched sibling is preferable to
an identical twin, particularly in the acute lymphocytic leukemias, since it appears that a mild graft versus host reaction is also somewhat of a graft versus leukemia reaction and
may help prevent recurrence. Younger patients do better than
older ones, patients in good condition and in complete remission do better than those in relapse, and those in first
remission, at least in ANNL, and perhaps also in ALL, appear
to do better. Thomas et al.[53] report 12 out of 19 (63%) such
ANNL patients in remission 15-36 months post-transplant, and
there have been no relapses after 12 months. Similarly, CMLs
in the chronic state do better than those in the acute blast
crisis, although occasional cases which have been reinduced
into a temporary remission also do well.

     Preliminary results from the transplant group at MSKCC so
far show 16 out of 27 ANNL (59%) patients in first or second
complete remission living with no evidence of disease 2-19

months with a median of seven months post-transplant.[45]
Although it is likely that better chemotherapeutic regimens
may soon approach or surpass these figures, transplantation
in the ANNL patient under 40 appears at present to be a viable alternative to a long course of consolidation and maintenance therapies.

MARKERS

A great deal of effort has been spent in trying to correlate various features of the diseases, either clinical or
morphologic, with prognosis. A more complete discussion of
these prognostic determinants will be presented by Drs. Freireich and Miller later in the program. In children with ALL,
those in the 2-7 years age group appear to have a better
prognosis than either those younger or older than this. With
adult AML, it generally appears that the younger patient has
a better response. Another important factor in children's
ALL is the WBC, as initial WBCs under 10,000 are associated
with a good prognosis, whereas those over 50,000 show much
shorter remissions. Morphologically, the French-American-
British (FAB) classification seems to be of value in determining both prognosis and form of treatment. ALL is divided
into L-1, L-2, and L-3, with the small lymphocytic type, L-1,
being associated with a better prognosis. Fortunately, this
makes up over 80% of childhood ALL, with L-2 and L-3 being
respectively 15% and 1%.

The terminal deoxynucleotidyl transferase (TdT), a DNA-
polymerizing enzyme, is of great value in differentiating the
lymphoid leukemias from the myeloid and monocytic since it is
high in the former and low in the latter.

Immunologic markers divide ALL into T-cell, which forms
rosettes with sheep erythrocytes and against which specific
antisera can be raised, B-cell, with demonstrable surface
immunoglobulins, and null-cell, which lacks both of these
markers and is usually particularly high in TdT. The null-
cell group make up about 75% of the children's ALL, and at
least 60% have, in addition, a common ALL antigen. These
common antigen null-cells are associated with other determinants of good prognosis. Patients with T-cells often have a
high white count, sometimes with mediastinal involvement, and
have a shorter remission duration. The B-cells have the
poorest prognosis of all. Fortunately, they make up only
about 3% of the childhood ALL.

One of the oldest markers is the Ph+ chromosome in CML,
which has been used with some success to determine the

effectiveness of intensive therapy for CML in destroying the
leukemic cells. Unfortunately, the present techniques for
karyotyping are cumbersome and expensive and not sensitive
enough to show a very small percentage of surviving Ph+
cells. Attempts are being made to find monoclonal antibody
to the Ph+ cell which, if successful, might provide an im-
munofluorescent test of great sensitivity.

These markers and other prognostic indicators are of considerable value in determining the type of therapy, particularly for those leukemias for which present therapy is
adequate, and for those which require more aggressive treatment. TdT has been particularly valuable also in the acute
blast crisis of CML in separating those which are acute lymphoid from those which are acute myeloid types. The former
respond, at least temporarily, reasonably well to vincristine
and prednisone, whereas the latter require more strenuous
treatment with perhaps some combination such as AMSA, ara-C,
and thioguanine.

IN VITRO STUDIES

A great deal of work has been done with relatively short-
term cultures of bone marrow from normal and leukemia individuals, and much has been learned about the factors necessary for the growth of normal and leukemic myelopoiesis.
These studies have considerable importance in leukemia, particularly if it can be demonstrated that some of these leukemic cells retain some of the responsiveness to the hematopoietic regulators so important in the growth and differentiation of normal cells. Recent studies by Moore and his
group[41] have shown the feasibility of relatively long-term
cultures of mouse marrow, and now such cultures of the human
marrow, both normal and leukemic, should give a better opportunity to study the effect of regulators on the leukemic
cell. Of particular interest has been the demonstration by
Broxmeyer[9] and others that marrows from leukemic patients,
particularly those with acute leukemia in relapse, have a
leukemia-associated inhibitory activity (LIA) which is inhibitory to myeloid and macrophage colony formation. This LIA
has now been shown to be acidic isoferritin which inhibits
normal myeloid and macrophage growth, and which may be a normal hematopoietic regulator. It does not inhibit the growth
of leukemic cells, however, and although it may not be produced directly by the leukemic cell, the leukemic state appears somehow to stimulate its production since it is present
in high concentrations in the marrow of acute leukemics in

relapse and present only to a low degree in marrows of normal individuals or of acute leukemic patients in remission.

Permanent cell lines of human leukemic cells such as
CCRF-CEM from a child with T-cell leukemia, K562 from a patient with the acute stage of CML, and HL-60 from a patient
with promyelocytic leukemia, are all very useful in screening
new cytotoxic agents and compounds capable of stimulating
differentiation such as the retinoids. Studies of Kaplan et
al.[34] using conditioned media containing human serum have
demonstrated that it may be possible with these special techniques to get non-EBV-infected permanent cell lines started
with a greater degree of regularity, particularly those of
the lymphoid and histiocytic types. Burkitt's tumor cell
lines, infected as they usually are with EB virus, grow with
a much higher degree of regularity in permanent culture.
Leukemic cell lines free of this virus have been difficult
to grow in the past, but Kaplan et al. reported success with
cultures obtained from two of three patients with ALL using
their technique.[34]

PROSPECTS

Finally, there are many areas in leukemia research which
seem promising for further study. These include:

1. The development of new compounds with different mechanisms of action and without cross-resistance to conventional
agents.

2. Careful clinical pharmacology to determine the best
schedule of new and existing agents to avoid toxicity and
maximize therapeutic effect.

3. Development of better combination therapy by mechanism
of action, kinetic, and animal-model studies.

4. Intensive search for markers as determinants for best
form of therapy, and to give more precise quantitation of
the presence of leukemic cells, perhaps by immunofluorescence
with monoclonal antibodies.

5. Improved assay techniques for sensitivity of a given
patient's leukemic cells to a particular agent, either cytotoxic or maturation-promoting, by either *in vitro* or *in vivo*
techniques initially using intracerebral inoculation in the
nude mouse.

6. Search for new compounds or combinations which will
induce remission in ANNL without causing dangerous marrow
toxicity, as can be done in ALL with vincristine and prednisone.

7. Better therapy for the ANNL occurring after prolonged

palliative or adjuvant chemotherapy or radiotherapy, and for the blast crisis of CML.

   8. Study of maturation factors such as the retinoids *in vivo* as well as *in vitro*, particularly in acute promyelocytic leukemia since Breitman et al.[7] have shown that both the permanent line HL-60 and fresh APL marrows can be caused to mature by exposure to easily attainable levels of cis retinoic acid. These factors should also be studied in CML in the chronic stage at which time it may really be a preneoplastic state. Parenthetically, such a study is getting underway at the present time in the South-West Oncology Group. There is also a possibility, although it would seem less likely, that compounds of this sort might act to prevent relapses in other types of acute leukemia once a complete remission is induced with standard cytotoxic regimens. Retinoids or similar compounds might also be used along with adjuvant therapy in an attempt to prevent the induction of acute leukemia by such potentially leukemogenic therapy.

   9. Attempts to abrogate the LIA of acidic isoferritin on the normal elements in leukemic marrow.

   10. Further studies on the role of immunotherapy in leukemia not only with new agents, but also to determine with some of the older agents the time when immunotherapy should be given in relation to chemotherapy, either before or during therapy, or after a remission has been achieved.

   11. Wider application of bone marrow transplant by *in vitro* treatment of non-HLA-identical marrows to prevent GVH reaction. This, obviously, would make bone marrow transplants available to a much broader segment of the leukemias.

   With the increasing understanding of the leukemic process at both the basic and clinical levels, the large number of drugs with antileukemic activity already available, and the increasing development of new agents, there will be an ever accelerating number of new combinations and new forms of treatment which will speed the day when most leukemias can be controlled and patients are able to look forward to a normal life span.

REFERENCES

1. Arlin Z, Gee T, Kempin S, et al: Treatment of acute leu-
    kemia in relapse with AMSA in combination with cytosine
    arabinoside (ara-C) and 6-thioguanine (6TG). Proc Amer
    Soc Clin Onc 21:438, 1980.
2. Armstrong JG, Dyke RW, Fouts PJ, et al: Hodgkin's dis-
    ease, carcinoma of the breast, and other tumors treated
    with vinblastine sulfate. Cancer Chemother Rep 18:49,
    1962.
3. Bernard J: Acute leukemia treatment. Cancer Res 27:
    2565, 1967.
4. Bernard J, Marie J, Salet J, & Cruciani C: Essai de
    traitement des leucemies aigues de l'enfance par l'as-
    sociation aminopterin-cortisone. Bull Mem Soc Med
    Hopitaux 16:621, 1951.
5. Bernard J, Weil M, Boiron M, et al: Acute promyelocytic
    leukemia: Results of treatment by daunorubicin. Blood
    41:489-496, 1973.
6. Bonadonna G, Modfardini S, De Lena M: Phase I and pre-
    liminary phase II evaluation of adriamycin (NSC-123,127).
    Cancer Res 30:2572, 1970.
7. Breitman TR, Selonick SE, Keene BR, et al: Induction of
    differentiation of the human promyelocytic cell line
    HL-60 by retinoic acid. Proc Amer Assoc Cancer Res
    21:44, 1980.
8. Brock N, Wilmanns H: Wirkung eines zyklischen n-lost-
    phosphamidesters auf experimentell erzeugte tumoren der
    ratte: Chemotherapeutische wirksamheit und pharmakolo-
    gische eigenschaften von B518 ASTA. Dtsch Med Wochen-
    schr 83:453, 1958.
9. Broxmeyer HE, Grossbard E, Jacobsen N, & Moore MAS:
    Persistence of inhibitory activity against normal bone-
    marrow cells during remission of acute leukemia. New
    Engl J Med 301:346-351, 1979.
10. Burchenal JH: Long-term survivors in acute leukemia and
    Burkitt's tumor. Cancer 21:595-599, 1968.
11. Burchenal JH, Ciovacco K, Kalaher K, et al: Antileuke-
    mic effects of pseudoisocytidine, a new synthetic pyri-
    midine C-nucleoside. Cancer Res 36:1520-1523, 1976.
12. Burchenal JH, Murphy ML, Ellison RR, et al: Clinical
    evaluation of a new antimetabolite, 6-mercaptopurine,
    in the treatment of leukemia and allied diseases.
    Blood 8:965, 1953.
13. Burchenal JH, Murphy ML, & Tan CT: Treatment of acute
    leukemia. Pediatrics 18:643-660, 1956.

14. Burchenal JH, Purple JR, Bucholz E, & Straub PW: Poten-
    tiation of methyl-glyoxal bis(guanylhydrazone) by stil-
    bamidine in transplanted mouse leukemia. Cancer Chemo-
    ther Rep No. 29, 85089, 1963.
15. Clarkson BD: Personal communication.
16. Coltman C: Personal communication.
17. Ellison RR: Personal communication.
18. Ellison RR, Holland JF, Weil M, et al: Arabinosylcyto-
    sine, a useful agent in the treatment of acute leukemia
    in adults. Blood 32:507, 1968.
19. Evans JS, Musser EA, Bostwick L, & Mengel GD: The effect
    of 1-β-D-arabinofuranosylcytosine hydrochloride on mu-
    rine neoplasms. Cancer Res 24:1285, 1964.
20. Farber S, Diamond LK, Mercer RD, et al: Temporary remis-
    sions in acute leukemia in children produced by the
    folic acid antagonist, 4-aminopterylglutamic acid (Am-
    inopterin). New Engl J Med 238:787, 1948.
21. Frei E, Freireich EJ, Gehan, et al: Studies of sequen-
    tial and combination antimetabolite therapy in acute
    leukemia: 6-mercaptopurine and methotrexate. Blood
    18:431-454, 1961.
22. Frei E, Karon M, Levin RH, et al: The effectiveness of
    combinations of antileukemic agents in inducing and
    maintaining remission in children with acute leukemia.
    Blood 26:642-656, 1965.
23. Freireich EJ, & Frei E, III: Clinical studies of intra-
    venous methyl-glyoxal bis(guanylhydrazone) (CH$_3$GAG).
    Proc Amer Assoc Cancer Res 3:319, 1962.
24. Freireich EJ, Karon M, & Frei E: Quadruple combination
    therapy (VAMP) for acute lymphocytic leukemia of child-
    hood. Proc Amer Assoc Cancer Res 5:20, 1964.
25. Galton D: Clinical trials of p-(di-2-chloro-ethylamino)-
    phenylbutyric acid (CB 1348) in malignant lymphoma.
    Br Med J 2:1172, 1955.
26. Glidewell O: Personal communication.
27. George P, & Pinkel D: Central nervous system radiation
    in children with acute lymphocytic leukemia in remis-
    sion. Proc Amer Assoc Cancer Res 6:22, 1965.
28. Goodman L, Wintrobe M, Dameshek W, et al: Use of methyl-
    bis (B-chloroethyl)amine hydrochloride and tris (B-
    chloroethyl) amine hydrochloride for Hodgkin's disease,
    lymphosarcoma, leukemia, and certain allied and miscel-
    laneous disorders. JAMA 132:126, 1946.
29. Haddow A, & Timmis GM: Myleran in chronic myeloid leuke-
    mia: Chemical constitution and biological action. Lan-
    cet 264:207, 1953.

30. Haghbin M, Murphy ML, Tan CT, et al: A long-term clinical follow-up of children with acute lymphoblastic leukemia treated with intensive chemotherapy regimens. Cancer 46:241-252, 1980.
31. Hammond D, Chard RL, D'Angio GJ, et al: Pediatric malignancies, in Hoogstraten B (ed): Cancer Research: Impact of the Cooperative Groups. New York, Masson, 1980, pp. 1-24.
32. Heyn RM, Brubaker CA, Burchenal JH, et al: The comparison of 6-mercaptopurine with the combinations of 6-mercaptopurine and azaserine in the treatment of acute leukemia in children: Results of a cooperative study. Blood 15:350-359, 1960.
33. Henle W, & Henle G: EB virus and infectious mononucleosis. New Engl J Med 288:263-264, 1973.
34. Kaplan H, Goodenow R, Gartner S, et al: Biology and virology of the human malignant lymphomas. Cancer 43:1-24, 1979.
35. Karon M, Sieger L, Leimbrock S, et al: 5-azacytidine: A new active agent for the treatment of acute leukemia. Blood 42:359-365, 1973.
36. Kennedy BJ, Yarbro JW: Metabolic and therapeutic effects of hydroxyurea in chronic myeloid leukemia. JAMA 195:1038-1043, 1966.
37. Legha SS, Bodey GP, Keating MJ, et al: Early clinical evaluation of actidinylamino-methanedulfon-m-anisidide (AMSA) in patients with advanced breast cancer and acute leukemia. Proc Amer Soc Clin Onc 20:416, 1979.
38. Leventhal BG, Levine AS, Graw RG, et al: Long-term second remissions in acute lymphatic leukemia. Cancer 35:1136-1140, 1975.
39. Li MC, Hertz R, & Spencer DB: Effect of methotrexate therapy upon choriocarcinoma and chorioadenoma. Proc Soc Exp Biol Med 93:361, 1956.
40. Look T, Dahl G, Rivera G, et al: Effective remission induction of refractory childhood acute non-lymphocytic leukemia (ANNL) with the combination of VP16-123 (VP16) and 5-azacytidine (5AZ). Proc Amer Soc Clin Onc 21:435, 1980.
41. Moore MAS: Humoral regulation of granulopoiesis. Clin in Haemat 8:287-309, 1979.
42. Murphy ML, Tan CT, Ellison RR, et al: Clinical evaluation of chloropurine and thioguanine. Proc Amer Assoc Cancer Res 2:36, 1955.
43. Oettgen HF, Burkitt D, & Burchenal JH: Malignant lymphoma involving the jaw in African children: Treatment with methotrexate. Cancer 16:616, 1963.

44. Oettgen HF, Clifford P, & Burkitt DP: Malignant lymphoma involving the jaw in African children: Treatment with alkylating agents and actinomycin-D. Cancer Chemother Rep 28:25, 1963.
45. O'Reilly R: Personal communication.
46. Pinkel D: Five-year follow-up of "total therapy" of childhood lymphocytic leukemia. JAMA 216:648-652, 1971.
47. Pinkel D: Treatment of acute lymphocytic leukemia. Cancer 43:1128-1137, 1979.
48. Sather H: Personal communication.
49. Sykes MP, Karnofsky DA, Philips FS, et al: Clinical studies on triethylenephosphoramide and diethylenephosphoramide: Compounds with nitrogen mustard-like activity. Cancer 6:142, 1953.
50. Tan CT, & Aduna NS: Preliminary clinical experience with leurocristine in children. Proc Amer Assoc Cancer Res 3:367, 1962.
51. Tan C, Tosaka H, You KP, et al: Daunomycin, an antitumor antibiotic in the treatment of neoplastic disease. Cancer 20:333, 1967.
52. Tan C, Wollner N, King O, et al: Adriamycin, a new antibiotic in treatment of childhood leukemia and other malignant neoplasms. Proc Amer Assoc Cancer Res 11:79, 1970.
53. Thomas ED, Buckner CD, Clift RA, et al: Marrow transplantation for acute nonlymphoblastic leukemia in first remission. New Engl J Med 301:597-599, 1979.
54. Weinstein HJ, Mayer RJ, Rosenthal DS, et al: Treatment of acute myelogenous leukemia in children and adults. New Engl J Med 303:473-478, 1980.
55. Whiteside JA, Philips FS, Dargeon HW, & Burchenal JH: Intrathecal amethopterin in neurological manifestations of leukemia. Arch Intern Med 101:279, 1958.

TREATMENT OF GRANULOCYTIC LEUKEMIAS.

Jean BERNARD, Marise WEIL, Claude JACQUILLAT

Institut de Recherches sur les Leucémies et les Maladies du
Sang - Hopital Saint-Louis - 75475 PARIS CEDEX 10 - FRANCE

INTRODUCTION
In 1947, acute granulocytic leukemia was not only a fatal,
but also an irreversible and fulminant disease with a mean
duration of about 1,5 months.
In 1947, too, the achievement of the first complete remission
by exchange transfusion proved that symptoms of leukemia
could be reversed by treatment.
Achievement of remissions became then the first aim of hema-
tologist.
Aminopterin, corticosteroïds, 6-mercaptopurine which were the
first available drugs were more active in acute lymphocytic
leukemias (60% C.R.) than in acute granulocytic leukemias
(10 % C.R.). An in 1965, the mean duration of APL was still
29 days. However, at this time some improvement was already
achieved by the combination of methyl GAG and 6-MP (4). But
the modern period of the treatment of AGL opens between 1963
and 1966 with the discovery and the use of Cytarabine and
Daunorubicin (12, 21).

Progress since this time has been associated with improvement
in the administration of the drugs or their derivatives, especially in their use in combination and with improvement in
understanding and managing the complications (1).

MATERIAL AND METHODS
We have treated in our department of hematology 1 238 cases
of acute granulocytic leukemias. Repartition of age and sex
is shown on table I. All cytological examinations have been
performed in Dr. FLANDRIN's laboratory. May Grunwald Giemsa,
peroxidase stainings and specific esterase reactions have
been done in all patients. Since 1977, many patients have
had cytogenetic examinations in Dr. BERGER's laboratory.

The 3 types of classification which have been used are shown
on table II.

From the onset, we have stratified patients according to 3
subgroups. Acute myelocytic leukemias (AML), acute promyelocytic leukemias (APL), acute monoblastic leukemias (AMonoL).

SEX - AGE

	SEX		AGE		
	M	F	< 20	≥20	
A.M L.	510	483	311	682	993
A.P.L.	69	59	20	88	108
A Mono L.	67	70	51	86	137

Table 1

THE 3 TYPES OF CLASSIFICATION OF A.G.L.

CYTOLOGY 1960	FAB 1976	CYTOCHEMESTRY Peroxydases	Specific Esterases 1970	CYTOGENETIC 1977
A.M.L.	M_1 M_2	+ +		t (8 ; 21) or others A.M.L.
A.P.L.	M_3 M_4	+ +		t (15 ; 17) t (15 ; 17) ___ M_3 variants
A Mono L	M_5 M_6	+ +	+	Long arm of 11

Table 2

This tratification was based on morphological and an clinical characteristics (6,14). More recently, the FAB classification confirmed this stratification but recognized in addition other subtypes according to the level and the morphology of blasts differenciation (2).
Cytochemistry was useful under two circumstances : 1. Peroxidase activity was sometimes observed within cells apparently devoid of granulation on cytologic smears ; 2. it authentified acute monoblastic leukemias by the specific fluorid inhibited ASD Acetate esterase reaction. More recently cytogenetic findings resulted in some striking correlation between M_3 and the translocation (t15 ; 17), between M_2 and the translocation (t 8 ; 21) (30), between the long arm of chromosome 11 and the monoblastic (M_5) subtype (31). In addition, the presence of the translocation (t15 ; 17) led to the identification of M_3 variants (3).
In addition to these subtypes, some conditions include various disorders with uncertain limits and these have been described under various terms namely preleukemic syndrom, smoldering leukemia, refractory anemia with an excess of myeloblasts in the bone marrow, oligo leukemia. The distintion between oligo leukemias and some A.M.L. with differentiation (M_2) is not easy. Whenever peripheral cytopenias become dangerous for the patients, they must be considered and treated as A.M.L.. Otherwise, specially in elderly people it is better to wait since some stability may be observed in this condition. Since we are not sure that all patients with oligo leukemias have been homogeneously diagnosed, we shall exclude these cases from our analysis.
Acute granulocytic leukemia is probable a disease for which study of etiology is most rewarding. It is difficult in our material to assess with ascertainty the proportion of professional exposure to benzen or to radiation. 35 cases were diagnosed in patients previously treated by combined chemo- and radiotherapy for Hodgkin's disease.
Some othe patients heve been treated by combined radiotherapy and chemotherapy for ovarian cancer or breast cancer or by malphelan for myeloma.
Many of these secundary leukemias are preceded by a preleukemia phase and do not fit well within any category of the FAB classification. They were entered into our studies only when they were typical A.M.L., or M_3 (1 patient) or M_5 (1 patient). All these cases, whether treated or untreated, have a poor prognosis.

Since treatments have been different for A.M.L., A.P.L. (M_3)
and AMonol (M_5) we shall considere our results separatly for
these 3 subtypes.

RESULTS

A) Acute myelocytic leukemias. Table 3 shows the progress
achieved through the successive studies. Before DNR, incidence and duration of C.R. were poor despite improvements
achieved by Ara-C and by the combination of Ara-C, M.GAG,
6-MP and Prednisone. Between 1966 and 1971, DNR or various
combinations with DNR (Asparaginase, Methotrexate, short
courses of Ara-C) were given for induction and reinduction.
From 1971 to 1974, Rubidazone was given for 5 consecutive
days instead of Daunorubicin (22). During all that time,
maintenance treatment remained unchanged and included daily
6-MP, weekly MTX and periodic reinduction courses. Thus,
whereas improvement in induction rate could be ascribed to
the better availability of granulocytes transfusions as well
as to the remplacement of DNR by Rubidazone, the increase
in survivals over 3 years without relapse could be regarded
as an argument for the advantage of Rubidazone over DNR in
A.M.L.
However the 7-3 DNR Ara-C combination for induction and the
monthly cyclic courses for maintenance, first proposed by
Holland and the CALGB (20) were an indeniable improvement
since with such treatments, the relapse free survival rate
reaches 35 %. In 1976, we initiated protocol LAM 76 to compare combinations of Ara-C and DNR to Ara-C and Rubidazone.
More recently, we activated protocol LAM 79 which compares
Ara-C, Rubidazone, 6-MP and M. GAG to Ara-C, Rubidazone,
VCR and Prednisone. It is too early to have any opinion on
these quadruple combinations.
None of our protocols includes CNS prophylaxis in A.M.L.. Our
experience of meningitis in A.M.L. is the following. 7 pts
had initial meningeal involvement, 9 had simultaneous hematologic and meningeal relapses, only 3 had primary meningeal
relapses. High initial WBC count (9 pts) and undifferentiated
cells (no granulation on Romanovski stains but peroxidase po-
sitivity)(5pts) were frequently observed in these patients.

Prognosis factors in A.M.L. have already been studied by
others (11, 13, 18, 32) or by us (9, 33). Age and sex influence rate of C.R. Initial count of WBC and of platelets influence their durations. The clinical correlations of the various

PERCENTAGE OF C.R. AND OF LONG TERM C.R. ACCORDING TO PROTOCOLS IN 933 PATIENTS WITH A.M.L.

		No.Patients	C.R.		N .pts and % C.R. at 3 years	
Before AraC		276	61	22 %	7	14 %
AraC	Before 1966	31	8	26 %	2	33 %
Quadruple		48	20	42 %	2	18 %
DNR or combin. DNR	1966-1971	400	185	46 %	18	14 %
Rubidazone	1971-1974	67	38	57 %	7	23 %
DNR + AraC 3 - 7 + intermit.	1974-1976 11 LAM 74 CALGB 7521	81	47	58 %	12	36 %
DNR AraC Rubidazone ARC	14 LAM 76 1976 - 1979	90	56	62 %	2	30 % ✗
Rubidazon e - AraC	1980					
Rubidazon e + AraC + MGAG + 6 MP Rubidazon e + AraC + VCR						

Table 3   ✗ actuarial percentage

275

subtypes of the FAB classification are not yet known. Results
of induction according to these subtypes in recent homogeneously treated patients are shown on table 4.

Cytogenetic studies have been carried out successfully in
25 patients. In 9 cases all mitosis were normal, in 4 cases
all were abnormal, in 12 cases there was a mixture of normal
and abnormal mitosis : one of this patient had a secundary
A.M.L. (Hodgkin disease treated by combined chemotherapy and
radiotherapy 4 years prior to A.M.L.). We did not found the
translocation (t 8 ; 21) which is observed in about 9 % of
M_2 A.M.L. and which would have a relatively good prognosis in
contrast to other cytogenetic abnormalities (29). The implications of the poor prognosis heralded by abnormal chromosomes
in relation to persistence of normal clonogenic cells and in
relation to kinetic behaviour of leukemic clones are under
study.

B) Acute promyelocytic leukemias. Before Daunorubicine, APL
deserved to be considered as "very acute leukemias" (5) ;
short remissions had been observed only in 3 children ; all
other patients died within the first 6 weeks from hemorrhages.
Table 5 indicates our progress.

For reasons which have never been clearly understood, DNR is
specially active on this variety and 46 % C.R. were achieved
in the first 31 patients (7). Analysis of remissions deaths
showed that half of them occured within the first 5 days of
treatment at a time of maximum cellular lysis : the thrombo-
plastic activity of malignant promyelocytes explains the
link between cellular lysis and DIC which has been recognized
as the main factor of these hemorrhages. Now these hemorrhages are prevented in almost all patients by the simultaneous
onset of Daunorubicine 2 mg/kg for 5 consecutive days, heparin 1,5 mg/kg and high doses platelets transfusions, 8 units/
m2 every 12 hours. This triple combination is considered as
an emergency treatment in our department.
Induction results according to age are shown on table 6.
There is a continuous increase in the incidence of induction
deaths with years of age. Otherwise, initial WBC count, initial platelets count have no influence. Initial fever in our
experience has no predictive value except when it is associated with pulmonary infections.
Duration of C.R. according to treatment is shown of figure 1.
For patients treated after DNR, the rate of C.R. is over 46 %
at 3 years for all patients.

CORRELATION BETWEEN FAB CLASSIFICATION AND INDUCTION RESULTS IN PROTOCOL 14 LAM 76

	C.R.	P.R.	Failures	Induc. Death	Total
M_1	11 (52,38 %)	1	6	3	21
M_2	17 (77.27 %)	2	3		22
M_3		1			1
M_4	11 (50 %)	1	4	6	22
M_4Eo	6				6
Erythrol.	4		1		5 / 77 pts

Table 4

ACUTE PROMYELOCYTIC LEUKEMIAS

	C.R.	Failures	Induction deaths	Total
Before Daunorubicine	3 (8 %)	9	24	36
Daunorubicine	13 (46 %)		15	31
Daunorubicine and systemat. Heparin	33 (75 %)		11	44

Table 5

277

	≤ 10	≤ 20	≤ 40	≤ 60	> 60
Total	8	6	19	30	9
C.R. % C.R.	7 (87 %)	5 (83 %)	13 (72 %)	18 (62 %)	3 (33 %)
Resistance	-	-	-	-	-
Induc. death	1	1	6	12	6

Table 6

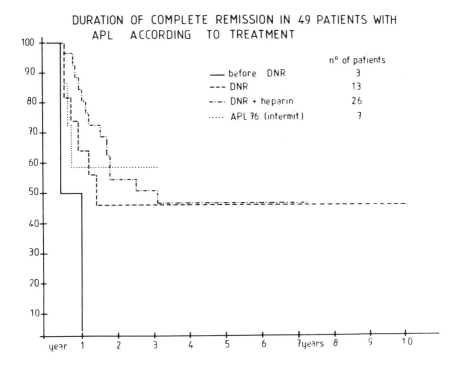

DURATION OF COMPLETE REMISSION IN 49 PATIENTS WITH APL ACCORDING TO TREATMENT

n° of patients

—— before DNR 3
--- DNR 13
-·-· DNR + heparin 26
····· APL 76 (intermit.) 7

Fig. 1

278

Since 1976, we have replaced continuous maintenance with rein-
ductions by monthly courses of Ara-C combined to DNR, 6-MP
or Cyclophosphamide. This strategy did not prevent the frequent first year relapses.
Age and sex, initial WBC and platelets counts do not influence duration of C.R. in A.P.L. Cytogenetic examinations
(table 7) were performed in 8 of these patients ; in 5 cases
translocation (t 15 ; 17) was observed : 3 patients died in
induction, 1 had a 10 months remission and the 5th is in C.R.
for 11 months. For the 3 patients without cytogeneric abnormality, results were the following : 1 induction death, 1
22 months survival, 1 patient in C.R. for more than 24 months.
In addition, this translocation (t 15 ; 17) was observed in
4 other patients not identified as A.P.L. at the first examination. These variants are characterized by high WBC count
(mean 117.000/mm3) and differ from other A.P.L. by their cytologic morphology : most cells are devoid of granulations
at the Romanovski stain but are strongly peroxidase positive.
Less than 5 % of the cells are hypergranular with "fagot"
Auer bodies. The translocation was present in all cells. Prognosis was very poor since a short C.R. (4 months) was achieved in but one patient.
It is possible that cytogenetic studies will help to recognize intermediates between M2 type and the typical M3 type that
we have exclusively considered as A.P.L. up to now (3).

In typical A.P.L., hematologic relapses may reproduce the
initial cytologic picture with hypergranular cells : in other
patients, cells are undifferenciated at relapses : in these
2 categories survival after relapses in short (median 2
months) ; 4 patients died in C.R. from infections (2 pts),
suicide (1 pt), liver fibrosis probably due to Methotrexate
(1 pt).
We may conclude that we still ignore the prognostic parameters of typical A.P.L. but we may suspect that factors related to drug activation are especially important in this disease.

C) Acute monoblastic leukemias. 137 patients have been diagnosed as AMonol. by cytologists but since 1970 the diagnosis
 was confirmed by cytochemistry (14, 28). Over all results
are shown on table 8.
Before 1970, various treatments had been tried and prognostic
was poor in most patients. In 30 pts treated by DNR or its
combination, a high rate of induction deaths were observed :

A.P.L.

CYTOGENETIC DATA

	A.P.L. M$_3$		Variant (?)
t (15 ; 17)	5 3 : death during induction 1 : 10 m C.R. 1 : 10 m C.R.	4	3 : induction deaths 1 : 4 m C.R.
no cytogenetic abnorm.	3 1 : induction death 1 : > 22 m C.R. 1 : > 24 m C.R.		

Table 7

RATE OF C.R. ACCORDING TO TREATMENT IN ACUTE MONOBLASTIC LEUKEMIA

	C.R.	P.R.	Failures	Induc. deaths	Total
Before 1970	8 (19 %)	2	18	14	42
DNR or combinations with DNR	12 (40 %)	2	5	11	30
Rubidazone	42 (73 %)	1	5	9	57
Combinat. with Rubidazone	7 (87 %)			1	8

Table 8

280

some were due to early renal failure due to hyperuricemia
and possible lysosomial nephropathy. Because of its progressive action, Rubidazone in 1972, brought a significant improvement of the induction treatment(8). However in 1975 and in
1976, we insisted on the shortness of C.R., on the relatively
high incidence of leukemic meningitis and of skin and gums
infiltrations. Since 1976, CNS prophylaxis (skull irradiation
and 6 intrathecal Methotrexate injections) is undertaken once
C.R. is achieved. In addition intermittent monthly courses
combining Ara-C to Rubidazone, 6-MP, Cyclophosphamide or VCR
has replaced continuous maintenance.

Despite the progress that are reflected on the survival figures for all patients (fig. 2), too many relapses occur during
the first year. Therefore in our last protocol, we try to in-
tensify induction treatment by adding to Rubidazone, Ara-C
and VM 26 or Ara-C, 6-MP and M.GAG. Results are not yet available. We have already indicated that there was no prognostic
factor for induction results. As shown on figure 3, initial
WBC counts have a significant influence on remissions durations in acute monoblastic leukemia. Duration of C.R. are
also influenced by age and children have a worse prognosis
than adults. This may be related to the fact taht 64 % children (18 / 28) had over 20.000 WBC/mm3 in contrast to 46 %
adults (19 / 41).
Cytogenetic studies have been performed in 8 patients. Abnormalities of the long arm of chromosome 11 were observed in 5
of the 6 patients who had "undifferentiated" monoblasts and
in none of the 2 who had differenciated cells (table 9).

LONG TERM REMISSION
It has been claimed (Powles) that there were no cures in
acute granulocytic leukemias and that bone marrow allograft
was the only chance for relapse free survival. We have gathered the records of the 71 patients who had at least 3 years
relapse free survival. Their evolution after 3 years is summarized on table 10.

A conservative approximation would be that once C.R. is
achieved the rate of 3 years disease free survival is 25 % in
A.M.L., 45 % in A.P.L. and 30 % in AMonol. Among these patients 80 % of A.M.L. , 100 % of A.P.L. may be cured. Our
experience of 3 years C.R. in AMonoL is too recent for long
term predictions. These data are summarized on table 11.

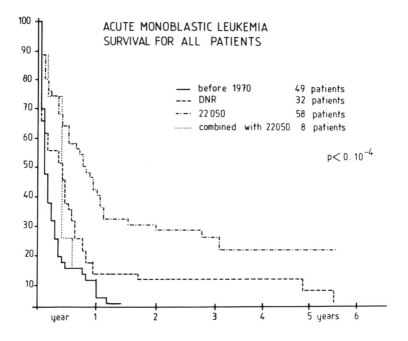

Fig. 2

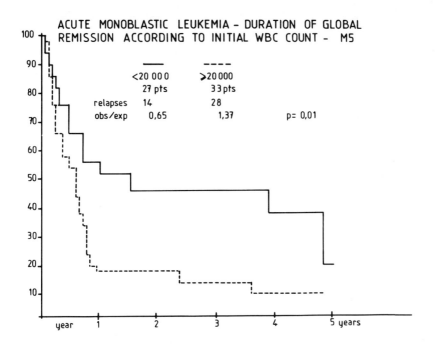

Fig. 3

CYTOGENETIC ABNORM. IN A MONO L

ABNORMAL LONG ARM OF CHROMOSOME 11

M$_5$1	5	1
M$_5$2	-	2

Table 9

LONG TERM RESULTS IN A.G.L. (71 patients)

	No. at 3 years	Late relapses	Remission death	Still surviving
A M L	49	9	3	37
A P L	16	-	1	15
A mono L	6	1		5
Total	71	10	4	57

Table 10

PROBABILITY FOR CURES IN AML, APL and A mono L

	Rate of 3 years relapse free survival	Probability for cure
A.M.L.	30 %	80 %
A.P.L.	45 %	100 %
A mono L	30 %	?

Table 11

284

DISCUSSION

These results are both useful and poor with so many patients
still dying. To obtain better results, 3 ways of research
may be explored :
1°) the first way, the most orthodox is the way of chemotherapy : a) by the preparation of new drugs belonging to
series already known (new anthracyclins , new Ara-C),
or really new (Amsa, ellipticins) ,
b) by a better knowledge of the mechanism of this effect,
c) by a better use of the drugs according to the variety
of the disease as suggested by Freireich.
We strongly believe in the specificity of the treatment,
in the importance of efforts in these direction. Already
the effects of DNR in A.P.L. of Rubidazone in AMonol are
good models. And the recent progress of cytogenetic
studies support this hypothesis.

2°) the second way is represented by the methods, different
from chemotherapy and already tried. Immunotherapy is
unfortunately a failure for the present time. But it may
be hoped that a better knowledge of the immunology of
leukemia will inspire in the future new development. Bone
marrow transplantation is at the present time, very promising.
Dr. Thomas will to morrow discuss his remarkable results.
It will be very important in the near future to compare
the results of chemotherapy the results of bone marrow
transplantation not in general but in each prognostic
group of A.M.L.
It will be important to increase the possibilities of
bone marrow transplantation, using HLA non compatible
donors, and to diminish the dangers of GVH.

 3°) But a third way exists, the way of unexpected,
unexplored fields. We must not forget our ignorances.

The leukemic cell is immortal and anarchic. But we do not
know the biophysic, biochemical basis of anarchy, of
immortality. We do not what are, where are the quiescent
cells described or postulated by Bessis and myself 20 years
ago.
The truth, the complete victory may come from these unexpected fields. A good rule, a good direction for researchs has
been given by our poet Paul Claudel "Ne cherche pas l'eau,
cherche la soif". Do not seek water, seek thirst.

REFERENCES

1 - BALKWILL F.R., OLIVER R.T.D.
Remission in acute leukemia. Lancet, 1979, 2,n°8149
pp 961-962

2 - BENNET J.M., CATOVSKY D., DANIEL M.Th.,FLANDRIN G.,
GALTON D.A., GRALNICK H.R., SULTAN CI. Proposale for
the classification of the acute leukaemia (FAB cooperative group). Brit. J.Haemat., 1976, 33, 4, 452-458

3 - BENNET J.M., CATOVSKY D., DANIEL M.Th., FLANDRIN G.,
GALTON D.A.G., GRALNICK H.R., SULTAN C1. A variant form
of hypergranular promyelocytic leukaemia (M3). Brit.J.
Haemat., 1980, 44, 1, 169-170

4 - BERNARD J., BOIRON M., JACQUILLAT Cl., WEIL M.,
Premiers résultats de l'association de Methyl-glyoxal
bis (Guanyl Hydrazone) et de 6 Mercaptopurine dans le
traitement des leucémies de la série granulocytaire
Presse Med., 1964, 72, 807

5 - BERNARD J., BOIRON M., LORTHOLARY P. et al.
The very acute leukemias. Cancer Res., 1965, 25, 457-459

6 - BERNARD J., MATHE G., BOULAY J., CEOARA B. et CHOME J.
La leucose aigue à promyélocytes. Etude portant sur
20 observations. Schweiz. Med. Wschr., 1959, 89, 604

7 - BERNARD J., WEIL M., BOIRON M., et al. Acute promyelocytic leukemia ; results of treatment by Daunorubicin
Blood, 1973, 41, 489-496

8 - BERNARD J., WEIL M., FLANDRIN G. et al. Clinical study
of acute monoblastic leukemia.
Proc. Am. Soc. Clin. Oncology, 1975, 16, 201

9 - BERNARD J., WEIL M., JACQUILLAT Cl., Prognostic factors
in human acute leukemias, in Fliedner TM, Perry S (eds).
Advances in the Biosciences Pergamon Press, 1975, vol14
pp 97-121

10 - BESSIS M. et BERNARD J. Remarquables resultats du traitement par exanguino-transfusion d'un cas de leucémie
aigue. Bull. Mém. Soc.Med.Hôp. Paris, 1947,63,28 et 871.

11 - CURTIS J.E.,TILL J.E., et al. Comparison of out-comes
and prognostic factors for two groups of patients with
acute myeloblastic leukemia. Leukemia Research, 1979
3,n°6, pp 409-416

12 - ELLISON R.R., HOLLAND J.F,, WEIL M., JACQUILLAT Cl.,
BOIRON M., BERNARD J., SAWITSRI A., ROSNER F., QUSSOF R.
SILVER R.T., KARANAS A., CUTTNER J., SPURR C.L., MAYES
D.M., BLON J., LEONE L.A., HAURANI F., KYLE R.,
HUTCHISON J.F., FORCIER R.J. and MOON J.H. Arabinosyl
Cytozin, a useful agent in the treatment of acute leu-
kemia in adults. Blood, 1968, 32, 507

13 - ELLISON R.R., WALLACE H.J., MOAGLAND H.D. et al. Prognostic parameters in acute myelocytic leukemia as seen
in the acute leukemia group B, in Fliedner TM, Perry S
(eds). Advances in the Biosciences. Pergamon Press, 1975
vol 14, pp 51-59

14 - FLANDRIN G., DANIEL M.Th., BLANCHET P. et al. Les leucémies aigues monocytaires. Situation clinique et pro-
nostique actuelle à la lumière des techniques de déter-
mination des estérases spécifiques. Nouv. Rev, Fr.
Hématol., 1969, 9, 65-86.

15 - FREIREICH E.J., Grounds for optimism in treating acute
granulocytic leukemia (adult acute leukemia). A look at
the data. Arch. Int. Med., 1976, 136, n° 12, 1375-1376

16 - FREIREICH E.J., KEATING M.F., GEHAN E.A., Mc URADIN K.R.
BODEY J.P. and SMITH T. Therapy of acute myelogenous
leukemia.   1978, 42, 874

17 - GALE R.P., Advances in the treatment of acute myelogenous leukemia. New England J.Med., 1979, 300, 21,1189-99

18 - GALTON D.A.G. Can remission duration be prolonged in
acute myeloid leukaemia ? Stragegies in clinical hematology. Ed.by R. GROSS K.P. HELLRIEGEL Berlin, Springer
Verlag, 1979, 55-62

19 - GUTTERMAN J.U., HERSH E.M., RODRIGUEZ V. et al. Chemo-
     immunotherapy of adults acute leukemias. Lancet, 1974,
     2, 1405-1409

20 - HOLLAND J.F., GLIDEWELL O., ELLISON R.R., COREY R.,
     SCHWARTZ J., WALLACE J., HOAGLAND C., WIERNIK P., RAI K.
     BEKESI G., CUTTNER J. Acute myelocytic leukemia. Arch
     Inter. Med., 1976, 136, 1377-1381

21 - JACQUILLAT Cl., BOIRON M., WEIL M., TANZER J., NAJEAN Y.
     BERNARD J., Rubidomycin, a new agent active in the treat-
     ment of acute leukemia. Lancet, 1966, 11, 27

22 - JACQUILLAT Cl., WEIL M., GEMON M.F., IZRAEL V., SCHAISON
     G., BOIRON M., BERNARD J. Treatment of acute myeloblas-
     tic leukemia with RP 22 050. Brit. Med. J., 1972, IV,468

23 - PEGORARO L., ABRAHM J., COOPER R.A., LEVIS A., LANGE G.
     MEO P. and ROVIEKA Q. Differentiation of human leukemias
     in response to 12-0 Tetradecanoyl phorgol. 13. Acetate
     in vitro. Blood, 55, 5, 859-862

24 - POWLES R. Immunotherapy for acute myelogenous leukemia
     using irradiated and unirradiated leukemia cells.
     Cancer, 1974, 34, 1558-1562

25 - POWLES R.L., MOGENSTERN G. et al. The place of bone-
     marrow transplantation in acute myelogenous leukaemia.
     Lancet, 1980, n° 8177, 1047-1050

26 - SACHS L. Control of growth and differentiation in normal
     and malignant white blood cells. E.W. GELFAND H.M. DOSCH
     Bio. of immunodeficiency, New York Kraven Press, 1980
     15-23

27 - THOMAS E.D.L. Marrow transplantation for acute leukemia.
     Cancer, 1978, 42, n° 2, suppl. 895-900.

28 - TOBELEM G., JACQUILLAT Cl.,CHASTANG Cl., AUCLERC M.F.
     LECHEVALLIER T., WEIL M., DANIEL M.Th. , FLANDRIN G.
     HAROUSSEAU J.L., SCHAISON G., BOIRON M. and BERNARD J.
     Acute monoblastic leukemia. A clinical and biological
     study of 74 cases. Blood., 1980, 55, 71-76

29 - 1st International Workshop on chromosomes in leukemias. Chromosomes in acute non lymphocytic leukaemias. Brit. J. of Haemat., 1978, 34, 311

30 - 2 nd Internat. Workshop on chromosomes in leukemias. Cytogenetic, morphologic and clinical correlations in acute non lymphocytic leukemia with t (8 q- ; 21 q t). Cancer Genet. Cytogenet. , 1980, 2.

31 - 2nd Internat. Workshop on chromosomes in leukemias. Morphological analysis of A.P.L. (M3) and t (8 ; 21) cases. Cancer Genet. Cytogent., 1980, 2

32 - VAUGHAN W.P., KARP J.E. et al. Long chemotherapy free remissions after single-cycle timed-sequential chemotherapy for acute myelocytic leukemia. Amer. J. Med., 1980 68, n° 3, 859-865

33 - WEIL M., JACQUILLAT Cl., GEMON-AUCLERC M.F., CHASTANG Cl. IZRAEL V., BOIRON M, BERNARD J. Acute granulocytic leukaemias. Treatment of the disease. Arch. Intern. Med., 1976, 13, 1389-1395

Prognostic Factors in Acute Leukemia

Emil J Freireich, M.D*, Edmund Gehan, Ph.D**,
Michael Keating, M.D*, Kenneth McCredie, M.D*, and
Gerald P. Bodey, M.D*

*Department of Developmental Therapeutics
**Department of Biomathematics
The University of Texas System Cancer Center
Houston, Texas

Complete hematological remissions were observed rarely in adults with acute leukemia prior to 1967. The discovery of the antileukemic activity of the anthracycline antibiotics and cytosine arabinoside has been followed by progressive improvement such that over two-thirds of the patients treated achieve remission in virtually every center in the country. The patients who fail to respond to chemotherapy are benefited little if at all. The survival post diagnosis of these patients is extremely unfavorable and approximates the survival of patients treated prior to 1967. Further progress in chemotherapy can be approached in two ways. We can continue to pursue new treatments in patient groups assigned either at random or by some stratification procedure to a proposed new treatment and to conventional treatment and continuously seek to select treatments which are most effective for the average patient. This method is both inefficient and ineffective. It is clear to every experienced therapeutic scientist that there are obvious differences between the groups of patients who respond to therapy and those who do not. What has in the past been lacking is an objective quantitive method for evaluating those factors which influence the probability of response and converting that knowledge into a form which can influence the choice of treatment for patients. In this paper we will discuss the use of multivariate statistical methods to create logistic regression equations which allow estimates of probability of response for each patient. Having constructed such models, it becomes necessary to prospectively evaluate the model and, should the model prove to be effective at predicting responsive patients, it should then be extremely useful in prescribing treatment. Patients with a high probability of response to conventional treatment should receive conventional treatment, while patients who have low probabilities of response would have a better chance of response to a proposed new treatment, and this could be compared to the expectations derived from the model.

To generate a data base for construction of a model, we have studied a group of 325 consecutive patients treated at our center between March, 1973, and March, 1977. For this group of patients, the porportion who achieved a complete remission was 65%. A total of 21 separate factors were found to be significantly predictive for response. However, there was significant interaction between variables and therefore a stepwise regression analysis was conducted to identify the contribution of each variable additional to the most highly correlated variables.

TABLE 1

LOGISTIC REGRESSION ANALYSIS
RELATING REMISSION AT ONE YEAR TO PRE-TREATMENT CHARACTERISTICS

CHARACTERISTIC	REGRESSION COEFFICIENT	MAX. LOG LIKELIHOOD	P	PROBABILITY OF 1 YR. CR FAVORABLE*	UNFAVORABLE**
Constant	.002	-99.80			
Eos./promyelocytic	-2.209	-94.65	<.01	.88	.45
Days to <10% infilt.	- .865	-90.82	<.01	.64	.24
AML	1.828	-86.55	<.01	.62	.21
Differentiation ratio	1.197	-82.37	<.01	.62	.33

This analysis revealed six variables which significantly contributed information to improving the prediction of response. The six variables are listed in the order in which they appeared in the stepwise regression. With this data, it becomes possible to construct a logistic regression equation, as a linear function of the patient characteristics. The model can be validated first by calculating probability of response for each patient who contributed data to the model, that is, the original 325 patients. Table 2 shows groupings of patients according to the predicted probability of response and these predictions are compared to the observed outcomes, and there is noted to be an excellent correspondence. The chi-square statistic is nowhere near statistical significance.

TABLE 2

OBSERVED RESPONSE RATES BY PREDICTIONS BASED ON MODEL
FOR THE 325 PATIENTS FROM WHICH THE MODEL WAS DERIVED

Predicted Prob. of CR	Number of Patients	Number Responding (%)		Expected No. Responding
0 - .19	33	5	(15)	4.0
.20 - .39	52	14	(27)	15.9
.40 - .59	60	32	(53)	32.4
.60 - .79	58	45	(78)	42.4
.80 - 1.0	97	85	(88)	86.2

$$X^2 = .65$$
$$P = .96$$

The model can then be evaluated prospectively. For the next 107 patients to enter our institution, similar chemotherapy was administered. The probability of response was computed prior to the administration of therapy and the predictions were compared to outcomes as shown in Table 3.

TABLE 3

COMPARISON OF OBSERVED AND PREDICTED RESPONSES
WHEN THE REGRESSION MODEL WAS APPLIED TO
107 RECENTLY TREATED PATIENTS

Predicted Prob. of CR	Number of Patients	Number Responding (%)		Expected No. Responding
0 - .19	14	3	(21)	1.9
.20 - .39	18	5	(28)	5.4
.40 - .59	21	11	(52)	11.2
.60 - .79	25	20	(80)	18.3
.80 - 1.0	29	25	(86)	25.7

$$X^2 = .83$$
$$P = .94$$

Cox's Test of Agreement Between Observed and Predicted Probabilities

Translation:	T = 64.0	E(T) = 62.5	P = .73
Dispersion:	T = 7.6	E(T) = 8.2	P = .79

The data reveal that the model functioned in an outstanding fashion, showing excellent correspondence between predictions and outcomes. Thus, this methodology has been validated and should prove effective for assigning new treatment. In our clinic, patients with a probability of response estimated to be less than .40, that is, an average of 20% of patients predicted to respond to treatment, are given candidate new therapy, and the outcomes are evaluated by comparing results to the predictions. In contrast, favorable patients with predicted probabilities above .40, that is, an average probability of .70, receive conventional treatment since the probability of response is so favorable.

When patients achieve complete remission, there is again a wide spectrum of outcomes. Almost half the patients relapse within the first year following onset of complete remission. A quarter remain disease free for more than two years, and between 15 and 20% have prolonged survivorship beyond three years. A significant question in cancer treatment is the choice of appropriate treatment for a patient in remission. It has been established that bone marrow transplantation, as support for total body radiation and cyclophosphamide chemotherapy, is highly effective when administered to patients in relapse. Further, without further therapy the majority of patients will recur promptly. Thus, treatment in remission is clearly indicated. Conventional maintenance chemotherapy again can be highly effective in some and virtually ineffective in others. We therefore applied similar analysis to the generation of a model for prediction of the duration response for patients who achieve remission.

In this instance, the factors which appear are substantially different from those features which predict for probability of response (Table 4). Again, application of this model to the data base from which it derived shows excellent correspondence (Table 5). However, when the data is plotted as a survival curve, there is substantial overlap between prognostic groupings. In an effort to refine this model, we examined the impact of variables measured at the outset of remission on ability to predict for different phases of the remission, that is, probability of remaining in remission at one year, two years, and three years (Table 6). We found that variables which were effective for predicting overall duration of response were primarily predicting the long term survivors and were relatively ineffective at making predictions about relapse during the first year of remission. We attempted to improve the model by limiting the distance between the measurement of the variable and its predicted outcome. Therefore, a model was generated for predicting probability of relapse during the first year of remission.

TABLE 4

SUMMARY OF REGRESSION ANALYSIS RELATING
LENGTH OF RESPONSE TO PATIENT CHARACTERISTICS

Characteristic	P	Log-Likelihood	Fav.	Relative Risk Unf.	Ratio
LDH	<.001	-437.506	.66	1.31	1.98
Fibrinogen	.001	-432.464	.71	1.52	2.14
Co.to CR	.004	-428.426	.79	1.80	2.28
AML	.081	-426.909	.83	1.54	1.86
Time to Halv. Leuk. Cells	.031	-424.570	.66	1.42	2.15
Age	.056	-422.749	.93	2.10	2.26

TABLE 5

TEST OF FIT OF REGRESSION MODEL
OBSERVED AND PREDICTED MEDIAN LENGTH OF CR

Predicted Median (wks)	Total Number Observed	Number Relapses	Observed Median (wks)
<28	43	37	23
28 - 35	43	24	43
36 - 55	42	26	51
≥56	41	17	80

TABLE 6

FACTORS PREDICTIVE FOR REMISSION DURATION AT VARIOUS
INTERVALS IN A.M.L.

	1 YR.	2 YR.	3 YR.
1. LDH	N.S.	.04	< .01
2. FIBRINOGEN	N.S.	< .01	< .01
3. MORPHOLOGY A. PRO. L.	N.S.	< .01	< .01
4. CHANGE IN LEUK. INFILTRATE	< .01	.05	.06

We had published a model for prediction of long term survivorship in people who are still in remission at one year, and
we decided that the choice of treatment early in remission
should be designed to assure that patients remain in remission for one year, at which time either late intensification
or a chemotherapy change could be undertaken and new prognostic variables identified. When the model was generated to
detect probability of relapse during the first year of complete remission, we discovered new variables which became
important (Table 7). This model, when applied to the data
base from which it derives (Table 8) shows improved correspondence. Thereafter, patients who were predicted to have
greater than a .40 probability of remaining in remission for
one year received conventional treatment, whereas the patients
predicted to have a less than .40 or an average of a .20 probability of remaining in remission were given developmental

therapy in remission.

TABLE 7

STEPWISE LOGISTIC REGRESSION ANALYSIS OF
RESPONSE DATA RELATED TO PRE-TREATMENT CHARACTERISTICS

Characteristic	Regression Coefficient	Significance Level	Log- Likelihood	% Reduction in Log- Likelihood
(Constant)	.541		-201.49	
Age	-.786	<.01	-183.53	36
Cytogenetics	1.503	<.01	-171.93	23
PHA	-1.615	<.01	-162.01	20
Temperature	-1.029	<.01	-156.13	12
Serum Creatinine	-.937	.01	-153.02	6
Hemoglobin	1.008	.06	-151.22	4

Regression Equation:

$$\log_e \left(\frac{p}{1-p} \right) = .541 - .786 \,(\text{age} - 2.54) + 1.503 \,(\text{cyto.} - 1.85)$$
$$-1.615 \,(\text{PHA} - .19) - 1.029 \,(\text{temp.} - 1.34)$$
$$-.937 \,(\text{creat.} - 1.16) + 1.008 \,(\text{Hgb} - 1.11).$$

Favorable Characteristics: Age <20, Metaphases present, No PHA, Temp. <101°F, Creat. <1.4, Hgb $\geq$ 12

TABLE 8

COMPARISON OF OBSERVED ONE YEAR REMISSION RATES TO PREDICTIONS BASED ON REGRESSION MODEL

PREDICTED PROBABILITY OF 1 YEAR CR	TOTAL NUMBER OBSERVED	NUMBER IN CR AT 1 YEAR	(%)
<.20	15	2	(13)
.20-.39	56	15	(27)
.40-.59	23	15	(65)
.60-.79	37	27	(73)
$\geq$.80	13	12	(92)

SUMMARY

We have created a logistic regression model for predicting probability of response to Adriamycin, ARA-C, Vincristine
Prednisone combination chemotherapy in adult acute leukemia.
We have tested this model prospectively in 107 consecutive
patients and shown an excellent correspondence between prediction and outcome. This demonstrates that this form of
clinical investigation should prove highly useful in the
future. Models have been created for predicting duration of
response and, while these models have proven useful, we have
generated refined models for predicting relapse during the
first year of remission and have shown an improved selectivity as a result of these models. These studies demonstrate
that it should be possible to use these objective quantitative techniques to investigate new therapies in patients who
have the lowest probability of benefit from conventional
treatment and therefore the highest potential for benefit to
balance the increased risk of developmental therapy. With
improved knowledge of new treatment, it becomes necessary to
evaluate such treatments in more favorable patients only at a
time when the benefit/risk ratios make this desirable. This
technique for conducting clinical research should greatly
improve the efficiency and the effectiveness of clinical
investigation and perhaps more important permit the physician
to prescribe conventional or developmental therapies in an
informed and ethical manner.

REFERENCES

1. Keating, M.J., Smith, T.L., Gehan, E.A., McCredie, K.B.,
    Bodey, G.P. and Freireich, E.J: Prediction of remission
    in adult acute leukemia: Generation of a model. Sub-
    mitted to Cancer, 1980.
2. Smith, T.L., Gehan, E.A., Keating, M.J. and Freireich,
    E.J: Prediction of remission in adult acute leukemia:
    Prospective test of predictive models. Submitted to
    Cancer, 1980.
3. Freireich, E.J, Gehan, E.A., Speer, J.F., Heilbrun, L.,
    Smith, T.L., Bodey, G.P., McCredie, K.B., Rodriguez, V.,
    Hart, J.S. and Burgess, M.A.: The usefulness of multiple
    pretreatment patient characteristics for prediction of
    response and survival in patients with adult acute leu-
    kemia. IN T.M. Fliedner and S. Perry (eds.), Advances
    in the Biosciences 14. Pergamon Press (New York), 1973,
    pp. 131-144.

4. Gehan, E.A., Smith, T.L., Freireich, E.J, Rodriguez, V., Speer, J. and McCredie, K.B.: Prognostic factors in acute leukemia. Seminars in Oncology 3:271-282, 1976.
5. Keating, M.J., Smith, T.L., Gehan, E.A., McCredie, K.B., Bodey, G.P., Spitzer, G., Hersh, E.M., Gutterman, J.U. and Freireich, E.J: Factors related to length of complete remission in adult acute leukemia. Cancer 45: 2017-2029, 1980.
6. Freireich, E.J and Gehan, E.A.: The limitations of the randomized clinical trial. Methods in Cancer Res. 17: 277-310, 1979.

RESULTS OF INTENSIVE TREATMENT OF
ACUTE LYMPHOBLASTIC LEUKEMIA IN
ADULTS

BAYARD CLARKSON, M.D., PETER SCHAUER, M.D.,
ROLAND MERTELSMANN, M.D., TIMOTHY GEE, M.D.,
ZALMEN ARLIN, M.D., SANFORD KEMPIN, M.D.,
MONROE DOWLING, M.D., PEGGY DUFOUR, M.A.,
CONSTANCE CIRRINCIONE, M.S., AND
JOSEPH BURCHENAL, M.D.

Hematology/Lymphoma Service
Department of Medicine and
Department of Biostatistics
Memorial Sloan-Kettering Cancer Center
New York, New York   10021

Supported in part by grants awarded
from the National Cancer Institute
CA-05826; CA-08748; CA-19117.
The American Cancer Society, ACS-CH-6J
and 6K and The United Leukemia Fund.

Reprint Requests:
Bayard Clarkson, M.D.
Memorial Sloan-Kettering Cancer Center
1275 York Avenue
New York, New York   10021

The treatment of acute lymphoblastic leukemia (ALL) in children has improved greatly in recent years. Complete remission
rates of 90% or higher are now the rule, and in several large
series where there has been a sufficiently long follow-up,
it has been estimated that one third (8) to one half (9) of
the children will remain in continuous remission indefinitely
and can be considered cured.

There has been less progress in the treatment of ALL in
adults. Because this type of leukemia is relatively infrequent
in adults, there are fewer reports on modern treatment
programs, but the results are invariably worse in adults than
in children (10,11,14,16). Several years ago, we also reported
poorer results in adults than in children with ALL who were
treated with a similar regimen (L-2 protocol) which was

initiated in 1969 (7). In adults the complete remission rate
was 79%, the median duration of remission 2 years, and the
median survival 2½ years, whereas in children the complete
remission rate was 98% and their median remission duration
has still not been reached 11 years after beginning the
study (9). Treatment was discontinued after 3 years and all
patients have now been off therapy for 4 years or longer.
Only 6 of the 29 adults (21%) who started on the L-2
protocol have remained in continuous remission, whereas 40 of
the 75 children (53%) are still in continuous remission (9).
Although the results in children treated with the L-2
protocol were markedly better than in children treated with
previous regimens at our Center, the results in adults with
ALL were not much better than in our own experience during
the preceding decade, except for a higher incidence of long
term continuous remissions (21% with L-2 protocol vs. 9% in
our historical control series).

To try to improve the treatment of both children and
adults, a new multiple drug protocol for ALL (L-10 protocol)
was designed in 1973, and from July 1973 to April 1977 all
previously untreated patients with ALL seen at Memorial
Hospital were entered on this new protocol. Whereas the
initial results of the L-10 in adults appeared better than
those of the L-2, because some relapses nevertheless occurred
early during the course of treatment with the L-10, in 1977
the L-10 protocol was modified (L-10M) to try to correct its
presumed deficiencies and prevent early relapse. From May 1977
to December 1979, all previously untreated adults with ALL
were entered on the L-10M protocol. Children continued to be
treated with the L-10 protocol until 1978, and the comparative
results of the L-2 and L-10 protocols in children have recently
been reported (9).

MATERIALS AND METHODS

Patient Population
    All previously untreated or minimally pretreated patients
aged 15 or older referred to Memorial Sloan-Kettering Cancer
Center in whom the diagnosis of ALL was confirmed were entered
on the L-2 (n=29), L-10 (n=34), or L-10M (n=38) protocols
according to the chronological sequence described above.
There was no patient selection and no previously untreated
nor minimally pretreated patients with a diagnosis of ALL
were excluded for any reason. The clinical and hematologic
characteristics of the cohorts of patients entered on the 3
protocols were very similar.

    In the case of patients entered on the L-2 and earlier
patients entered on the L-10, the diagnosis of ALL was based

on standard morphological criteria for identification of
lymphoblasts on stained smears of blood and bone marrow
aspirates together with generally accepted cytochemical
criteria. The slides of all patients on all protocols have
been reviewed retrospectively to confirm the morphological
diagnosis of ALL. Most patients entered on the L-10 and L-10M
protocols also had cell surface marker studies and measurement
of deoxynucleotidyl transferase for confirmation of the
diagnosis (15).

Treatment Protocols
    The strategic considerations underlying the designs and
detailed descriptions of the L-2 (2,3), L-10 (1,4,9) and
L-10M (5) protocols have been reported previously. The
protocols are shown schematically in Figures 1-6.
    There are 3 main differences between the L-2 and L-10
protocols. 1) The first is that the L-10 has a more prolonged
consolidation phase, with three 5-day courses of intravenous
methotrexate (MTX) alternating with the three courses of
arabinosylcytosine (Ara-C) and 6-thioguanine (TG) which was
used for consolidation in the L-2. 2) Secondly, the intensity
of chemoprophylaxis for central nervous system (CNS) leukemia
was increased. Adults treated with the L-2 received no CNS
prophylaxis after the consolidation phase (7). On the L-10
all patients received intrathecal (IT) MTX on day 4 and at
the end of induction. After completing remission induction
patients whose pretreatment WBC was greater than 20,000/mm^3
and who were therefore at high risk of developing CNS leukemia
had a subcutaneous Ommaya reservoir implanted, and all
subsequent injections of MTX were given into the ventricle (5).
Use of the intraventricular Ommaya reservoir has been shown
to facilitate repeated administration of drugs and allows
better drug distribution in the subarachnoid space. It also
avoids the possibility of inadvertent injection of drug into
the epidural space instead of the subarachnoid space as may
pccur when drugs are given repeatedly via lumbar puncture.
During the consolidation phase of the L-10, adults were given
3 to 5 additional injections of MTX and they continued to
receive 2 intrathecal or intraventricular injections of MTX
every 8 weeks throughout the maintenance phase for 3 years.
    3) The third major difference between the L-2 and the L-10
protocols is that the L-10 maintenance program was completely
redesigned in an attempt to eradicate residual disease. This
phase of the treatment includes relatively high doses of
several cell cycle non-specific drugs (i.e., adriamycin,
dactinomycin, BCNU and cyclophosphamide) to try to eliminate
long-term dormant leukemic cells (1,6,13). A total of 8 drugs
are administered in a sequential schedule and the sequence is

INTENSIVE "L-2" TREATMENT PROTOCOL FOR ACUTE LYMPHOBLASTIC LEUKEMIA

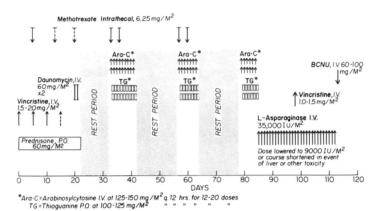

Fig. 1. L-2 induction and consolidation schedules as employed
in adults with ALL.

INTENSIVE CHEMOTHERAPY FOR ACUTE LYMPHOBLASTIC LEUKEMIA AND LEUKOSARCOMA IN CHILDREN
(L-2 PROTOCOL)

Part II

REMISSION MAINTENANCE THERAPY

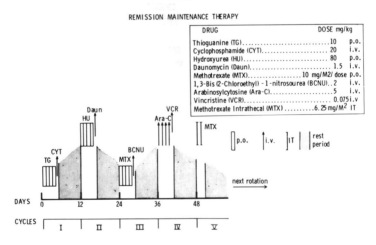

Fig. 2. L-2 maintenance schedule which was continued for 3
years. Intrathecal methotrexate was given to children but not to adults during maintenance.

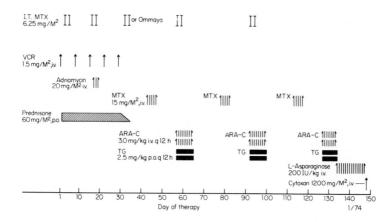

Fig. 3. L-10 induction and consolidation schedules. An
Ommaya reservoir was implanted and intraventricular
methotrexate administered in patients whose initial
WBC was greater than 20,000/mm³.

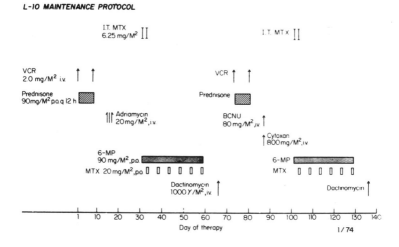

Fig. 4. L-10 maintenance or attempted "eradication" schedule;
this was continued for 3 years and left unchanged in
the L-10M protocol.

305

L-10M INDUCTION

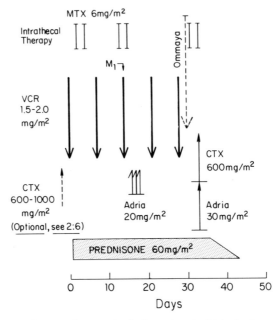

Fig. 5. L-10M induction schedule. An initial dose of cyclo-phosphamide (CTX) was given in patients with bulky tumor masses if there were no contraindications.

L-10M CONSOLIDATION

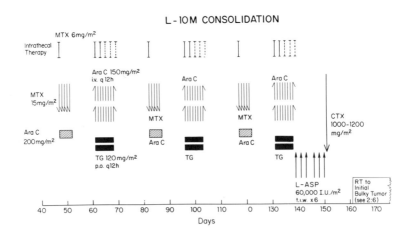

Fig. 6. L-10M consolidation schedule. Radiotherapy (RT) was given at the end of the consolidation to sites of initial bulky tumor masses. The dose of L-asparaginase (L-ASP) was reduced in patients if poorly tolerated.

repeated approximately every 20 weeks. After 1 to 2 weeks rest after consolidation, therapy is resumed with high doses of prednisone plus vincristine, followed by adriamycin. This is followed by a 28-day course of 6-mercaptopurine (6-MP) and MTX. A single injection of dactinomycin is administered after this "cytostatic" course of antimetabolite therapy. Prednisone and vincristine are then again administered for a short period and then cyclophosphamide and BCNU are given in combination. A second course of 6-MP and MTX followed by a dose of dactino-mycin completes the 20-week sequence. Rest periods of 1-2 weeks are inserted between the therapeutic sequences to allow regeneration of normal hematopoietic cells. The adults were treated for 3 years with this attempted "eradication" program. Since the induction and consolidation phases lasted about 6 months, the total duration of treatment was about 3½ years.

After the L-10 had been in effect for about 3½ years, preliminary analysis showed that some patients had early relapses of their disease despite good adherence to the protocol. At the time of this analysis, 4 relapses had occurred within 2 to 5 months after attaining a remission (M1) marrow; all of these were in patients who initially presented with high WBCs (48,000 to 113,000/mm^3) and who had clinical evidence of rapidly progressive leukemia. One of the 4 patients was 73 years old and, although she briefly attained an M1 marrow, she was unable to tolerate the treatment and relapsed before even reaching the consolidation phase. However, the other 3 patients all rapidly attained remissions and received the full course of treatment prescribed by the protocol. In protocols calling for multiple drugs in rapid sequence, if there is an ineffective therapeutic component included in the sequence which allows regrowth of the leukemic population, it may be difficult to identify which component is the "weak link" even if serial marrow exami-nations are performed frequently. However, the timing of relapse in 2 of these patients led us to suspect that the component in which methotrexate was given alone during the consolidation phase might be a weak link. The protocol was designed for previously untreated patients whose leukemic cells had had no prior exposure to methotrexate, and it had been assumed that primary resistance to moderately high doses of this drug was unlikely. However, because marrow relapse occurred almost immediately after the methotrexate sequence in these patients, this assumption was apparently erroneous.

Because of these early relapses, in May 1977 we modified the L-10 protocol by introducing 4 changes (L-10M protocol). 1) The first was to add 1 or 2 intravenous doses of cyclo-phosphamide to produce initial reduction in the leukemic cell

mass. The first injection of cyclophosphamide was given as
the initial treatment in patients with large mediastinal
masses or other bulky lymphadenopathy providing there were no
contraindications such as extreme thrombocytopenia, septicemia
associated with severe neutropenia, bilateral ureteral
obstruction or other conditions causing inadequate urinary
output. The second injection of cyclophosphamide was given
later in combination with adriamycin to further reduce the
leukemic cell mass prior to beginning the consolidation phase
with the antimetabolite sequences. 2) Secondly, vincristine
and prednisone were inserted in the middle of the consolidation
phase to try to prevent relapses during this phase. 3) The
third change was that after remission induction, radiotherapy
was administered to areas of originally bulky tumor masses,
such as an enlarged spleen or contiguous lymph node masses
whose largest dimension exceeded 5 cm. 4) The fourth change
was to administer a continuous intravenous infusion of Ara-C
together with the intravenous MTX during the condolidation
phase to try to overcome the (presumed) weak link. Experience
had already shown that the limiting toxicity of MTX when
given alone in the dosage schedule employed in the L-10 was
stomatitis rather than marrow suppression, and it was therefore felt that the additional hematotoxic effects of Ara-C
could be safely tolerated. The maintenance or eradication
phase of the protocol was left unchanged.

Criteria of Response
    Complete remissions were defined according to conventional
criteria as previously described (4,7). The duration of
remission was measured from the time of the first normal (M1)
marrow until the first sign of hematologic or CNS relapse.
Kaplan-Meier projections were used to measure remission
duration and survival (12).

                            RESULTS

    Because of space limitations, the results can only be
briefly summarized here; a detailed report including analysis
of possible prognostic factors will be published elsewhere.

TABLE I

Comparative Results of L-2, L-10 and
L-10M Protocols in Adults with ALL

	L-2	L-10	L-10M
# Entered	29	34	38
# CR	23 (79%)	29 (85%)	32 (84%)
# PR	0	1	1
# Died During Induction	3	3	2
# Failed	3	1	3
# Died in CR	0	0	1
# Censored	--	3	--
# Relapsed on Protocol	17	11	9
# Continuous CR	6 (21%)	15 (44%)	22 (58%)

The results are summarized in Table I. The patients listed
as partial remissions (PR) achieved marrow remissions, but
had persistent lymph node enlargement. Deaths during induction
therapy resulted from leukopenia and sepsis. One patient on
the L-10M delivered a child during induction and subsequently
died of post partum complications while in complete remission
(CR); in the analysis she was included as a disease-related
death. Patients listed as failures had persistence of lymphoblasts in the marrow after completing 5 to 6 weeks of therapy.
  Because the results were similar with the L-10 and L-10M
protocols, they have been combined for evaluating remission
duration (Fig. 7) and survival (Fig. 8). Three of the 29
patients on the L-10 who achieved complete remissions were
censored from evaluation of remission duration at the time
they began maintenance treatment because they returned to
their homes in foreign countries at this point and received
less intensive maintenance therapy which was quite different
than that called for by the protocol. Although these 3
patients eventually relapsed at 16, 23, and 35 months and
subsequently died, since they were still in continuous CR
at the time of breaking protocol they were included as
responders in the remission and survival duration curves up
to the time of censor. None of the patients on the other
protocols were censored. Thus of the patients achieving CR
and who were evaluable in that they followed the protocols
26% (6/23) on the L-2, 58% (15/26) on the L-10 and 69%
(22/32) on the L-10M remain in continuous remission. The
approximate median follow-up times for the 3 protocols are 9
years for the L-2, 5 years for the L-10 and 2 years for the
L-10M.

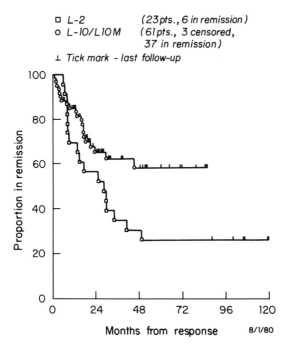

REMISSION DURATION
L-2 vs. L-10/L-10M

□ *L-2*   *(23 pts., 6 in remission)*
○ *L-10/L10M*   *(61 pts., 3 censored,*
                37 in remission)
⊥ *Tick mark - last follow-up*

Proportion in remission

100
80
60
40
20
0

0   24   48   72   96   120

Months from response   8/1/80

Fig. 7. Remission duration of patients achieving complete remissions on L-10 and L-10M protocols compared to those on L-2 protocol.

310

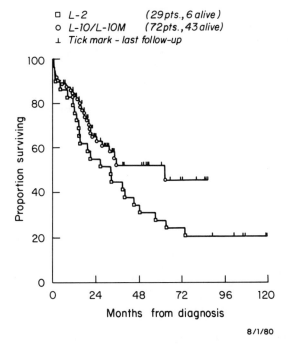

Fig. 8. Duration of survival of all patients entered on
L-2 and L-10/L-10M protocols.

311

As is evident in Fig. 7, most of the 20 patients who
relapsed on the L-10 or L-10M protocols did so during the
consolidation phase or during the early part of the maintenance phase (the one patient who died in CR is also included
as a relapse in this analysis). The most likely explanation
for these early relapses and for the failures is (relative)
primary resistance of the leukemic cells to the cytotoxic
drugs. Pretreatment pulse ^{3}H-thymidine labeling indices of
the marrow leukemic cells revealed no significant cytokinetic
differences between the leukemic populations in these
patients compared with those who remained in durable
remissions. So far no patients have relapsed during the third
year of maintenance and only one has relapsed after completing all therapy. The bone marrow was the site of first
relapse in 15 of the 20 patients and nearly simultaneous bone
marrow and CNS relapse occurred in an additional 3 patients.
The incidence of isolated CNS relapse has been low, occurring so far in only 2 of the 61 patients achieving remission
on the L-10 or L-10M, thus supporting our previously reported
contention that chemoprophylaxis alone without cranial or
craniospinal irradiation is effective in preventing meningeal
leukemia (5). No cases of isolated relapse in testicular or
other extramedullary sites have yet been observed in this
series of adults with ALL.

The major serious toxicity encountered with the L-10 and
L-10M protocols was sepsis associated with leukopenia during
induction; this occurred in about 65% of patients. Moderate
or severe alopecia occurred in all patients. Transient
meningismus due to intrathecal MTX, severe vincristine-
induced neuropathy or ileus and corticosteroid-induced psy-
chosis or hyperglycemia also occurred, but the incidence of
each was less than 10%. Hepatitis occurred in 9 patients,
herpes zoster in 3, and pneumocystitis carinii pneumonia in
3, the latter complication developing in all 3 patients as
prednisone was tapered after induction. After prophylactic
trimethoprim and sulfmethoxazole therapy was instituted
during this period no further cases of pneumocystitis
occurred. To date no patients have developed leukoencephalopathy or symptomatic cardiomyopathy. One man fathered a child
4 months after therapy was discontinued. The infant was born
with multiple congenital abnormalities and died shorter after
birth.

Factors of Prognostic Importance

Multiple clinical features and hematologic parameters are
currently being analyzed for prognostic significance and the
results will be reported elsewhere when the analysis is
completed. Factors so far identified which have a statis-

tically favorable prognosis are age below 25 years, female
sex, WBC below 15,000/mm^3 and normal serum albumin level.
High serum uric acid or lactic dehydrogenase levels, normal
hemoglobin value (as opposed to low hemoglobin) were unfavorable parameters, but were not statistically significant.
Bulky mediastinal masses, lymph node enlargement and hepatomegaly or splenomegaly were not of prognostic importance.
Of 59 patients whose leukemic cells were studied for surface
markers, 11 (19%) had T-cell ALL and 7 of these patients
(64%) remain in continuous remission. Neither the pretreatment pulse ^{3}H-thymidine labeling index of the leukemic cells
nor the level of terminal deoxynucleotidyl transferase in the
bone marrow were of prognostic significance.

DISCUSSION

These studies demonstrate that it is possible to achieve
complete remissions in about 85% of unselected adults with
ALL with intensive multi-drug chemotherapy. Although the
follow-up is still relatively short, it appears that about
half of the patients will remain in continuous remission
after treatment is discontinued after 3½ years. The results
in adults with the L-10 protocol are similar to those in
children treated with the same protocol (9), but unlike the
children in whom the results with the L-2 and L-10 protocols
were similar, the more intensive L-10 or L-10M protocols
cause improved remission duration and survival in adults as
compared with the L-2. Prolonged intraventricular or intrathecal chemoprophylaxis appears to be as effective in
preventing meningeal leukemia as cranial irradiation and
does not cause late complications such as leukoencephalopathy
or cognitive disorders (5,9).

The L-10/L-10M protocols are admittedly complicated and
arduous regimens to follow for both patients and physicians
in that they require multiple hospital admissions during
induction and consolidation and cause significant toxicity.
However, until some simpler and less toxic but equally
effective regimen can be devised, this protocol or a similar
type of intensive multi-drug regimen appears to be the best
treatment presently available for adults with ALL. Possibly
improvements can be made in choice of drugs and in their
dosage and sequencing, although our own efforts to improve
the L-10 (i.e., L-10M) have so far not succeeded in improving
the results. We are currently comparing a new protocol (L-17)
which includes a more intensive but abbreviated consolidation
phase with the existing L-10M protocol, but it is much too
soon to evaluate the results.

No series has yet been reported in which patients with ALL

in their first remission have received marrow ablative cytotoxic drugs and total body irradiation followed by bone
marrow transplantation from histocompatible (non-identical)
sibling donors. The results of marrow transplantation in
patients with ALL in second or later remissions do not appear
to be as good as in patients who receive primary treatment
with the L-10 or L-10M, but of course this is not a fair
comparison. Patients who relapse during intensive treatment
with regimens such as the L-10/L-10M can frequently be reinduced into remission, but the second remissions are usually
short both in adults and in children and most patients die
of their disease within a year. On the other hand, 8 of the
12 children who relapsed after completing the L-2 protocol
had long second remissions (8+ to 60+ months) and it is
possible they will become long survivors (9). So far only 1
adult has relapsed after completing the L-10 or L-10M
protocols and, although a second remission was reinduced, he
again relapsed and died about a year later.

Trials are currently in progress in Seattle with bone
marrow transplantation in children with ALL in their first
remission who have unfavorable prognostic features at
diagnosis, and it will be of great interest to see whether
the results will be better than with the L-2 or L-10 protocols
in this poor prognosis group of children. We have not yet been
able to identify a clearly unfavorable prognostic pattern in
adult ALL which would permit selection of such patients for
bone marrow transplantation in first remission. Younger
patients tolerate the intensive therapy and transplant
procedure better than older patients, but the former also
do better on intensive chemotherapy alone. Hopefully ways
will soon be found to avoid the formidable hazards still
associated with bone marrow transplantation (e.g., graft-
versus-host disease and interstitial pneumonia), and such
developments should then allow a comparative study of
intensive therapy followed by bone marrow transplantation
versus intensive chemotherapy alone in young adults with ALL
in first remission.

The L-10/L-10M protocols were specifically designed with
curative intent (1,4). It is too soon to know if this
objective has been achieved, but the remission duration curve
of the L-10 appears to be reaching a plateau after 4 years
and no relapses have yet occurred after 4 years on the L-2
protocol which has the longest follow-up (median=9 years)
(Fig. 7). Although these results represent a distinct improvement in the treatment of ALL, the treatment fails to
eradicate the leukemic populations in about half of both
adults and children who are still dying of their disease.
It is unlikely that even more intensive cytotoxic chemo-

therapy can be tolerated without rescuing the patients with bone marrow transplantation, but this appraoch to treatment is presently limited to younger patients with suitable donors and further improvements will depend on development of ways to prevent the serious complications associated with transplantation. Other possible approaches to improving the treatment of ALL include development of more selective leukemocidal drugs or of monoclonal antibodies with clear leukemic specificity, learning how to trigger long-term dormant leukemic cells (6) into the proliferative cycle in order that they will be more vulnerable to cytotoxic therapy, or developing procedures to force leukemic stem cells to differentiate and thereby lose their unlimited proliferative potential. Possibly some of these approaches can be coupled with autologous transplantation of normal stem cells obtained from the marrow or blood during remission to rescue patients after marrow ablation, provided that a reliable way can be found to selectively destroy any residual leukemic cells in the autograft. Hopefully one or more of these or other experimental approaches will become sufficiently advanced during the next few years to allow successful clinical application and lead to further improvements in the treatment of ALL.

REFERENCES

1. Arlin, Z.A., Fried, J., and Clarkson, B.: Therapeutic
    role of cell kinetics in acute leukemia. Clinics in
    Hematology 7: 339-362, 1978.
2. Clarkson, B., and Fried, J.: Changing concepts of
    treatment in acute leukemia. In: Medical Clinics in
    North America (Krakoff, I.H., ed.), Vol. 55, Philadelphia,
    London, Toronto, W.B. Saunders, Co., pp. 561-600, 1971.
3. Clarkson, B.: Cell cycle kinetics: Clinical applications.
    In: Antineoplastic and Immunosuppressive Agents for the
    Handbook of Experimental Pharmacology. (Johns, D. and
    Sartorelli, A.C., eds.), Berlin, Heidelberg, New York,
    Springer-Verlag, pp. 157-193, 1974.
4. Clarkson, B., Dowling, M.D., Gee, T.S., Cunningham, I.B.,
    and Burchenal, J.H.: Treatment of acute leukemia in
    adults. Cancer 36: 775-795, 1975.
5. Clarkson, B., Haghbin, M., Murphy, M.L., Gee, T.S.,
    Dowling, M.D., Arlin, Z.A., Kempin, S., Posner, J.,
    Shapiro, W., Galicich, J., Dufour, P., Passe, S., and
    Burchenal, J.H.: Prevention of central nervous system
    leukemia in acute lymphoblastic leukemia with prophylactic
    chemotherapy alone. In: International Symposium on the
    CNS Complications of Malignant Disease, 1978 (Monograph),
    MacMillans, 1979, pp. 36-58.
6. Clarkson, B., Chou, T-C., Strife, A., Ferguson, R.,
    Sullivan, S.,Fried, J., Kitahara, T., and Oyama, A.:
    Duration of the dormant state in an established cell
    line of human hematopoietic cells. Cancer Res. 37: 4506-
    4522, 1977.
7. Gee, T.S., Dowling, M.D., Haghbin, M., and Clarkson, B.:
    Acute lymphocytic leukemia in adults and children.
    Differences in responses on a single therapeutic regimen.
    Cancer 37: 1256-1264, 1976.
8. George, S.L., Aur, R.J.A., Mauer, A.M., and Simone, J.V.:
    A reappraisal of the results of stopping therapy in
    childhood leukemia. New Engl. J. Med. 300: 269-273, 1979.
9. Haghbin, M., Murphy, M.L., Tan, C.C., Clarkson, B., Thaler,
    H.T., Passe, S., and Burchenal, J.H.: A long-term clinical
    follow-up of children with acute lymphoblastic leukemia
    treated with intensive chemotherapy regimens. Cancer 46:
    241-252, 1980.
10. Henderson, E.S.: Treatment of acute leukemia. Sem. Hematol
    6: 271-319, 1969.
11. Jacquillat, C., Weil, M., Gemon, M-F., Auclerc, G.,
    Loisel, J-P., Delobel, J., Flandrin, G., Izrael, V.,

Bussel, A., Dresch, C., Weisgerber, C., Rain, D., Tanzer, J., Najean, Y., Boiron, M., and Bernard, J.: Combination therapy in 130 patients with acute lymphoblastic leukemia (protocol 06 LA 66-Oaris). Cancer Res. 33: 3278-3284,1973.

12. Kaplan, E.L., and Meier, P.: Non-parametric estimation from incomplete observations. J. Amer. Statis. Assoc. 53: 457-481, 1958.

13. Kuo, A.H., Yataganas, X., Galicich, J.H., Fried, J., and Clarkson, B.: Proliferative kinetics of central nervous system (CNS) leukemia. Cancer 36: 232-239, 1975.

14. Lister, T.A., Whitehouse, J.M.A., Beard, M.E.J.,Brearley, R.L., Wrigley, P.F.M., Iliver, R.T.D., Freeman, J.E., Woodruff, R.K., Malpas, J.S., Paxton, A.M., and Crowther, D.: Combination chemotherapy for acute lymphoblastic leukemia in adults. British Medical Journal 1: 199-203, 1978.

15. Mertelsmann, R., Koziner, B., Filippa, D.A., Grossbard,E., Incefy, G., Moore, M.A.S., and Clarkson, B.: Clinical significance of TdT, cell surface markers and CFU-c in 297 patients with hematopoietic neoplasias. In: Modern Trends in Human Leukemia III (Neth, R., Gallo, R.C., Hofschneider, P.-H., and Mannweiler, K., ads.), Springer-Verlag, Berlin-Heidelberg, New York, pp. 131-138, 1979.

16. Willemze, R., Hillen, C., Hartgrink-Groeneveld, C.A., and Haanen, C.: Treatment of acute lymphoblastic leukemia in adolescents and adults: A retrospective study of 41 patients (1970-1973). Blood 46: 823-834, 1975.

CHILDHOOD LEUKEMIAS

Denis R. Miller, M.D.

Enid A. Haupt Professor and Chairman,
Department of Pediatrics
Memorial Sloan-Kettering Cancer Center
New York, N.Y.

Leukemia is the second leading cause of death in children accounting for approximately 35 percent of all deaths related to malignancies. Acute lymphoblastic (ALL) or undifferentiated leukemia (AUL) accounts for 80 to 85 percent of the childhood leukemias; acute nonlymphoblastic leukemias (ANLL) comprise the remaining 15 to 20 percent. Yearly, in the U.S., 2500 children are diagnosed with leukemia, of whom 2100 have ALL/AUL.

The recent advances in the biology, prognosis, and treatment of childhood leukemias, as well as impediments to cure, will be reviewed in this article.

CLINICAL PROGNOSTIC FACTORS IN ALL

The presenting clinical and laboratory features of a large series of children with ALL are presented in Tables 1 and 2. These features are key determinants of successful response to induction therapy, complete continuous remission, and survival.[4]

Univariate and multivariate statistical methods have documented the prognostic importance of the leukemic cell burden, the degree of adenopathy, the age of the patient, sex, the level of hemoglobin, hepatosplenomegaly, the presence or absence of central nervous system disease at diagnosis, lymphoblast morphology based upon French-American-British (FAB) classification,[2] immunoglobulin levels at diagnosis, and the rapidity of response of the bone marrow to initial therapy.[4,9,10] The treatment regimen itself is prognostic. Stratification at the time of patient entry on study or in the analysis of treatment results is now standard practice in the evaluation of all prospective trials.

Supported by a grant from USPHS-NCI (CA23742) and the Heckscher Foundation.

TABLE 1
Presenting Clinical Findings in Children with ALL

Clinical Features	Percent	Clinical Features	Percent
Age (yrs)		Hepatosplenomegaly	
<1.5	6	None	32
1.5-3	18	Moderate	55
3-10	54	Marked	13
>10	22	WBC ($\times 10^9$/liter)	
Sex		<10	53
Male	57	10-49	30
Female	43	>50	17
Race		Hemoglobin (gm/dl)	
White	89	<7	43
Non-white	11	7-11	45
Fever	61	> 11	25
Hemorrhage	48	Platelets ($\times 10^9$/liter)	
Bone pain	23	<20	28
Lymphadenopathy		20-99	47
None	50	>100	25
Moderate	43	Blasts in bone marrow (%)	
Marked (>3 cm)	7	25-64	25
Mediastinal mass	7	65-94	50
Central nervous		>95	25
system disease	4		

TABLE 2
*Presenting Immunological and Morphological
Features in Childhood ALL*

Feature	Percent
Lymphoblast cell surface markers	
Common ALL	65
T-cell ALL	15-20
B-cell ALL	<5
"Null" ALL	10
Lymphoblast morphology (FAB)	
L_1	84
L_2	15
L_3	1
Immunoglobulins G,A,M	
Normal	82
Decreased (1 or more classes)	18

Many factors are interrelated or interdependent. Accordingly, multivariate analysis using the Cox regression[9] model of a current large scale Childrens Cancer Study Group trial has established the weighted contribution of individual factors in predicting the duration of remission (Table 3) and survival (Table 4).

TABLE 3
*Predictors of Disease-Free Survival**

Variable	Significance Level (P-value)
Log WBC	.002
Hemoglobin	.005
IgM	.005
Splenomegaly	.007
Age^2	.014
Day-14 marrow	.029
Sex	.036
IgG	.070
Morphology	.090

*Platelet count, CNS disease at diagnosis, nodal enlargement, mediastinal mass status, race, IgA, and hepatomegaly were not significant predictors of DFS in this multivariate analysis.

TABLE 4
Predictors of Survival by Multivariate Analysis

Variable	Significance Level (P-value)
Log WBC	.001
IgG	.009
Age	.038
Morphology	.048
IgM	.067
CNS disease at diagnosis	.089
Hemoglobin	.159

Certain factors (eg. FAB morphology, IgG) are predictive of survival but are of borderline significance in predicting disease-free survival. In part, these seemingly disparate findings relate to the importance of FAB morphology and IgG in predicting response to induction therapy (Table 5), in which both factors are highly significant. Failure to achieve a complete remission is invariably associated with early death.

TABLE 5
Univariate Predictors of Induction Failure

Variable	% Failure	Significance Level (P-value)
CNS disease at diagnosis	18.8	.0001
L2 morphology	12.5	.0001
L3 morphology	30.0	.0001
PAS <40% positive	8.9	.007
IgG decreased	8.6	.009
Age >10 yrs	7.7	.01
WBC >20,000/μl	6.2	.09
Down's syndrome	13.3	.09
All patients	4.5	

Except for sex, these prognostic factors lose their significance after two years of complete continuous remission. Both sexes have equal success in achieving complete remission. The difference in relapse rates appears 9 to 12 months from initial remission with accentuation after discontinuation of therapy. The poorer prognosis in males is partially the result of testicular relapses.

Prognostic factors identify subsets of patients at high risk of early relapse and death or with a particularly high probability of prolonged disease-free survival and potential cure. Favorable and unfavorable clinical factors defining groups with good, average, or poor prognosis are presented in Table 6. On the basis of these and similar analyses, children in the poor prognostic groups are currently being treated more intensively than children with a more favorable prognosis. Whether more aggressive and toxic therapy will improve the dismal outlook for patients in the unfavorable prognostic groups is still undetermined. Less intensive but equally effective therapy for children with a good prognosis is desirable, if toxicity and complications are reduced and if survival is not compromised.

TABLE 6
Newly-Defined Prognostic Groups from CCG 141

| Factor | Prognostic Group | | |
	Good	Average	Poor
WBC x10^9/liter	<20	20–100	>100
Age, yrs	2–10	>10	<1
"Lymphoma" syndrome*	0	0–2	3 or more
Hgb, gm/dl	<10		>10
Liver,spleen,nodes	not markedly enlarged		markedly enlarged
Mediastinal mass	absent	absent	present
CNS disease at Dx	absent	absent	present
FAB morphology	L_1	L_1	L_2^+
Ig classes decreased	0–1	0–3	0–3
BM day 14	M_1,M_2	$M_{1,2,3}$	$M_{1,2,3}$
% all patients	28.1	50.8	21.1
48 mos CCR	92.1	55.0	45.7

*Lymphoma syndrome = 3 or more features, Hgb >10 gm/dl, markedly enlarged liver, spleen or nodes, and mediastinal mass. +L_2 = $\geq$25% L_2 lymphoblasts.

BIOLOGICAL CLASSIFICATION OF CHILDHOOD ALL

Recently reported morphologic, histochemical, biochemical[3] cytogenetic, and immunologic[5] studies have clearly demonstrated the heterogeneity of childhood ALL. The continued study

of these biologic markers may provide the future foundations
for specific chemotherapy and immunotherapy.

Cytomorphologically, three distinct subgroups in ALL have
been identified using the FAB classification. L_2 morphology
is associated with a significantly lower rate of induction of
complete remission and higher relapse and death rates. However, there is no relationship between lymphoblast morphology
and conventional cell surface markers except for L_3 morphology
associated with B-cell ALL. Excellent reviews of the diagnostic role of cytochemistry in ALL and ANLL are available[11]
and are beyond the scope of this presentation. Their prognostic utility is less certain however.

Terminal deoxynucleotidyl transferase (Tdt) is an enzyme
found in most T-, common, and null cell ALL, and serves as a
differentiation marker. Since Tdt is not found in mature and
well-differentiated lymphocytes, raised levels of Tdt during
presumed remission may permit the detection of residual leukemic cells and refine the current, albeit inaccurate, definition of remission. Similarly, determination of adenosine
deaminase, 5' nucleotidase, hexosaminidase, and glycophorin A
may aid in further subclassifying leukemias.

Preliminary reports suggested that increased cytoplasmic
receptors of glucocorticoids was associated with common ALL,
steroid responsiveness, and improved prognosis. These receptors are found in most hematopoietic cells and their true
therapeutic and prognostic utility remains to be determined.

A small percentage (<5) of children with apparent ALL have
the Ph^1 (Philadelphia) chromosome and are in the acute blast
phase of chronic myelogenous leukemia. The presence of Tdt
and lymphoid cell surface characteristics demonstrates the
lymphoid derivation of the blasts. In most children with ALL,
specific chromosomal anomalies are not characteristic and a
wide range of karyotypic abnormalities (aneuploidy, hyperdi-
ploidy, pseudodiploidy) have been identified. To date, karyotypic abnormalities in ALL, unlike in ANLL, are of no prognostic importance.

Flow cytofluorometry with the dye acridine orange measures
the DNA/RNA content of a large sample of individual leukemic
cells.[1] The presence of aneuploidy, the proportion of leukemic
cells in the various stages of the cell cycle, and therapy-
induced cytoreduction and cell kill can be determined with
this technique. Rare cases of biphenotypic (ALL/ANLL) and
other indeterminant acute leukemias can be classified more
accurately with these newer investigational tools. To date,
cell kinetic data--labelling index, mitotic index, proportion
of cells in S phase--are not prognostic.

At least 5 phenotypic groups of ALL have been identified:
approximately 15 to 20 percent are T-cell ALL; 1 to 5 percent

are B-cell ALL; 75 percent of non-T, non-B lymphoblasts (65 percent of the total) react with antibody made against non-T, non-B leukemic cells, and are designated common ALL (cALL); approximately 20 percent of ALL patients have blast cells with the characteristics of cALL plus cytoplasmic IgM, and are designated pre-B ALL; and the remaining 10 to 15 percent is true null-cell ALL. As in cALL and B-ALL, null cells may possess the Ia(DR) antigen.

The availability of monoclonal antibodies directed against specific surface antigens of ALL should refine the current immunologic classification.

Preliminary reports indicate that cell surface markers are of prognostic importance. Multivariate analysis of large numbers of patients will be required to determine whether or not immunologic markers are significant independent variables. Remissions are difficult to obtain in B-cell ALL and therapy designed for non-Hodgkin's lymphoma may be more effective. This approach is also under investigation for T-cell ALL, a disease with distinctive clinical features--higher median age, high initial white blood cell count, high male:female ratio (>3.0:1), "lymphoma syndrome", and high incidence of extra-medullary relapse.

TREATMENT OF ALL[7,8,13]

Induction and Consolidation Therapy

The objectives of induction therapy are to destroy rapidly a large proportion of leukemic cells to preserve normal hema-topoietic cells, and to restore quickly normal hematopoiesis. Prompt induction of complete remission is essential. Children in whom there is less than 50 percent reduction in bone marrow lymphoblast infiltrate by day 5 or more than 25 percent lym-phoblasts in the bone marrow by day 14 of induction therapy, have a significantly higher rate of hematologic relapse and death. Alternative methods of induction therapy must be con-sidered for slow responders or non-responders to induction therapy. Complete remission rates of 90 to 98 percent are achieved with combinations of vincristine, prednisone, plus either an anthracycline (daunomycin or adriamycin) or L-asparaginase and are superior to induction with prednisone and vincristine.

Consolidation therapy or reinduction therapy immediately after achieving complete remission has not been beneficial in most reported series. More recently, however, consolidation with intravenous and intrathecal methotrexate, cyclophospha-mide, and L-asparaginase as reported by SWOG or consolidation and reinduction either immediately after consolidation or after three months of maintenance therapy (Berlin-Frankfurt-

Muenster Group) appear to be superior to standard maintenance without consolidation in children with a poor prognosis.

CNS Prophylaxis

The CNS sanctuary, if unprotected, will become the site of isolated extramedullary relapse in over 50 percent of children in whom the rate of CNS relapse is 4 percent per month for the first 24 months, declining thereafter to 1 percent per month. With currently effective prophylactic regimens, isolated CNS relapse in patients with a good and poor prognosis is 5 percent and 10 percent or higher, respectively, regardless of therapy. The risk of CNS leukemia is directly proportional to the initial white blood cell count, conversely proportional to age and platelet count at diagnosis, and higher in T-cell ALL. The results of current regimens are shown in Table 7. Recent studies have demonstrated the inferiority of IT MTX if given only during induction, the effectiveness of 1800 rads of cranial radiation plus IT MTX, and IT MTX alone if given throughout the maintenance phase.

TABLE 7
CNS Prophylaxis in Childhood ALL

Regimen	Isolated CNS Relapse Rate (Percent)	Institution or Group
IT MTX x6	40	CCSG
IT MTX, induction and maintenance	5-8	SWOG,MSKCC
C-S radiation: 2400 rads	5-8	CCSG,SJCRH
1800 rads	6	CCSG
Cranial radiation:		
1800 rads+IT MTX x6	4-13	CCSG
2400 rads+IT MTX x5 or 6	0-7	SFCC,SJCRH
IV MTX+IT MTX x3	10	CALGB
IMFRA	8	Wayne State

Late effects of CNS prophylaxis, particularly the combination of cranial radiation and IT MTX, have been documented. These include leukoencephalopathy, mineralizing vasculopathy, abnormalities on CT scan, neuropsychologic dysfunction, postradiation somnolence syndrome, pituitary dysfunction, blindness and CNS malignancies.

The risk:benefit ratio of CNS prophylaxis must be seriously considered in modifying effective regimens particularly in patients at high risk of CNS relapse. Although IT MTX alone appears to be effective in good prognosis patients, the CNS relapse rate of 10 percent or higher in poor prognosis patients mandates more effective regimens.

Maintenance Therapy

Ideally, maintenance or continuation therapy regimens are designed to control the disease, prevent the development of drug-resistant clones, and prevent bone marrow and extramedullary relapses without inducing bone marrow aplasia and severe immunosuppression. Although the efficacy of maintenance therapy has been established, a beneficial role of any intensive regimen in use during the past decade has not been established, particularly for poor prognosis patients. A great deal of effort has been expended in designing variations of a "standard" program consisting of daily 6-mercaptopurine, weekly methotrexate, and periodic pulses of vincristine and prednisone. Experimental regimens employed intensive continuous, intermittent, and cyclic therapy. Despite these manipulations, adding agents merely increased morbidity and toxicity without significantly affecting duration of remission and survival.

RETRIEVAL THERAPY

Bone Marrow Relapse

The median survival following isolated bone marrow, testicular, and CNS relapse for patients on therapy is 10 months, 18 months, and 20 months, respectively. Thus, bone marrow relapse on therapy is one of the most unfavorable prognostic factors. Although second, or even more remissions can be achieved with intensive reinduction programs, subsequent remissions are progressively shorter, toxic effects are compounded, and marrow reserves are depleted. The combined hazards of opportunistic infections and hemorrhage are invariable the cause of death.

Basic problems relating to early relapse include growth characteristics of the leukemic clone or a subpopulation that is unaffected by therapy, persistence of leukemic cells resulting from drug resistance or their presence in protected pharmacologic sanctuaries, the inadequacy of the current definition of remission and the inability to identify residual leukemic cells with any degree of precision or sensitivity.

Investigational new drugs or new combinations and dosage schedules are reserved for patients refractory to conventional therapy. New agents undergoing active trials in children include deoxycoformycin, an inhibitor of adenosine deaminase; polyinosine-cytidine, an inducer of interferon; MAMSA, an arthracycline-like agent; and the combination methotrexate and vindesine. Developmental therapeutics and the pharmacology of new agents are presented in detail elsewhere in this Symposium.

Extramedullary Relapse

Children experiencing an isolated extramedullary relapse should receive not only specific local therapy but also reinduction therapy to prevent bone marrow relapse. CNS relapse can be effectively treated with an additional course of cranial radiation (1800 rads) plus spinal radiation (1000 rads), if high-dose methotrexate was not used previously. Reinduction therapy with IT MTX alone or in combination with cytosine arabinoside, with or without hydrocortisone, is effective. At MSKCC, intrathecal MTX and cytosine arabinoside, neuraxis radiation, 600 rads, and intraventricular methotrexate via an Ommaya reservoir have been effective for disease control.

Isolated testicular relapses occur in 10 to 15 percent of males on therapy and 10 to 30 percent of boys off therapy after three years or more of disease-free survival. Effective therapy employs bilateral testicular irradiation (1800 to 2400 rads) including the inguinal canal, as well as iliac and paraortic nodes, if their involvement is detected by lymphangiography, CT scan, sonography, or exploratory laparotomy.

Because occult testicular disease is being reported in 8 to 33 percent of boys completing three years of treatment, bilateral open wedge testicular biopsies are recommended prior to cessation of therapy. Prophylactic gonadal radiation in high risk boys has its advocates, but earlier testicular biopsies should help resolve this controversial issue.

Duration of Therapy and Cure

The singular statistic dramatizing the improved prognosis in childhood ALL is the 5-year disease-free survival of 60 percent. The question of duration of therapy is under active investigation today. When therapy was arbitrarily or randomly discontinued after two to three years of complete continuous remission, 10 to 15 percent of patients relapsed, usually within 12 months after cessation of therapy. Few, if any, relapses occurred four years after discontinuation of therapy, suggesting that this fortunate subset is cured. Unfortunately exceptions have occurred with late relapses reported as long as six years after therapy was stopped. Long-term follow-up of "cured" children with ALL will be required to determine the true curability of this disease. We know little about the true incidence of delayed adverse late effects on the central nervous system, second malignancies, endocrinopathies, growth failure, liver dysfunction, sterility, and congenitally-deformed offsprings of cured leukemic patients.

EXPERIMENTAL MODALITIES

Immunotherapy

Mathe and coworkers in France, and Ekert in Australia, suggested that immunotherapy with BCG prolonged the duration of remission in ALL. However, controlled studies from Britain, the United States, and Belgium showed no superiority of immunotherapy over conventional chemotherapy.

Bone Marrow Transplantation

Early attempts at bone marrow transplantation from HLA-identical, MLC-compatible donor to end-stage patients in relapse were associated with a disease-free survival of 15 percent. The projected survival at two years is 50 percent for patients transplanted in remission. Death from nonleukemic causes (graft-vs-host disease, interstitial pneumonia) and the recurrence rate of leukemia were also decreased significantly in patients transplanted in remission. For these reasons,bone marrow transplantation during remission in patients experiencing at least one relapse has been advocated and is under active study. Serious consideration must be given to this procedure in poor prognosis patients in first remission.

FUTURE ENDEAVORS

Clinical and laboratory research in childhood ALL in the 80's will attack a number of key issues and obstacles to cure. Among the most pressing and challenging are 1) the specific clinical and biologic characteristic of poor prognosis patients; 2) redefinition of the term "complete remission" using more sensitive laboratory tests to detect residual leukemic cells; 3) designing the least toxic, most effective regimens for children with a good prognosis (exclusion of radiation therapy and prolonged immunosuppressive maintenance therapy are two areas worthy of study); and 4) the biologic determinants of sanctuaries and pharmacologic resistance.

The past decade of clinical research in childhood ALL has resulted in overall improvement in rates of complete remission, duration of remission, and survival. Well-defined clinical and laboratory features have permitted a more precise and meaningful classification of ALL, now recognized as a heterogeneous disease with many phenotypes. Efforts in the 80's will explore the biology of leukemia. Future progress will depend upon our ability to apply the newly-derived knowledge to innovative therapeutic strategies.

ACUTE NON-LYMPHOCYTIC LEUKEMIA[6,13]

Progress in the treatment of childhood ANLL has been frustratingly slow and is at least 10 to 12 years behind ALL. Complete remissions are achieved in only 60 to 75 percent of patients. Early deaths caused by infection or hemorrhage, or

both, occur in 10 to 15 percent of children. The median duration of complete remission is about one year and the proportion
of patients surviving at 12,24,36 and 48 months is 55,32,21 and
18 percent, respectively. The obstacles to the successful
treatment of ANLL are formidable and are related to 1) the necessity of eradicating the malignant hematopoietic stem cell to
achieve a complete remission; 2) the significantly lower rate
of induction of complete remission compared to ALL; 3) inadequate or ineffective maintenance therapy; and 4) the rapid development of drug resistance.

The morphologic, histochemical, biochemical, and immunologic markers of childhood ANLL are similar to the disease in
adults and will not be reviewed further. The FAB classification
(M1 to M_6) for ANLL is useful in the pediatric population. Except for the poor prognosis in erythroleukemia (M_6), the prognostic significance of FAB subtypes in childhood ANLL is not
established. Unfavorable prognostic indicators for induction
failure include age (<5 or >10 yrs), black race, CNS disease
at diagnosis, gingival hypertrophy, WBC >100x10^9/liter, decreased bone marrow cellularity, and an abnormal karyotype. Predictors of early relapse include age, Hispanic ethnic background, high initial white blood cell count, and chromosomal
abnormalities. Black race, the presence of CNS disease, gingival hypertrophy, infection and disseminated intravascular
coagulation, a low platelet count (<25x10^9/liter), and a high
initial WBC (>100x10^9/liter) are unfavorable prognostic factors
for survival.

Successful induction regimens in children include the bi-
weekly cyclic combination of cytosine arabinoside and either
daunomycin or adriamycin. Generally, two to six cycles are
required to induce remission requiring 28 to 84 days. The prolonged period of bone marrow aplasia poses the gravest threat
to children with ANLL and the greatest challenge to the pediatric oncologist. Massive blood component support, granulocyte
transfusions, broad spectrum antimicrobials, anticoagulation
therapy for DIC, and intensive metabolic support for hypercalcemia and hyperkalemia are often required in each patient.
Children with 5÷15 percent myeloblasts in the bone marrow at
completion of induction do as well as children with <5 percent
blasts in the bone marrow. Accordingly, caution must be ex-
ercised in administering repeated courses of induction therapy.

Maintenance regimens are less effective and their true
role is uncertain. Cyclic maintenance, intermittent reinduction and continuous moderate intensity programs are under investigation. An effective, albeit uncontrolled, induction and
maintenance regimen in use at the Sidney Farber Cancer
Institute[13] yielded a complete remission rate of 70 percent and

a *projected* two year survival in patients achieving a complete remission of 50 per cent. These results translate to a two-year overall survival of 35 percent.

Bone marrow transplantation in first remission offers the best chance for long-term survival in childhood ANLL. It is anticipated that over 50 to 60 percent of children transplanted in remission will have long-term remissions and the best chance for cure. This approach is under active investigation by the CCSG and its collaborating centers.

REFERENCES

1. Andreeff M, Darzynkiewicz Z, Sharpless TK et al: Discrimination of human leukemia subtypes by flow cytometric analysis of cellular DNA and RNA. Blood 55:282-293, 1980.
2. Bennett JM, Catovsky D, Daniel MT et al: Proposals for the classification of the acute leukemias. Br J Haematol 33: 451-457, 1976.
3. Coleman MS, Greenwood MF, Hutton JJ et al: Serial observations on terminal deoxynucleotidyl transferase and lymphoblast surface markers in acute lymphoblastic leukemia. Cancer Research 36:120-126, 1976.
4. Hammond D, Sather H, Honour RC et al: The relative importance of clinical and biological predictors of outcome in the treatment of acute lymphocytic leukemia,in"Cell Markers in Acute Leukemia,"National Cancer Institute, March, 1980.
5. Kersey J, LeBien T, Hurwitz et al: Childhood leukemia-lymphoma: Heterogeneity of phenotypes and prognoses. Amer J Clin Pathol 72:746-752, 1979.
6. Kobrinsky NL, Robison LL, Nesbit ME: Acute nonlymphocytic leukemia. Pediatr Clin N Amer 27:347-360, 1980.
7. Mauer AM:Therapy of acute lymphoblastic leukemia in childhood. Blood 56:1-10, 1980.
8. Miller DR: Acute lymphoblastic leukemia. Pediatr Clin N Amer 27:269-291, 1980.
9. Miller DR, Leikin S, Albo V et al: The use of prognostic factors in improving the design and efficiency of clinical trials in childhood leukemia. Cancer Treat Rep 64:199-210, 1980.
10. Robison L, Sather H, Coccia PF et al: Assessment of the interrelationship of prognostic factors in childhood acute lymphoblastic leukemia. Am J Pediatr Hem/Onc 2:5-13, 1980.
11. Shaw MT: The cytochemistry of acute leukemia:A diagnostic and prognostic evaluation. Semin Oncol 3:219-228, 1976.
12. Simone J: The treatment of acute lymphoblastic leukaemia. Br J Haematol 45:1-4, 1980.
13. Weinstein HJ, Mayer RJ, Rosenthal DR et al:Treatment of acute myelogenous leukemia in children and adults. New Engl J Med 303:473-478, 1980.

The Chronic Leukemias

GEORGE P. CANELLOS, M.D.

Chief
Division of Medical Oncology
Sidney Farber Cancer Institute
Boston, Massachusetts

A. Chronic Granulocytic Leukemia

Although chronic granulocytic leukemia (CGL) is a rare disease a study of its pathogenesis has contributed to our understanding of stem cell physiology. The Philadelphia chromosome abnormality, although consistent through the course of the disease, represents a translocation from the 22 to the 9 position. It is apparent that rarer variants of translocation to other chromosomes might occur and that the abnormality may not be as strictly confined to cells of erythroid, myeloid and megakaryocyte origin. Whether a lymphoid cell line is also involved is a matter of current investigation and debate. The terminal phase of the disease has been described as a blastic transformation or metamorphosis. Although most therapeutic maneuvers are known to be ineffective, the fact that a minority of patients may have blast cells with morphologic, enzymatic, and surface membrane marker characteristics compatible with acute lymphoblastic leukemia is reflected in the response of these patients to antilymphoblastic chemotherapy - Vincristine and Prednisone. Allogeneic bone marrow transplantation has been disappointing but recently, Fefer and co-workers have demonstrated that identical twin marrow can be safely and successfully transplanted to patients in the chronic phase following ablation with Cyclophosphamide, Dimethyl Myleran and total body irradiation to 920 rads. It is encouraging that this program has effectively eliminated the Philadelphia chromosome from periods varying between 24 and 36 months. Identical twin transplantation in the blastic phase has been a disappointment and has reflected the refractoriness of blastic leukemia at that stage. In any transplantation experience, a long-term cure is hard to assess since it will require several

years of follow-up to be assured that the last Ph$_1$ chromosome
bearing cell has been eradicated. It has been estimated that
it will take 6.3 years to achieve a 100% Philadelphia chromosome positive metaphases in the marrow before there is an
elevation in the leukocyte count above 10,000/mm^3.

Allogeneic transplantation in the chronic phase would
expose the patient to the hazards of graft versus host disease and interstitial pneumonia, etc. Although it seems that
the chronic phase leukemia would be easier to eradicate. The
use of autologous marrow or peripheral stem cells offers an
attractive alternative. However, the basic problem of elimination of refractory blast cells remain unsolved, especially
in light of the identical twin blastic transformation
experience at Seattle. The use of intensive therapy to eliminate or diminish the percentage of Philadelphia positive
metaphases represents another potential for long-term control
of the disease. If the marrow could be returned to a Ph
negative status, these cells could be cryopreserved for subsequent transplantation. The optimal regimen is unknown but
must lie somewhere between the L-5 protocol (Memorial) and
the chemo-radiotherapy ablation program of Seattle. The
availability of an antiserum specific for the Philadelphia
chromosome bearing cell lines would be of great assistance
in cell sorting and in the use of immunologic techniques to
eradicate residual leukemic cells.

B.   Chronic Lymphocytic Leukemia

The diagnostic criteria for chronic lymphocytic leukemia
include the finding of absolute lymphocytosis with 15,000/mm^3
with 40 to 50% lymphocytes in the bone marrow. These minimal
criteria only, however, are often associated with a very prolonged natural history. Since CLL has a median age of approximately 60 years and can be associated with secondary abnormalities of immunoglobulin synthesis, the risk of intensive
therapy should be weighed against the benefits. The majority
of CLL patients will have a disorder of B lymphocyte proliferation. These cells characteristically stain faintly for
surface immunoglobulins as opposed to B cell lymphomas such
as nodular lymphoma. The use of a staging classification
that predicts survival is essential in determining criteria
for therapy and the results of new therapeutic programs. A
commonly used staging scheme is that of Rai where Stage 0 is
associated with a median survival in excess of 150 months and
consists of only the minimum diagnostic criteria. Stage I
patients have lymphocytosis plus lymphadenopathy only and
depending on the series of median survival varies from 60 to
100 months. Stage II is characterized by lymphocytosis and

splenomegaly and/or hepatomegaly with or without lymph node enlargement. The median survival varies from 45 to 70 months. Stage III includes lymphocytosis, but an anemia of <10 grams in females and <11 grams in males. Hepatosplenomegaly and lymphadenopathy may not be present. The median survival is approximately 24 months. Stage IV includes those with a platelet count of <100,000. The median survival is the same as in the Stage III, approximately 24 months. Males seem to have a more unfavorable prognosis. A rare occurrence of T cell CLL should be noted in that it has a short natural history with a rather high incidence of skin involvement and poor response to therapy. Radiation therapy can be effectively used to control locally enlarged lymph nodes. The vast majority of patients who require therapy systemic control of their disease which will often be associated with constitutional symptoms such as weight loss and fever.

Irradiation has been used in the past for systemic control including techniques for extracorporeal irradiation of peripheral blood; mediastinal or thymic irradiation; fractionated total body irradiation; intravenous P32; and splenic irradiation. All of these techniques can effect the shrinkage of enlarged organs and decrease of leukocyte count. No one technique has emerged superior. It is controversial whether mediastinal irradiation is useful. One report in the literature condemns it as potentially extremely toxic. Both extracorporeal irradiation and intensive leukophoresis can reduce blood counts to relatively low levels without significant change in organomegaly. It takes approximately 3 to 4 months before the count returns to its previous level. Fractionated total body irradiation from 100 to 400 rads appears to act like a systemic chemotherapeutic agent in that it can achieve an improvement in all manifestations of the disease. It is associated with the risk of bone marrow suppression. Complete remissions are rarely achieved in the treatment of CLL but total body irradiation (TBI) can achieve complete disappearance of all clinical manifestations of the disease, although a small fraction of lymphocytes will remain in the marrow aspirate or biopsy. Cell surface marker studies may even note that lymphocytes containing monoclonal immunoglobulins will disappear from the peripheral blood and marrow. TBI has also been reported to increase the abnormally low serum immunoglobulins which is rarely seen with any other mode of treatment. It is difficult to interpret the effect on survival since patients in the Stage 0 and Stage I seem to have had the best responses.

Cytotoxic chemotherapy can be effectively used in the treatment of CLL with Chlorambucil and Cyclophosphamide being

the principal cytotoxic agents. Regardless of the schedule
of administration, daily or oral, biweekly or monthly,
approximately half of the patients will achieve hematologic
and clinical benefit. The doses vary from 6 to 12 mgs. a day
up to 20 to 30 mgs. biweekly or monthly. It is unclear
whether the addition of Prednisone will improve survival but
it appears to enhance the hematologic benefit. Prednisone
itself used as a single agent rarely achieves the quality of
remission seen with chemotherapy or radiation. Corticosteroids are indicated for the treatment of autoimmune phenomena
and may allow for an improvement in hematologic abnormalities
associated with advanced chronic lymphatic leukemia. The use
of combination chemotherapy such as might be used for myeloma
achieves a high order of response, but it is hard to determine whether it will be superior to the former. The M2 protocol which includes Cyclophosphamide, BCNU, Vincristine,
Prednisone, and Melphalan is currently under investigation.
Complete remissions have been achieved in less than 15% of
cases, but they have not been long lasting.

New modalities of treatment should be compared in trials
where there is stratification according to stage. At the
present time, chronic lymphatic leukemia like nodular lymphocytic lymphoma is extremely difficult to eradicate by intensive therapy.

CHRONIC GRANULOCYTIC LEUKEMIA
References

1. Canellos GP: Chronic granulocytic leukemia. Medical
    Clinics of North America 60:1001-1008, 1976.
2. Canellos GP: The treatment of chronic granulocytic
    leukaemia, in Canellos GP (ed): The Lymphomas. East
    Sussex, England, W.B. Saunders, 1977, pp 113-128
3. Doney K, Buckner CD, Sale GE, et al.: Treatment of
    chronic granulocytic leukemia by chemotherapy, total
    body irradiation and allogeneic bone marrow transplanta-
    tion. Exp Hematol 6:738-745, 1978.
4. Fialkow PJ, Jacobson RJ, Papayannopoulou : Chronic
    myelocytic leukemia: Clonal origin in stem cell common
    to the granulocyte, erythrocyte, platelet and monocyte/
    macrophage. The Amer J. of Med 63:125-130, 1977.
5. Goldman JM, Spiers ASD, Catovsky D, et al.: Use of cryo-
    preserved buffy coat cells as a bone marrow autograft
    for patients with chronic granulocytic leukemia in trans-
    formation. Blood 52:251, 1978.
6. Janossy G, Greaves MF, Sutherland R, et al.: Comparative
    analysis of membrane phenotypes in acute lymphoid leuke-
    mia and in lymphoid blast crisis of chronic myeloid
    leukaemia. Leukemia Research 1:289-300, 1977.
7. Kamada N, Uchino H: Chronologic sequence in appearance
    of clinical and laboratory findings characteristic of
    chronic myelocytic leukemia. Blood 51:843-850, 1978.
8. Marks SM, Baltimore D, McCaffrey R: Terminal transferase
    as a predictor of initial responsiveness to vincristine
    and prednisone in blastic chronic myelogenous leukemia.
    The New Eng J of Med 298:812-814, 1978.
9. Rosenthal S, Canellos GP, Whang-Peng J, et al.: Blast
    crisis of chronic granulocytic leukemia. The Amer J
    of Med 63:542-547, 1977.

CHRONIC LYMPHOCYTIC LEUKEMIA
References

1. Binet JL, Leporrier M, Dighiero G, et al.: A clinical
    staging system for chronic lymphocytic leukemia.
    Cancer 40:855-864, 1977.
2. Curtis JE, Hersh EM, Freireich EJ: Leukapheresis therapy
    of chronic lymphocytic leukemia. Blood 39:163-174,
    1972.
3. Hansen MM: Chronic lymphocytic leukemia: Clinical
    studies based on 189 cases followed for a long time.
    Scand J Haemat 18:3-286, 1973.
4. Johnson RE, Ruhl U: Treatment of chronic lymphocytic
    leukemia with emphasis on total body irradiation. Int
    J Radiat Oncol Biol Phys 1:387-397, 1976.
5. Knospe WH, Loeb V, Jr., Huguley CM, Jr.: Bi-weekly
    chlorambucil treatment of chronic lymphocytic leukemia.
    Cancer 33:555-562, 1974.
6. Koziner B, Kempin S, Gee T, et al.: Cell-marker analysis
    of complete remissions in chronic B-cell leukemias.
    The Lancet 1:158, 1979.
7. Phillips EA, Kempin S, Passe S, et al.: Prognostic fac-
    tors in chronic lymphocytic leukaemia and their implica-
    tions for therapy. Clinics in Haematology 6:203-222,
    1977.
8. Rai KR, Sawitsky A, Cronkite EP, et al.: Clinical
    staging of chronic lymphocytic leukemia. Blood 46:219-
    234, 1975.
9. Sawitsky A, Rai KR, Aral I, et al.: Mediastinal irradia-
    tion for chronic lymphocytic leukemia. The Amer J of
    Med 61:892-896, 1976.
10. Sawitsky A, Rai KR, Glidewell O, et al.: Comparison of
    daily versus intermittent chlorambucil and prednisone
    therapy in the treatment of patients with chronic
    lymphocytic leukemia. Blood 50:1049-1059, 1977.
11. Silver RT: The treatment of chronic lymphocytic leukemia.
    Seminars in Hemat 6:344-356, 1969.

Solid Tumors 1

Current Views on the
Primary Treatment of Breast Cancer

GIANNI BONADONNA, PINUCCIA VALAGUSSA
and UMBERTO VERONESI

Istituto Nazionale Tumori, Milan, Italy

Cancer of the breast is today one of the most serious problems
of clinical and research oncology. It is the leading cause of
death of women in many countries and there is great uncertainty as to whether the emphasis should be on prevention, detection or treatment. From the therapeutic point of view, breast
cancer remains at the center of innumerable disputes regarding
the treatment strategy, although the recent experience has dem
onstrated the importance of multidisciplinary approach. This
review will attempt to outline the most important recent
achievements in the curative treatment of primary breast cancer.

The objective in the treatment of primary breast cancer
are twofold: (1) to increase survival and cure rates through
earlier diagnosis and more effective therapy, and (2) to improve the quality of life by the application of conservative
treatments in selected patients and by post treatment reabi-
litation. In the direction of first objective, important results were recently obtained by a rational use of adjuvant che
motherapy and better selection of patients to be treated with
endocrine manipulations. To reach the second objective, trials
are still in progress; however the results of some of them
clearly indicate that mutilating surgery is not required for
patients with tumor of limited dimensions.

* This work was supported in part by Contract NO1-CM-33714
with the Division of Cancer Treatment, National Cancer Institute, NIH, Bethesda, Maryland.

Reprints requests: Gianni Bonadonna, M.D., Istituto Nazionale
Tumori, Via Venezian, 1, 20133 Milano, Italy.

IMPROVEMENT OF SURVIVAL

Prognostic Factors

   In recent years, innumerable observations have confirmed
that the classical approach based only on anatomical principles (radical mastectomy with or without postoperative irradia
tion) has reached a plateau in the cure rate of primary breast
cancer. In most patients the reasons for primary treatment
failure are due to the progressive growth of distant micrometastases present prior to diagnosis. Following local-regional
modality, the course of the disease bears no geographical restrictions as clearly outlined by the studies of NSABP [13] and
Milan Institute [26] carried out through the analysis of prospec
tive randomized series. In particular, the curves of primary
treatment failure have indicated a pattern of progressive relapse rate so that at 10 years from optimal surgery the relapse-free survival (RFS) was about 50%. Furthermore, the histologic status of axillary lymph nodes represented the single
most useful prognostic factor (Table 1). While the RFS was in-

Table 1. Current Prognostic Parameters for
Primary Operable Breast Cancer

AXILLARY NODES	10-yr RFS	
Negative (N-)		72-75%
Positive (N+)		23-24%
1-3		33-35%
> 3		13-16%
ESTROGEN RECEPTORS	3-yr RFS	
ER+		78-82%
ER-		35-40%
HISTOLOGIC GRADING	10-yr Surv.	
Low		55-60%
High		20-25%
VASCULAR INVASION	Visceral Recurr.*	
Yes		43%
No		4%

* From Nime et al., Am. J. Surg. Path., 1977

versely proportional to the size of primary tumor (T) only in
patients with N+ (T_1: 50.2%; T_2: 24.1%; T_{3a}: 17.6%), both RFS
and total survival were not affected by menopausal status.
Finally, in N+ patients the incidence of local-regional recurrence (particularly chest wall and homolateral supraclavicular

area) was highest during the first 3 years from mastectomy (81.4%) and within the subsequent 24 months, this was followed by distant metastases in 60.3%. [26]

In more recent years, other prognostic factors have been considered. Although for some of them their relative importance requires more precise delineation in given subsets, they are now being utilized in the stratification parameters of prospective randomized studies. Of particular interest is the estrogen receptor (ER) assay on the primary tumor. As recommended by the Consensus Meeting on "Steroid Receptors in Breast Cancer" held at NCI on June 27-29, 1979, the most reliable and reproducible methods for cytosol ER assay appear to be sucrose density gradient sedimentation analysis and multiple point, dextran charcoal assay analyzed by Scatchard plot. The controversy concerning the quantitative criteria to classify tumors as ER positive or negative is not completely settled but most investigators class as ER+ tumors containing more than 10 fmol/mg cytosol protein. Despite lack of quality control in reported observations, there is ample evidence that, at least during the first 3 years from surgery, the RFS was higher in women with ER+ tumors compared to women with ER- tumors (Table 1). It is interesting to point out that in N- patients with ER- tumors the 3-year RFS curve appears very similar to that of N+ patients. [8] The clinical aggressiveness of ER- tumors is largerly explained by the observation of higher proliferative activity (high labeling index, high grade tumor histology) compared to ER+ tumors. It is therefore recommended that each primary breast cancer should be assayed for ER so that the information will not only be available when needed at the time of disseminated disease, but it will also help in the selection of high risk N- patients who could be candidate for adjuvant chemotherapy.

Multimodality approach

Current multimodality strategy finds its rationale in the above reported clinical findings after single modality as well as in the experimental animal data. As summarized by Schabel, [23] the effectiveness of surgical adjuvant chemotherapy decreases as (1) the tumor staging is advanced prior to surgery; (2) the interval from surgery to start of effective chemotherapy is increased; (3) the drug doses are reduced. Other experimental findings derived from the same research group [23] and providing the scientific basis for administering adjuvant chemotherapy in humans can be summarized as follows: (1) tumor cell population growth kinetics indicates that the fraction of viable cells undergoing active replication is inversely related to population size; (2) first order cell-kill

kinetics characterizes effective drug cell kill of tumor cells;
(3) surgical adjuvant chemotherapy is both dose-responsive and
related to the body burden of metastatic tumor at the time of
drug treatment.

From the clinical point of view, after the initial attempts
with short-term (perioperative) single agent chemotherapy [7]
the multimodality approach for operable breast cancer was re-
vitalized in 1972 when the National Cancer Institute launched
two large-scale randomized trials through the NSABP group and
the Milan Cancer Institute. The trials were very similar in
terms of patient selection, surgical treatment and follow up
studies. They differed only in the type of drugs utilized
(NSABP: single agent chemotherapy with l-phenylalanine mustard
or l-PAM; Milan: combination chemotherapy with cyclophosphamide, methotrexate and fluorouracil or CMF). The publication of
the early results [2,11] dramatically generalized the physician
interest and the public attention on adjuvant chemotherapy as
a potentially important weapon to improve the cure rate of pri
mary breast cancer. Numerous randomized and non randomized
trials were then mounted all over the world to confirm or to
attempt to improve the results of l-PAM and CMF. The body of
data which has accumulated in only five years is already immense to be adequately reported within a limited space; for
this reason, the readers are advised to consult some of the re
cent review publications [5,7,18,22] to which we will refer
throughout the text. Table 2 outlines some of the current drug
regimens utilized in the adjuvant situation. They can be
roughly subdivided into four main subgroups, i.e. with and
without prednisone, with and without adriamycin. Ongoing studies can also be schematically subdivided into ten subgroups,
i.e. with and without concomitant surgical control group, with
single agent (l-PAM) versus combination chemotherapy (CMF,
CMFV, CMFVP, CFP), with and without postoperative irradiation,
with and without hormones (tamoxifen), with and without immune
stimulation (BCG, C. Parvum, levamisole, Poly A-Poly U). Since
the final evaluation of an adjuvant trial will take many years
of follow up, the results of many studies are still too premature to provide a meaningful answer to the practicing oncologist concerning the relative merits of a given adjuvant regimen. In fact, the reports contain actuarial RFS and total survival projections of 2 to 3 years, with many patients being
under follow up for less than that period and some still under
active treatment. [7] Only a few trials meet the three classical
criteria of (1) adequate control of an experience with surgery
alone; (2) adequate follow up time for RFS and overall survival and (3) adequate number of patients in critical subsets. In
spite of these limitations, the few available series with N+

Table 2. Some of the Drug Combinations
being Utilized in Adjuvant Therapy

| Acronym | Response in advanced breast ca. | | Treatment duration in an adjuvant setting |
	CR+PR %	Duration median in mos.	
CMFVP	51	8	2 yr or 9 mos.
CMFP	68	8	12 cycles
CMF	53	8	24, 12 or 6 cycles
CFP	52	8.5	10 cycles
AC	78	12	8 cycles
FAC+BCG	76	12	2 yr
CMF(P)—>AV	60	12	CMF(P) 6 cycles —> AV 4 cycles

C=Cyclophosphamide; M=Methotrexate; F=Fluorouracil;
V=Vincristine; P=Prednisone; A=Adriamycin.

and followed for a minimum of 3 to a maximum of 6-7 years have
so far provided encouraging results to sponsor a NCI Consensus
"Conference on Adjuvant Chemotherapy of Breast Cancer" (July
14-16, 1980). The essential therapeutic findings are summarized in Table 3. The findings of the CMF adjuvant program carried out in Milan [3,21] confirmed the initial observations [2] on
the usefulness of combination chemotherapy in improving both
RFS and total survival rates. Furthermore, (1) local-regional
recurrence was less after mastectomy plus CMF (8.7%) compared
to mastectomy alone; (2) CMF-induced amenorrhea failed to influence the RFS; (3) the rate and the duration of response to
second-line treatment were comparable in patients relapsing
after mastectomy vs those relapsing after mastectomy plus CMF;
(4) there was no increased incidence of secondary tumors.

Important additional findings were provided by the analysis
of dose level [3] and of ER status. [4] The frequency of complete
plus partial remission in advanced disease and the improvement
of RFS and total survival rates in the adjuvant setting, respectively, were directly proportional to the level of dose
administered. This observation indicated that a relationship
of dose to response existed in the treatment of human breast
cancer. For comparative dose levels ($\geq$ 85%, 84-65%, < 65%)
there was no difference in the RFS and total survival between

Table 3. Essential Findings of Adjuvant Studies
with Follow Up $\geq$ 3 Years

Adjuvant therapy	Results
CMF (12 or 6 cycles) Milan Cancer Inst.	Significant improvement of 5-yr RFS and total survival vs controls. No difference between pre and postmenopausal patients receiving comparative dose levels of CMF. No influence on results by ER status. No increased incidence of second neoplasms.
PAM and PAM+FU NSABP Group	Significant improvement of 5-yr RFS and total survival in premenopausal patients with 1-3 nodes given PAM compared to controls. Significant improvement at 4 yr in postmenopausal patients with > 3 nodes given PAM+FU compared to PAM alone.
CFP $\pm$ RT Mayo Clinic	Improved 4 yr results over historical controls. Combination chemotherapy is superior to PAM especially in premenopausal women. Postoperative RT failed to influence the results.
AC $\pm$ RT Univ. Arizona	Improved 4 yr results over historical controls. Preliminary evidence of a dose-response effect. Lower RFS in patients given postoperative RT.
FAC + BCG $\pm$ RT M.D. Anderson Hosp.	Improved 4 yr RFS and total survival over historical controls. Best available results in women with > 3 nodes. No influence of postoperative RT. The role of BCG remains unsettled.

pre and postmenopausal women. Furthermore, as shown in Table 4, within each dose level the results were related to the number of axillary nodes and within each nodal group the 5-year RFS was dose related. Adjuvant treatments started in N+ patients with low-dose regimens were found ineffective also by Senn et al. and by Hubai et al. [18] In untreated breast cancer the ER status per se was not confirmed to be an important predictor for chemotherapy response.[4] This held true both in advanced and operable breast cancer with N+ treated with CMF. In fact, at 3 years after radical mastectomy the RFS was similar for ER+ and

for ER- tumors, regardless of menopausal status. The results
for ER+ tumors were not substantially different when the two
levels of fmoles (> 5 or > 10) were considered. In particular,
for ER+ and ER- tumors the RFS was comparable both in the two
major nodal subgroups and in patients with and without CMF-
induced amenorrhea. The latter finding definitely ruled out
the hypothesis that in premenopausal women the therapeutic effect of CMF was largerly related to chemical castration.

Table 4. Percent 5-Year RFS Related to CMF Levels

% of optimal drug dose	Premenopause			Postmenopause		
	Total	Nodes 1-3	Nodes > 3	Total	Nodes 1-3	Nodes > 3
Level I ($\geq$ 85%)	79.1	86.0	64.4	75.3	83.2	59.9
Level II (84-65%)	55.7	68.1	32.8	55.9	67.3	37.7
Level III (< 65%)	45.5	55.9	23.3	48.9	57.9	27.1
Control	43.4	48.5	26.8	49.3	50.8	40.5

From the results of other research institutions taking part
to the Consensus Meeting and quoted in Table 3, there is no
clear evidence for a predominant effectiveness of adjuvant
chemotherapy in pre vs postmenopausal women. On the contrary,
the available findings would strongly support the evidence
that also in an adjuvant setting and regardless of the drugs
in the regimen, combination chemotherapy is superior to single
agent chemotherapy, such as 1-PAM. [22] Furthermore, the role of
adriamycin in the combination could be very important at least
in certain subsets. The findings reported by the M.D. Anderson
with FAC plus BCG [22] in women with > 3 nodes appear, for the
time being, superior to all other results reported in this sub
group. Available results on adjuvant hormonal treatment are
still too preliminary, although there is an emerging evidence
from the Cleveland [18] and the NSABP groups that the administra
tion of tamoxifen can favourably influence the 2-3 years RFS
of women with ER+ tumors. The results of the Toronto trial [18,
22] with ovarian radiation and prolonged administration of pred
nisone yielded favorable results in the subgroup of premenopausal women $\geq$ 45 years. The same cautious consideration applies to the various forms of adjuvant immune stimulation. The
true efficacy of BCG, C. Parvum and tumor cell vaccine remains,
at present, unsettled for a number of reasons (e.g. lack of
randomized studies, short-term follow up). Available findings

failed to indicate an improvement of results by adjuvant MER[30] or levamisole [14] when combined with chemotherapy compared to the results obtained with chemotherapy alone. The provocative results of Lacour et al. [17] who have claimed an improved 5-year RFS after adjuvant Poly A-Poly U need to be confirmed in women not subjected to adjuvant castration.

CONSERVATIVE THERAPY

Alternatives to Halsted Mastectomy

As mentioned before, a redefinition of the basis for the primary treatment of breast cancer is in progress and follows present understanding of tumor biology. The possibility that the classical Halsted mastectomy could not represent the treatment of choice for all breast carcinomas has been raised long time ago by isolated pioneers. [5,27] Unfortunately, the limited number of patients treated with unconventional surgery and, most important, the lack of prospective randomized trials have posponed for more than 30 years the possibility to bring before surgeons the convincing evidence that alternatives to the Halsted mastectomy do indeed exist. In the past few years, the increasing awareness that breast cancer represents a heterogeneous group of neoplasms and that cancer in general is often a systemic disease resulted in the development of new scientific, rather than emotional basis for breast cancer surgery. As demonstrated by the studies of Fisher et al., [10,12] there is no orderly pattern of tumor-cell dissemination that could be based on mechanical considerations; therefore, variations in local-regional therapy are unlikely to affect survival substantially. Considering the tumor spread, Halsted mastectomy appears inadequate to alter the incidence of systemic recurrence while it seems an excessively mutilating procedure particularly for women with neoplasms of limited dimensions.

The concept that the "radical" extirpation of a breast tumor is not directly proportional to the extent of surgery has been proven by two large prospective randomized multicentric trials. The first study [16,29] was performed by an international group and failed to show the superiority of the extended radical mastectomy over the classical Halsted operation. The second study was carried out by members of the NSABP group [10,12] and the results indicated that in clinically node negative patients (40% of whom had histologically positive nodes), three distinctly different regimens - radical mastectomy, total (simple) mastectomy plus local-regional irradiation or total mastectomy and removal of nodes that later became clinically positive - yielded no substantial difference in the overall incidence of treatment failure, the incidence of distant metasta ses or total survival. Similarly, in clinically node positive women, treatment by radical mastectomy or total mastectomy plus local-regional radiotherapy yielded no substantial difference on the basis of the aforementioned criteria. The above mentioned results, as well as data from other series, indicated at the Consensus-development Conference on "The Treatment of Primary Breast Cancer: Management of local disease" sponsored by NCI on June 5, 1979 [24] that total mastectomy with axillary dissection can be regarded as a satisfactory alternative to the Halsted radical mastectomy in women with Stage I or Stage II disease. Therefore, this procedure should be recognized as the current standard treatment. The axillary dissection is performed for the purpose of staging as well as for therapeutic benefit.

The evolution of breast cancer surgery, which has abandoned the keystone of the halstedian principles of tumor management, i.e. the importance of en-bloc dissection, as well as advances in clinical radiation therapy and radiotherapeutic equipment, have open the way to the study and application of conservative treatments in properly selected patients. Other important concomitant factors working on the new line of understanding are represented by the detection through mammography of an increasing number of tumors of limited dimensions (< 2 cm) and by women awareness of the relative merits of alternative procedures.

Conservative Surgery

The definition of conservative surgery should be limited to procedures preserving at least part of the breast. It does not seem appropriate to consider as conservative treatment that removing the totality of one breast, as total gastrectomy, cystectomy or pneumonectomy cannot be defined as conservative procedures. [5,27]

Conservative treatment by surgery alone consists of two types of operation. [5,27] The partial mastectomy proposed by Crile [9] consists of a large resection of the breast with at least 2 cm of normal tissue removed around the tumor edges. The incision may be radial to the nipple or transverse, the pectoralis fascia is removed en-bloc and the reconstruction allows a cosmetically acceptable breast. The second operation consists in the same type of large breast resection with simultaneous axillary dissection. The lymph node dissection may be performed en-bloc with the primary tumor if this is located in the outer upper quadrants, or in discontinuity for tumor in other quadrants. This second type of operation is that currently performed in the randomized trial conducted by the NSABP group. [5,10,27] At the Cancer Institute of Milan, U. Veronesi et al. [28] have devised the technique of quadrantectomy which

provides a more precise and quantitative description of the
operation. The resection of the mammary tissue comprises an
entire quadrant of the breast together with the overlying skin
and the corresponding portion of the fascial sheet of the
pectoralis major. The operation includes a simultaneous axillary dissection which, whenever possible, is performed en-bloc
and in continuity with the breast quadrantectomy. Many conservative surgical treatments are supplemented by postoperative
radiotherapy, with doses varying from 25-30 Gy. In the Milan
trial [5,27,28] radiotherapy is delivered to the residual breast
tissue and consists of 50 Gy with high-energy irradiation
through two opposing tangential fields, and a boost of 10 Gy
to the skin sorrounding the scar with orthovoltage equipment.
Radiotherapy starts 15-20 days after surgery and is completed
within six weeks.

Comprehensive reviews of all past and ongoing trials were
recently published elsewhere. [5,27] Briefly, the Helsinki trial
(not randomized) published by Mustakallio and Rissanen as well
as the Toronto trial (not randomized) reported by Peters where
the conservative approach consisted of local tumor excision
followed by postoperative radiotherapy, yielded 5 and 10-year
survival rates which were almost superimposable to those of
radical mastectomy $\pm$ irradiation. The only trial where conservative treatment yielded lower survival rates as well as
higher incidence of local and axillary recurrence compared to
radical mastectomy plus irradiation was the randomized study
of the Guy's Hospital. [5] The main reason for this unsuccessful
trial was probably due to the low dose of postoperative irradiation (35 Gy) delivered to the axilla.

The two most important contemporary trials are those designed by the Milan Cancer Institute [5,27,28] and the NSABP group.
[5,10,12] Figure 1 shows the schema of the Milan trial which applies to T_1 N_{0-1a} M_0 patients, i.e. with tumors less than 2 cm
in diameter. The study was activated in September 1973 and
from January 1975 radiotherapy to lymph node regions was discontinued while all patients with N+ were given 12 cycles of
adjuvant CMF chemotherapy. [28] As of May 1980, a total of 701
evaluable patients were accrued (Halsted group 349, conservative group 352). The details of study patients and of treatment results will be published separately. Sufficit for this
review to show in Table 5 the comparative summary of 5-year results. The lack of difference in both RFS and total survival
between the two treatment groups allows to conclude for the
first time that through a large randomized series there is no
clinical justification to perform Halsted mastectomy for breast
cancers of small dimensions. Figure 2 shows the schema of the
NSABP trial. For the time being, this is the only randomized

Fig. 1. Conservative Treatment of Breast Cancer
Milan Trial

$T_1 N_{0-1a}$

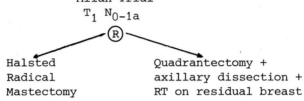

Halsted	Quadrantectomy +
Radical	axillary dissection +
Mastectomy	RT on residual breast

Accrual period: Sept. 1973 - May 1980
Total entered : 701 patients

N-: No further therapy
N+: Sept. 73-Dec. 75 (R) : No further therapy vs postop. RT
    Jan. 76-May 80 CMF x 12 cycles

Table 5. Milan Trial. 5-Yr Results
(Data are in percent)

	RFS	Surv.
Halsted	83.0	89.7
Conservative	82.7	88.5
N-	87.8	92.6
N+	67.5	78.8
Outer quadrants	83.2	91.8
Others	82.0	84.8
Premenopause	84.4	89.7
Postmenopause	81.1	89.3

Fig. 2. Conservative Treatment of Breast Cancer
NSABP Trial

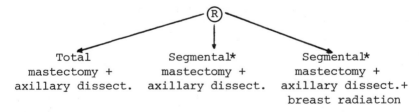

Total	Segmental*	Segmental*
mastectomy +	mastectomy +	mastectomy +
axillary dissect.	axillary dissect.	axillary dissect.+
		breast radiation

N+: Adjuvant chemotherapy (1-PAM+FU)

* Total mastectomy for tumor in ipsilateral breast.

controlled trial in the United States and Canada evaluating
the biologic and the clinical importance of tumor multicentricity. In fact, women who have undergone segmental mastectomies
are divided into two groups, one will receive breast irradiation, and the other will not. At the time of this writing, the
NSABP is still accruing patients, and so far more than 600 women were randomized.

Curative radiotherapy

The conservative management of breast cancer utilizing radical irradiation either alone or following gross removal of
the primary tumor by lumpectomy was pioneered by Baclesse more
than 40 years ago. [1] Since the early European studies, reports
on the efficacy of radiotherapy without mastectomy in the primary management of breast cancer are appearing in the literature with increasing frequency. [5,6,15,19,20,25] The principles
of radical radiotherapy for primary breast cancer can be summarized as follows: (1) the gross tumor mass should be surgically removed (lumpectomy); (2) the treatment volume includes
the entire breast as well as the axillary, supraclavicular and
internal mammary nodes; (3) supervoltage equipment is utilized
and treatment should be carefully planned; (4) the dose consists of 45-50 Gy to the areas of subclinical disease plus an
optional boost of 10-20 Gy to the tumor area. Some radiation
therapists [5,15] utilized implants with iridium-92 instead of
the boost technique with external beam. Larger doses (> 60 Gy)
are required for the local control of bulky tumors.

Table 6 summarizes the therapeutic results of the most important large European and American series. Some of the data
are still unpublished and they were kindly provided by the
investigators. In spite of different policies utilized in patient selection, staging procedures and radiotherapeutic techniques, available results are remarkably consistent, and for
primary tumors less than 3 cm total survival appears comparable to that obtained with Halsted mastectomy ± postoperative
irradiation. All radiation therapists have stressed the prognostic importance of tumor size. For tumor larger than 3 cm
and/or in the presence of clinical N_{1b} axillary nodes survival
rates were lower compared to less advanced cases. However,
also in these groups the results appear comparable to those re
ported by radical surgery. For tumors less than 3 cm the incidence of local recurrence was less than 10% and this was not
obviously correlated with the dose (with and without boost,
with and without iridium-92 implant). Women requiring salvage
surgery for recurrent or residual disease were higher in the
series of Calle et al. [6] and Spitalier et al. [25] compared to
the other series. [15,19,20] Cosmetic results were good to

Table 6. Percent 5-Year Results After Primary Radiotherapy with or without Surgical Excision

Author	Total Pts/ surgical excision	Clinical stage		RFS (%)	Total survival (%)	Surgery*** after RT (No. Pts)
Pierquin	303/70	T_1-T_2-T_3 (N_0-N_1)	T_1	82	92	
			T_2	75	81	25
			T_3	54	70	
Calle	953/204	T_1-T_2-T_3 (N_0-N_1)	T_1 N_0	92	92	
			T_2 N_0-N_1	79	79	441
			T_3 N_0-N_1	58	58	
Spitalier	1644/528	T_1-T_2-T_3 (N_0-N_1)	T_1 N_0	83	84	
			T_1 N_1	66	71	427
			T_2 N_{0-1}			
			T_3 N_{0-1}	37	45	
Hellman	184/166	I and II	I	95**	96	
			II	91**	68	7
Prosnitz	293*	I and II	I	87	91	
			II	62	77	12

*   Exact No. with prior surgical excision not available.
**   Local control.
*** Mainly mastectomy for persistent or recurrent disease.

excellent in more than 75% of cases, and were influenced by
(1) the location and extent of the biopsy procedures; (2) the
time-dose factors of radiation therapy, and (3) the technique
of irradiation. [5,15] Radiation sequelae were rare (< 10%) and
consisted primarily in rib fractures followed by radiation
pneumonitis, excessive fibrosis, limitation of motion and
brachial plexus injury (sensory).

FUTURE DEVELOPMENTS

The past decade has witnessed a fondamental evolution in
the treatment approach for breast cancer. The evolution has
been primarily based on new concepts of tumor biology and natural history as well as on prospective randomized trials.
While the emerging results seem to support the proposed new
strategy, several problems appear connected with the future
development of both conservative and multimodality treatments.

Various forms of conservative approach are now cautiously
entering the common treatment practice for selected patients.

From the surgical point of view, the number of unsolved
questions can be summarized as follows: (1) limits of indication to perform quadrantectomy or segmental resection. The
first Milan trial was limited to women with tumors less than
2 cm in diameter because it was believed that the progress in
conservative treatments should be obtained with the minimum
risk for the patients on study. Future trials will consider
tumor of larger size but the question is whether cosmetic results will be acceptable also in women with small breast
having tumors $\geq$ 3 cm; (2) the real need of axillary dissection.
Although the NSABP study [5,10,12] failed to demonstrate either
a benefit or disadvantage for the removal of axillary nodes on
incidence of distant metastases or survival, the information
on the histologic status of regional lymph nodes is of considerable importance for planning adjuvant treatment. There are
two more reasons to perform the axillary dissection, which is
per se a non disfigurating procedure. The first one is that
tumor burden is further reduced and the second one is that
surgery avoids very careful follow up with patients self-
examining the axilla frequently, thereby perpetuating a condition of anxiety; (3) the multicentricity of breast cancer.
Since 25% of patients with cancer in one breast also have
microfoci of carcinoma in the opposite breast, the risk of
developing a second breast cancer applies indeed to both remaining breasts. However, it is extremely rare to observe two
or more clinically overt primary cancers in the same breast
and synchronous bilateral tumors are an uncommon event; [5,10]
[27] (4) the risk of delayed concerogenesis connected with the
irradiation of the homolateral breast tissue. At present, this
risk is difficult to evaluate, and may be balanced by the potential sterilizing effect of radiotherapy on the occult micro
foci. Here too, the answer will come from appropriate randomiz
ed studies, such as that of NSABP. [10] In conclusion, a more
modulated surgical strategy appears advisable according to the
extent of disease and perhaps also in relation to some of the
new biologic parameters such as ER, labeling index and tumor
grading (Table 7).

   The results of curative radiotherapy suggest that this modality in experienced hands and with appropriately selected pa
tients could be an alternative to mastectomy. The published re
sults demonstrate both good local control probability with satisfactory cosmetic results. Thus, the potential of primary
radiotherapy should not be ignored and the alternative to surgery can be discussed with the patient. The problem connected
with curative radiotherapy are dealing with (1) patients selec
tion; (2) technique of irradiation and (3) better information
on the status of axillary nodes. As far as patient selection

Table 7. Proposed Modulated Strategy Related to Tumor Extent

Tumor Extent	Local-Regional treatment	Adjuvant therapy
$T_1 N_{0-1}$	Quadrantectomy + axillary dissection + RT on residual breast	High-risk groups Yes
$T_2 N_{0-1}$	Total mastectomy + axillary dissection	
$T_3 N_{0-1}$	Total mastectomy + axillary dissection or Halsted mastectomy	Low-risk groups No
$T_{1-3} N_2$	Halsted mastectomy	

is concerned, it appears that the potential of curative radiotherapy decreases considerably with tumors greater than 3 cm
in diameter. In these cases, gross tumor excision must preceed
radiotherapy if more extensive surgery is refused. The technical modifications include boost therapy to the site of local
primary lesion, either with external beam or with iridium
implantation. Clinicians should also be aware that, at the
present moment, the correct application of the appropriate
radiotherapeutic technique is still limited to a few centers.
Finally it is desirable, through adequate sampling, to know
the histological status of axillary nodes in order to select
the patients who may be candidate for adjuvant therapy.

As far as multimodality treatment (i.e. local-regional and
systemic therapy) is concerned, some of the trials have established the efficacy of adjuvant chemotherapy in terms of significant increase of RFS and survival. While the optimal adjuvant therapy (regimen, schedule, duration) in N+ patients has
not yet been achieved, current information on CMF suggests
that multiple drug regimens at full dose are necessary both in
pre and postmenopausal women to achieve clinical benefit.
Therefore, chemotherapy should always be administered through
schedules which allow for continuous full dose treatment (e.g.
CMF every 3 weeks injecting all drugs intravenously). [3] Today,
the administration of adjuvant chemotherapy can be prescribed
to high risk patients by or under the supervision of a physician experienced in the use of cytotoxic drugs. Ongoing and fu
ture controlled trials will provide the answer to the many unsolved questions [7] such as (1) the possibility of lesser surgi

cal procedures in patients candidate to systemic adjuvant ther
apy; (2) the impact of different regimens on long-term survival; (3) long-term morbidity, including psychosocial problems;
(4) the role of hormonal manipulations in patients with ER+ tu
mors; (5) the actual efficacy of Poly A-Poly U immune stimulat
ion in various subsets; (6) the role of adjuvant chemotherapy
in high-risk groups with N- (e.g. ER- tumors).

REFERENCES

1. Baclesse F: Roentgen therapy as the sole method of treat-
    ment of cancer of the breast. Am J Roentgenol Radium Ther
    Nucl Med 62:311-319, 1949
2. Bonadonna G, Brusamolino E, Valagussa P, et al: Combina-
    tion chemotherapy as an adjuvant treatment in operable
    breast cancer. N Engl J Med 297:405-410, 1976
3. Bonadonna G, Valagussa P: Dose-response effect after CMF
    chemotherapy in breast cancer. N Engl J Med, 1980 (in
    press)
4. Bonadonna G, Valagussa P, Tancini G, Di Fronzo G: Estrogen
    receptors status and response to chemotherapy in early and
    advanced breast cancer. Cancer Chemother Pharmacol 4:37-41,
    1980
5. Bonadonna G, Veronesi U (Ed.): Breast cancer. Semin Oncol
    5:341-468, 1980
6. Calle R, Pilleron JP, Schlienger P, Vilcoq JR: Conservati-
    ve management of operable breast cancer. Ten years expe-
    rience at the Foundation Curie. Cancer 42:2045-2053, 1978
7. Carter SK: Surgery plus adjuvant chemotherapy - A review
    of therapeutic implications. I. Breast cancer. Cancer
    Chemother Pharmacol 4:147-163, 1980
8. Cooke T, George D, Shields R, Maynard P, Griffiths K:
    Oestrogen receptors and prognosis in early breast cancer.
    Lancet 1:995-997, 1979
9. Crile G, Esselstyn CB, Hermann RE, Hoerr SO: Partial
    mastectomy for carcinoma of the breast. Surg Gynecol Obstet
    136:929-933, 1973
10. Fisher B: Breast cancer management. Alternatives to radi-
    cal mastectomy. N Engl J Med 301:326-328, 1979
11. Fisher B, Carbone P, Economou SG, et al: Phenylalanine
    mustard (L-PAM) in the management of primary breast cancer.
    A report of early findings. N Engl J Med 292:117-122, 1975
12. Fisher B, Redmond C, Fisher ER, et al: The contribution of
    recent NSABP clinical trials of primary breast cancer
    therapy to an understanding of tumor biology. An overview
    of findings. Cancer 1980 (in press)
13. Fisher B, Slack N, Katrych D, Wolmark N: Ten year follow
    up results of patients with carcinoma of the breast in a

co-operative clinical trial evaluating surgical adjuvant chemotherapy. Surg Gynecol Obstet 140:528-534, 1975

14. Forastiere AA, Hakes TB, Tallos P, et al: CMF ± levamisole (L) breast adjuvant chemotherapy: analysis of results after 3.5 years. Proc Am Soc Clin Oncol 21:402, 1980

15. Hellman S, Harris JR, Levene M: Radiation therapy of early carcinoma of the breast without mastectomy. Cancer 1980 (in press)

16. Lacour J, Bucalossi P, Caceres E, et al: Radical mastectomy versus radical mastectomy plus internal mammary dissection. Five-year results of an international cooperative study. Cancer 37:206-214, 1976

17. Lacour J, Lacour F, Spira A, et al: Adjuvant treatment with poly adenylic-poly uridylic acid (Poly A-Poly U) in operable breast cancer. Lancet 2:161-164, 1980

18. Mouridsen HT, Palshof T (Ed.): Breast Cancer-Experimental and Clinical Aspects. Oxford: Pergamon Press Ltd, 1980

19. Pierquin B, Owen R, Maylin C, et al: Radical radiation therapy of breast cancer. Int J Radiat Oncol Biol Phys 6:17-24, 1980

20. Prosnitz LR, Goldenberg IS, Packard RA, et al: Radiation therapy as initial treatment for early stage cancer of the breast without mastectomy. Cancer 39:917-923, 1972

21. Rossi A, Bonadonna G, Valagussa P, Banfi A, Veronesi U: CMF adjuvant program for breast cancer: five-year results. Proc Am Soc Clin Oncol 21:404, 1980

22. Salmon SE, Jones SE (Ed.): Adjuvant Therapy of Cancer II. New York: Grune & Stratton, 1979

23. Schabel FM Jr: Rationale for adjuvant chemotherapy. Cancer 39:2875-2882, 1977

24. Special Report. Treatment of Primary Breast Cancer. N Engl J Med 301:340, 1979

25. Spitalier J, Brandone H, Ayme Y et al: Cesiumtherapy of breast cancer. A five-year report on 400 consecutive patients. Int J Radiat Oncol Biol Phys 2:231-235, 1977

26. Valagussa P, Bonadonna G, Veronesi U: Patterns of relapse and survival following radical mastectomy. Analysis of 716 consecutive patients. Cancer 41:1170-1178, 1978

27. Veronesi U: Surgical approach to breast cancer of limited extent. In press

28. Veronesi U, Banfi A, Saccozzi R, et al: Conservative treatment of breast cancer: a trial in progress at the Cancer Institute of Milan. Cancer 39:2822-2826, 1977

29. Veronesi U, Valagussa P: Inefficacy of internal mammary nodes dissection in breast cancer surgery. Cancer 1980 (in press)

30. Weiss R, Tormey D, Glidewell O, Falkson G, Perloff M, Leone L, Holland JF: Evaluation of postoperative chemoim-

munotherapy in mammary carcinoma. Proc Am Ass Cancer Res 20:244, 1979

Chemotherapy for Advanced
Breast Cancer

IRWIN H. KRAKOFF, M.D.

Director
Vermont Regional Cancer Center
University of Vermont
Burlington, VT 05401

In spite of advances in surgical techniques, radiotherapy techniques, and attempts at early detection, the overall outlook for breast cancer is still not good. It has been noted[3] that for patients with involvement of the axillary lymph nodes by breast cancer, the five year recurrence rate is 67%. For patients with four or more positive nodes, the recurrence rate is 80%. For patients with axillary node involvement and large primary lesions, the figures are still worse, with five year recurrence rates as high as 94%. Even with no involvement of the axillary lymph nodes by cancer, the recurrence rate is 21% at five years and 30% at ten. We can conclude that the prospect for long-term survival of patients with localized breast cancer is no better than 70% overall, and for those with regional node metastases it is substantially worse.

Adjuvant chemotherapy, as has been discussed earlier in this Symposium,[1] has clearly prolonged the disease-free period following mastectomy and now appears to be prolonging survival as well; it is a reasonable anticipation that long-term survival will also be improved, i.e. that adjuvant chemotherapy will effect an increase in cure rates. Nevertheless there remains and will continue to be a distressingly large number of patients who develop locally recurrent or metastatic disease. Adjuvant chemotherapy may even complicate the treatment of those patients who develop recurrences since their prior exposure to the best available anti-tumor drugs may severely limit the therapeutic options.

Nevertheless, there are increasingly effective measures for the treatment of recurrent breast cancer. The available measures are not curative; i.e. most patients who develop metastatic breast cancer will die of it unless there is some intervening cause of death. However, significant palliation can often be achieved, and recently there is evidence that the best chemotherapy can produce some prolongation of survival. Complete remissions in breast cancer, as in most other solid tumors, are uncommon. Partial remissions (by definition more than 50% regression of tumor) are occurring with increasing frequency.

SYSTEMIC THERAPY

Hormone Therapy: Hormone therapy is still the most confusing of the therapeutic measures available to treat breast cancer. It may be accomplished by the administration of exogenous hormones or by surgical ablation of the ovaries, adrenals, or pituitary. Responses to therapy differ in premenopausal and postmenopausal patients, and these groups should, therefore, be considered separately.

Premenopausal patients are, for practical purposes, those who are within one year of cessation of menstrual periods. In that group, oophorectomy is effective in approximately one-third of patients. The average duration of response in those patients is approximately nine months. Patients who respond to oophorectomy and then later develop recurrent disease may have a second response to adrenalectomy or hypophysectomy. Patients who fail to respond to oophorectomy rarely respond to additional endocrine organ ablation. Although there have been attempts to improve the outlook of premenopausal patients by performing oophorectomy at the time of mastectomy, current conventional wisdom does not endorse that procedure. In several large studies,[6] "prophylactic" oophorectomy was seen to prolong the disease-free interval somewhat, but in those patients who developed recurrences there was a compensatory decrease in the period from recurrence to death, and thus no overall improvement in survival.

Postmenopausal patients, as one would expect, are rarely benefitted by oophorectomy. Approximately one-third of such patients may respond to adrenalectomy or hypophysectomy probably as a result of the removal of residual low levels of estrogen. That, however, is not entirely clear, and it may be that the removal of prolactin and growth hormone resulting from hypophysectomy also play a role in response to hypophysectomy. The administration of exogenous estrogen is effective in approximately one-third of postmenopausal patients. As a rule of thumb, the longer postmenopausal a patient is, the more likely she is to enjoy a response from estrogens. If estrogens are to be used, they should be given in large doses, i.e. 15mg daily of diethylstilbestrol or 3mg daily of ethinylestradiol. Responders who subsequently relapse may respond again to adrenalectomy or hypophysectomy. Non-responders are much less likely to respond to those ablative procedures. For all of those endocrine manipulations, responses occur most frequently in patients who are more than five years postmenopausal.

The recent development of a group of synthetic "anti-estrogens" provides an appealing alternative to the administration of exogenous hormones.[8] These compounds are free of some of the disturbing side effects of estrogen (e.g. fluid retention) and produce similar response rates. Among that group of compounds, tamoxifen is superior to nafoxidine or clomiphene since it does not produce the side effects which occur with those other compounds. It is usually administered in a dose of 10mg twice daily and its effects do not appear to be dose dependent, i.e. no better activity is observed with increasing doses. As is the case with natural hormones, response to tamoxifen appears related to the presence of estrogen receptors in the tumor.

A slightly different approach to hormonal manipulation is in the use of aminoglutethimide to produce so-called medical adrenalectomy.[5] This compound inhibits the endogenous synthesis of estrogen by the adrenal and in extra-glandular tissues. It is effective in approximately one-third of patients which is similar to the response rate produced by adrenalectomy; the duration and quality of responses is also similar to those produced by adrenalectomy. The full role of aminoglutethimide in the therapy of breast cancer has not yet been established. However, it appears that it may predict a response to

adrenalectomy or hypophysectomy and further may
spare patients a major surgical procedure.

The entire area of hormonal therapy in breast
cancer has been influenced by the development over
the last several years of assays for estrogen receptors.[7] The procedure has been simplified so that it
can now be performed in many good clinical biochemistry laboratories. In essence the procedure determines the level of a specific protein on the cell
surface which is capable of binding estrogens.
There is a high degree of correlation between the
presence of estrogen receptors and the response to
endocrine therapy of all kinds. It has been widely
reported that 55 to 60% of patients whose tumors
contain estrogen receptors will respond to either
additive or ablative hormonal therapy. Less than
10% of those patients whose tumors do not contain
estrogen receptors will respond. Thus, although
this procedure does not increase the cure rate or
response rate of hormonal manipulation, it identi-
fies those patients who are most likely to respond
and thus spares the probable non-responders the
burden of unnecessary surgery or prolonged hormonal
therapy. The addition of the progesterone receptor
determination can further refine this predictive
ability; approximately 75% of those patients whose
tumors demonstrate receptors for both hormones will
respond to hormonal manipulation. Of those estrogen receptor positive patients whose tumors are
negative for progesterone receptors, it appears that
only about 20% will respond. Thus, the utilization
of hormone receptors can be an extremely useful tool
in determining the likelihood of response to endocrine therapy. It is important now to have the
hormone receptor determination done on the primary
tumor at the time of initial surgery. Even though a
certain percentage of patients will be cured by primary surgery, those who are not may develop their
recurrences in anatomical areas which are not accessible to biopsy of sufficient tissue to perform the
estrogen receptor determination. Thus, failure to
have that determination at the time of initial
surgery may require that a patient later participate
in the "statistical game" of probable response since
the biologic indication may not be available to her.
A further benefit of the estrogen receptor determination is in the general estimation of overall

prognosis. In general, estrogen receptor posi-
tivity is a good prognostic sign; patients in that
category have a longer overall disease-free interval and longer survival than do patients whose
tumors are estrogen receptor negative.

Chemotherapy: Breast cancer is responsive to a
large number of diverse chemotherapeutic agents.
However, as noted above, breast cancer, as is the
case with other solid tumors, contains cells which
are biologically heterogeneous and complete responses are therefore rare in patients treated with
single drugs. Partial responses do occur with
single agents; the frequency of response to various
conventional chemotherapeutic agents is from less
than 10% to as much as 45%.

Single Agents in
Advanced Breast Cancer

Drug	Response Rate (%)
Chlorambucil	20
Cyclophosphamide	32
Melphalan	23
Nitrogen Mustard	34
Arabinosyl Cytosine	11
5-Fluorouracil	28
Methotrexate	33
Adriamycin	45
Hydroxyurea	19
Vinblastine	20
Vincristine	20
Prednisone	18

(Summary Data)

The heterogeneity of breast cancer as in the
case of other solid tumors makes combinations of
drugs more likely to be effective than are single
agents. With some solid tumors discussed elsewhere
in this Symposium, the limited successes of single
agent chemotherapy have led to effective combination

chemotherapy with very high rates of complete responses and an increasing incidence of long-term
remission (probable cure) in systemic disease produced by chemotherapy alone. Combination chemotherapy in breast cancer was shown to be effective
in 1963.[4] In 1969, striking results were reported
with a five-drug regimen.[2] Although there were
variations in the reported response rates, many
different trials have now confirmed the activity of
a variety of therapeutic regimens; combination
chemotherapy appears to be producing overall response rates of about 50%. Complete responses are
still disappointingly few, although they are seen
more frequently than with single drugs. In other
solid tumors it is the complete remission which is
necessary for prolonged survival and this is probably true in breast cancer also.

Combination Chemotherapy
in
Advanced Breast Cancer

Drugs	Response Rate % CR + PR	CR
CMF	55	11
CMF-VP	53	11
CAF	66	15
CAF-VP	58	13
AV	52	16

(Summary Data)

Combinations of endocrine therapy and chemotherapy have not yet been fully evaluated. The data
from several trials presently suggest that the addition of endocrine therapy to chemotherapy does not
add to response rates. A case could be made, on
theoretical grounds, that endocrine therapy, by reducing the number of actively proliferating cells,
may indeed reduce the response to cytotoxic chemotherapy. This point, too, is not yet fully established, and the precise role of combined treatment
with endocrine and cytotoxic drugs remains to be
established.

PALLIATIVE THERAPY

In our enthusiasm to achieve long-term and complete remissions it is important to bear in mind
that more limited objectives may also have important
therapeutic legitimacy. Many of the complications
of progressive breast cancer can be and should be
treated vigorously. Locally recurrent disease involving the chest wall can be painful, disfiguring,
and esthetically unpleasant. When extensive, such
lesions become infected and contribute to the increasing debility of patients. Local X-ray therapy
to the chest wall may result in good local healing
which even if not curative, can substantially increase quality of survival.

Patients with pleural metastases may be afflicted with recurrent extensive pleural effusion.
Although not curative, the instillation of a poly-
functional alkylating agent (nitrogen mustard or
thiopeta), radioactive phosphorus, or tetracycline
may produce sclerosis of the pleura so that pleural
effusion does not recur.

The patient with cerebral metastases can
appear moribund from advancing disease. The administration of adrenal-corticosteroids can markedly and rapidly improve the functional state of such
patients and the delivery of radiotherapy to the
entire head can result in further and prolonged
improvement.

Hypercalcemia, a consequence of bony involvement by metastatic tumor, can be relieved acutely
by the administration of adrenal-corticosteroids,
by the administration of mithramycin which has a
direct pharmacologic effect on calcium metabolism,
or by X-ray therapy to the offending osseous lesion.

In the same vein, a pathologic fracture can be
a catastrophic episode in the course of a patient
with metastatic cancer. Attention to bone pain and
a detailed attempt to evaluate the structural integrity of the affected bone should be made. The
administration of X-ray therapy to the painful lesion can result in healing, even though metastatic
disease is progressing elsewhere. For a bone which
appears to be in imminent danger of fracture, prophylactic nailing can be accomplished with little
morbidity and very brief hospitalization. Waiting

Irwin H. Krakoff

until the fracture has occurred presents a much more complicated problem.

The list of complications which can occur in the course of progressive breast cancer could be an encyclopedia of medicine. It is important to address each issue with a careful analysis of the problem and a careful evaluation of the legitimate goal of possible treatment. It is extremely important in our management of patients with advanced breast cancer, or indeed any other kind of cancer, to recognize that by appropriate active intervention with a problem, we may restore a patient to a good, functional status even though that patient will ultimately succumb to advancing cancer.

It is important also to remain aware that breast cancer or other cancers do not confer immunity to other disease. Careful attention and identification of the cause of symptoms can lead to recognition of infection, cardiac failure, hyperthyroidism, and many other non-cancerous problems; the correction of these can restore a patient to good, functional health even in the presence of advanced cancer.

The striking success of multidisciplinary management of some solid tumors should serve to encourage us that our limited success in breast cancer to date can be expected to be replaced by increasingly better results as we understand better the biology of the disease and as we have available to us more effective drugs to be used in more effective ways.

REFERENCES

1. Bonadonna, G. This Symposium
2. Cooper, R.G. Combination chemotherapy in hormone resistant breast cancer. Proc. Am. Assoc. Cancer Res., Am. Soc. Clin. Onc. 10:15, 1969. abstract.
3. Fisher, B., Slack, N., Katrych, D., and Wolmark, N. Ten-year follow-up results of patients with carcinomas of the breast in a co-operative clinical trial evaluating surgical adjuvant chemotherapy. Surg. Gynec. Obstet. 140:528-534, 1975

4. Greenspan, E.M., Fieber, M. Lesnick, G., Edelman, S. Response of advanced breast carcinoma to the combination of the antimetabolite, methotrexate, and the alkylating agent, Thio-Peta. J. Mt. Sinai Hosp. 30:246-67, 1963.
5. Harvey, H.A., Santen, R.J., Osterman, J. et al. A comparative trial of transsphenoidal hypophysectomy and estrogen suppression with aminoglutethimide in advanced breast cancer. Cancer 43:2207-2214, 1979.
6. Kennedy, B.J., Mielke, P.W., Jr., and Fortuny, I.E. Therapeutic castration versus prophylactic castration in breast cancer. Surg. Gynec. Obstet. 118:524, 1964.
7. McGuire, W.L., Carbone, P.P., Sears, M.E., and Escher, G.C. Estrogen receptors in human breast cancer: an overview in McGuire, W.L., Carbone, P.P. and Vollmer, E.P., eds. Estrogen receptors in human breast cancer. New York. Raven Press. 1975, pp. 1-7.
8. Tagnon, H.J. Antiestrogens in the treatment of breast cancer. Cancer 39:2959, 1977.

CHEMOTHERAPY OF OVARIAN CARCINOMA

W. Michael Hogan, M.D.
Robert C. Young, M.D.

Medicine Branch
National Cancer Institute, NIH
Bethesda, Maryland

INTRODUCTION

Among the malignant neoplasms involving the female reproductive tract, ovarian cancer has long given rise to the greatest pessimism among clinicians. The American Cancer Society estimates that 17,000 new cases will be diagnosed in 1980 and 11,200 women will die of the disease (6% of all female cancer deaths) (6). According to data from the Third National Cancer Survey, roughly one woman in 70 will develop this disease during her lifetime, and only 25% of these women will be diagnosed at a time when the disease is confined to the ovary. Epidemiologic factors responsible for these distressing statistics are poorly understood. Combined modality treatment including radical surgery, whole abdominal irradiation, and single agent chemotherapy have, in the past, done little to influence the seemingly inexorable downhill course of patients afflicted with this malignancy. The cachectic patient with bulky abdominal and pelvic masses, large effusions, and small bowel obstruction continues to be a difficult management problem. Nevertheless, there are recent indications that progress is being made in the care of these patients.

In recent years, a renewed interest in ovarian cancer has lead to a better understanding of its natural history and pattern of spread as well as an increased awareness of the importance of thorough operative staging. Recent reports have re-emphasized the role of cytoreductive surgery and the "second-look" procedure and defined several important prognostic factors. At the same time, chemotherapy has assumed an increasingly important role in the overall treatment of the disease. Formerly used as second line treatment for radiation therapy failures, chemotherapy is now widely used as a primary modality of treatment for patients with advanced disease and also as an adjuvant to surgery for early stage disease. The discussion which follows summarizes recent developments in the chemotherapy of ovarian cancer. Exciting advances in drug sensitivity testing and new and unique techniques for drug delivery are also briefly presented.

ADJUVANT THERAPY - EARLY STAGE (I & II) DISEASE
     With the exception of Stage Ia(i) and Ib(i), well dif-
ferentiated tumors, for which careful staging followed by
surgical excision results in long term survival rates exceeding 90%, the optimal treatment of ovarian cancer confined to
the pelvis remains undetermined (12,27). It is clear that the
traditional approach of surgery with or without postoperative
pelvic irradiation results in significant failure rates even
when complete tumor removal appears to have been accomplished
(2). In view of recent reports establishing the frequency of
occult abdominal metastases and unsuspected para-aortic nodal
involvement, the failure of local therapy is not surprising
(34,36). It is now apparent that patients with Stage II and
high-risk Stage I disease are at risk for failure throughout
the abdominal cavity. Adjuvant therapy, if it is to succeed,
must obviously encompass this entire area.
     Systemic chemotherapy and whole abdominal irradiation are
two approaches which have the potential to eradicate micrometastases throughout the area at risk; unfortunately, institutional bias has limited the number of randomized trials
which have sought to evaluate the relative merits of these two
forms of treatment. There are, nevertheless, several published
studies which deserve comment.
     A large trial carried out at the MD Anderson Hospital
compared postoperative whole abdominal irradiation with a
pelvic boost (70 patients) and single agent melphalan chemotherapy (79 patients) in patients with early ovarian cancer
(41,43). The study prospectively randomized 43 patients with
Stage I disease. There was no significant difference in five
year disease-free survival between the group treated with
irradiation (85%) and the group treated with melphalan (90%).
The percentage of patients with unilateral ovarian involvement
was roughly equal in the two groups (71% and 68%) but there
was no stratification according to histologic grade.
     Another study attempting to define appropriate post-
operative treatment for Stage I disease was carried out by the
Gynecologic Oncology Group (GOG) (21). This study prospectively
randomized Stage Ia and Ib patients to receive pelvic irradiation (5000 rads/5-6 weeks), melphalan (0.2mg/kg/day for 5 days
every 4 weeks for 18 courses), or no further treatment. The
highest recurrence rate occurred in patients treated with
postoperative pelvic irradiation (36%). There is no statistical
difference in the recurrence rate between the control (21%)
and melphalan (7%) treated groups. Survival statistics among
the subgroups are not different to date but, in view of our
knowledge of the behavior of this tumor, it is likely that
recurrence rates will eventually be reflected in differences

in survival. Unfortunately, the large number of patients
excluded from this study on the basis of protocol violations
and the fact that patients were neither rigorously staged nor
stratified by histologic grade makes the study difficult to
interpret.

Two well designed Ovarian Cancer Study Group (OCSG)-GOG
protocols comparing postoperative L-PAM with observation in
Stages Ia and Ib, grade 1 and 2 disease, and L-PAM versus 32P
in Stage I patients with ascites, positive washings, capsular
rupture, or poorly differentiated lesions should help to
define the optimal treatment of Stage I patients (54). Patients
are admitted to these protocols only after extensive operative
staging and they are stratified by the important known
prognostic factors. One hundred and two patients have thus
far been randomized on these trials. Survival information is
not yet available.

Two recent studies have addressed the problem of postoperative treatment in Stage II disease. The MD Anderson
study, referred to previously, included 66 Stage II patients
with residual tumor nodules less than 2 cm in diameter.
Again, there was no significant difference in survival (58%
versus 55%) when L-PAM treatment was compared with pelvic and
abdominal irradiation. The patients were not stratified by
grade and no distinction was made between patients with complete tumor removal and those with minimal residual disease.

Conflicting results have been reported by Dembo et al.
from the Princess Margaret Hospital in a prospective randomized
trial of pelvic irradiation, pelvic plus abdominal irradiation,
and pelvic irradiation followed by chlorambucil (11). While
there was no overall difference in survival between the treatment groups, those Stage II patients (35) who had a completed
total abdominal hysterectomy and bilateral salpingo-oophorectomy
(BSOH) followed by whole abdominal irradiation had improved
actuarial 5 year survival (79%) over those treated with
pelvic irradiation alone (46%) or pelvic irradiation followed
by chemotherapy. It is difficult to completely reconcile the
differing results from these two studies. It should be noted,
however, that the Princess Margaret study employed a method of
whole abdominal irradiation which included the domes of the
diaphragm and did not use liver shielding (10). It must also
be noted that the patient population in the Princes Margaret
study did not undergo rigorous pretreatment surgical staging.
Only the patients having a complete BSOH showed any benefit
and 64% of those were said to be completely free of disease
after surgery. When one considers the OCSG data, indicating
that up to 40% of Stage II patients can be demonstrated to
have disease extension outside the pelvis on careful restaging

(55), it is apparent that the Princess Margaret study, at least to some degree, compares minimal residual Stage III patients treated with aggressive irradiation with a group treated with single agent chemotherapy. It is possible that the use of combination chemotherapy, rather than a single alkylating agent would provide superior results in this group of patients and eliminate the survival advantage for the irradiated group. The data from the National Cancer Institute (NCI) showing Hexa-CAF superior to L-PAM in achieving surgically-confirmed complete remissions in a subgroup of Stage III and IV patients with minimal disease (8 of 8 versus 2 of 11, $p <$ .001) supports this idea (56). It is obvious that additional studies comparing the effectivenss of combination chemotherapy and new techniques of whole abdominal irradiation are needed to clearly define the best form of adjuvant therapy in Stage II and high risk Stage I disease.

THERAPY OF ADVANCED (STAGE III & IV) DISEASE

Single alkylating agent chemotherapy has been the most widely used treatment for patients with bulky residual disease in recent years. Previous reviews indicate that response rates of 33% to 65% can be anticipated with this form of therapy. Median survivals of all treated patients range from 10 to 14 months with median survivals of 17-22 months in those responding to treatment. Overall five year survivals range from 0% to 9% but 16% to 22% of responders are alive at 5 years (51). Over the years the most extensive experience has been with melphalan, establishing this agent as the standard in ovarian cancer chemotherapy to which new drugs and combinations must be compared.

A number of non-alkylating agents have also demonstrated activity in ovarian cancer (45). Adriamycin, hexamethylmelamine, and cis-platinum are of particular interest (13,47,53). In a randomized prospective trial, adriamycin and hexamethylmelamine achieved response rates of 29 and 33% compared to 30% for L-PAM (42). Hexamethylmelamine and cis-platinum are, in addition, the only drugs to date that have been useful as second line agents in patients failing initial therapy with alkylating agents (22,50). The relatively high response rates to various single agents from differing drug classes has provided the impetus for today's interest in combination chemotherapy (14).

A wide variety of drug combinations have been introduced in the past five years. Overall response rates vary from 22% to 91% with complete remission rates of 10 to 69%. Most published reports are single arm studies, and many have dealt with previously treated patients. Few combinations have been studied in randomized trials where differences in patient age,

performance status, histologic grade, and amount of postoperative disease residual have been taken into consideration
in assessing response rates. In many studies, in fact, it is
probable that patient characteristics have a more important
influence on survival than the chemotherapy regimen being
tested. In addition, complete clinical responses are not
always surgically confirmed and long term follow up is often
limited. It is often not clear whether the reported response
rates will eventually translate into an increased long term
survival. Despite these problems in interpreting much of
todays literature, several well designed studies have provided
useful information.

It is now apparent that combination chemotherapy can
significantly increase response rates over those achieved with
single agents. This was initially demonstrated in studies at
the NCI employing the Hexa-CAF regimen (hexamethylmelamine,
cyclophosphamide, methotrexate, and 5-fluorouracil)(52), at
the Mayo Clinic using AC (adriamycin-cyclophosphamide)(16),
and subsequently in a GOG prospective trial randomizing non-
optimal Stage III patients to receive AC, alkeran-hexamethyl-
melamine, or alkeran alone (30). The NCI data shows an increase
in overall median survival from 17 months to 29 months in
addition to a higher overall response rate (76% versus 54%)
and more complete responses (33% versus 16%). Although these
reports are encouraging, it is apparent that the improved
results obtained with combination in comparison to single
agents are most obvious for patients with minimal residual
disease. In the Hexa-CAF study, for example, the overall
response rate in patients with residual tumor nodules less
than 2 cm in diameter was 84% compared to 53% for patients
with greater than 2 cm residual disease. Indeed the Mayo
Clinic data showed a therapeutic advantage for the combination
of cytoxan and adriamycin only in the group with minimal
residual disease.

Histologic grade may also influence the response rate to
single agent versus combination chemotherapy. Analysis of the
NCI data indicate that patients with modified Broders grade 2
or 3 lesions were the ones who appeared to benefit the most
from the Hexa-CAF combination. The median survival of the
grade 2 and 3 patients treated with the combination was increased by approximately 10 months over that of a similar
group treated with L-PAM. The generally good outcome of grade
1 patients and the poor response of grade 4 did not seem to be
significantly altered by choice of chemotherapy (31).

Following the establishment of cis-platinum as an active
agent in previously treated patients, it has been included in
a number of combination chemotherapy programs currently in

progress (4,5,17,20,46,48). These combinations have not been
in use long enough to fully evaluate their effect on survival
in comparison with currently established combination treatments or single agents. The percentage of complete responses
(up to 69%), however, is encouraging since it is this group
that has the potential for cure. The Princess Margaret group
recently presented preliminary information on a randomized
prospective trial comparing single agent melphalan with Hexa-
CAF and the PAC regimen (cis-platinum, adriamycin, and cyclophosphamide) in 67 untreated patients with Stage III and IV
epithelial ovarian cancer (44). Although there is a trend
favoring the PAC regimen, there is no statistical difference
in survival among the three groups at one year. Unfortunately,
only patients with bulky residual disease after surgery were
included in this trial so results can not be easily compared
to previous studies from the Mayo Clinic (AC) or from the NCI
(Hexa-CAF) which included patients with bulky, as well as
minimal residual disease. Future results from this trial, a
GOG study comparing PAC with AC and the current NCI trial of
CHEX-UP (cyclophosphamide, hexamethylmelamine, 5-FU, and cis-
platinum) will hopefully further define the role of platinum
containing combinations.

GERM CELL AND MALIGNANT OVARIAN STROMAL TUMORS
        Malignant tumors derived from ovarian germ cells include
the dysgerminoma, endodermal sinus or yolk sac tumor, malignant teratoma, and choriocarcinoma. Although they represent
only about 10% of all ovarian tumors, they are especially
common in children, accounting for approximately 60% of ovarian
tumors in patients less than 20 years of age (28).
        The endodermal sinus tumor (yolk sac tumor) and immature
(malignant) teratoma accounted for only 22% and 13% respectively of all germ cell tumors in the AFIP series (25). They
are of importance, however, since they represent particularly
aggressive lesions which, prior to the use of combination
chemotherapy, were almost invariably fatal. In a recent
review of 150 cases, Gallion et al. found the overall two year
survival for Stage I pure endodermal sinus tumors to be 27%
(18). Survival with immature teratoma is closely related to
the grade of the tumor. In a review of the AFIP data survival
is almost 100% in grade 0 lesions, but decreases to approximately 30% with grade 3 tumors (29). Surgery alone is
ineffective even when disease is confined to one ovary and
abdominal irradiation with or without single agent chemotherapy
has added little to the poor survival figures associated with
these lesions. Reports from the Gynecologic Oncology Group
(39) and the MD Anderson Hospital (7,9), however, have shown

that aggressive triple agent chemotherapy can dramatically alter the outlook for patients with these neoplasms. Combinations employing methotrexate, actinomycin-D, and cyclophosphamide (MAC), and actinomycin-D, cyclophosphamide, and 5-FU (AcFuCy) have been used, but the largest experience is with the VAC regimen (vincristine, actinomycin-D, and cyclophosphamide). Of 21 patients with aggressive germ cell tumors reported by Cangir et al. (7) from the MD Anderson Hospital, 14 who had second look operation following two years of VAC chemotherapy had no evidence of malignancy. In a report from the same institution dealing specifically with immature teratomas, Curry et al. noted 10 of 12 patients surviving from 16 to 68 months (9). Eight of these patients were seen for recurrence, and all had either Stage III or IV disease when seen at MD Anderson.

The study from the Gynecologic Oncology Group yielded similar results (39). Of 16 patients with previously untreated yolk sac tumor, embryonal carcinoma, or mixed tumor in whom complete surgical resection was followed by treatment with VAC or AcFuCy, 7 are disease free from 14 to 47 months. Of 11 patients with advanced or recurrent disease, 6 are disease free from 19 to 49 months. In the same series 12 patients presented with pure malignant teratoma. Nine of these patients are living without disease from 10 to 37 months following combination chemotherapy (VAC or MAC).

Presently, most patients with germ cell lesions are being treated with combination chemotherapy for one to two years prior to second look laparotomy. A recent report from Duke University, however, suggests that three courses may be adequate, at least for patients with Stage I disease (8). The number of patients in this series was small and 11 of 26 patients received some form of postoperative irradiation, in addition to chemotherapy. Further controlled trials are needed before this approach to the adjuvant treatment of early stage disease can be advocated.

Chemotherapy has only rarely been employed in the treatment of dysgerminoma since, historically, radiation therapy has played a primary role even for advanced and recurrent disease. Two patients with recurrent pure dysgerminoma treated at MD Anderson with AcFuCy had responses lasting 6 and 15 months (24). Creasman recently reported using short term triple agent chemotherapy (3 courses of MAC) in six patients with primary "anaplastic" dysgerminoma. Five of these patients had Stage IA disease and all are NED from 3 to 36 months. One patient was treated for advanced (Stage III) disease with MAC and is NED at 7 months. This patient, however, also received pelvic and abdominal irradiation (8).

Malignant tumors of the ovarian stroma (granulosa-theca cell and Sertoli-Leydig cell) are rare lesions which demonstrate a low incidence of malignant behavior. Experience with chemotherapy in the treatment of these lesions is, therefore, limited. Single agent chemotherapy does not appear to be particularly effective. Among 27 patients with granulosa cell tumors treated with various single alkylating agents at the MD Anderson Hospital and Mayo Clinic, 5 had objective responses (38,26). Three patients in the Mayo Clinic series received 5-FU as a second line agent, but there were no responses. A single patient showed a partial response to actinomycin-D after failing cytoxan. DiSaia et al. recently reported a complete response induced by adriamycin in a patient with a recurrent granulosa cell tumor after failing abdominal irradiation and chemotherapy with melphalan and 5-FU. Remission was sustained for one year (15). Barlow et al. reported a complete response of in a patient with a Stage III granulosa cell tumor treated with adriamycin and bleomycin (3). At MD Anderson Hospital, the AcFuCy combination was administered to two patients with optimal Stage III lesions following surgery. Both patients are NED at 27 and 35 months (38). Lastly, in a recent preliminary report from the GOG, 3 complete responses and 1 partial response was obtained in 9 patients with measurable advanced or recurrent tumors of the ovarian stroma treated with AcFuCy (40).

It is clear that combination chemotherapy has improved, significantly, the outlook of patients with aggressive germ cell tumors of the ovary. More effective combinations are needed, however, for patients with advanced and recurrent germ cell and ovarian stromal tumors.

CURRENT INVESTIGATION

Recent developments in the areas of cell culture and clinical pharmacology have provided information of particular interest to physicians involved in the care of ovarian cancer patients.

In 1977, Hamburger and Salmon reported the development of a soft agar technique which allows culture of human tumor progenitor (stem) cells (19). Previously, studies by Roper and Drewinko had shown that in vitro colony formation, which reflects a cell's ability to reproduce, provided the only relevent criterion by which to assess cell lethality (35). With the report of Hamburger and Salmon, a method was made available by which drug sensitivity could be determined in vitro on this basis.

Ovarian cancer stem cells have been easily grown in the soft agar system and data on 65 ovarian cancer patients has

recently been published (1). Forty of these patients underwent 95 clinical drug trials subsequent to in vitro sensitivity
testing. The predictive accuracy of the assay for complete
and partial remissions was 62% and the accuracy of the assay
for predicting drug resistance was 99%. It is apparent that
the assay is particularly helpful in eliminating drugs from
consideration which are unlikely to benefit the patient. To
date, the stem cell technique has been applied mostly in the
selection of second and third line therapy for patients with
recurrent disease. It, perhaps, has greater potential for
selecting primary treatment, adjunctive chemotherapy, and as a
screening mechanism to evaluate new drugs for potential
cytotoxic effect in ovarian cancer. Salmon has reported
preliminary results of such in vitro phase II trials demonstrating the potential activity of AMSA, pentamethylmelamine, and
vindesine (37).

In addition to confirming the high rate of successful
ovarian cancer colony growth when cells are obtained from
malignant effusions, investigators at the NCI have been able
to grow colonies in 92% of cytologically malignant washings
(32). When high volume washings (1500-2000ml) were used,
sufficient colony growth was obtained to allow in vitro drug
sensitivity testing. These results are important since they
demonstrate that specimens can be obtained from patients
without malignant effusions or readily biopsiable tumor. This
may have important implications in the selection of adjuvant
chemotherapy for patients with early stage disease. By using
a chronic indwelling peritoneal dialysis catheter (Tenckhoff),
it may also be possible to obtain sequential samples for drug
testing. The emergence of drug resistance might then be
predicted before clinical relapse is detected.

The unique tendency of ovarian cancer to remain confined
to the intrabdominal space has suggested a new pharmacologic
approach to treatment. The pharmacologic basis for this
technique has been described by Jones et al. (23). Initial
studies at the NCI have utilized the Tenckhoff catheter to
administer methotrexate, 5-FU and, more recently, adriamycin
in a large volume (2 liters) of peritoneal dialysate. Studies
utilizing the stem cell assay system, noted dose dependent
adriamycin resistance in a group of ovarian cancer patients
who had relapsed while undergoing therapy with non-adriamycin
containing regimens (49). Eight patients who were shown to be
resistant to adriamycin at in vitro drug concentrations of 1
ug/ml were sensitive when the drug concentration was raised to
10 ug/ml. Although this drug concentration is not achievable
clinically by conventional methods of drug delivery, concentrations
in this range can be achieved with intraperitoneal administration.

A preliminary report indicated that 2 of 3 patients who
demonstrated in vitro sensitivity to high dose adriamycin in
the stem cell assay had objective reduction in ascites without
concomitant adverse systemic effects (33). This "belly bath"
approach may have its greatest utility in Stage III patients
with minimal residual disease or as a surgical adjunct in
early stage disease.

CONCLUSION
        It is apparent that the problem of ovarian cancer has
stimulated a great deal of interest among physicians from
various disciplines. A number of carefully designed prospective clinical trials recently implemented are beginning to
answer some of the longstanding questions regarding the optimal
management of this neoplasm. Although progress in the management of this disease has been slow, one can anticipate that
continued systematic investigation of established and innovative modes of therapy will have a beneficial impact on the
survival of patients with ovarian cancer.

1. Alberts DS, Salmon SE, Chen HSG, et al.: In vitro
clonogenic assay for predicting response of ovarian cancer to
chemotherapy. Lancet 2:340-342, 1980.
2. Bagley CM, Young RC, Canellos GP, DeVita VT: Treatment
of ovarian carcinoma: possibilities for progress. N Eng J Med
287:856-862, 1972.
3. Barlow JJ, Piver MS, Chuang JT, et al.: Adriamycin and
bleomycin alone and in combination in gynecologic cancers.
Cancer 32:735-743, 1973.
4. Bruckner HW, Cohen CJ, Deppe G, et al.: Chemotherapy
of gynecological tumors with platinum II. J Clin Hem and Onc
7:619-632, 1977.
5. Bruckner HW, Ratner LH, Cohen CJ et al: Combination
chemotherapy for ovarian carcinoma with cyclophosphamide,
adriamycin and cis-dichlorodiammineplatinum (II) after failure
of initial chemotherapy. Cancer Treat Rep 62:1021-1023, 1978.
6. Cancer Facts and Figures 1980. American Cancer Society
Publication, New York.
7. Cangir A, Smith J, VanEys J: Improved prognosis in
children with ovarian cancer following modified VAC (Vincristine
sulfate, dactinomycin, and cyclophosphamide) chemotherapy.
Cancer 42:1234-1238, 1978.
8. Creasman WT, Fetter BF, Hammond CB, Parker RT: Germ
cell malignancies of the ovary. Obstet Gynecol 53:226-230, 1979.
9. Curry SL, Smith JP, Gallagher HS: Malignant teratoma
of the ovary: prognostic factors and treatment. Am J Obstet
Gynecol 131:845-849, 1978.
10. Dembo AJ, Van Dyke J, Japp B et al: Whole abdominal
irradiation by a moving-strip technique for patients with
ovarian cancer. Int J Rad Onc Biol Phys 5:1933-1942, 1979.
11. Dembo AJ, Bush RA, Beale FA, et al: Ovarian carcinoma:
improved survival following abdominopelvic irradiation in
patients with a completed pelvic operation. Am J Obstet Gynecol
134:793-800, 1979.
12. Dembo AJ, Bush JF, Sturgeon FG: Postoperative radiotherapy in ovarian cancer stages I and II, In Van Oosterom AT,
et al. (eds). Therapeutic Progress in Ovarian Cancer, Testicular
Cancer, and the Sarcomas. The Hague/Boston/London, Martinus
Nijhoff, 1980, pp. 13-26.
13. dePalo GM, DeLena M, DiRe F et al.: Melphalan versus
adriamycin in the treatment of advanced carcinoma of the ovary.
Surg Gynecol Obstet 141:899-902, 1975.
14. DeVita VT and Schein PS: The use of drugs in combination
for the treatment of cancer. Rationale and results. N Eng J
Med 288:988-1006, 1973.
15. DiSaia PJ, Saltz A, Kagan AR, Rich W: A temporary
response of recurrent granulosa cell tumor to adriamycin.
Obstet Gynecol 52:355-358, 1978.

16. Edmonson TH, Fleming TR, Decker DG et al.: Different chemotherapeutic sensitivities and host factors affecting prognosis in advanced ovarian carcinoma versus minimal residual disease. Cancer Treat Rep 63:241-247, 1979.

17. Ehrlich CE, Einhorn CH, Williams D, Morgan J: Chemotherapy for stage II-IV epithelial ovarian cancer with cis-dichlorodiammine-platinum (II), adriamycin, and cyclophosphamide. A preliminary report. Cancer Treat Rep 63:281-288, 1979.

18. Gallion H, VanNagell JR, Powell DR et al.: Therapy of endodermal sinus tumor of the ovary. Am J Obstet Gynecol 135: 447-451, 1979.

19. Hamburger AW and Salmon SE: Primary bioassay of human myeloma stem cells. Science 197:461-463, 1977.

20. Holland JF, Bruckner HW, et al.: Cis-platinum therapy of ovarian cancer, in Van Oosterom AT et al. (eds), Therapeutic Progress in Ovarian Cancer, Testicular Cancer and the Sarcomas, The Hague/Boston/London, Martinus Nijhoff, 1980, pp. 41-52.

21. Hreshchyshyn MH, Norris GH, Park R, et al.: Postoperative treatment of resectable malignant and possibly malignant epithelial ovarian tumors with radiotherapy, melphalan or no further treatment. Abstract 9W57. Proc of XII Int Cancer Congress 157, 1978.

22. Johnson BL, Fischer RI, Bender RA, et al.: Hexamethylmelamine in alkylating agent-resistant ovarian carcinoma. Cancer 42:2157-2161, 1978.

23. Jones RB, Myers CE, et al.: High volume intraperitoneal chemotherapy ("belly bath") for ovarian cancer: pharmacologic basis and early results. Cancer Chemother Pharmacol 1:161-166, 1978.

24. Krepart G, Smith JP, Rutledge F, Delclos L: The treatment for dysgerminoma of the ovary. Cancer 41:986-990, 1978.

25. Kurman RJ and Norris HJ: Malignant mixed germ cell tumors of the ovary. A clinical and pathologic analysis of 30 cases. Obstet Gynecol 48:579-589, 1976.

26. Malkasian GD, Webb MJ, Jorgensen EO: Observations on chemtherapy of granulosa cell carcinomas and malignant ovarian teratomas. Obstet Gynecol 44:885-888, 1974.

27. Munnell EW: The changing prognosis and treatment in cancer of the ovary. Am J Obstet Gynecol 100:790-805, 1968.

28. Norris HJ and Jensen RD: Relative frequency of ovarian neoplasms in children and adolescents. Cancer 30:713-719, 1972.

29. Norris HJ, Zirkin HJ, Benson WL: Immature (malignant) teratoma of the ovary. A clinical and pathologic study of 58 cases. Cancer 37:2359-2372, 1976.

30. Omura GZ, Blessing JA, Buchsbaum WJ, et al.: A randomized trial of melphalan versus melphalan plus hexamethylmelamine versus adriamycin plus cyclophosphamide in advanced ovarian adenocarcinoma Proc Am Soc Clin Oncol 20:358, 1979.

31. Ozols RF, Garvin AJ, Costa J, et al.: Advanced ovarian cancer: correlation of histologic grade with response to therapy and survival. Cancer 45:572-581, 1980.

32. Ozols RF, Willson JKV, Grotzinger KR, Young RC: Cloning of human ovarian cancer cells in soft agar from malignant effusions and peritoneal washings. Cancer Res 40:2743-2747, 1980.

33. Ozols RF, Young RC, Speyer JL, et al.: Intraperitoneal (IP) adriamycin (ADR) in ovarian carcinoma (OC). Proc Am Soc Clin Oncol 21:425, 1980.

34. Piver MS, Barlow JJ, Lele SB: Incidence of sub-clinical metastasis in stage I and II ovarian carcinoma. Obstet Gynecol 52 100-104, 1978.

35. Roper PR and Drewinko B: Comparison of in vitro methods to determine dry induced cell lethality. Cancer Res 36:2182-2188, 1976.

36. Rosenoff SH, DeVita VT, Hubbard S, Young RC: Peritoneoscopy in the staging and follow-up of ovarian cancer. Semin Oncol 2:223-228, 1975.

37. Salmon SE, Soehnlen B, Alberts DS: New drugs in ovarian cancer: In Vitro phase II screening with the human tumor stem cell assay, In Van Oosterom AT et al (eds), Therapeutic Progress in Ovarian Cancer, Testicular Cancer and the Sarcomas, The Hague/Boston/London, Martinus Nijhoff, 1980, pp. 113-128.

38. Schwartz PE and Smith JP: Treatment of ovarian stromal tumors. Am J Obstet Gynecol 125:402-411, 1976.

39. Slayton RE, Hreshchyshyn MM, Silverberg SG et al.: Treatment of malignant ovarian germ cell tumors: response to vincristine, dactinomycin, and cyclophosphamide (preliminary report). Cancer 42:390-398, 1978.

40. Slayton RE, Johnson G, Brady L, Blessing J: Radiotherapy (RT) and chemotherapy (CT) in malignant tumors of the ovarian stroma (MTOS). Proc Am Soc Clin Oncol 21:430, 1980.

41. Smith JP, Rutledge F, Delclos L: Postoperative treatment of early ovarian cancer: a random trial between postoperative irradiation and chemotherapy. Natl Cancer Inst Monogr 42:149-153, 1975.

42. Smith JP: Report of the ovarian cancer contract. NCI Jan. 1, 1976.

43. Smith JP: Treatment of ovarian cancer, in Umezawa, et al (eds). Advances in Cancer Chemotherapy. Japan Sci Soc Press Tokyo/Univ. Park Press, Baltimore, 1978, pp. 493-503.

44. Sturgeon JFG, Fine S, Bean HA, et al.: A randomized trial of melphalan alone versus combination chemotherapy in advanced ovarian cancer. Proc Am Soc Clin Oncol 21:422, 1980.

45. Tobias JS, Griffiths CT: Management of ovarian carcinoma: Current concepts and future prospects. N Eng J Med 294:818-823 and 877-882, 1976.

46. Vogl SE, Berenzweig M, Kaplan GH, Moukhtar M, Bulkin W: The CHAD and HAD regimens in advanced ovarian cancer: combination chemotherapy including cyclophosphamide, hexamethylmelamine, adriamycin, and cis-dichlorodiammine platinum (II). Cancer Treat Rep 63:311-317, 1979.

47. Wharton JT, Rutledge F, Smith P, et al.: Hexamethylmelamine: an evaluation of its role in the treatment of ovarian cancer. Am J Obstet Gynecol 133:833-844, 1979.

48. Williams CJ, Stevenson KE, Buchanan RB, Whitehouse JMA: Advanced ovarian carcinoma: a pilot study of cis-dichlorodiammineplatinum (II) in combination with adriamycin and cyclophosphamide in previously untreated patients and as a single agent in previously treated patients. Cancer Treat Rep 63:1745-1753, 1979.

49. Willson JKV, Ozols RF, Grotzinger KR, Young RC: New sources of clonogenic human ovarian cancer cells for drug sensivity studies. Proc Am Assoc Cancer Res 21:175, 1980.

50. Wiltshaw E and Kroner T: Phase II study of cis-dichlorodiammineplatinum (II) (NSC-119875) in advanced adenocarcinoma of the ovary. Cancer Treat Rep 60:55-60, 1976.

51. Young RC, Hubbard SP, DeVita VT: The chemotherapy of ovarian cancer. Cancer Treat Reviews 1:99-110, 1974.

52. Young RC, Chabner BA, et al.: Advanced ovarian adenocarcinoma. A prospective clinical trial of melphalan (L-PAM) versus combination chemotherapy. N Eng J Med 299:1261-1266, 1978.

53. Young RC, Von Hoff DD, Gormley P et al.: Cis-dichlorodiammineplatinum (II) in the treatment of advanced ovarian cancer. Cancer Treat Rep 63:1539-1544, 1979.

54. Young RC: A strategy for effective management for early ovarian cancer, in Jones SE and Salmon SE (eds). Adjuvant Therapy of Cancer II, New York, Grune and Stratton, 1979, pp. 467-474.

55. Young RC, Wharton JT, et al.: Staging laparotomy in early ovarian cancer. Proc Am Soc Clin Oncol 20:399, 1979.

56. Young RC: Unpublished data, 1979.

Combined Modality Approach for Brain Tumors

William R. Shapiro, M.D.

Head, George C. Cotzias Laboratory of Neuro-Oncology
Memorial Sloan-Kettering Cancer Center
New York, NY 10021

Introduction.

Cancer affects the nervous system frequently. Primary tumors of the central nervous system (CNS) are the second most common cancer in children and primary brain tumors in adults are more common than Hodgkin's disease. In 1977 there were approximately 11,000 new cases of primary CNS cancer and 8,800 deaths. Of the 690,000 new cases of cancer in the United States in 1977, 385,000 patients died; 50,000 of these deaths were directly associated with metastatic cancer to the nervous system mostly from lung cancer, breast cancer, malignant melanoma, lymphomas and leukemias.

Prior to 1969 there was little emphasis on treating patients with primary brain tumors or those who suffered metastatic brain tumors as complications of their systemic cancer[21]. Since then, neurologists, neurosurgeons and oncologists have taken an increasingly active role in managing patients with brain tumor. Organized efforts have been directly against primary brain tumors with the advent of multiple center studies under the Brain Tumor Study Group (BTSG) of the National Cancer Institute, and the Radiation Therapy Oncology Group (RTOG). Through such efforts, the survival of patients with malignant glioma has more than doubled in the last 10 years.

The 1970's also saw the development of the computerized axial tomographic scanner (CT scan), a product of the space age that has produced a breakthrough in the diagnosis of patients with brain tumor. With greater safety than was possible before the CT scanner, patients with headache or seizures that might be produced by brain tumor can be diagnosed at an earlier stage. While the earlier diagnosis of brain tumor has not by itself meant prolonged survivorship, it has reduced the residual post-operative deficit. The CT scanner has even made possible needle biopsy for diagnosis[11].

The scanner has also permitted a more direct evaluation of the tumor itself as the patients are treated and thus has permited more precise follow-up.

We shall review the multimodality therapy studies published in this decade. The tumors under discussion are primary brain tumors, i.e., glioblastoma multiforme and malignant astrocytoma (grades III or IV). We shall not discuss metastatic brain tumors or lesser grade astrocytomas. Finally we shall review recent laboratory studies on brain tumors that are likely to impinge on therapy.

Brain Tumors as Cancer.

When a patient develops systemic cancer, his body must deal with a "cancer burden" consisting of a population of cancer cells in the blood or bone marrow (leukemia) or in a solid, single mass or in multiple metastatic masses (carcinoma). For the average adult it is thought that a 1 kg burden of systemic tumor is lethal; this amount of tumor is equivalent to 1×10^{12} cells. In contrast, a brain tumor shares its space with the brain which already occupies 1200 cc in the small confines of the skull and in this confined space 100 grams of tumor, equivalent to 1×10^{11} cells, is almost always lethal. Patients presenting with neurological symptoms usually have tumors 30 to 60 grams in size. To cure any cancer, it is necessary to reduce the tumor bulk to a size that the body's natural immune mechanisms can suppress and eventually kill. In general, this is thought to require a reduction of tumor size to approximately 0.0001 gram or 1×10^5 cells. Assuming an initial malignant brain tumor burden of 100 grams or 1×10^{11} cells, a subtotal surgical resection might remove 90% of the tumor, reducing it to 10 grams or 1×10^{10} cells. A "total resection" might reduce the tumor to 1 gm, equal to 1×10^9 cells to be treated by subsequent radiation and chemotherapy. It is thought that radiation therapy can kill 2 logs of brain tumor cells. It is then left for chemotherapy to reduce the population of cells 2 more logs to 0.0001 gm or 1×10^5 cells. Such a scenario is rarely played out, however, because in all instances therapy falls short of these theoretic goals. The surgeon is rarely able to do a total resection and often must be satisfied with removing 30-40% of the tumor. Radiation therapy can reduce tumor bulk and prolong survival, but only at the cost of some brain damage especially at radiation doses of 6000 rads. The currently available chemotherapeutic agents produce only a 1 log net cell kill, permitting the tumor to grow at a rate faster than it can be killed by the drugs. Thus, present day multi-modal therapy can treat the brain tumors but cannot cure them. However, therapy permits patients to live longer and with a better quality of life. This therapy is based on considering brain tumors as a problem in cancer and their therapy as a problem of killing cancer cells.

Surgical Considerations.

Even after 75 years of experience resecting primary brain tumors (the past 20 using corticosteroid hormones that have reduced surgical mortality to 1-2%), the role of surgery in the treatment of primary malignant brain tumors remains controversial. No one disagrees that only surgery permits a pathological diagnosis to be established during life. However, many physicians consider that our current methods of radiological diagnosis including the CT scan permit a diagnosis of malignant brain tumor without the necessity for operation, thus avoiding the risks of surgery. Such a view denies a role for surgery as "cancer" therapy. There is evidence that surgical removal of tumor bulk can prolong survival and permit the patient to return to an active life for a year or longer. In one retrospective study[7] patients undergoing extensive surgical resection survived more than a year while all patients who had minimal resection or needle biopsy died within a year. Our experience is similar; patients undergoing surgical resection for malignant brain tumor appear to do better than those not operated on. If the surgeon confines his resection to the tumor itself, he rarely induces a new major neurological defect. On the contrary, patients are frequently able to return to a fully active life without the need for large doses of corticosteroid hormones to ameliorate incapacitating symptoms. No controlled study, however, has compared the overall efficacy of surgical versus wholly non-surgical therapy in the management of malignant glioma. We now recognize five surgical goals that on the whole favor an active role for the neurosurgeon: (1) establish a diagnosis; (2) provide symptomatic relief especially by reducing intracranial pressure; (3) prolong life enough to permit anticancer therapy, specifically radiation treatment and early chemotherapy which requires a minimum of 8 to 10 weeks; (4) remove tumor bulk as a form of anticancer treatment; (5) increase the sensitivity of tumor cells to chemotherapy and radiation by reducing tumor bulk.

Radiation Therapy.

The proper portals and doses of radiation therapy in the treatment of brain tumor remains controversial. It has been demonstrated that larger radiation portals more reliably include more tumor than do smaller portals[9]. The BTSG reported in a controlled study that whole brain radiation

therapy increases the survival of patients over that which
follows surgery alone[26] (see below). Furthermore, data
from the BTSG show that patients receiving 5500 to 6000 rads
live significantly longer than those receiving 5000 rads or
less[29]. However, there is good evidence in experimental
animals that doses of 6000 rads produce damage to the normal
brain[12]. What is still not certain is the extent of such
damage in patients and how it may be made worse by associated
chemotherapy. Limited pathological observation suggests that
damage can occur in the setting of radiation and chemotherapy[3] and patients undergoing such treatment may show defi-
cits in cognitive function[6]. The incidence of such complications, i.e., the ratio of the number of patients who eventually develop the complication to those at risk, remains to
be determined since most patients with this disease die in
the first two or three years.

Chemotherapy.
        Chemotherapy of CNS neoplasms shares with chemotherapy
of systemic cancer the problem of tumor sensitivity, but in
addition requires two other important considerations. The
first is the microenvironment of the tumors--the blood-brain
barrier. Drugs that are too large, ionized or lipid insoluble may not readily enter the normal regions of the brain.
Secondly, the absence of a lymphatic system in the brain
means that fluid produced by malignant brain tumors adds to
the mass effect of the tumor in the form of cerebral edema,
increasing symptoms and signs. Cerebral edema can be effectively treated with corticosteroid hormones but the resulting
improvement in symptoms adds to the complexity of evaluating
chemotherapy results. With respect to evaluation, survival
time in adjuvant studies remains the best measure of the
effectiveness of new forms of treatment. Evaluating phase II
studies requires measurements of both patient response and
tumor shrinkage. Unfortunately, patient response is also a
function of the residual damage following surgery, the effect
of cerebral edema and its treatment, and is highly dependent
on the location of the tumor (large, bulky tumors in the
frontal lobe produce few symptoms, small tumors lying deep
near the thalamus produce major symptoms). Thus, clinical
changes are only a rough measure of tumor response. Evaluating tumor size itself has been made easier by the CT scan
and attempts to use this device in the longitudinal evaluation of such patients are now underway.
        The first major controlled trial of BCNU in the treat-
ment of glioblastoma multiforme was that undertaken by the
BTSG[26]. The study divided patients post-operatively into
four groups that received (1) no further specific anti-cancer

therapy, (2) BCNU, (3) radiation therapy 5000-6000 rads whole head, or (4) combined BCNU and radiation therapy. The median survival time of the group of patients who received no therapy beyond that of surgery (control) was 14 weeks; that of patients receiving BCNU 18.5 weeks; patients receiving radiation therapy 36 weeks (P = 0.001), and for combined radiation therapy and BCNU, 34.5 weeks (P = 0.001). The 14-week median survival of the surgical group represents the best available information as to the value of initial surgery in the treatment of glioma. Furthermore, the 36-week median survival achieved in the radiation therapy group was the first demonstration of the value of radiation in a controlled study. BCNU did not add significantly to the median survival of the group receiving radiation alone but at 18 months there was a significant difference in the survival of the 4 groups. Nineteen percent of the patients receiving BCNU and radiation therapy in addition to their surgery were alive at 18 months, but in none of the other groups did more than 4% of the patients live that long.

In 1972 the BTSG evaluated methyl-CCNU in another 4-arm study[28]. In preliminary results the median survival time of patients who received methyl-CCNU was 27 weeks, radiation therapy alone 37 weeks, methyl-CCNU plus radiation therapy 43 weeks, and BCNU plus radiation therapy 52 weeks. The last figure was significantly different from that of the methyl-CCNU alone (P = 0.001) and close to being significantly different from that of radiation therapy alone (P = 0.08). Thus, the combination of BCNU and radiation therapy appeared to be effective in the treatment of malignant gliomas, producing a one-year median survival. The 18-month survival figure exceeded 30%.

In another phase III study, the BTSG treated all patients with 6000 rads of whole brain radiation therapy[27]. In addition, patients received either (1) BCNU in order to validate the best previous arm, (2) procarbazine, a drug which had been demonstrated in uncontrolled studies to be effective; (3) high dose corticosteroid hormones (methyl prednisolone 400 mg/m^2/day for 7 days out of every 28) to test the oncolytic capacity of such compounds; or (4) a combination of BCNU and high dose methyl prednisolone. This study has been closed to accrual and preliminary results show that the patients in the group receiving radiation plus medrol survived a significantly shorter time than patients in any of the other three groups, indicating that corticosteroid hormones are not chemotherapeutic in the treatment of malignant glioma.

That the nitrosoureas, especially BCNU and CCNU, are effective agents has also been demonstrated in smaller but supporting studies, both in this country and in Europe, as have a number of newer agents including dianhydrogalactitol (DAG) and combination chemotherapy with nitrosoureas and hydroxyurea (see reviews by Shapiro[18],[19]).

The available chemotherapy is still only minimally effective, and for a cure better agents must be found. However, for patients with malignant glioma, the multimodality approach of surgery, radiation and chemotherapy has more than doubled survival and such increased survival has been accompanied by improved or stable quality of life. Like cancer in general, the problem of brain tumor is one of finding an effective non-toxic chemotherapy. As noted[14], 20 years were required before childhood leukemia was brought under control and perhaps a similar time will be required for malignant brain tumor.

Research Topics in Chemotherapy of CNS Neoplasms.

In addition to the clinical chemotherapy studies reported above, a number of laboratory investigations in the last ten years have yielded new therapeutic approaches and have improved our knowledge of the biology of brain tumors. These laboratory efforts are likely to make important contributions to the management of these patients and as such deserve review.

Radiosensitizers.

In both in vitro and in vivo experimental systems, hypoxic cells have been shown to be more resistant than well oxygenated cells to killing by low linear energy transfer (LET) radiation. It requires about three times the dose of X-rays to kill the same fraction of hypoxic cells as required to kill oxygenated cells. Tumor cells thought capable of surviving hypoxia may become radioresistant if not killed by the usual low LET radiation. Measures designed to circumvent hypoxia in radiation therapy of brain tumors include irradiation under hyperbaric oxygen, neutron irradiation and electron affinic hypoxic cell radiosensitizers. Radiation sensitizing agents serve as substitutes for oxygen, are not metabolized and can diffuse into hypoxic regions of a tumor. They increase radiosensitivity of the hypoxic cells without a corresponding sensitization of normal cells. The two available compounds are both nitroimidazoles: metronidazole (Flagyl, a 5-nitroimidazole derivative) and misonidazole (Ro-07-0582, a 2-nitroimidazole derivative). Urtasun et al[30] gave metronidazole to glioma patients radiated with 3000 rads and found their survival was equal to that of patients receiving 6000 rads without metronidazole. Misonidazole can be used at lower dosage producing an oxygen enhancement ratio of 1.5-2.0 based on concentrations obtained in patients after oral administration[25]. A number of different protocols have been developed at various doses of misonidazole and at various radiation therapy doses. A phase III trial is currently under way by the BTSG combining whole head radiation therapy with misonidazole, and the drug is also under investigation by other groups in the United States and in Europe.

In Vitro and Animal Model Drug Testing for Human Brain Tumor Chemotherapy.

The last decade has seen a variety of animal brain tumor models designed to test potentially useful chemotherapeutic agents. Recently two new systems have been devised for drug testing. The first uses an in vitro model system with human gliomas similar to a system reported for other cancers[17]. Kornblith and Szypko[3] used cultures of human malignant gliomas in a microcytotoxicity assay to test several doses of BCNU, and similar studies were performed by Rosenblum et al[16] using a clonogenic cell assay. In vivo testing of human gliomas has been reported by Shapiro et al[23] and Shapiro and Basler[22], who grew the gliomas in the brains or subcutaneous tissues of athymic nude mice. Chemotherapy testing demonstrated differences in chemosensitivity to BCNU and procarbazine among a series of patients' tumors. One implication of these results is the possibility that human tumors and specifically human gliomas are heterogeneous in composition, composed of different cell populations whose chemosensitivities differ and whose growth in vitro and in vivo may also differ. Recent work at Memorial Sloan-Kettering Cancer Center by Shapiro et al[24] and Rankin et al[15] appears to have confirmed this concept. These studies demonstrated that human brain tumors consist of many karyotypically different cells. With appropriate statistical analysis the subpopulations for each tumor could be grouped into 3 to 21 clonal populations. The clonal populations had phenotypic differences in growth rate and response to chemotherapeutic agents. Such studies imply the need for multiple therapeutic regimens to treat multiple inherently resistant cell populations. The work confirms that of other investigations in animal systems[5] and supports the notion that studies of the basic biological nature of cancer requires an awareness of the inherent heterogeneity of tumors and the rapidity with which such tumors change in vitro and in vivo.

The Blood-Brain Barrier and Brain Tumor Chemotherapy.

Levin[10] has raised questions about the value of available chemotherapy in the treatment of malignant brain

tumors based on studies of computer modeling of the rat 9L
tumor. Blood flow, capillary permeability and drug exposure
data suggested that while lipid-soluble drugs that cross normal blood-brain barrier may penetrate into most regions of a
brain tumor, cells distant from tumor capillaries, for example, those in necrotic regions, may not be exposed to enough
drug to prevent the emergence of resistant cells. Water
soluble drugs that cannot cross the blood-brain barrier are
unlikely to penetrate into regions of a tumor where cells are
actively dividing because of their slow diffusion. New
chemotherapeutic agents must be designed that can circumvent
the problems of blood flow dependency and relative capillary
impermeability. The blood-brain barrier within a tumor is
substantially altered and permits the entry of a variety of
water-soluble molecules, e.g., methotrexate[20]. Problems
of entry, however, persist along the growing edge of the
tumor and into very small tumors. Studies by Blasberg et
al[2] in animals suggest that the blood-brain barrier along
the edge of a tumor is variably broken down and is intact in
very small tumors. Another approach to the problem of the
blood-brain barrier is the possibility of purposely disrupt-
ing it using hyperosmotic agents. This was done in normal
dogs by Neuwelt et al[13] and was examined in tumor-bearing
animals by Hasegawa and colleagues[4] who determined the
penetration of methotrexate into rats with carcinomatous
meningitis with and without hyperosmolar intracarotid mannitol. A small increase in survival was associated with the
additional effectiveness of the methotrexate afforded by better drug entry. However, when the blood-brain barrier was
opened in solid brain tumor- bearing animals given methotrexate, no improvement in survival occurred, and it was not possible to show increased methotrexate concentration in the
tumor itself, but only in the normal brain around the
tumor[1]. The whole problem of the blood-brain barrier and
chemotherapy remains an important area still under active
investigation.

Conclusions.
    The chemotherapy of brain tumors remains in its adoles-
cence. Randomized prospective protocols demonstrate the definite but modest effectiveness of nitrosoureas. Combination
chemotherapy programs in centers around the world suggest
greater efficacy than programs of single drug treatment. New
approaches under active investigation include radiation sensitizers and combination chemotherapy. The need to test
human tumors directly either in vitro or in immunodeficient
animals in vivo has also been recognized.

REFERENCES

1. Allen JC, Hasegawa H, Mehta BM, et al: Influence of intracarotid mannitol on intracerebral methotrexate (MTX) concentrations surrounding experimental brain tumors. Proc Am Assoc Cancer Res 20:286, 1979.

2. Blasberg RG, Gazendam J, Patlak CS, et al: Changes in blood-brain barrier transfer parameters induced by hyperosmolar intercarotid infusion and by metastatic tumor growth, in Eisenberg H, Suddith, R (eds): Cerebral Microvasculature: Investigations of the Blood-Brain Barrier. New York, Plenum (in press).

3. Berger PC, Mahaley MS, Dudka L, et al: The morphologic effects of radiation administered therapeutically for intracranial gliomas. Cancer 44:1256-1272, 1979.

4. Hasegawa H, Allen JC, Mehta BM, et al: Enhancement of CNS penetration of methotrexate by hyperosmolar intracarotid mannitol or carcinomatous meningitis. Neurology 29:1280-1286, 1979.

5. Heppner GH, Shapiro WR, Rankin JK: Tumor heterogeneity, in Humphrey, GB (ed): Pediatric Oncology (in press).

6. Hochberg FH, Slotnick B: Neuropsychologic impairment in astrocytoma survivors. Neurology (Minneap) 30:172-177, 1980.

7. Jelsma R, Bucy PC: Glioblastoma multiforme: its treatment and some factors affecting survival. Arch Neurol 20:161-171, 1969.

8. Kornblith PL, Szypko PE: Variations in response of human brain tumors to BCNU in vitro. J Neurosurg 48:580-586, 1978.

9. Kramer S: Tumor extent as a determining factor in radiotherapy of glioblastomas. Acta Radiol Therap 8:111-117, 1969.

10. Levin VA: Current trends in brain tumor therapy, in Paoletti P, Walker MD, Butti G, Knerich R (eds): Multidisciplinary Aspects of Brain Tumor Therapy. Elsevier/North Holland Biomedical Press, 1979, pp 165-172.

11. Maroon JC, Bank WO, Drayer, BP, et al: Intracranial biopsy assisted by computerized tomography. J Neurosurg 46:740-744, 1977.

12. Nakagaki H, Brunhart G, Kemper TL et al: Monkey brain damage from radiation in the therapeutic range. J Neurosurg 44:3-11, 1976.

13. Neuwelt EA, Maravilla KR, Frenkel EP, et al: Osmotic blood-brain barrier disruption. J Clin Invest 64:684-688, 1979.

14. Posner JB, Shapiro WR: Brain tumor: Current status of therapy and its complications. Arch Neurol 32:781-784, 1975.

15. Rankin JK, Yung WA, Shapiro WR: Isolation, karyotype and clonal growth of heterogeneous subpopulations of human malignant gliomas. Submitted to Cancer Res.

16. Rosenblum ML, Vasquez DA, Hoshino T, et al: Development of a clonogenic cell assay for human brain tumors. Cancer 41:2305-2315, 1978.

17. Salmon SE, Hamburger AW, Soehnleu B, et al: Quantitation of differential sensitivity of human-tumor stem cells to anticancer drugs. New Eng J Med 298:1321-1327, 1978.

18. Shapiro WR: Brain Tumors, in Pinedo HM (ed), Cancer Chemotherapy 1979, Amsterdam, Excerpta Med, 1979, pp 451-472.

19. Shapiro WR: Brain Tumors, in Pinedo HM (ed), Cancer Chemotherapy 1980, Amsterdam, Excerpta Med, 1980 (in press).

20. Shapiro WR, Allen JC, Mehta B, et al: Pharmacodynamics of entry of methotrexate into brain of humans, monkeys and a rat brain tumor model, in Paoletti P, Walker MD, Butti G, Knerich R (eds): Multidisciplinary Aspects of Brain Tumor Therapy. Elsevier/North Holland Biomedical Press, 1979, pp 135-142.

21. Shapiro WR, Ausman, JI: Chemotherapy of brain tumors: A clinical and experimental review, in Plum, F (ed): Recent Advances in Neurology. Philadelphia, FA Davis, 1969, pp 149-235.

22. Shapiro WR, Basler GA: Chemotherapy of human brain tumors transplanted into nude mice, in Paoletti P, Walker MD, Butti G, Knerich R (eds): Multidisciplinary Aspects of Brain Tumor Therapy, Elsevier/North Holland Biomedical Press, 1979, pp 309-316.

23. Shapiro WR, Basler GA, Chernik NL, et al: Human brain tumor transplantation into nude mice. J Natl Cancer Inst 62:447-453, 1979.

24. Shapiro WR, Rankin JK, Yung WA, et al: Heterogeneity of chemotherapy in nude mice and in vitro clones of human gliomas. Cancer Treat Rep (in press).

25. Sheline G, Wasserman T, Wara W, et al: The role of radiosensitizers in therapy of malignant brain tumors, in Paoletti P, Walker MD, Butti G, Knerich R (eds): Multidisciplinary Aspects of Brain Tumor Therapy, Elsevier/North Holland Biomedical Press, 1979, pp 197-207.

26. Walker MD, Alexander E Jr, Hunt WE, et al: Evaluation of BCNU and/or radiotherapy in the treatment of anaplastic gliomas. A cooperative clinical trial. J Neurosurg 49:333-343, 1978.
27. Walker MD, Strike TA: An interim analysis of methylprednisolone, procarbazine, BCNU or BCNU plus methylprednisolone in the treatment of malignant glioma. Proc Am Assoc Cancer Res 20:200, 1979.
28. Walker MD, Strike, TA: The treatment of malignant glioma in controlled studies, in Paoletti P, Walker MD, Butti G, Knerich R (eds), Multidisciplinary Aspects of Brain Tumor Therapy. Elsevier, North-Holland Biomedical Press, 1979, pp 267-274.
29. Walker MD, Strike TA, Sheline GE: An analysis of dose-effect relationship in the radiotherapy of malignant gliomas. Int J Rad Onc Biol Phys 5:1725-1731, 1979.
30. Urtasun R, Band P, Chapman JD, et al: Radiation and high-dose metronidazole in supratentorial glioblastomas. New Eng J Med 294:1364-1367, 1976.

Management of Local and Regional Melanoma

UMBERTO VERONESI

Chairman

W.H.O. International Melanoma Group

The two major problems in melanoma management
are: 1) the role of elective dissection of regional
lymphnodes in stage I and 2) the role of adjuvant
therapy in stage II.

Stage I: Immediate or delayed dissection of regional
lymphnodes.
When planning treatment of stage I melanoma of the
skin the decision whether regional lymphnodes should
or should not be removed, is the more difficult to
take. The two opposite approaches in support and
against elective dissection were modified by new
methods of histologic classification and most authors
agree that immediate dissection of clinically uninvolved regional nodes has not to be performed for
thin lesions with excellent prognosis. However, the
concept of "thin lesion" or "low risk patient"still
varies: according to Wanebo et al. (12) elective
dissection may be avoided only in level I and II
melanomas thinner than 0.9 mm; Breslow (2) Balch
et al.(1) suggested the opportunity of an immediate node dissection for primary melanomas thicker
than 1.5 mm, Cascinelli et al.(3)indicated
elective node dissection only in melanoma level V.
Moreover preliminary results of two prospective
randomized clinical trials have shown the inefficacy
of immediate node dissection in stage I melanoma of
the limbs as regards long-term survival, independent
ly of Clark's level or degree of thickness. The WHO
multicentric international study on 553 patients
with stage I melanoma patients showed identical
results whether or not an elective regional dissection
was performed (8,9)   . Identical conclusions were
reached by Sim et al.(7) in a prospective randomized

391

clinical trial carried on at the Mayo Clinic.
    In the WHO international trial 553 cases of
malignant melanoma of the extremities with clinically uninvolved regional lymphnodes were accrued
from 1967 to 1974.
    Patients with a primary melanoma originated only
on limbs were selected because these are the sites
where the first lymphatic hasin is easily identifiable. Cases with maximum diameter more than 5 cm or
with fixation to muscular fascia were excluded.
Cases with satellite nodules were included provided
that nodules were in an area no more than 5 cm in
diameter comprised that of primary melanoma. Patients
who were never treated or those who had been submitted to an excisional biopsy of primary melanoma
less than four weeks before final treatment were ad
mitted into the study. A quarterly follow up
examination was done in patients submitted to
immediate regional lymphnode dissection during the
first 5 years after treatment. In the same period the
follow up was done monthly in patients submitted
only to wide excision of primary. From the sixth
year the follow up was at six month interval. The
elapsing time between diagnosis of suspected regional
lymphnode metastases and node dissection was never
longer than 30 days.
    As regards the surgical technique, the primary
melanoma was generously excised with the patient
in general anesthesia. The skin was incised not less
than 3 cm from the visible margins of the tumor (or
of the area including the satellite nodules) in all
directions;skin incision was made not less than 3
cm from the wound in all directions in cases that
had been previously subjected to excision biopsy.
The incision extended 1-2 cm down into the subcutaneous fat and the underlying area of muscular
fascia was removed in depth. In the case of tumors
occurring on the fingers or toes, disarticulation
was performed at metacarpo or metatarso-phalangeal
level for the distal phalanges and at the level of
the carpometacarpal or tarsometatarsal joint for the
proximal phalanges. In any case the distance between
the margin of the melanoma and the skin incision
line was never less than 3 cm.
    In lower limb melanomas inguino-iliac node
dissection was performed, including the inguino-
crural, external iliac and obturator node groups.

In upper limb melanomas the operation was an axillary
dissection up to the subclavian muscle with en-bloc
removal of the lymph nodes and the small pectoral
muscle. No patient received adjuvant treatments.

Patients were randomized into two groups:
1) patients to be submitted to wide excision and
immediate regional node dissection and 2) patients
to be submitted to wide excision only.   Cases
were stratified by Centre. Most of patients (81.4%)
were females, the age group most frequently affected
was between 45 and 59 years, 88.6% of the 553 cases
were never treated for their melanoma and the great
majority of melanomas (82.8%) arose on lower limbs.
Among the 267 cases which were submitted to elective
node dissection 54   (20.2%) showed the presence
of occult metastases at the histologic examination
of the regional lymphnodes. Out of the 286 cases
treated with excision only of the primary melanoma
  64   (22.3 %) were operated on in the subsequent
years for the appearance of metastases in regional
lymphnodes. Most of the delayed dissections of
regional nodes occurred in the first three years
from the excision of the primary (Table 2).

The actuarial computed survival observed in
the two groups of patients is given in graph 1:
results obtained in the 286 patients treated with
wide excision of primary melanoma and regional node
dissection at the time of appearance of regional
node metastases are similar to those observed in the
267 patients submitted to wide excision of primary
and elective node dissection.

To assess whether some groups of patients may
benefit from immediate node dissection, survival of
different subsets according to type of treatment
given, has been evaluated. Table 3 shows 10-year
actuarial computed survival by clinical criteria.
There are no conditions in which the elective node
dissection improve the prognosis compared to the
simple excision of primary melanoma.
Sixty three patients had an excisional biopsy of
their melanoma within four weeks before final treatment. It is worth noting to stress that this
procedure does not worse survival and that also in
this case immediate lymph node dissection does not
achieve better results than wide excision of primary
and node dissection delayed at the time of appearance

Table 1   -   TRIAL 1 DESIGN

$$T_{1-3}N_0M_0$$

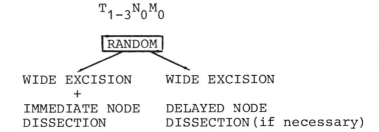

RANDOM

WIDE EXCISION   WIDE EXCISION
     +
IMMEDIATE NODE   DELAYED NODE
DISSECTION   DISSECTION (if necessary)

Table 2

	No.	occult metastases
EXCISION AND IMMEDIATE DISSECTION	267	54 (20.2%)

	No.	delayed dissections for metastases
EXCISION ONLY	286	64 (22.3%)

Graph 1

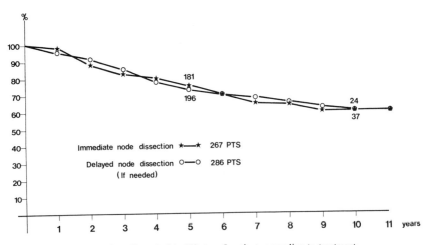

- Overall survival in 553 stage I patients according to treatment.

394

of regional node metastases.

Breslow's and Clark's methods of classification
are the key factors in the assessment of prognosis:
irrespectively of treatment this series confirms
that this two classifications are those that sub-
divide best patients with different prognosis.

As regards levels of invasion 325 melanomas
have been considered evaluable; 165 of these patients
have been submitted to immediate regional dissection.
The very limited number of cases classified level I
and II does not allow a statistical evaluation of
survival: however all patients were alive with no
evidence of disease at the end of the observation
period irrespectively of treatment. The crucial
levels are level III and IV. The level III group is
constituted by 90 patients; 45 of these have been
submitted to elective regional node dissection;
table 4 shows that immediate or delayed node dissect
ions achieve very similar results. The same results
were observed in 197 cases of level IV, 92 of which
have been submitted to wide excision of primary and
delayed node dissection, when necessary. As regards
level V the too limited number of patients does not
allow a good statistical evaluation, however four out
of the 9 level V patients are living with no
evidence of disease after immediate node dissection,
and six of the 14 cases submitted to wide excision
and delayed node dissection are alive with no
evidence of disease at the same period.

Maximum tumor thickness has been evaluated in
338 cases: 188 patients have been submitted to wide
excision and immediate node dissection. The efficacy
of elective node dissection has been evaluated in
two clusters of thickness up to 3.5 mm and over this
value, in order to have subgroups of a good numerical
consistence: the cut at 3.5 mm has been done because
this value is very close to the mean one.

There is no difference in survival in
patients submitted to wide excision and immediate
node dissection compared to the observed in
patients submitted to wide excision and delayed node
dissection, whether thickness is less or more than
3.5 mm.

In conclusion there is a good evidence that in
stage I melanoma of the limbs delayed dissection is
as effective as the immediate one in the control of

Table 3 — 10-year Survival (%)

	Excision + immediate dissection	Excision only
Males	49.5	48.7
Females	62.4	62.0
Age < 47 yr	64.9	68.7
>47 yr	54.5	51.9
Ø < 1.5 cm	67.9	64.8
>1.5 cm	42.7	46.4
Satellite		
Absent	59.4	59.5
Present	33.7	42.3

Table 4

10-year Survival (%)

	Excision+ immediate dissection	Excision only
Clark's level III	68.7	66.2
Clark's level IV	55.6	55.7

the disease if the patient can kept under strict
clinical control. If the surgeon is not sure that
the patient will stay under a quarterly follow up,
the immediate dissection is compulsory at least
for melanomas thicker than 2 mm.

Stage II: The role of adjuvant chemotherapy and
immunostimulation

Patients operated on for malignant melanoma and
with positive regional nodes are considered at high
risk of recurrence, and in fact only 15% survive for
five years. A severe prognosis is also reported for
patients with negative regional nodes but with the
primary melanoma originating in the skin of trunk
when the histologic level - according to Clark's
classification - is from 3 to 5.

For these high risk groups of patients, in 1974
the W.H.O. Collaborating centres for Evaluation of
Methods of Diagnosis and Treatment of Melanoma have
designed a multicentric controlled study, with the
aim of verifying the effectiveness of an adjuvant
treatment after radical surgery: the intent of the
trial is to investigate the effect of prolonged
chemotherapy, immunotherapy, or chemo-immunotherapy
on the disease free interval and on the survival in
melanoma patients with minimal residual disease.

For this protocol, Clinical Trial n.6, outlined
in Table 5, dacarbazine (DTIC, DIC,NSC-45388)has
been chosen as chemotherapy, since its specific and
widely experienced activity against advanced melanoma;
BCG has been adopted as a specific immunostimulant,
due to the report evidencing a decrease in recurrence
and increase in survival in a pilot series after
surgery and adjuvant BCG compared with historical
controls treated with surgery alone. (6 ˜)

According to the W.H.O. Trial n.6, the patients
must have adequate surgical treatment. The primary
melanoma must be removed with at least 3 cm cutaneous
incision in healthy tissue, and the incision must
reach in depth an area of the muscular fascia that
corresponds to the skin removed. The regional lymph
nodes are removed according to the classic criteria.

The treatments are as follows (Table 5)
-dacarbazine is administered by intravenous bolus,
at the dose of 200 mg/m^2 daily for 5 consecutive

Table 5

OUTLINE OF CLINICAL TRIAL No.6

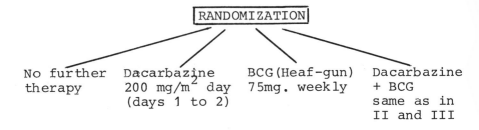

	RANDOMIZATION		
No further therapy	Dacarbazine 200 mg/m^2 day (days 1 to 2)	BCG (Heaf-gun) 75mg. weekly	Dacarbazine + BCG same as in II and III

Table 6

No. Evaluable patients

Controls	157
DTIC	188
BCG	173
DTIC + BCG	178
TOTAL	696

days, every 4 weeks;
- BCG is applied through the multipuncture Heaf-gun
technique (4 shoots at 2 mm depth), at the weekly
dose of 75 mg (moist weight) using as sites of
administration the base of the four limbs - except
the operated limb - in clockwise rotation, until a
positive cutaneous reaction (at least erythema plus
infiltration) is produced: thereafter patients
receive a vaccination every 4 weeks;
- when dacarbazine and BCG are given in association,
the doses are the same and the timing of BCG starts
from the 5th day of dacarbazine.
Courses of all adjuvant treatments are repeated every
4 weeks for 2 years or until relapse occurs.
       From June 1974, 792 patients have been registered
but 90 of them (11%) are inelegible according to the
protocol requirement, and 6 patients have received
fully inadequate treatments.
       No difference is detectable in distribution of
cases according to the stratification parameters.
       The per cent relapse free at 36 maonths in
relation to treatments and to stratification parameters is shown in Table 7 and 8.
The actuarial analysis indicates that in general the
per cent difference remains superior in the adjuvant
groups compared to surgery alone, being however
statistically significant only if the adjuvant dacarbazine versus the untreated controls is compared.
       However, this apparently favourable effect on
the relapse free period, at present, is not reflected
in the survival: in fact, as it is shown in Table 7
and 8 no difference in survival is detectable in
the adjuvant treated as compared with the untreated
controls, either considering the stage II (N+) or
the stage I(N-, trunk) patients.
       As regards the site of first relapse, no
difference in the patterns of either local or distant
site of metastases (including brain localizations)is
detectable among the 4 groups.
       As to toxicity, treatments have been well
tolerated by the majority of patients. As usual, a
short duration of gastrointestinal phenomena (nausea
and vomiting, during 1-2 days) is reported in dacarbazine treated cases. The drug-related myelosuppression, being mild and always reversible, has
not been able to significantly modify the planned
treatment.

Table 7

| | 3-YEAR RESULTS (%) (N+ patients) | |
	RFS	SURV
Controls	18	32
DTIC	38	49
BCG	38	44
DTIC + BCG	29	49

Table 8

| | 3-YEAR RESULTS (%) (Trunk N- patients) | |
	RFS	SURV
Controls	59	62
DTIC	72	77
BCG	41	65
DTIC + BCG	46	70

The skin reactions due to BCG administration have been easily managed. Only few cases of systemic effects such as fever of liver toxicity have been of clinical relevance.

No differences in toxicity (additive or subtractive) are at present associated with the use of combined chemotherapy and immunotherapy.

Upon relapse, the response rate is very poor in the previously dacarbazine $\pm$ BCG treated patients, either to nitrosourea, or higher dacarbazine doses or other phase II drugs. A 20% objective response rate is, however, obtainable with dacarbazine in the controls or in the adjuvant BCG treated patients.

The data are too preliminary to allow any conclusion. However, it seems that the adjuvant treatment both with chemotherapy and immunostimulation does not modify the prognosis of stage II malignant melanoma in a significant extent.

The clinical results are, however, the expression of a true preliminary and not fully assessed evaluation which need to be furthermore largely reviewed before definitive judgement. This will be realized in 1981.

The following Institutes of the group took part in the WHO trial 1 and/or 6 described in this report: Abteilung für Klinische Immunologie, Medizinische Hochschule, Hannover (Federal Rep.Germany) - Cancer Research Centre of the U.S.S.R. Academy of Medical Sciences, Moscow (U.S.S.R.) - Fondazione Pascale, Naples (Italy) - Herzen State Oncological Institute, Moscow (U.S.S.R.) - Het Nederlands Kankerinstituut, Amsterdam (The Nederlands) - Hospital A.C.Camargo, Sao Paolo (Brazil) - Hospital de Clinicas "M.Quintela", Montevideo (Uruguay) - Instituto Nacional de Cancer, Rio de Janeiro (Brazil) - Instituto Nacional de Enfermedades Neoplasticas, Lima (Perù) - Institut Gustave Roussy, Villejuif (France) - Institut Jules Bordet, Brussels (Belgium) - Institut Paoli Calmett, Marseille (France) - Institute of Oncology, Beograd (Yugoslavia) - Istituto Nazionale Tumori, Milan (Italy) Norwegian Radium Hospital, Oslo (Norway) - Oncological

Research Institute, Sofia (Bulgaria) - Oncological Institute,
Cracow (Poland) - Oncological Institute, Gliwice
(Poland) - Oncological Institute, Warsaw (Poland) -
Oncological Institute, Brno (Czechoslowakia) - Petrov
Research Institute of Oncology, Leningrad (U.S.S.R.)
State Institute of Oncology, Budapest (Hungary) -
University of Glasgow, Western Infirmary, Glasgow
(United Kingdom) - University of Sydney, dept. of
Surgery, Sydney (Australia).

REFERENCES

1. Balch M.C. et al.: Tumor thickness as a guide
    to surgical management of clinical stage I
    melanoma patients. Cancer 43:883-888, 1979
2. Breslow A.: Tumor thickness, level of invasion
    and node dissection in stage I cutaneous melanoma.
    Ann.Surg.182:572-575, 1975
3. Cascinelli N., Balzarini G.P., Fontana V.,et al.:
    Long terms results of surgical treatment of
    melanoma of the limbs. Tumori 62:233-242, 1976
4. Clark WH Jr., From L., Bernardino E.A., Mihm M.
    C.Jr.: The histogenesis and biologic behavior
    of primary human malignant melanomas of the skin.
    Cancer Res.29: 705-727, 1969
5. Comis R.L., Carter S.K.: Integration of Chemo
    therapy into Combined Modality Therapy of Solid
    Tumors.IV.Malignant Melanoma. Cancer Treat.Rev.
    1:285-304, 1974
6. Gutterman J.U., McBride C., Freireich E.J., et
    al.: Active Immunotherapy with BCG for Recurrent
    Malignant Melanoma. Lancet i:1208-1212, 1973.
7. Sim F.H., Taylor W.F., Ivins J.C., Pritchard D.J.,
    Soule E.H.: A prospective randomized study of
    the efficacy of routine elective lymphadenectomy
    in management of malignant melanoma. Cancer 41:
    498, 1978
8. Veronesi U,, Adamus J., Bandiera D.C., et al.:
    Inefficacy of immediate node dissection in stage
    I melanoma of the limbs. New Engl.J.of Medicine

297:627-630, 1977
9.   Veronesi U., Adamus J., Bandiera D.C., et al.:
     Stage I melanoma of the limbs. Immediate versus
     delayed node dissection. Tumori 66:373-396, 1980
10. Veronesi U., Bajetta E., Cascinelli N., et al.:
     New trends in the treatment of malignant mel-
     anoma. Int.Adv.Surg.Oncol. 1:113-116, 1978
11. Veronesi U., Beretta G.; Controlled study for
     prolonged chemotherapy, immunotherapy, and
     chemotherapy plus immunotherapy as an adjuvant
     to surgery in malignant melanoma (Trial 6):
     Preliminary report. In "Recent results in cancer
     Research", Vol.68, Ed.by G.Bonadonna, G.Mathé,
     S.E.Salmon. Springer-Verlag, Berlin , pag.375-
     379, 1979
12. Wanebo H.J., Fortner J.G., Woodruff J., et al.:
     Selection of the optimum surgical treatment of
     stage I melanoma by depth of microinvasion:
     use of the combined microstage technique (Clark
     Breslow). Ann.Surg. 182:302-313, 1975.

Chemotherapy of Adult

Soft Tissue Sarcoma

H.M. PINEDO

Head of Div.of Biochemical Pharmacology
& Head of Dept.of Oncology
Netherlands Cancer Institute & Free University Hospital
Amsterdam, The Netherlands

VIVIEN H.C. BRAMWELL

Senior Registrar, Cancer Research Campaign
Dept.of Medical Oncology, Manchester University
& Christie Hospital & Holt Radium Institute,
Manchester, England

Introduction

Soft tissue sarcomas are primary mesenchymal tumors located outside the skeleton and comprise many histological subtypes. They tend to metastasise by haematogenous routes predominantly to the lung. The main treatment is local surgical resection of the primary tumor or amputation of the extremity. The main prognostic criteria are the size of the primary tumor and the histological grade, which are more important than the histological subtype of the tumor. These findings have led to a new clinical staging system, based on the TNM classification, in which these two main prognostic criteria have been taken into consideration[37].

While chemotherapy has had a great impact on survival of children with rhabdomyosarcomas[30], the results of chemotherapy in adult sarcomas have not improved during the past 5 years, and are still dismal, with the exception of the small percentage of patients in whom a complete remission is achieved[43]. An initial enthusiasm has been dampened by failure to reproduce the high response rates achieved in early studies of combination chemotherapy. In this chapter we will discuss: 1) single agent activity in advanced disease, 2) combination chemotherapy in advanced disease, 3) adjuvant chemotherapy, 4) pre-operative intra-arterial chemotherapy, and 5) attempt to make a summary and conclusions of existing experience as a basis for new possibilities.

Single Agent Chemotherapy in Advanced Disease

Adriamycin

Adriamycin is the most effective agent in adult soft tissue sarcoma.   Reported responses range from 9-79%[26], depending on the dose administered, the extent of previous treatment and the number of patients in the series.   A mean response rate of 27% in 357 patients has been reported[9].   For a long time there has been evidence that changes in schedule and dose influence the response rate[24], 75 mg/m^2/3 wks giving higher response rates than doses $\leq$50 mg/m^2 given at intervals exceeding 4 wks.   This dose response relationship has been reconfirmed in recent years.   The low response rate of 13% in a study using 60 mg/m^2/3 wks (Table 1) may be partly related to the fact that most patients had received prior treatment[39].   The high dose required for adriamycin to be active creates problems when combinations with other myelosuppressive drugs are attempted.   One may have to resort to the use of protective environments[33], unless bone marrow sparing drugs such as DTIC, which show synergism with adriamycin, become available[9, 10]. In addition to the problem of myelosuppression, there is also that of cardiotoxicity after prolonged administration of the drug.

TABLE 1
Variations in Dose and Schedule of Administration of
Adriamycin as a Single Agent in Soft Tissue Sarcoma[†]

Dose and Schedule	No.of Patients	Response Rate (CR)	Ref.
0.4mg/kg/days 1,2,3,8,9,10 then 0.4mg/kg/wk	36*	39% (8%)	22
0.4mg/kg/days 1,2,3,8,9,10 then q 2 wks starting day 15	41ɵ	17% (2%)	7
1 mg/kg/wk until toxicity then 0.5 mg/kg/wk	35*	26% (9%)	5
60 mg/m^2 q 3 wks	63Φ	13% (3%)	39
70 mg/m^2 q 3 wks	39*	28% (8%)	34

*not specified whether patients received prior chemotherapy (PC); ɵ14 received PC; Φmost received PC; †only studies including more than 30 patients.

The latter hazard has triggered a number of studies investigating various schedules of administration (Table 1).   It appears that adriamycin retains its activity when given weekly[5-7, 22].
Again, there is a correlation between dose and effect.   Although a weekly schedule seems less cardiotoxic, myelosuppression is not reduced.   Adriamycin by continuous infusion is also active, producing a 57% response rate in 21 patients[41].   However, all patients received DTIC concomitantly, and some, vincristine and cyclophosphamide in addition.

A second approach is to find an anthracycline analog which is at least as effective as adriamycin, but which causes less heart damage.   Several analogs are waiting to be incorporated in Phase II studies[41].   The only analog adequately evaluated which has shown activity in sarcomas is carminomycin, with a 27% response rate[25].

Dimethyl Triazeno Imidazole Carboxamide (DTIC)

Although the single agent activity of DTIC was as low as 16% in 61 patients reviewed from the literature[26], the increased response rate to the combination of adriamycin + DTIC[9] as compared to either of these two drugs alone makes re-evaluation of the activity of this drug unnecessary.

Methotrexate

Methotrexate has been studied in both conventional doses and high doses with leucovorin rescue.   Several regimens with low doses have been applied in non-pretreated patients[42, 45], but it is not clear from the data which is most effective.   However, the drug did show activity with response rates of approximately 30%.
Responses (8 in 24 patients) have also been observed with high dose regimens (50-300 mg/kg)[12, 13].

The EORTC Soft Tissue and Bone Sarcoma Group performed a Phase II study in heavily pre-treated patients and observed no responses in 22 evaluable patients (manuscript in preparation).
There is a need to confirm the data on conventional dose methotrexate with a larger number of non-pretreated patients on a fixed regimen.   There is at present insufficient data to show any advantage of high dose over low dose methotrexate.

Other Agents

Few data are available on the single agent activity of vincristine, actinomycin D and cyclophosphamide as single agents.   Results appear to be disappointing[26].

In 42 pre-treated patients on a 5 day regimen of cisplatin every 3 weeks, Samson et al observed 3(7%) partial responses[38], while the EORTC group, using a single high dose schedule, observed no responses in 17 patients[4].   In contrast to these findings, 3 responses were observed in a small series of 13 patients[14].

The reports on vindesine are inconclusive.   Although no responses have been observed in broad Phase II studies, recently Magill et al reported 5 (16%) responses in 32 sarcoma patients[21]. Additional studies with this drug are required.

A high cumulative response rate of 77% in 53 patients from two series has been observed with the combination of ICRF-159 and radiotherapy[11,31].   A controlled trial comparing this combination with radiotherapy alone is needed.

Other drugs which have been studied (each in more than 20 patients) and which have shown a response rate of less than 10% are dianhydrogalactitol, gallium nitrate, Baker's antifol, pyrazofurin, VM-26, chlorozotocin and cytembena[41], ICRF-159 (without radiotherapy), maytansine[3], AMSA, DCNU[21], CCNU, cycloleucine, 5-azacytidine, piperazinedione and hexamethylmelamine[22]. Unfortunately, many of these drugs have been evaluated in heavily pre-treated patients.

Combination Chemotherapy in Advanced Disease

Adriamycin + DTIC (adriamycin 60mg/m^2 on day 1, and DTIC 250mg/m^2 on days 1-5) has been the backbone of many combinations. The SWOG reported a 42% response rate to ADIC with 11% complete responders[9].   The cumulative response rate in 192 patients reported in the literature[26] is even higher with 47% of the patients responding.   While initially the SWOG response rates for CYVADIC (ADIC + cyclophosphamide and vincristine) ranged up to 59%, in a more recent study by the same group, the response rate dropped to 51%[44].   The EORTC, in their randomised protocol comparing two schedules of these same 4 drugs, has found a response rate of 37% for CYVADIC[28].   One difference between the two CYVADIC regimens which may account for the difference in response rates is the longer interval of 4 weeks between each cycle in the EORTC study compared with 3 weeks in the SWOG study.   Patients in the cycling arm of the EORTC protocol, who received CTX/VCR and ADIC alternately at 4 weekly intervals, showed a response rate of 23% which is significantly lower than that of the full regimen[28]. In a more recent analysis, the response to the cycling regimen was even lower, being only 14% of the evaluable patients (Table 2)

TABLE 2
Combinations including Adriamycin in Soft Tissue Sarcoma*

Combination	No. of patients	CR	PR	Overall	Ref.
		Response rate(%)			
ADM/CTX/MTX	100	–	–	36	18
ADM/MeCCNU	53	9	30	39	32
ADM/MeCCNU/VCR	42	–	–	26	20
ADM/ACD/VCR/HDMTX–CF	34	–	–	44	20
ADM/ACD/VCR/HDMTX/DTIC/CLB	33	–	–	27	20
ADM/CTX/VCR	38	3	10	13	34
ADM/CTX/VCR/MDMTX/ACD	40	5	22	27	45
ADM/DTIC	192	13	34	47	26
ADM/DTIC/VCR	86	9	38	47	9
ADM/DTIC/VCR/CTX(q 3 wks)	119	17	34	51	44
ADM/DTIC/VCR/CTX(q 4 wks)	84	17	21	38	EORTC
ADM/DTIC/VCR/CTX(q 4 wks, cycling)	77	5	9	14	EORTC
ADM/DTIC/VCR/CTX/HDMTX–CF	38	11	16	27	19
ADM/DTIC/VCR/ACD	224	12	28	40	44

*Only regimens studied in more than 30 patients; ADM = adriamycin
CTX = cyclophosphamide, MTX = methotrexate, MeCCNU = methyl
CCNU, VCR = vincristine, HDMTX = high dose MTX, MDMTX =
medium dose MTX, CLB = chlorambucil, ACD = actinomycin D.

It seems therefore, that cyclophosphamide and vincristine do
not add much to the effect of ADIC, but they do increase the overall
toxicity.   This makes ADIC the best treatment available at present.

Although the combination of adriamycin plus methyl CCNU did
result in a response rate of 39% in one study[32], the same combination including vincristine resulted in a response rate of 26%[20]
which is similar to that of adriamycin alone.   Methyl CCNU given
as a single agent has shown no activity[26].

Recently, it was shown in a randomised study that actinomycin
D has no place in combination therapy[2], which correlates with its
lack of activity as a single agent.   The combination of adriamycin,
cyclophosphamide and methotrexate (ACM) has given a 36% response
rate, while that of vincristine, high dose methotrexate, adriamycin
and actinomycin D gave a response rate of 44%.   Considering the
lack of activity of actinomycin D, cyclophosphamide and vincristine,
the latter studies indicate that methotrexate may indeed be an
effective agent.

One of the interesting observations of the EORTC study was the
fact that survival of partial responders was identical to that of
patients with stabilisation of disease (median survival of 56 weeks),
both groups doing significantly better than those patients with progressive disease (Fig.1).   This observation accounts for the identical survival curves of the two treatment arms (median survival
45 weeks), despite the presence of a significant difference in complete plus partial response rates. Thus, the difference in complete
response rate (Table 2) did not alter the overall survival curves
significantly due to the relatively long survival of patients with
stable disease.   It also appeared that more than 3 cycles, sometimes up to 6 cycles, might be required to achieve a response[27].

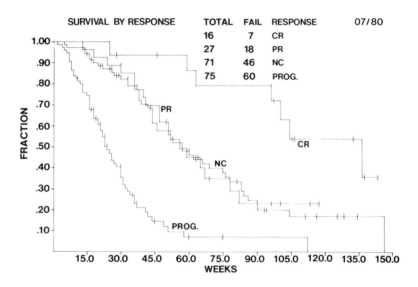

Fig.1.   EORTC Study 62761 for Advanced Sarcomas.
Survival by type of response.

Response rates are significantly higher in patients with
advanced inoperable disease than with metastatic disease[43,45].
The London study[45] observed an overall response rate of 26% in
metastatic disease and 57% for inoperable or locally recurrent
tumour.   An analysis of 53 patients who achieved a complete remission on adriamycin-containing regimens supports this observation
[43].   The median duration of remission and survival of 15 patients
with advanced local disease was 23 and 39 months, while that of 38
patients with metastases was 11 and 27 months, respectively.

Conversion of a partial remission to a complete remission by surgery seemed to improve the prognosis significantly. In the majority of cases relapse occurs at the original site of disease and so in future studies we should consider surgery or radiotherapy at the original site of disease after achieving a response.

Adjuvant chemotherapy

Patients with soft tissue sarcoma have a high rate of local recurrence after excision of the tumor.   Although the incidence of local recurrences can be reduced by post-operative adjunctive radiotherapy[35, 36], many patients still develop metastatic disease. In a randomised study at the NCI investigating the role of post-operative local radiotherapy, all 49 patients received adjuvant chemo-therapy consisting of adriamycin, high dose methotrexate with leucovorin and cyclophosphamide.   Disease-free survival and overall survival were significantly improved compared with histor-ical controls. (Fig.2).   72% of the patients remain free of disease (median follow up 38 months)[35, 36].   These results have prompted the same centre to initiate a randomised study which includes a control arm, without chemotherapy, in order to clearly define the role of adjuvant chemotherapy.

SOFT TISSUE SARCOMA SURVIVAL

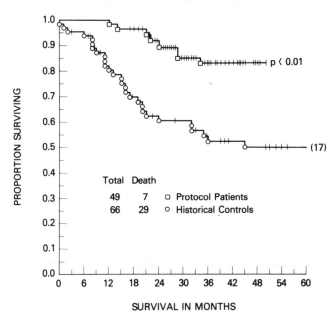

Figure 2

A second study with 61 evaluable patients used a regimen including adriamycin, actinomycin D, vincristine, high dose methotrexate with leucovorin, DTIC and chlorambucil (ALOMAD) given over
10 weeks following surgery[40]. The patient population, however,
was heterogeneous with 19 patients undergoing surgery for the
primary tumor, 8 for a local recurrence and 34 patients receiving
pre- or post-operative radiotherapy in addition to chemotherapy, or
chemotherapy after resection of pulmonary metastases. Although
there was no treatment-free control group and the drug regimen is
relatively ineffective in advanced disease (Table 2), the results are
encouraging; 74% of the patients remaining free of disease (median
follow-up 16 months).

Recently a small study in which 19 patients received postoperative radiation therapy plus combination chemotherapy consisting of adriamycin, cyclophosphamide and DTIC has been reported[1].
Again there was no concurrent control group without chemotherapy.
Survival at 18 months was 55% for historical control patients
matched for stage and histology, and 95% for study patients; 79% of
the treated patients were continuously disease-free.

The results of these three adjuvant studies suggest that adjuvant
chemotherapy given concomitantly with or following radiotherapy
after removal of the tumor is of benefit to the patient. Nonetheless,
in view of the recent improvements in diagnostic procedures, surgical technique and radiation therapy, we should await the results
of randomised trials with large numbers of patients at the NCI[35]
and in the EORTC[29] (more than 100 patients on study) which contain
a control arm without chemotherapy. Until these data confirm the
value of adjuvant chemotherapy there is no indication to give this
type of treatment on a routine basis.

Pre-operative Chemotherapy

As already stated, local recurrence after surgery for the
primary tumour used to be a significant problem in patients with
soft tissue sarcomas. This problem has now been partly solved
by post-operative radiation therapy. Considering the good responses to chemotherapy achieved in patients with locally advanced
primary tumors[43, 45], there might be a place for pre-operative
regional intra-arterial or systemic chemotherapy for the primary
tumor. Isolation perfusion of the limb with adriamycin using a
tourniquet results in a tenfold increase in drug concentrations in
all tissues of the perfused limb[8, 16]. However, there is a risk of
wound complications, severe tissue damage, sepsis and even death,

particularly in less experienced hands. Response rates of over
80% have been observed[15, 16, 23]. Although pre-operative perfusion
should not be used on a routine basis, the technique should be considered in locally advanced disease, only eradicable by amputation.
Apart from a few case reports[17] there is little information on
systemic pre-operative chemotherapy. Such a combined modality
approach would give information on the sensitivity of the tumor to
chemotherapy (allowing the most efficient use of the limited number
of effective chemotherapeutic agents available) and might eliminate
micrometastases at an early stage, thereby improving the prognosis
of patients with soft tissue sarcomas.

Summary, Conclusions and Suggestions for the Future

The results of treatment of advanced soft tissue sarcomas are
still poor. Complete responders on chemotherapy benefit most
from the treatment, with a median survival of 2.5 years. Patients
with a partial response or stable disease show an identical median
survival which is in excess of one year. In future studies more
attention should be given to data on patients with stable disease.
Patients with progressive disease have a median survival of
around 6 months which approximates to that of patients receiving
no treatment. There are several ways to attempt to improve survival. One approach is to study the effect of aggressive surgery
and/or radiation therapy in patients with a partial response with the
aim of converting a partial remission into a complete remission.
This would involve about 25% of all patients. A measure that might
improve survival of complete responders is excision of tissue,
where feasible, from sites involved by tumor prior to chemotherapy,
as it has been shown that these are the commonest sites of relapse.
Another approach, is to perform further Phase II studies in the hope
of finding new effective drugs, preferably non-myelosuppressive
and non-cardiotoxic, which may be combined in full doses with adriamycin. However, these trials should be limited to patients who
have received no more than two drugs previously. Marrow sparing
drugs could be combined with anthracyclines, while non-cardiotoxic
active anthracyclines should replace adriamycin. Other agents
which show an additive effect with adriamycin, such as DTIC, offer
a great advantage. In this respect, a trial of adriamycin plus cisplatin is worthwhile, despite its poor activity as a single agent. The
role of hypoxic sensitisers in combination with radiotherapy should
also be critically assessed.

Pre-operative chemotherapy, both systemically and locally needs to be studied further as the response rate in primary tumors is relatively high and valuable information could be obtained on the sensitivity of the tumor. The same drugs could then be used in an adjuvant setting after post-operative local radiotherapy. However, all these types of studies should include control groups of patients.

REFERENCES

1. Antman, K, Blum, R, Corson, J, et al. Effective adjuvant chemotherapy for localised soft tissue sarcoma. Proc Amer Assoc Cancer Res 21:141, 1980

2. Baker,L, Benjamin, R, Fine, G, et al. Combination chemotherapy in the management of disseminated soft tissue sarcomas. A South West Oncology Group (SWOG) study. Proc Amer Soc Clin Oncol 20:378, 1979

3. Borden, E, Ash, C, Rosenbaum, C, Lerner, H. Phase II evaluation of dibromodulcitol (DBD), ICRF-159 and Maytansine in sarcomas and mesotheliomas. Proc Amer Soc Clin Oncol 21:479, 1980

4. Bramwell, VHC, Brugarolas, A, Mouridsen, HT, et al. EORTC Phase II study of Cisplatin in Cyvadic-resistant soft tissue sarcoma. Eur J Cancer 15:1511-1513, 1979

5. Chlebowski, RT, Paroly, WS, Pugh, RP, et al. Adriamycin given as a weekly schedule without a loading course: clinically effective with reduced incidence of cardiotoxicity. Cancer Treatm Rep 64:47-51, 1980

6. Creagan, ET, Hahn, RG, Ahmann, DL, et al. A clinical trial with adriamycin (NSC-123127) in advanced sarcomas. Oncology 34:90-91, 1977

7. Cruz, AB, Thames, EA, Aust, JB, et al. Combination chemotherapy for soft tissue sarcomas: a Phase III study. J Surg Oncol 11:313-323, 1979

8. Didolkar, MS, Kanter, PM, Baffi, RR, et al. Comparison of regional versus systemic chemotherapy with adriamycin Ann Surg 187:332-336, 1978

9. Gottlieb, JA, Baker, LM, O'Bryan, RM, et al. Adriamycin (NSC-123127) used alone and in combination for soft tissue sarcomas. Cancer Chemother Rep 6:271-282, 1975

10. Griswold, DP, Laster, WR, Schnabel, FM. Therapeutic potentiation by adriamcyin and 5-(3,3-demethyl-1-triazeno)-imidazole-4-carboxamide against B16 melanoma, C3H breast carcinoma, Lewis lung carcinoma and leukaemia L1210. Proc Amer Assoc Cancer Res 14:15, 1973

11. Hellman, K, Ryall, RDH, MacDonald, E, et al. Comparison of radiotherapy with and without razoxane (ICRF-159) in the treatment of soft tissue sarcomas. Cancer (Philad) 41:100-107, 1978

12. Isacoff, WH, Eilber, F, Cowe, L, et al. A Phase II clinical trial with high dose methotrexate therapy and leucovorin rescue. Cancer Treatm Rep 62:1295-1304, 1978

13. Karakousis, CP. High dose methotrexate in metastatic sarcomas. Proc Amer Soc Clin Oncol 19:401, 1978

14. Karakousis, CP, Holtermann, DA, Holyoke, ED. Cis-Dichlorodiammineplatinum (II) in metastatic soft tissue sarcomas Cancer Treatm Rep 63:2071-2075, 1979

15. Karakousis, CP, Lopez, R, Catane, R, et al. Intra-arterial adriamycin in the treatment of soft tissue sarcomas. J Surg Oncol 13:21-17, 1980

16. Krementz, ET, Carter, RD, Sutherland, CM, et al. Chemotherapy of sarcomas of the limbs by regional perfusion. Ann Surg 185: 555-564, 1977

17. Lokich, JJ. Pre-operative chemotherapy in soft tissue sarcoma. Surgery Gynaecology & Obstetrics 148:512-516, 1979

18. Lowenbraun, S, Moffit, S, Smalley, R, et al. Combination chemotherapy with adriamycin, cyclophosphamide and methotrexate (ACM) in metastatic sarcomas. Proc Amer Soc Clin Oncol 18:186, 1977

19. Lynch, G, Magill, GB, Golbey, RN. Combination chemotherapy of soft part sarcomas with CYOMAD(S-7). Proc Amer Ass Cancer Res 20:116, 1979

20. Magill, GB, Golbey, RN, Krakoff, IH. Chemotherapy combinations in adult sarcomas. Proc Amer Soc Clin Oncol 19:332, 1977

21. Magill, GB, Sordillo, P, Gralla, R, Golbey, RN. Phase II trial of DVA, AMSA and DCNU as single agents in adult sarcomas. Proc Amer Soc Clin Oncol 21:362, 1980

22. Mitts, DL, Gerhardt, H, Armstrong, D, et al. Chemotherapy for advanced soft tissue sarcomas: results of Phase I and II cooperative studies. Texas Medicine 75:43-47, 1979

23. Norton, DL, Eilber, FR, Weisenburger, TH. Limb salvage using preoperative intra-arterial adriamycin and radiation therapy for extremity soft tissue sarcomas. Aust NZJ Surg 48:56-59, 1978

24. O'Bryan, RM, Luce, JK, Talley, RW, et al. Phase II evaluation of adriamycin in human neoplasia. Cancer, 32:1-8, 1973

25. Perevodchikova,NI, Lichnitser, MT, Gorbunova, VA.   Phase I clinical study of carminomycin: its activity against soft tissue sarcomas.   Cancer Treatm Rep 61:1705-1707, 1977

26. Pinedo, HM, Kenis, Y.   Chemotherapy of advanced soft tissue sarcoma in adults.   Cancer Treatm Rev 4:67-86, 1977

27. Pinedo, HM, Van Ooosterom, AT.   Treatment of advanced soft tissue sarcomas in adults: past, present and future, in Van Oosterom, AT, Muggia, FM, Cleton, FJ (eds): International course on recent advances in the treatment of ovarian and testicular cancer and of soft tissue and bone sarcomas.   The Hague, Nijhoff, 1980, pp 425-438

28. Pinedo, HM, Vendrik, CPJ, Bramwell, VHC, et al.   Re-evaluation of the CYVADIC regimen for metastatic soft tissue sarcoma.   Proc Amer Soc Clin Oncol 20:346, 1979

29. Pinedo, HM, Vendrik, CPJ, Bramwell, VHC, et al.   Evaluation of adjuvant therapy in soft tissue sarcoma: a collaborative multidisciplinary approach (EORTC protocol, 62771).   Eur J Cancer 15:811-820, 1979

30. Pinedo, HM, Voute, PA.   Combination chemotherapy in soft tissue sarcomas, in Tagnon, HJ, Staquet, MJ (eds): Recent advances in cancer treatment.   New York, Raven Press, 1977

31. Rhomberg, WU.   Radiotherapy combined with ICRF-159 (NSC-129943).   Int J Radiat Oncol Biol Phys 4:121-126, 1978

32. Rivkin, S, Gottlieb, JE, Thigpen, T, Elsebai, I.   Methyl CCNU -adriamycin in metastatic sarcomas.   Proc Amer Soc Clin Oncol 19:331, 1978

33. Rodriguez, V, Bodey, GP, Freireich, EJ.   Increased remission rate and prolongation of survival in patients with soft tissue sarcomas treated with intensive chemotherapy on a protected environment-prophylactic antibiotic programme (PEPA)   Proc Amer Soc Clin Oncol 18:320, 1977

34. Rosenbaum, C, Schoenfeld, D.   Treatment of advanced soft tissue sarcoma.   Proc Amer Soc Clin Oncol 18:287, 1977

35. Rosenberg, SA, Kent, H, Costa, J. et al.   Prospective evaluation of the role of limb sparing surgery, radiation therapy and adjuvant chemotherapy in the treatment of adult soft tissue sarcomas.   Surgery 84:62-69, 1978

36. Rosenberg, SA, Sindelar, WF.   Surgery and adjuvant radiation-chemo-immunotherapy in soft tissue sarcomas: results of treatment at the National Cancer Institute, in Van Oosterom, AT, Muggia, FM, Cleton, FJ (eds): International course on recent advances in the treatment of ovarian and testicular cancer and of soft tissue and bone sarcomas. The Hague, Nijhoff, 1980, pp 397-412

37. Russell, WO, Cohen, J, Enzinger, F, et al. A clinical and pathological staging system for soft tissue sarcoma. Cancer (Philad) 40:1562-1570, 1977

38. Samson, MK, Baker, LH, Benjamin, RS, et al. Cis-Dichlorodiammine platinum (II) in advanced soft tissue sarcoma and bony sarcomas: A Southwest Oncology Group Study. Cancer Treatm Rep 61:2027-2029, 1979

39. Savlow, ED, Knight, E, MacIntyre, JM, Wolter, J. Comparison of adriamycin with cycloleucine in the treatment of sarcomas. Cancer Treatm Rep, in press

40. Sordillo, P, Magill, GB, Howard, J, Golbey, RB. Adjuvant chemotherapy of adult soft part sarcomas with "ALOMAD". Proc Amer Soc Clin Oncol 19:353, 1978

41. Stewart, DJ, Benjamin, RS, Baker, L, et al. New drugs for the treatment of soft tissue sarcoma, in Van Oosterom, AT, Muggia, FM, Cleton, FJ (eds): International course on recent advances in the treatment of ovarian and testicular cancer and soft tissue and bone sarcomas. The Hague, Nijhoff, 1980, pp.453-479

42. Subramanian, S, Wiltshaw, E. Chemotherapy of sarcoma. Lancet, 1: 686-693, 1978

43. Yap, BS, Sinkovics, JG, Benjamin, RS, Bodey, GP. Survival and relapse patterns of complete responders in adults with advanced soft tissue sarcomas (STS). Proc Amer Soc Clin Oncol 20:352, 1979

44. Yap, BS, Baker, LH, Sinkovics, JG, et al. Cyclophosphamide vincristine, adriamycin and DTIC (CYVADIC)combination chemotherapy for the treatment of advanced sarcomas. Cancer Treatm Rep 64:93-98, 1980

45. Wiltshaw, E, Harmer, C, McKinna, A. Soft tissue sarcoma: treatment of advanced disease in the Royal Marsden Hospital, in Van Oosterom, AT, Muggia, FM, Cleton, FJ (eds): International course on recent advances in the treatment of ovarian and testicular cancer and of soft tissue and bone sarcoma. The Hague, Nijhoff, 1980, pp.413-423

Lymphomas

ADVANCES IN THE TREATMENT
OF MALIGNANT LYMPHOMAS: AN OVERVIEW

SAUL A. ROSENBERG, M.D.

PROFESSOR OF MEDICINE AND RADIOLOGY
STANFORD UNIVERSITY
STANFORD,CALIFORNIA

INTRODUCTION

The understanding and management of patients with malignant lymphomas has been a major advance of modern medicine of the last 10-20 years. These advances have transformed Hodgkin's disease from a predominantly fatal illness to a curable one for the great majority of patients diagnosed in 1980. Among the more heterogeneous group of patients with the so-called non-Hodgkin's lymphomas, curative treatment programs have been developed for several of the ten or so major clinicopathological entities now recognized, and excellent palliation is available for virtually all patients who cannot be cured.

Based upon these advances, there is great promise that new treatment methods will be developed over the next decade which will not only result in more patients being cured, but with a reduced morbidity of the treatment programs.

Details of some of the advances of therapy will be reviewed by others in this volume. This report will provide an overview of the subject and discussion of several areas of interest not reviewed elsewhere.

HISTOPATHOLOGIC CLASSIFICATIONS AND TERMINOLOGY

It was of great importance for pathologists to have developed reproducible and accepted classifications of the malignant lymphomas. This included the clear separation of Hodgkin's disease from the lymphomas other than Hodgkin's disease, the so-called non-Hodgkin's lymphomas. The concepts and proposal of Lukes and Butler were an improvement over the Jackson and Parker system and were modified and recommended for use at the important Rye conference in 1965. This rather simple accomplishment was one of several very significant contributions of that conference which, along with a similar conference in Paris in 1965, provided much of the bases for the productive clinical research of Hodgkin's disease which followed.

The four Rye subgroups (Table I) not only allowed the separation of patients with Hodgkin's disease into four meaningful prognostic groups, but provided correlations of disease sites and extent, as well as sex and age variables not previously appreciated. In recent years, with the progressive improvement of treatment results for all clinical settings of Hodgkin's disease, the prognostic value of the Rye histopathologic types is being lost. But this fact does not diminish the importance of the Rye classification since the natural history and behavior of the subtypes remains significant and future selection of treatment programs may well be determined by these factors.

Table I

HODGKIN'S DISEASE
HISTOLOGIC CLASSIFICATIONS

JACKSON AND PARKER	LUKES AND BUTLER	RYE
PARAGRANULOMA	LYMPHOCYTIC AND HISTIOCYTIC NODULAR	LYMPHOCYTE PREDOMINANCE
GRANULOMA	NODULAR SCLEROSIS	NODULAR SCLEROSIS
SARCOMA	MIXED CELLULARITY	MIXED CELLULARITY
	DIFFUSE FIBROSIS	
	RETICULAR	LYMPHOCYTE DEPLETION

The Rappaport classification of the non-Hodgkin's lymphomas provided a similar stimulus for the other lymphomas. The clarification of the histologic features of the nodular lymphomas and the separation of these diseases into 8 to 10 different pathologic entities was of very great value.

The previous use of three major subgroups (Table II) was greatly improved upon with the Rappaport system and was responsible for the significant advances in the clinical investigations which followed.

Table II

NON-HODGKIN'S LYMPHOMAS
HISTOLOGIC CLASSIFICATIONS

1930-1965	RAPPAPORT	MODIFIED RAPPAPORT
GIANT FOLLICLE LYMPHOMA	NODULAR OR DIFFUSE	NODULAR
LYMPHOSARCOMA	LYMPHOCYTIC, WELL DIFFERENTIATED	LYMPHOCYTIC, POORLY DIFFERENTIATED
RETICULUM CELL SARCOMA	LYMPHOCYTIC, POORLY DIFFERENTIATED	MIXED, LYMPHOCYTIC AND HISTIOCYTIC
	MIXED, LYMPHOCYTIC AND HISTIOCYTIC	HISTIOCYTIC
	HISTIOCYTIC	DIFFUSE
	UNDIFFERENTIATED	LYMPHOCYTIC, WELL DIFFERENTIATED ± PLASMACYTIC FEATURES
		LYMPHOCYTIC, POORLY DIFFERENTIATED
		MIXED, LYMPHOCYTIC AND HISTIOCYTIC
		HISTIOCYTIC
		LYMPHOBLASTIC ± CONVOLUTED CELL TYPE
		UNDIFFERENTIATED BURKITT'S TYPE

The Rappaport terminology and proposal has gradually been modified since its original description in 1965 and most clinicians and investigators now employ a modification of the Rappaport system which recognizes several limitations of the original proposal and acknowledges several important clinical entities. As emphasized by Lukes and his colleagues, the Rappaport system and terminology was not based upon modern concepts of the immune system and *in vitro* lymphocyte transformation. This has led to various new proposals to change the terminology of the modified Rappaport system and to propose new systems based upon the normal T (thymus) and B (bursal) lymphocyte system. This difficult but important subject is reviewed briefly elsewhere in this volume and extensively in the literature. It will be important for pathologists and clinicians to agree with the appropriate changes in the Rappaport system so that confusion can be minimized and clinical investigations not hindered.

DIAGNOSTIC METHODS

One of the most important clinical advances of the past 20 years was the development and widespread use of bipedal lymphography. This technique enlightened investigators in better appreciating the distribution, pattern, and extent of the lymphomas. It allowed recognition of previously occult involvement in the para-aortic and iliac lymph node regions and recognition of incomplete regression following therapy and early recurrence and extension of the disease to these sites.

This great advance in diagnostic ability stimulated the use of other available methods to detect lymphomatous involvement at the onset of the disease, such as the full utilization of tomography of the chest for patients with Hodgkin's disease and bone marrow biopsy, especially for patients with advanced Hodgkin's disease and for all patients with the non-Hodgkin's lymphomas.

Exploratory laparotomy with splenectomy was developed by the Stanford group as a by-product of a clinical trial of the treatment of Hodgkin's disease with radiotherapy fields confined to the sites of documented involvement. This surgical diagnostic approach identified otherwise occult involvement of the spleen as an important clinical problem and also demonstrated the virtual uniform association of hepatic Hodgkin's disease with splenic involvement. This provided further insight into patterns of Hodgkin's disease and helped establish that the disease was usually unicentric in its origin and spread via orderly and relatively predictable patterns along lymphatic channels. These observations made a very significant impact on the development of radiotherapy programs and, subsquently, combined modality therapy programs which have resulted in the curability of the majority of patients with the diseases.

Exploratory laparotomy and splenectomy were rapidly employed in the diagnostic approach to patients with the non-Hodgkin's lymphomas. In some diseases, enlightenment was also the result in that some of the Rappaport subgroups were often found to have widespread involvement of mesenteric and other abdominal lymph nodes, the spleen, liver and bone marrow. Paradoxically, this widespread involvement was found in patients who had the Rappaport histologic subtypes with the most favorable natural histories and prolonged survival. These were patients with the relatively small cell lymphocytic subtypes, both nodular and diffuse.

In contrast, patients in the poorer prognostic groups with large cell or histiocytic lymphomas, usually of diffuse architectural types, only rarely (10% or less) had occult disease in the abdomen or bone marrow discovered at exploratory laparotomy.

This information, gained initially in the setting of clinical trials of the therapy of malignant lymphomas, had a significant impact on the understanding of the disease and the proper selection of treatment programs.

STAGING OF THE LYMPHOMAS

During the 1960's, an acceptable and useful staging system was developed at the Rye (1965), Paris (1965), and Ann Arbor (1971) Conferences, (Table III)

Table III

LYMPHOMA STAGING SYSTEMS

PETERS, AND OTHERS	RYE, PARIS (1965)	ANN ARBOR (1971)
I	I	I
II	II	II
III	III	III
	IV	IV
A OR B	A OR B	A OR B
		E AND S
		CS AND PS

These international meetings of active investigators in this field provided stimulating and productive interactions by individuals from multiple disciplines with the common goal of improving the understanding and treatment of the malignant lymphomas. By providing a common language, not only for histopathologic subgroups but for a clinical staging system, the stage was set for the productive clinical studies of the next 10-15 years.

PHASE III CLINICAL TRIALS

It is important to appreciate that the advances in the management of the lymphomas would not have taken place if several research centers had not undertaken carefully planned, disciplined clinical trials with well-conceived plans and endpoints. In some instances, these were uniform new treatment programs not previously tested and, in other instances, were randomized clinical trials. These prospective studies helped to challenge the previous pessimism of clinicians responsible for the treatment of patients with the malignant lymphomas, because the results were based upon adequate numbers of well-defined prospective groups, rather than anecdotal and retrospective studies which could not be properly evaluated and accepted.

INTERDISCIPLINARY STUDIES AND CARE

Among the most significant advances responsible for the improved treatment results of patients with the malignant lymphomas has been the development of interdisciplinary research and patient care groups. The constructive interaction and collaboration of pathologists, radiotherapists, medical oncologists, surgeons, and oncology nurses have expanded and complemented the skills of each participant to the benefit of the patient and the study. The demonstration that physicians and colleagues from different disciplines can share, productively, in patient care and clinical trials has been extended to other oncologic problems and undoubtedly will continue in the future.

FUTURE CHALLENGES

The details of the therapeutic advances, as well as the morbidity and complications of therapy are reviewed elsewhere in this volume. Not all types of non-Hodgkin's lymphomas are treated as successfully as those with Hodgkin's disease. However, it can be predicted that these too will gradually be controlled and cured with currently available treatment methods. A current challenge is to develop methods of therapy with less acute and long term toxicity without reducing the very good cure rates which are possible. This will require new methods of discipline in quantitating morbidity - physical, emotional, and socioeconomic. Too little attention has been paid to these problems in the past.

It may be that recent dramatic developments in immunology, with the development of hybridoma monoclonal antibodies or genetic engineering with the production of specific molecules for diagnosis and therapy, will revolutionize the management of patients with these diseases. The most important advances, however, must await the understanding of the precise etiology of these neoplasms and their prevention or reversal.

Until that time, however, there is justifiable reason to be proud and optimistic because Hodgkin's disease and many of the other lymphomas have been transformed from predominantly fatal disorders to predominantly curable diseases. As significant as the achievements of the last decade have been, those of the next decade promise to be even greater.

Changing Concepts and Classification
of the Lymphomas-A Common Language

COSTAN W. BERARD, M.D.

Chairman
Division of Pathology
St. Jude Children's Research Hospital
Memphis, Tennessee

Between September 1976 and June 1980 a large-scale study of
the classification of non-Hodgkin's lymphomas was performed
at four major institutions. Financial support was provided
by the Division of Cancer Treatment of the United States'
National Cancer Institute. Complete clinical records and
histopathologic sections of initial diagnostic biopsies
were collected for 1175 patients at the Milan Tumor Institute, the University of Minnesota, Stanford University, and
Tufts University. Detailed forms of clinical data for analysis by computer were prepared for all cases by clinical
principal investigators at each of the participating institutions. All histologic sections were reviewed and classified independently by a panel of six "expert" pathologists
and a counterpart group of six "control" pathologists.
    Each of the cases was classified according to six systems:
Rappaport System (11-13), Dorfman System (2,3), Kiel System
(4,5), British System (1), World Health Organization System
(9,10), and Lukes System (6-8). The "expert" pathologists,
each of whom was required to classify the cases according
to only his/her own system, were, respectively: Dr. Henry
Rappaport, Duarte, California; Dr. Ronald Dorfman, Stanford,
California; Dr. Karl Lennert, Kiel, West Germany; Dr.
Kristin Henry, London, England; Dr. Gregory O'Conor,
Bethesda, Maryland; and Dr. Robert Lukes, Los Angeles,

California. The "control" pathologists, each of whom was
required to classify the cases according to all six systems,
were: Dr. Costan Berard, Bethesda, Maryland; Dr. Robert
Hartsock, Pittsburgh, Pennsylvania; Dr. Gerhard Krueger,
Cologne, West Germany; Dr. Koji Nanba, Hiroshima, Japan;
Dr. A.H.T. Robb-Smith, Woodstock, England; and Dr. Martin
Sacks, Beer-Sheba, Israel.

To assess reproducibility as well as comparability of the
various systems, twenty per cent of the cases were selected
at random and reviewed and classified a second time by each
of the twelve pathologists. Detailed statistical analyses
of the results have been completed and discussed by all
participating clinicians and pathologists. Although each of
the systems had merit, as applied by either the "expert"
pathologists or the "control" pathologists, none was clearly
superior to the others. The "control" pathologists were
able to use all six systems with comparable facility, and
there were no important differences in reproducibility between the various systems.

Based on this massive international effort, the investigators reached consensus on a new Working Formulation of Non-
Hodgkin's Lymphomas for Clinical Usage - Recommendations of
an Expert International Panel (Table 1). The Formulation,
with detailed clinicopathologic analyses and appropriate
microscopic descriptions and illustrations, will soon be
disseminated. Hopefully it will be found throughout the
world to be clinically relevant, scientifically accurate,
readily usable, and highly reproducible.

TABLE 1
A Working Formulation of Non-Hodgkin's Lymphomas for
Clinical Usage
Recommendations of an Expert International Panel

Low Grade

Malignant lymphoma, small lymphocytic
Malignant lymphoma, follicular, predominantly small cleaved
 cell
Malignant lymphoma, follicular, mixed small cleaved and
 large cell

Intermediate Grade

Malignant lymphoma, follicular, predominantly large cell
Malignant lymphoma, diffuse, small cleaved cell
Malignant lymphoma, diffuse, mixed small and large cell
Malignant lymphoma, diffuse, large cell

High Grade

Malignant lymphoma, large cell, immunoblastic
Malignant lymphoma, lymphoblastic
Malignant lymphoma, small non-cleaved cell

Miscellaneous

Composite malignant lymphoma
Mycosis fungoides
Extramedullary plasmacytoma
Unclassifiable
Other

REFERENCES

1. Bennett, M.H., Farrer-Brown, J., Henry, K., and Jeliffe,
    A.M.: Classification of non-Hodgkin's lymphomas.
    Lancet 2:405-406, 1974.
2. Dorfman, R.F.: Classification of non-Hodgkin's lympho-
    mas. Lancet 1:1295-1296, 1974.
3. Dorfman, R.F.: The non-Hodgkin's lymphomas. In The
    Reticuloendothelial System: IAP Monograph No. 16, J.W.
    Rebuck, C.W. Berard, and M.R. Abell, Eds., Baltimore,
    Williams and Wilkins, 1975, pp. 262-281.
4. Gerard-Marchant, R., Hamlin, I., Lennert, K., et. al.:
    Classification of non-Hodgkin's lymphomas. Lancet 2:
    406-408, 1974.
5. Lennert, K., Mohri, N., Stein, H., and Kaiserling, E.:
    The histopathology of malignant lymphoma. Br. J.
    Haematol. (Suppl.) 31:193-203, 1975.
6. Lukes, R.J. and Collins, R.D.: Immunologic characteri-
    zation of human malignant lymphomas. Cancer 34:1488-
    1503, 1974.
7. Lukes, R.J. and Collins, R.D.: A functional classifica-
    tion of malignant lymphomas. In The Reticuloendothe-
    lial System: IAP Monograph No. 16, J.W. Rebuck, C.W.
    Berard, and M.R. Abell, Eds., Baltimore, Williams and
    Wilkins, 1975, pp. 213-242.
8. Lukes, R.J. and Collins, R.D.: New approaches to the
    classification of the lymphomata. Br. J. Cancer
    (Suppl. II) 31:1-28, 1975.
9. Mathe, G.: Workshop for the classification of non-
    Hodgkin's lymphoma. Biomedicine 22:466-467, 1975.
10. Mathe, G., Rappaport, H., O'Conor, G.T., and Totloni,
    H.: Histological and cytological typing of neoplastic
    diseases of hematopoietic and lymphoid tissues. In WHO
    International Histological Classification of Tumors,
    No. 14, Geneva, World Health Organization, 1976.
11. Nathwani, B.N., Kim, H., and Rappaport, H.: Malignant
    lymphoma, lymphoblastic. Cancer 38:964-983, 1976.
12. Rappaport, H.: Tumors of the hematopoietic system. In
    Atlas of Tumor Pathology, Section III, Fascicle 8,
    Washington, D.C., Armed Forces Institute of Pathology,
    1966, pp. 97-161.

13. Rappaport, H. and Braylan, R.C.: Changing concepts in the classification of malignant neoplasms of the hematopoietic system. In The Reticuloendothelial System: IAP Monograph No. 16, J.W. Rebuck, C.W. Berard, and M.R. Abell, Eds., Baltimore, Williams and Wilkins, 1975, pp. 1-19.

Chemotherapy of Lymphoma

STEPHEN E. JONES, M.D.

Professor of Medicine
Chief, Section of Hematology-Oncology
University of Arizona Cancer Center
Tucson, Arizona

INTRODUCTION

The last decade has seen remarkable progress in the drug treatment of lymphoma. Many forms of Hodgkin's disease (HD) and malignant lymphoma (ML) which were once viewed as incurable if they presented in advanced stages or if they recurred after radiotherapy can now be considered potentially curable with presently available combination chemotherapy programs. A list of these lymphomas is presented in Table 1.

The definition of "cure" for an individual patient implies a durable complete remission (CR) free of signs of lymphoma and for groups of patients implies survival and relapse-free survival curves which demonstrate a clear "plateau". Follow-up in some series and with some programs is necessarily brief due to the newness of the treatment. Nonetheless, for all of the lymphomas without a question mark listed in Table 1 there has been convincing evidence of curability from one source with confirmation by at least one other report. Question

TABLE 1

Lymphomas Which Can Be Cured With Chemotherapy

Hodgkin's disease (all subtypes)
Malignant lymphoma
    Diffuse large cell (DH)
    Diffuse undifferentiated (DU)
    Nodular (follicular) large cell (NH)
    Nodular (follicular) mixed (NM)
    Lymphoblastic (?)
    Diffuse mixed (?)

marks are listed for lymphoblastic lymphoma and diffuse mixed
cell lymphoma due to the lack of confirmatory series at this
time. Thus, the majority of patients with lymphoma will have
types which are amenable to potential cure with appropriate
chemotherapy.

The first step in realizing cure of lymphoma is the initial
achievement of a complete remission (CR). This concept is
well established [11, 13, 14, 27]. Definitions of CR have
changed over the last decade and are now generally based on
careful reevaluation of the patient who has achieved a clinical complete response. Repetition of initially abnormal tests
such as lymphangiography, computed tomographic (CT) scanning,
bone marrow and liver biopsies and even laparotomy have
revealed that about 10% of patients with HD and 20% of those
with ML will still harbor occult disease and, therefore,
require additional treatment [13, 14]. Attainment of a carefully
documented CR followed by no further therapy has provided the
critical information about the curability of many types of
lymphoma[2, 11, 27].

It is not possible in this brief review to include or even
mention all of the chemotherapy programs which have been or
currently are being tested. Instead, I have chosen to limit
my discussion to a relatively few programs which illustrate
some of the progress and remaining challenges of chemotherapy
of lymphoma.

Hodgkin's Disease

One of the most important treatment advances in HD was the
development of the 4-drug combination known as MOPP (nitrogen
mustard, vincristine, procarbazine and prednisone)[10]. DeVita
and associates have recently summarized the first 15 years of
experience with MOPP which is curative in about 70% of patients who achieve a CR[11]. CR rates vary with several prognostic factors but in general 50-80% of patients with recurrent or advanced stages of HD can achieve a CR with the MOPP
regimen.

There have been many efforts to make substitutions in the
basic MOPP schedule either to improve the results or to less-
en the toxicities associated with this intensive regimen.
Recently Lewis and DeVita have reviewed some of these other
regimens [20]. None have appeared to be superior to MOPP,
although the British chlorambucil-based 4-drug regimen and a
CCNU-based 4-drug regimen appear to have less gastrointestinal
toxicity than MOPP [7, 18].

The question remains whether there is now any approach to
drug therapy for HD which is superior to MOPP. Two programs

appear to be likely candidates. In a series of sequential clinical trials in the Southwest Oncology Group (SWOG), we demonstrated that the addition of low-dose bleomycin to MOPP (MOPP-LDB) improved the CR rate and survival over MOPP alone[6]. Based on these results we initiated a clinical trial in 1974 comparing MOPP-LDB to the same combination with adriamycin (the then new active anthracycline) substituted for half of the nitrogen mustard dose (MOP-BAP). This trial is now final and has demonstrated an overall superiority for the MOP-BAP regimen (76% CR rate) compared to a 67% rate for MOPP-LDB (p=0.09)[15]. This effect of the addition of adriamycin to MOPP-LDB was manifested primarily in prognostically more favorable subgroups of patients (those without B symptoms or bone marrow involvement and those with higher initial hemo-globins and higher performance status). This improved CR rate was also translated into survival benefit as well in the same favorable subgroups[15].

The second approach to improve the results of chemotherapy for HD involved the development of an effective 4-drug regi-men which contained agents other than those in MOPP. The most successful of these is the combination of adriamycin, bleomycin, vinblastine and DTIC (ABVD) developed at the Milan National Cancer Institute[25]. When compared to MOPP this regimen is equally active[4]. Moreover, this regimen is prob-ably the most active in MOPP-resistant patients and has been given the designation as a "non-cross resistant" combination.[20] Thus, it was logical to alternate courses of 2 non-cross-resistant regimens (MOPP/ABVD) and compare the results to MOPP. The results of such a trial, although still prelimin-ary, are impressive.[26] MOPP/ABVD produced an 87% CR rate in 32 evaluable patients with Stage IV HD compared to a 67% CR rate in 33 patients treated with MOPP (p=0.05). Relapse-free survival and survival are superior for MOPP/ABVD treated patients but longer follow-up of this important study is needed.

Although initially combination chemotherapy was most often employed to treat far-advanced stages of disease, there has been an increasing trend in recent years to employ effective regimens earlier in the disease. The very favorable results in asymptomatic patients in the original MOPP studies (100% CR rate in 23 patients)[11] and more recently in the SWOG study (MOP-BAP produced a 94% CR rate)[15] lend support to the view that chemotherapy is highly effective in more favorable patients and the results compare favorably to radiotherapy alone. Thus, the National Cancer Institute has initiated a clinical trial comparing MOPP to conventional radiotherapy for even earlier more favorable disease (Stage I and II HD).[9]

It would appear unlikely to me that either treatment would
prove superior to the other and any eventual decision regarding choice of these 2 treatments for early disease will
necessarily be based on their relative morbidities and late
effects (e.g., leukemia).

Another approach to early disease is to combine chemotherapy and radiotherapy, perhaps reducing the intensity or
duration of one or both modalities. Elsewhere in this Symposium Dr. Rosenberg has reviewed the Stanford experience
with combined modality therapy. This approach seems most
worthwhile for patients with limited HD with clinical or
pathologic features associated with a relatively high likelihood of relapse if radiotherapy alone is employed. These
high risk-features include a large mediastinal mass, the
presence of "B" symptoms, and, possibly extralymphatic
disease ("E"). Several studies indicate a marked reduction
in recurrence rates if chemotherapy is combined with radiotherapy for these "high-risk" patients[5, 19].

Nodular (Follicular) Lymphoma

The less common forms of nodular lymphoma (large cell and
mixed cell types) are potentially curable (Table 1) and,
hence, most oncologists feel that combination chemotherapy is
indicated in order to induce a CR and give each patient the
opportunity for cure. However, the choice of chemotherapy
for the most common type of nodular lymphoma (nodular lymphocytic or NLPD) remains highly controversial. The choices for
therapy for NLPD include deferred treatment until progression[24], single alkylating agents (e.g., chlorambucil), simple
combinations (e.g., cyclophosphamide, vincristine, and prednisone [COP]) or more aggressive combinations (e.g., CHOP
which includes adriamycin as well as the other agents in COP).
Representative CR rates for these programs are shown in
Table 2.

TABLE 2

CR Rates by Treatment for Nodular Lymphocytic Lymphoma

Treatment	% CR
Single Alkylating Agents	30-60%
COP	70-80%
CHOP	70-80%

Although CR rates are higher for combination therapy, to date it has not been possible to demonstrate improved survival or curability of these tumors with combination chemotherapy compared to single-agent treatment[22, 24]. Moreover, no other combination has yet proven to have any advantage compared to COP alone[16, 17].

Nodular lymphocytic lymphoma remains a challenge for selection of therapy. Moreover, despite the achievement of a CR, patients exhibit a pattern of continuous relapse once treatment is discontinued[2]. Since there is some evidence suggesting that even in patients with the favorable NLPD histology, attainment of a CR is associated with superior survival compared to partial response, my recommendation for therapy is COP rather than single-agent treatment.

Although it has been difficult to show any alteration in the natural history of nodular lymphoma dependent on treatment, there is now evidence suggesting that some biologic response modifiers may favorably affect these tumors. For instance, in a large controlled trial carried out by the Southwest Oncology Group, chemotherapy plus immunotherapy with BCG resulted in a significant prolongation of survival compared to 2 types of chemotherapy alone[17]. Preliminary evidence also suggests that interferon may be active in these lymphomas[21]. Further investigation into biologic response modifiers and their use, particularly in the more favorable nodular lymphomas, will be awaited with interest.

Diffuse Lymphomas

The majority of these lymphomas are poor prognostic types which may be cured with combination chemotherapy (Table 1). The most common of these, diffuse large cell lymphoma (DH), can be cured in 40-50% of patients with advanced stages of disease[8]. In general, the adriamycin-based regimens (e.g., CHOP) have CR rates superior to those of non-adriamycin based regimens[16]. For example, as part of a randomized clinical trial we compared COP+bleomycin to CHOP+bleomycin. Although the CR rates were only slightly higher for CHOP (49% vs 41%), complete remission duration and survival were clearly superior[16].

Recently several new approaches to the drug treatment of DH lymphoma have appeared. For purposes of comparison we have analyzed our experience at the University of Arizona with the CHOP regimen in 72 previously untreated patients (13 with Stage II disease and the remainder with Stage III or IV disease) and used this as a basis for comparing 3 other regimens: COMLA (cyclophosphamide, vincristine,

TABLE 3

Comparison of Selected Regimens Used
for Diffuse Large Cell (DH) Lymphoma

Regimen (Institution)	No. Treated	%CR	Reference No.
CHOP (Arizona)	72	72%	--
COMLA (Chicago)	48	60%	29
ProMACE-MOPP (NCI)	40	57%	12
M-BACOD (Boston)	51	77%	28

methotrexate with leucovorin rescue, cytosine arabinoside)
[29], ProMACE-MOPP (VP-16, cyclophosphamide, adriamycin, methotrexate with leucovorin rescue and prednisone plus MOPP consolidation)[12], and M-BACOD (high dose methotrexate with
rescue plus CHOP)[28]. The representative CR rates are shown
in Table 3. In terms of CR rates, the only regimen which
appears superior to CHOP is M-BACOD[28]. The difficulties and
expense in using high-dose methotrexate, however, will limit
the general use of this program. The proMACE-MOPP program
is also difficult and highly toxic (12% of the patients
reported died from toxicity)[12]. Long term follow-up of these
programs will be needed to assess their relative importance
compared to CHOP in the management of patients with DHL.

As in HD there is now greater interest in applying regimens which have proven to be curative for advanced forms of
diffuse lymphoma to patients with more limited disease.
Several trials have reported reduced recurrence rates and
improved survival with the use of adjuvant chemotherapy after
local radiotherapy. However, in the majority of these programs the regimens employed (e.g., COP) were less than
optimal. There are now 2 reports of the use of primary
chemotherapy employing adriamycin-based regimens (e.g., CHOP)
as initial therapy for Stages I and II DHL and this data has
been summarized recently[23]. In our experience 94% of
patients with Stage I or II DH achieved a CR compared to 56%
of patients with Stage III or IV disease. Thus, immediate
primary chemotherapy with effective regimens (e.g., CHOP) for
early disease offers great promise.

FUTURE PROSPECTS

Despite the advances in the chemotherapy of lymphoma, new
approaches for both HD and ML are required. Several investigational agents appear promising for use in new combinations:
m-AMSA, vindesine (another vinca alkaloid), new anthracyclines (e.g., dihydroxyanthracenedione), gallium nitrate,

platinum compounds, and methyl-GAG. The exploration of biologic response modifiers (e.g., BCG, interferon) is also in
its infancy and should have an impact on treatment of
lymphoma.

Another area for potential study is to develop methods of
modifying or limiting myelosuppression. Evidence exists suggesting a dose-response relationship in the treatment of lymphoma and conceivably better results could be achieved with
high-dose regimens. However, myelosuppression is the usual
dose-limiting factor. Lithium, which stimulates granulopoiesis, has been reported to reduce treatment-induced myelosuppression in leukemia and oat cell lung cancer . Lithium
needs to be evaluated in lymphoma. Isolation of patients
(e.g., protected environments) and administration of prophylactic antibiotics has reduced the infectious complications
of escalated dose treatment of lymphoma in one study and
needs to be evaluated further, particularly since survival of
patients treated at high dose levels appeared to be superior
to that achieved at lower doses[3]. Myelosuppression may also
be limited by autologous marrow infusion and this approach
will need to be investigated too.

SUMMARY

The past decade has seen marked progress in the chemotherapy of human lymphoma. Hodgkin's disease and many types
of other malignant lymphomas are now potentially curable with
drugs. Results in advanced stages have led to applications
in earlier stages with encouraging preliminary results. In
the next decade, development of new agents and new combinations, use of biologic response modifiers, and development of
methods to limit myelosuppression (e.g., Lithium, isolation
units, autologous bone marrow "rescue") should result in
equally remarkable progress in the treatment of lymphoma.

REFERENCES

1. Anderson, T: Lithium carbonate stimulation of granulo-
    poiesis in hematologic and oncologic disease. Ariz. Med.
    36:762-763, 1979.
2. Anderson, T., Bender, R.A., Fisher, R.I., et al: Com-
    bination chemotherapy in non-Hodgkin's lymphoma: Results
    of long-term followup. Cancer Treat. Rep. 61:1057-1066,
    1977.
3. Bodey, G.P., Rodriguez, V., Cabanillas, F., et al: Pro-
    tected environment-prophylactic antibiotic program for
    malignant lymphoma. Am. J. Med. 66:74-81, 1979.
4. Bonadonna, G., Zucali, R., Monfardini, S., et al: Com-
    bination chemotherapy of Hodgkin's disease with adriamy-
    cin, bleomycin, vinblastine, and imidazole carboxamide
    versus MOPP. Cancer 36:252-259, 1975.
5. Coltman, C.A., Fuller, L.A., Fisher, R., et al: Extended
    field radiotherapy versus involved field radiotherapy
    plus MOPP in Stage I and II Hodgkin's disease. In:
    Adjuvant Therapy of Cancer II (Jones, S.E., and Salmon,
    S.E., eds.), Grune & Stratton, New York, 1979, pp 129-136.
6. Coltman, C.A., Jones, S.E., Grozea, P.M., et al: Bleo-
    mycin in combination with MOPP for the management of
    Hodgkin's disease: Southwest Oncology Group experience.
    In Bleomycin: Current Status and New Developments (Car-
    ter, S.K., Crooke, S.T., and Umezawa, H., eds.), Aca-
    demic Press, New York, 1978, pp. 227-242.
7. Cooper, M.R., Pajak, T.S., Nissen, N.I., et al: A new
    effective four drug combination of CCNU, vinblastine,
    prednisone, and procarbazine for the treatment of
    advanced Hodgkin's disease. Cancer 46:654-662, 1980.
8. DeVita, V.T., Canellos, G.P., Chabner, B.A., et al:
    Advanced diffuse histiocytic lymphoma, a potentially
    curable disease. Lancet 1:248-250, 1975.
9. DeVita, V.T., Glatstein, E.J., Young, R.C., et al:
    Changing concepts: The lymphomas. In: Adjuvant
    Therapy of Cancer II (Jones, S.E., and Salmon, S.E.,
    eds.), Grune & Stratton, New York, 1979, pp. 173-190.
10. DeVita, V.T., Serpick, A.A., Carbone, P.P.: Combina-
    tion chemotherapy in the treatment of advanced Hodgkin's
    disease. Ann. Intern. Med. 73:881-895. 1970.
11. DeVita, V.T., Simon, R.M., Hubbard, S.M., et al: Cura-
    bility of advanced Hodgkin's disease with chemotherapy.
    Ann. Int. Med. 92:587-595, 1980.
12. Fisher, R.I., DeVita, V.T., Hubbard, S.M., et al: Pro-
    MACE-MOPP combination chemotherapy: treatment of dif-
    fuse lymphomas. Abstract. Proc. Am. Soc. Clin. Onc.
    21:468, 1980.

13. Herman, T.S., Jones, S.E.:Systematic restaging in the management of non-Hodgkin's lymphomas. Cancer Treat. Rep. 61:1009-1015, 1977.

14. Herman, T.S., Jones, S.E.: Systematic restaging in patients with Hodgkin's disease. A Southwest Oncology Group Study. Cancer 42:1976-1982, 1978.

15. Jones, S.E., Fisher, R.J., Jones, J., et al: Improved remission induction chemotherapy for patients with advanced Hodgkin's disease. Abstract Proc. Am. Soc. Clin. Onc. 21:464, 1980.

16. Jones, S.E., Grozea, P.N., Metz, E.N., et al: Superiority of adriamycin-containing combination chemotherapy in the treatment of diffuse lymphoma: A Southwest Oncology Group Study. Cancer 43:417-425, 1979.

17. Jones, S.E., Salmon, S.E., and Fisher, R: Adjuvant immunotherapy with BCG in non-Hodgkin's lymphoma: A Southwest Oncology Group controlled clinical trial. In: Adjuvant Therapy of Cancer II (Jones, S.E., and Salmon, S.E., eds.), Grune & Stratton, New York, 1979, pp. 163-172.

18. Kaye, S.B., Juttner, C.A., Smith, I.E., et al: Three Years' Experience with ChlVPP (A combination of drugs of low toxicity) for the treatment of Hodgkin's disease. Brit. J. Cancer 39:168-174, 1979.

19. Levi, J.A., Wiernik, P.H.: Limited extranodal Hodgkin's disease. Unfavorable prognosis and therapeutic implications. Am. J. Med. 63:365-372, 1977.

20. Lewis, B.J., DeVita, V.T.: Combination therapy of the lymphomas. Sem. in Hemat. 15:431-457, 1978.

21. Merrigan, T.C., Sikora, K., Breeden, J.H., et al: Preliminary observations on the effect of human leukocyte interferon in non-Hodgkin's lymphoma. N.E.J.M. 299:1449-1453, 1978.

22. Lister, T.A., Cullen, M.H., Beard, M.E.J., et al: Comparison of combined and single-agent chemotherapy in non-Hodgkin's lymphoma of favorable histologic type. B. Med. J. 1:553-557, 1978.

23. Miller, T.P., Jones, S.E.: Is there a role for radiotherapy in localized diffuse lymphomas? Cancer Chemotherapy Pharmacol. 4:67-70, 1980.

24. Portlock, C.S., Rosenberg, S.A.: Chemotherapy of the non-Hodgkin's lymphomas: the Stanford experience. Cancer Treat. Rep. 61:1049-1056, 1977.

25. Santoro, A., Bonadonna, G: Prolonged disease-free survival in MOPP-resistant Hodgkin's disease after treatment iwth adriamycin, bleomycin, vinblastine and dacarbazine (ABVD). Cancer Chemoth. Pharmacol. 2:101-105, 1979.

26.   Santoro, A., Bonadonna, G., Bonfante, V., et al: Non-
      cross resistant regimens (MOPP and ABVD) vs MOPP alone
      in Stage IV Hodgkin's disease. Abstract Proc. Am. Soc.
      Clin. Onc. 21:470, 1980.
27.   Schein, P.S., DeVita, V.T., Hubbard, S., et al: Bleo-
      mycin, adriamycin, cyclophosphamide, vincristine, and
      prednisone (BACOP) combination chemotherapy in the
      treatment of advanced diffuse histiocytic lymphoma.
      Ann. Intern. Med. 85:417-422, 1976.
28.   Skarin, A., Canellos, G., Rosenthal, D., et al: Therapy
      of diffuse histiocytic (DH) and undifferentiated (DU)
      lymphoma with high dose methotrexate and citrovorum
      factor rescue (MTX/CF), bleomycin (B), adriamycin (A),
      cyclophosphamide (C), oncovin (O), and decadron (D)
      (M-BACOD). Abstract Proc. Am. Soc. Clin. Onc. 21:463,
      1980.
29.   Stein, R.S., Collins, R.D., and Ultmann, J.E.: Diffuse
      histiocytic lymphoma (DHL): B-cell origin by Lukes-
      Collins criteria predicts favorable response to COMLA
      chemotherapy. Abstract Proc. Am. Soc. Clin. Onc. 21:
      469, 1980.

Radiotherapy of the Lymphomas

HENRY S. KAPLAN, M.D.

D'Ambrogio Professor of Radiology
Department of Radiology
Stanford University Medical Center
Stanford, California 94305

INTRODUCTION

The invention of several types of high energy apparatus
about twenty-five years ago ushered in the megavoltage era of
radiotherapy, [35] and opened the way to the development of
highly effective techniques for the treatment of Hodgkin's
disease and other lymphomas. The linear accelerator, which
produces megavoltage photons and electrons, [5] is superior to
other forms of megavoltage apparatus for the treatment of
patients with lymphomas because of its precision, versatility,
and performance characteristics. Megavoltage beams produce
their maximal ionization at a significant depth below the skin
surface, thus yielding a "skin-sparing effect" which excludes
cutaneous tolerance from consideration as a dose-limiting
factor. Linear accelerator photon beams have sharply defined
edges with relatively little lateral scatter, enabling treatment to be given in close proximity to vital structures, and
with significantly better hematological tolerance. Their high
penetration facilitates the delivery of tumoricidal doses to
neoplasms deep within the body, even in obese patients.
Finally, the very high output of linear accelerator photon

443

beams permits them to be used at long treatment distances,
thus enabling very large fields to encompass multiple chains
of lymph nodes in contiguity.

It had long been known that when lymph nodes involved by
Hodgkin's disease or other lymphomas were treated with sharply localized fields, the next site of involvement was frequently in adjacent lymph node chains. As megavoltage therapy
techniques evolved, treatment fields were gradually enlarged
to cover adjacent chains of lymph nodes in an attempt to
eradicate presumptive microscopic disease. [15] More precise
delineation of treatment fields required systematic studies
of the natural history and patterns of spread of different
types of lymphomas. Meticulous mapping of the sites of involvement, aided by the introduction of new diagnostic techniques such as lymphangiography and staging laparotomy with
splenectomy, revealed that the pattern of spread in Hodgkin's
disease is generally quite predictable, and tends to follow
lymphatic channels from a given involved node to other lymph
nodes in the same or other chains with which direct lymphatic
connections exist. [17,31] The patterns of spread in the non-
Hodgkin's lymphomas are less consistently predictable, and
spread to extra-lymphatic and distant sites is a much more
frequent manifestation; nonetheless, contiguous spread to
adjacent lymph node chains via lymphatic channels is observed
with high frequency in these lymphomas as well. [3] Unfolding
knowledge concerning the natural history of the lymphomas has
had an important influence on the development of radiotherapeutic field distributions and techniques. [18]

Concurrently, clinical investigations with megavoltage
photon beams began to explore progressively higher dose levels.
Analysis of the resultant body of data indicated that the
tumoricidal dose level for lymph nodes involved by Hodgkin's
disease was approximately 3,500-4000 rads delivered at a rate
of 1,000-1100/week. [16] Essentially the same dose level was

also consistently capable of eradicating disease in nodes involved by the nodular (follicular) and diffuse lymphocytic
lymphomas, whereas the diffuse large cell lymphomas ("histiocytic" lymphomas in the Rappaport classification) were somewhat more radioresistant and often required doses of 5,000
rads or more for eradication. [4] Modern megavoltage radiotherapy techniques permit the delivery of tumoricidal doses to
all lymph node chains above and below the diaphragm ("total
lymphoid" irradiation), thus permitting radiotherapy with
curative intent to be given even for disease of stage III
extent. [20]

It should be emphasized that the techniques involved are
among the most demanding in all radiotherapy, requiring meticulous dosimetry, careful delineation of treatment fields in
relation to the anatomical distribution of the relevant lymphatic tissues, precise beam alignment and field simulation
and frequent film verification of beam positioning. [23]
Dosimetry, beam alignment, and field shaping techniques are
beyond the scope of this presentation and are fully detailed
elsewhere. [19, 25, 26]

Radiation Techniques

Involved field treatment, as the name implies, is directed only at those lymph node chains or other lymphatic structures known to be clinically or pathologically involved by the
lymphoma. In extended field radiotherapy, adjacent lymph node
chains neighboring the involved regions are also treated.
Total lymphoid irradiation includes all of the major lymph
node chains and lymphatic structures both above and below
the diaphragm.

The mantle field is a complex, carefully shaped anterior
and posterior opposed field. [25] It encompasses the cervical
and supraclavicular, axillary, infraclavicular, mediastinal,
and hilar lymph nodes while shielding the lungs, the heart,
and the spinal cord with thick blocks of lead or low melting

point alloy. When the mediastinal nodes are uninvolved, as in most nodular lymphomas, this field may be reduced to a "mini-mantle" by shielding the mediastinal and hilar area. In the presence of large mediastinal masses or hilar lymph node involvement, pulmonary parenchymal micrometastases are likely to be present even when not clinically demonstrable. It is possible in these instances to treat one or both lungs through thin lead shields,[28] permitting the transmission of approximately 37% of the radiation dose, with the result that the lungs receive approximately 1650 rads in the same four week interval required to deliver a total of approximately 4,400 rads to the mediastinum. When pericardial effusions are present, the entire cardiac volume may be treated to a total dose of between 2,500 and 3,000 rads. The heart is then shielded with a lead block, the upper border of which is placed to permit continued irradiation of the subcarinal lymph nodes. The introduction of this subcarinal block technique has effectively eliminated the complication of radiation pericarditis.[19]

When very large mediastinal masses are present, continuous treatment to full dose during the usual 4 week interval would deliver high doses to large volumes of one or both lungs which could result in unacceptable degrees of pulmonary radiation reaction and fibrosis. Under these circumstances, modified fractionation techniques are valuable. Initial doses of 1,000 to 1,500 rads are delivered in 100-150 rad daily fractions, followed by a rest interval of several days to permit shrinkage of the mediastinal mass. A new mantle field is then delineated using wider lung blocks. The process may have to be repeated a third time to maximize protection to the lung. This "split course," shrinking field technique can achieve complete eradication of extremely large mediastinal masses with excellent preservation of pulmonary function.[19]

When the initial mediastinal mass is so large as to preclude
lymphangiography or staging laparotomy, these procedures can
be fitted in during the rest intervals between segments of the
split course mantle treatment, after adequate regression of
the mediastinal mass has occurred. When treatment must be
prolonged in this fashion, it is desirable to increase the
total dose to a total of 5,000 rads or more to compensate for
the longer elapsed treatment time.

Mantle field treatment may be accompanied by transient
nausea, dysphagia, esophagitis, and tracheitis, all of which
are usually mild and typically regress soon after the completion of treatment. Apical and paramediastinal pulmonary fibrosis usually develop within a few months after treatment but
are seldom associated with significant symptoms. Temporary
alopecia is typically seen in the occipital region of the
scalp. Skin reactions may occur along skin surfaces tangential to the X-ray beam, particularly in the supraclavicular
region and axillary folds. Late complications may include
hypothyroidism, L'hermitte's sign, rare thyroid cancers,
radiation pneumonitis and pulmonary fibrosis, and radiation
pericarditis. [19] The frequency of the latter complications
has been markedly reduced by refinements in treatment technique.

The Waldeyer field is intended to irradiate the preauricular lymph nodes in patients with Hodgkin's disease and the
lymphatic structures of the Waldeyer ring in patients with
non-Hodgkin's lymphomas. It is used almost routinely in the
latter group of patients, since the frequency with which they
develop involvement of the Waldeyer ring lymphatic tissues is
exceedingly high. In Hodgkin's disease, the use of this field
is limited to those patients with lymph node involvement in
the upper cervical region, who are known to be at risk of
spread of disease to the ipsilateral preauricular lymph node.

The lower margin of the Waldeyer field must be carefully
matched to the upper margin of the mantle field at approximately the lower edge of the mandible. When upper cervical
lymph nodes are massively involved, it is desirable to enlarge
the Waldeyer field to encompass these nodes through opposing
lateral fields. As the lymph nodes shrink, it is generally
possible to diminish the size of the Waldeyer field to its
usual dimensions while moving the upper edge of the mantle
field upward to continue the irradiation of the involved upper
cervical nodes. The superior margin of the Waldeyer field
usually traverses the sphenoid sinus, thus encompassing the
nasopharyngeal soft tissues. The anterior edge of the field
is generally placed just behind the last molar tooth, but may
have to be moved forward when relatively bulky masses are
present at the base of the tongue. The posterior edge of the
field is drawn through the midplane of the upper cervical
vertebrae, and thus encompasses the soft tissues of the posterior pharyngeal wall. The primary morbidity attributable to
Waldeyer field irradiation stems from injury to the salivary
glands and is manifested as xerostomia; it may be minimized
by limiting the radiation dose to approximately 3500 rads in
4 weeks.

The inverted Y field is carefully matched to the lower
margin of the mantle field near the level of the diaphragm.
It is designed to treat all of the subdiaphragmatic retroperitoneal structures in contiguity, from the diaphragmatic
level down to the femoral fossa. [26] Delineation of the inverted Y field is greatly aided by the placement of surgical
clips in the region of the splenic pedicle and at the sites of
excisional biopsy of lymph nodes in the paraaortic and celiac
chains at the time of staging laparotomy. Visualization of
the kidneys by intravenous urography is important to exclude
aberrant renal locations, absence of one kidney, or functional

abnormalities. Lymphangiographic opacification of the retroperitoneal lymph nodes is essential to assess the required
width of the field in the paraaortic and pelvic regions.

When splenectomy has not been performed, the upper end
of the inverted Y field must be extended laterally into the
left upper quadrant and shaped to cover the spleen, while
shielding as much of the left kidney as possible. Treatment
of the spleen diminishes hematologic tolerance, often making
it necessary to divide the inverted Y into two separate fields,
an upper paraaortic-splenic field and a lower pelvic field,
treated sequentially in 4-5 week intervals. When the spleen
is involved, micrometastases are frequently present in the
liver, even when liver biopsies at the time of staging laparotomy are negative. Under these circumstances, prophylactic
irradiation of the liver is indicated, and may be safely carried to doses of approximately 2,200 rads in 4 weeks, concurrently with paraaortic field treatment to 4400 rads, by use
of a 50% transmission lead block over the right lobe of the
liver.[34] This technique is well tolerated, except for transient increases in serum alkaline phosphatase levels which may
persist for a few months following treatment.

In young female patients, oophoropexy [30] and fixation of
the ovaries with metallic sutures permits wide, double thickness ovarian lead shields to be used which may preserve
menstrual function and even fertility [22] in patients requiring
high dose irradiation of the external iliac, inguinal, and
femoral lymph nodes. When the ovaries are properly positioned
as close to the midline as possible, this technique makes it
possible to limit ovarian dose to approximately 8-9 percent
of that delivered to the pelvic lymph nodes. In the male,
special lead devices have been designed to improve testicular
shielding. [19]

Involvement of the mesenteric lymph nodes is frequent in

the non-Hodgkin's lymphomas, especially those of nodular
histopathology,, and relatively uncommon in Hodgkin's disease.
When mesenteric lymphadenopathy is present or suspected, it is
necessary to modify the inverted Y technique to encompass the
mesenteric nodes. This cannot be safely accomplished simply
by widening the inverted Y field, since the kidneys would then
be exposed to unacceptable dose levels. A modified whole abdominal technique was devised at Stanford which involves a
combination of anterior-posterior opposed fields and lateral
opposed fields, [8] permitting the delivery of doses of 4400
rads to the mesenteric and paraaortic lymph node chains and
the splenic pedicle or spleen, and the prophylactic irradiation of the liver to doses of 1500 to 2200 rads, while limiting radiation dose to the kidneys to levels well within tolerance limits. This technique has proven highly effective and
extremely well tolerated in our experience.

Involvement of the epitrochlear and/or brachial lymph
nodes is not uncommon in the non-Hodgkin's lymphomas, particularly those of nodular type, and may also be observed in
patients with Hodgkin's disease in association with massive
ipsilateral axillary lymphadenopathy. Long narrow fields may
be delineated along the medial aspect of the upper arm to
treat the epitrochlear and brachial lymph node areas. It is
important to avoid overlap of the axillary field at the upper
end of the field. When actual involvement is present, the
dose levels employed are the same as those used for involved
lymph nodes elsewhere. When prophylactic treatment is given,
doses may be limited to 3000/3500 rads in about 4 weeks.

Several groups of investigators have now reported results
which compare favorably with those of chemotherapy in patients
with Stage III or IV non-Hodgkin's lymphomas of lymphocytic
type using whole body photon irradiation. [1,14] Patients may
be treated while seated on a chair, facing in opposite

directions for half of each treatment, or lying on their sides
on a gurney, with directions again reversed midway through
treatment. Treatment distances must be sufficiently great to
permit the entire body to be encompassed homogeneously within
the field. Compensators are used to correct for inhomogeneities
of dose distribution. Doses of 10 rads three times per week
or 15 rads twice per week are typically given and treatment is
usually carried to a total dose of approximately 150 rads in 5
weeks. When patients have had significant prior chemotherapy,
hematologic tolerance is often poor, and blood counts must be
closely monitored during whole body irradiation. Morbidity is
otherwise surprisingly mild in most patients. Although single
courses appear to be quite safe, patients treated with multiple courses of whole body photon irradiation have been reported
to develop acute leukemias. [24] We have found it desirable to
deliver local "boost" doses of radiotherapy to involved lymph
node regions, giving approximately 2000-3000 rads at a rate of
750 to 1000 rads per week following completion of the whole
body course.

Whole body electron beam irradiation has been an effective
treatment for mycosis fungoides and other cutaneous T cell
lymphomas. [10] Since 1972, we have used 4.0 MeV electrons
generated by a 10 MV linear accelerator. Peak ionization occurs in the first 4 mm. below the skin surface; depth dose
decreases rapidly thereafter, reaching 50% at a depth of 11.4
mm. A six field technique is used with patients standing on a
platform 10 feet from the linear accelerator window. The beam
is angled upward 15 degrees and downward 15 degrees from the
horizontal for half of each treatment (dual exposure technique.) [27] The anterior, posterior, and reciprocal four oblique
fields each receive equal dose fractions. Initially, total
doses of 800-1,000 rads were given; when it was ascertained
that the doses were well tolerated, but were often followed by

recurrence, dose levels were gradually increased. Currently,
patients receive a skin dose of 200 rads in each two day treatment cycle, during which all six fields are treated; total
doses of 3,000-3,600 rads are given at the rate of two cycles
per week. Areas such as the perineum and soles of the feet
which are not directly exposed to the electron beam are given
supplementary orthovoltage x-ray (120-250 Kvp) treatment to
doses of 2000 rads at 100 rads/day. The cornea and lens, and
in some cases the eyebrows and fingernails, are shielded with
lead. Acute morbidity is limited to transient erythema,
generalized cutaneous edema, and epilation. Minimal skin
atrophy or hyperpigmentation may be observed as late sequelae.

Treatment Results

Radiation therapy alone is the treatment of choice for
patients with Hodgkin's disease of stages I-A & I-B, II-A &
II-B, and most of those with pathological stage III-A or III_S-A.
In a consecutive series of patients treated at Stanford University Medical Center following staging with the aid of
lymphography and laparotomy with splenectomy, actuarial 10
year survival in stages I and II, with our without symptoms,
ranged between 83 and 86%; 65-74% of these patients were relapse-free at 10 years. [9,19] Adjuvant chemotherapy in pathologic stages III-A and III_S-A reduced initial relapse rates,
but failed to improve overall long-term survival. [13,19,32]
In view of its failure to improve survival, its almost ines-
capable effects on fertility in males, [36] and the demonstrated
hazard of late secondary leukemia or non-Hodgkin's lymphoma in
patients receiving both radiation therapy and combination
chemotherapy, adjuvant chemotherapy is not recommended in
these stages, except for patients with stage III-A or III_S-A
disease and extensive spleen involvement or multiple sites of
lymph node involvement. [13] In patients with disease of stage

III-B extent (and many of those with Stage IV), combined modality treatment with both radiotherapy and combination chemotherapy has yielded appreciably better survival than either
modality alone; an alternating sequence of the two modalities
is associated with improved hematologic tolerance and the
ability to deliver a greater fraction of planned drug and
radiation doses. [12] In a series of 28 consecutive patients
with PS III-B and III_S-B Hodgkin's disease treated with this
alternating technique at Stanford since 1974, actuarial survival at 5 years is an unprecedented 88.9% and relapse-free
survival is 72.8%. [13]

Radiation therapy has also demonstrated its curative
potential in the non-Hodgkin's lymphomas. In a randomized
clinical trial comparing involved field vs. total lymphoid
irradiation in a small series of patients with PS I or II
lymphomas of favorable histologic types, there was only one
death, due to intercurrent disease, during the last 5 years,
and only one patient, treated with the involved field technique, had relapsed. [6] In a larger series of patients with
PS I or II lymphomas of unfavorable histopathologic types,
total lymphoid irradiation yielded a 5 year survival rate of
70% and a relapse-free rate of 66.7%; neither result was improved by supplemental combination chemotherapy. [6] Total
lymphoid (including whole upper abdominal) irradiation alone
was used in a series of 68 patients with CS or PS III lymphomas treated at Stanford between 1961 and 1973. Only 17 of
these had diffuse histologic patterns; their 5 year survival
was 39%. The 51 patients with nodular patterns had 5 and 10
year survival rates of 75% and 65%, respectively, with corresponding relapse-free rates of 43% and 33%. [7] In patients with
stage IV "favorable" lymphomas randomized to single agent (SA)
chemotherapy or to multidrug chemotherapy (CVP) with or without subsequent total lymphoid irradiation, neither of the more

aggressive treatment regimens was found to be superior to continuous SA treatment. [29] A more recent randomized study of patients with stage III or IV "favorable" lymphomas, still in
progress, involves a comparison of SA, CVP, and whole body
irradiation (WBI) with involved field "boost" doses. Actuarial survival at 4 years is 84% for the entire group, but only
25% are relapse-free; once again, no significant advantage of
either CVP or WBI over SA treatment has emerged to date. [11]

Whole body electron beam irradiation is highly effective
in mycosis fungoides. Complete remissions were achieved in
51 (94%) of 54 patients who received total doses of 3,000 -
3,600 rads, vs. only 3 (18%) of 17 patients receiving doses of
800 - 1,000 rads. Of the 51 patients in the high dose group
who entered complete remission, 20 (39%) remained alive and
relapse-free 3 to 14 years after a single course of electron
beam therapy. [10]

Prognostic data cited in this paper are derived in part
from clinical trials conducted with the support of National
Cancer Institute grant CA-05838. These studies have involved
the collaborative assistance of many colleagues in the Divisions of Radiation Therapy, Medical Oncology, Diagnostic
Radiology, Surgical Pathology, General Surgery, and Nuclear
Medicine, to all of whom grateful acknowledgement is extended.

References

1. Carabell SC, Chaffey JT, Rosenthal DS, et al: Results of total body irradiation in the treatment of advanced non-Hodgkin's Lymphomas. Cancer 43: 994-1000, 1979.

2. Coleman CN, Williams CJ, Flint A, et al: Hematologic neoplasia in patients treated for Hodgkin's Disease. New Engl J Med 297, #23: 1249-1252, 1977.

3. Fuks Z, Glatstein E, and Kaplan HS: Patterns of presentation and relapse in the non-Hodgkin's lymphomata. Br. J Cancer 31 (Suppl. II): 286-297, 1975.

4. Fuks Z and Kaplan HS: Recurrence rates following radiation therapy of nodulat and diffuse malignant lymphomas. Radiology 108: 675-684, 1973.

5. Ginzton EL, Mallory KB, and Kaplan HS: The Stanford Medical linear accelerator - I. Design and development. Stanford Med. Bull. 15: 123-140, 1957.

6. Glatstein E, Donaldson SS, Rosenberg S, et al: Combined modality therapy in malignant lymphomas. Cancer Treat. Rep. 61: 1199-1207, 1977.

7. Glatstein E, Fuks Z, Goffinet DR, et al: Non-Hodgkin's lymphomas of stage III extent. Is total lymphoid irradiation appropriate treatment? Cancer 37: 2806-2812, 1976.

8. Goffinet DR, Glatstein E, Fuks Z, et al: Abdominal irradiation in non-Hodgkin's lymphomas. Cancer 37: 2707-2806, 1976.

9. Hoppe RT: Radiation therapy in the treatment of Hodgkin's disease. Sem. in oncology 7: 144-154, 1980.

10. Hoppe RT, Fuks Z, and Bagshaw, MA: The rationale for curative radiotherapy in mycosis fungoides. Int J Radiation Oncology Biol. Physics 2:843-851, 1977.

11. Hoppe RT, Kushlan P, Kaplan HS, et al: The treatment of advanced stage favorable histology non-Hodgkin's lymphoma: a preliminary report of a randomized trial comparing single agent chemotherapy, combination chemotherapy, and whole body irradiation. (Submitted for publication.)

12. Hoppe RT, Portlock CS, Glatstein E, et al: Alternating chemotherapy and irradiation in the treatment of advanced Hodgkin's disease. Cancer 43: 472-481, 1979.

13. Hoppe RT, Rosenberg SA, Kaplan HS, et al: Prognostic factors in pathological stage III-A Hodgkin's disease. Cancer 46: 1240-1246, 1980.

14. Johnson RE: Total body irradiation (TBI) as primary therapy for advanced lymphosarcoma. Cancer 35: 242-246, 1975.

15. Kaplan HS: The radical radiotherapy of regionally localized Hodgkin's disease. Radiology 78: 553-561, 1962.

16. Kaplan HS: Evidence for a tumoricidal dose level in the radiotherapy of Hodgkin's disease. Cancer Res 26: 1221-1224, 1966.

17. Kaplan HS: On the natural history, treatment and prognosis of Hodgkin's disease. Harvey lectures 1968-69. Academic Press, 1970.

18. Kaplan HS: Hodgkin's disease: unfolding concepts concerning its nature, management, and prognosis. Cancer 45: 2439-2474, 1980.

19. Kaplan HS: Hodgkin's Disease. (Ed. 2.) Cambridge: Harvard University Press, 1980.

20. Kaplan HS and Rosenberg, SA: Extended-field radical radiotherapy in advanced Hodgkin's disease: Short term results of 2 randomized clinical trials. Cancer Res 26(1): 1268-1276, 1966.

21. Krikorian JG, Burke JS, Rosenberg SA, et al: Occurrence of non-Hodgkin's lymphoma after therapy for Hodgkin's disease. New Engl J Med 300: 452-458, 1979.

22. Le Floch O, Donaldson SS, and Kaplan HS: Pregnancy following oophoropexy and total nodal irradiation in women with Hodgkin's disease. Cancer 38: 2263-2268, 1976.

23. Marks JE, Haus AG, Sutton HG, et al: Localization error in the radiotherapy of Hodgkin's disease and malignant lymphoma with extended mantle fields. Cancer 34: 83-90, 1974.

24. O'Donnell J, Brereton H, Greco F, et al: Acute myelocytic leukemia (AML) and acute myeloproliferative syndrome (AMPS) after therapeutic irradiation for non-Hodgkin's lymphoma. Proc Am Assoc Cancer Res 19: 60, 1978. (Abstract.)

25. Page V, Gardner A, Karzmark CJ, et al: Physical and dosimetric aspects of the radiotherapy of malignant lymphomas. I. The mantle technique. Radiol 96: 609-618, 1970.

26. Page V, Gardner A, Karzmark CJ: Physical and dosimetric aspects of the radiotherapy of malignant lymphomas. II. The inverted-Y technique. Radiol 96: 619-626. 1970.

27. Page V, Gardner A, Karzmark CJ: Patient dosimetry in electron treatment of large superficial lesions. Radiol 94: 635-641, 1970.

28. Palos B, Kaplan HS, and Karzmark, CJ. The use of thin lung shields to deliver limited whole-lung irradiation during mantle-field treatment of Hodgkin's disease. Radiol 101: 441-442, 1971.

29. Portlock CS, Rosenberg SA, Glatstein E, et al: Treatment of advanced non-Hodgkin's lymphomas with favorable histologies: preliminary results of a prospective trial. Blood 47: 747-756, 1976.

30. Ray GR, Trueblood HW, Enright LP, et al: Oophoropexy: a means of preserving ovarian function following pelvic megavoltage radiotherapy for Hodgkin's disease. Radiol 96: 175-180, 1970.

31. Rosenberg SA, and Kaplan HS: Evidence for an orderly progression in the spread of Hodgkin's disease. Cancer Res 26: 1225-1231, 1966.

32. Rosenberg SA, Kaplan HS, and Brown BW, Jr.: The role of adjuvant MOPP in the therapy of Hodgkin's disease: An analysis after ten years. Adjuvant therapy of cancer II, S.E. Jones and S.E. Salmon, eds., New York: Grune and Stratton, 1979, pp. 109-117.

33. Salzman JR, and Kaplan HS: Effect of splenectomy on hematological tolerance during total lymphoid radiotherapy of patients with Hodgkin's disease. Cancer 27: 471-478, 1971.

34. Schultz HP, Glatstein E, and Kaplan HS: Management of presumptive or proven Hodgkin's disease of the liver: a new radiotherapy technique. Int J Rad Oncol Biol Phys 1: 1-8 1975.

35. Schultz MD: The supervoltage story: Janeway lecture, 1974. Am J Roentgenol 124: 541-559, 1975.

36. Sherins RJ and De Vita VT: Effect of drug treatment for lymphoma on male reproductive capacity. Studies of men in remission after therapy. Ann Int Med 79: 216-220, 1973.

Late Effects of Lymphoma Treatment
The Consequences of Success

ARVIN S. GLICKSMAN, M.D.

Department of Radiation Oncology
Rhode Island Hospital
Section on Radiation Medicine
Brown University
Providence, RI

THOMAS PAJAK, Ph.D.

Cancer and Leukemia Group B
Scarsdale, NY

   With increasing frequency patients with Hodgkin's Disease
(HD) and other lymphomas are being successfully treated so
that the consequences of success are appearing in increasing
numbers. Fifteen years ago the standard textbook of medicine
characterized HD as a uniformly fatal illness with only a
rare survivor under unusual circumstances.(1) Now we can expect better than half of all patients with HD(2) to be cured
of this illness and 35-40% of Non-Hodgkin's Lymphoma (NHL)
patients to survive(3) intensive radiotherapy and chemotherapy. In growing numbers these survivors manifest some resultant morbidity associated with the achievement of cure. Just
about every organ system has some late sequela of either the
radiation, chemotherapy or both. In some instances the sequelae are extremely rare and in others it may account for as
many as 25 percent of the patients treated who survive. In
some instances the late effect may be minor and easily treatable; in other instances they may be extremely grave and life
threatening in themselves.

RESPIRATORY SYSTEM
Standard mantle therapy of 3500-4000 rads using a 4 MEV
Linear Accelerator will deliver approximately 500 rads to the
whole lung derived almost entirely from scatter and a small
amount of transmitted radiation through the blocks. Depen-

459

ding upon the size of the mediastinal disease and the generousness with which the hilar adenopathy is encompassed, symptomatic radiation effects on the lung can be expected to occur in no more than 5% of the patients.(4) However, if careful respiratory function studies are performed as many as 50% of the patients will show transient changes in total lung capacity, compliance and gas diffusion.(4a,5,6,7) These changes can be detected as early as 8 weeks after the completion of radiotherapy and usually disappear within 2 years. (8,9) When patients with pulmonary nodes have been treated with whole lung radiation with doses up to 2500 rads in 4 weeks (no inhomogeneity corrections having been applied), the risk of radiation induced lung disease increases with the dose. The use of a transmission block so that the dose is delivered at a rate of less than 100 rads a day will diminish the frequency with which radiation pneumonitis will be seen. (10)

The most important chemotherapeutic agent implicated in developing pulmonary changes is Bleomycin which appears to be dose dependent. Severe life threatening pneumonitis is associated with doses over 200 units per meter square.(11) In patients who are to receive both radiation and Bleomycin containing drug combination, the possibility exists that there will be increased pulmonary damage.

Other chemotherapeutic agents such as Cytoxan, BCNU and Actinomycin D can enhance radiation toxicity on the lung and recall prior exposure. MOPP therapy has been reported, on occasion, to induce pulmonary toxicity itself, but also, when associated with radiation. This may be due to the abrupt cessation of the steroid component of this combination rather than the Vincristine or Procarbazine toxicity on the lung directly.

CARDIOVASCULAR EFFECTS

Between 6 months and a year after mantle therapy with doses of 3500-4000 rads of irradiation, 10 to 15% of the patients may develop a pericardial rub. This is a dose related reaction. When the radiation is diminished to below 3000 rads the incidence falls considerably.(12,13) Acute pericarditis can develop during the course of radiation or as late as 4 or 5 years later. The disease is usually self limited but steroids can be helpful providing it is not precipitously discontinued. For patients who develop pericardial effusion and constrictive pericarditis a pleural-pericardial window or pericardial stripping may be life saving.(14,15,16)

In some cases, the process continues on to chronic pericardial disease(17) which may be appreciably more frequent than appreciated. Nine of 12 patients have been recently reported who had negative cardiac history and normal physical examinations. Echocardiographic abnormalities were detected in 10 of 12 patients who had been treated 10 to 16 years previously.(18)

Cases of premature myocardial infarction in patients who received radiation therapy to the chest have been reported. (19,20,21) While diffuse interstitial myocardial fibrosis has been seen in patients who have received doses in excess of 3500 rads to the heart, vascular changes are rare.(22) Intimal proliferation is a response to irradiation; these cells may be more sensitive to even modest changes in cholesterol levels and therefore are more apt to induce atheromatous changes.(23,24) Radiation can induce vascular changes in large vessels as well as in small arteries.(25) So called "pulseless" disease, the aortic arch syndrome,(26) as well as carotid artery disease(27) have been reported after radiation for HD and NHL.

Chemotherapeutic agents also produce cardiomyopathies. In a unique case report MOPP therapy induced a myocardial infarction like syndrome on 3 separate occasions in the same patient.(28) This must be an extremely rare event. Much more frequent and important is the myocardial injury associated with the Anthracyclines.(29) The particular injury produced by Adriamycin is clearly dose related and may be schedule related. As far as is currently known it is not reversible. Adriamycin and radiation injuries to the heart are additive rather than synergistic. Where it is anticipated that patients will receive both dose accommodations of each are necessary to prevent fatal cardiomyopathy.

HEPATOPATHOLOGIES

Ingold(30) and associates described the histopathology of radiation hepatitis which occurs when the entire liver received doses over 3000 rads. Little will be noted clinically although the liver scan and some enzymes may be abnormal,(31) or it may be severe, fulminating and fatal. For the most part this is transient although it can last as long as 2 years. In instances where lymphoma has involved the liver and radiation has been used, doses below 2500 rads are tolerable as in the experience of the Cancer and Leukemia Group B (CALGB) and the Memorial Sloan Kettering experience. The experience from Stanford indicated that doses over 3000 rads or 2000 rads plus radioactive gold can produce late hepatic fibrosis.

In another experience of the CALGB concurrent Vincristine with doses of radiation below 2000 rads was associated with severe and life threatening toxicity in 16 of 35 patients at risk.((32) Cassidy and co-workers(33) have also reported

this in children. A fatal radiation hepatitis has been reported in a patient following ABVD therapy and 2400 rads to
the liver. Another case of hepatitis associated with
Adriamycin has been reported at doses of radiation under
2500 rads of radiation.(34)

GENITOURINARY PROBLEMS

The serious nature of the late complications of irradiation of the kidneys at moderate doses is so well known to
radiotherapists that radiation nephritis is now an extremely
rare event.(35)   Kaplan reports that there was not one case
in 12,000 patients treated for HD at Stanford.(36)   In patients who have not had a splenectomy, the majority of the
left kidney may receive the full brunt of the irradiated dose
as was probably the case in the patient reported by Danforth
in 1975 (37) who was found 7 years subsequent to radiotherapy
to have total destruction of the left kidney. In patients
with abdominal presentation of NHL the dose to the kidney is
generally restricted to less than 1750 rads when abdominal
bath irradiation is given. Even in combination with the usu-
ual chemotherapeutic agents used for this disease, rarely is
radiation nephritis reported.(38)

Hemorrhagic cystitis from long-term Cytoxan therapy has
been frequently reported.(39,40,41) In one report examining
the records of over 19,000 cancer patients, Fairchild, et al
(42) found a nine-fold increase in bladder cancer in patients
who received Cyclophosphamide. Hemorrhagic cystitis has been
reported following a year of MOPP therapy, but this must be
very rare.(43)

Since many of the patients successfully treated for HD are
young and in the child-bearing period, attention must be giv-
en to attempts to preserve reproductive integrity. When
radiotherapy is used, the problem is somewhat different for
males and females and is age and dose dependent.(44)   In
males fractioned doses of radiation appear to be more de-
structive than single doses for sperm production.(45)   Peri-
aortic irradiation will result in 20-40 rads on the testis
from scatter. When pelvic radiation is added, the dose will
increase to as much as 300-400 rads unless special protective
devices are used. In most studies,(46,47)fractionated doses
of under 100 rads will produce temporary aspermia in 100% of
the patients, but recovery is expected approximately one year
later. With doses of 100-200 rads, temporary aspermia will
persist for two years. After doses of between 200-300 rads,
3 years may be required for recovery and over 5 years for
doses in excess of this, if it will occur at all. Serum FSH
levels will be elevated until the damaged seminiferous epithelium has been repaired and returns to normal function.

In females, fractioned doses of radiation can produce
temporary or permanent sterility, depending upon the dose
and age of the patient. A dose under 250 rads over a 4 week
period appears to have no permanent deleterious effects in
young women but can produce permanent sterilization in women
over the age of 40, while a dose of 250-500 rads is likely
to permanently steralize only about half of women under 40.
The remainder will have transient amenorrhea. Doses of 1000
to 3000 rads are likely to produce permanent sterility in
all women.

Preservation of ovarian function can be achieved by surgical procedures which place the ovaries in sites that are
likely to receive only scatter irradiation.(48) The midline
oophoropexy has been most widely used for this purpose, although the movement of the ovaries laterally to the iliac
fossa has been used in some institutions. With midline
oophoropexy and shielding during irradiation, approximately
two thirds of the women maintain normal ovarian function and
subsequent pregnancies are possible. To date, the offspring
appear to be normal as well.(49)

It is now clearly appreciated that chemotherapeutic effects on the gonads can be expected to be long term and, in
many instances, produce complete destruction of reproductive
potential.(50,51) In the male, Chlorambucil and Cyclophos-
phamide(52,53,54) have resulted in sterility and testicular
atrophy. Azospermia may persist for approximately 2 years
after intensive chemotherapy but return to normal function
could be anticipated.(55) Serum levels of testosterone and
LH were generally normal, but FSH elevation was observed
during the period of azospermia.(56) In prepubital boys
treated with Cyclophosphamide, no abnormalities of LH, FSH
or testosterone were found. MOPP therapy in prepubital boys
tested showed no change in serum gonadotropins, but pubes-
cent boys had moderate to severe gynecomastia, germinal a-
plasia, elevation in FSH and LH, and reduced testosterone
levels 2 years after combined chemotherapy.(57,58)

In young females, primary ovarian failure has been reported after single drug or combined chemotherapy. Elevated
FSH and LH were found in amenorrheic females previously
treated for HD, but this can be transitory and successful
pregnancies can occur.

Tetragenic effects of the low dose radiation have not
been clearly identified. However, when chemotherapy and
radiation have been used, Holmes and Holmes believe there is
a significant increase in fetal abnormalities in which either the father or the mother received chemotherapy and radiation treatment.(59,60) In men who wish to procreate, it

is advisable to advise the use of a sperm bank prior to the
onset of any treatment. This will preclude both the problem of azospermia or oligospermia and the tetragenic effects
of the treatments applied.

ENDOCRINE

Another serious, well-documented dysfunction of the endocrine system associated with the treatment of lymphoma is
the appearance of clinically significant thyroid dysfunction.
(61) Between 15-20% of the young patients treated for HD
have developed hypothyroidism.(62) However, at least 50% of
the patients who had radiation and lymphangiography have elevated TSH and another 20% may have an altered response to
Thyrotropin releasing hormone (TRH).(63) This is of major
concern because of the carcinogenic potential of prolonged
TSH elevation.(64) These patients require careful observation and exogenous thyroid replacement, even though they appear euthyroid, clinically. Incidental cases of thyroid
cancer have started to appear.(65) We have seen 1 case of
hyperthyroidism in a young girl who, two years later, developed thyroid carcinoma.(66) Thyroid dysfunction may be a co-
causal factor in the development of radiation pericarditis.

Pituitary function is temporarily altered during combined
chemotherapy which includes steroids. However patients do
not develop hypoadrenalism with abrupt withdrawal of steroids on MOPP therapy. Cushingoid appearance, and osteo-
porosis can occur. MOPP therapy has been found to depress
TSH and TSH response to TRH.(67) This does not decrease the
elevated TSH in patients who were treated by both radiotherapy and chemotherapy. However, no case of thyroid cancer in
a patient treated with both radiation and MOPP has yet been
reported.(68)

CNS PROBLEMS

Neurological sequelae of radiation, both acute and late
can occur. In the acute phase, the Lhermitte's syndrome can
occur with mantle therapy. This is characterized by an
electric shock on bending the head which can be extremely
frightening to the patient. It is transitory and does not
proceed to any serious, permanent sequelae.(69) Lhermitte's
syndrome has been reported to occur as frequently as 10-15%.

On the other hand, the late complications of radiation in
the CNS are much more devastating, irreversible, and un-
treatable. These late complications, particularly transverse
myelitis, have been reported with a frequency as high as 3%
and as low as .5%.(70,71) Occasionally, a single extremity
paresis has been reported. Careful attention to the physical
and technical application of adjacent fields can reduce the
possibility of an overdose of the spinal cord.(72) The 3 and

2 technique developed by Nisce and D'Angio at Memorial further diminishes the prospect of either a cold spot gap or an overlap hot spot in the area of the spinal cord.(73) Other technical considerations include treating each field every day and the use of a posterior cervical block in the mantle technique.(74)

Intrathecal Methotrexate, which is most frequently used in the management of acute lymphocytic leukemia, but is also a part of the treatment of some childhood lymphomas, has been reported to produce paraplegia.(75) This has been associated with abnormal cerebrospinal fluid dynamics and may also have been part of the problem of the diluent since preservative-free Methotrexate in close to 1000 children treated in CALGB Protocols has not resulted in a single case to date.(76)

Vincristine neurotoxicity has been well documented.(77) For the most part, it is transient, but long-term weakness has been noted in some cases. Decreased reflexes, paresthesias, motor weakness and constipation will occur with doses of 1 mg. per meter square and the severity of the neurotoxicity is dose related.

SKELETAL PROBLEMS

Soon after the discovery of X-ray, the impairment which it can produce in growing bone was appreciated.(78) Among the effects seen in young children receiving axial node irradiation and pelvic irradiation are diminished sitting height, in practically all growing children and scoliosis and kyphosis occasionally.(79,80) In the doses of radiation used in the management of lymphomas, osteonecrosis is not a problem. Dental problems, however, secondary to radiation effects on the mandible and maxilla will occur with malformation of the erupting permanent teeth. When the salivary glands are in the field, xerostomia, secondary to impaired saliva formation and changes in the consistency of saliva can contribute to severe dental decay if appropriate prophylactic and persistent oral hygiene measures are not instituted early after the radiotherapy.(81)

Late adverse effects on bone of combination chemotherapy have been reported. Avascular necrosis of the femoral head has been seen approximately 1 and 2 years after both MOPP and COPP.(82,83) It has been postulated that the steroid may be the responsible agent. Only 10 or so cases have been reported, but a larger number of unrecorded instances probably exists.(84,85)

HEMATOLOGIC PROBLEMS

As much as 75% of an adult marrow may be included in total nodal irradiation techniques; less in the child, because

of marrow activity in long bones. When orthovoltage techniques were used, Sykes and her colleagues showed that it
was unlikely that regeneration of marrow would occur in
doses above 3000 rads.(86,87) Experimental systems have indicated that mouse marrow will regenerate after 3000 rads in
9 to 12 months(88) and that some regeneration will be seen
using Fe 59 uptake studies, even after 4-5000 rads.(89)
However, this is not to be considered to indicate that the
marrow will function in a manner as if it had not been previously irradiated.(90,91,92) It is appreciably more difficult
to deliver MOPP therapy after total nodal irradiation. Most
patients will not tolerate full-dose chemotherapy and significant prolonged leukopenia and thrombocytopenia may occur.
Alternatively, using a combination of drugs, including
Nitrosurea it was found in the CALGB that there was unacceptable toxicity from the sequence of chemotherapy and
radiotherapy, although the alternate sequence was toxic but
manageable if the interval between chemotherapy and radiation therapy was long enough.(93) On the other hand, there
is extensive experience that salvage therapy with chemotherapy after radiotherapy can be accomplished in a large number
of cases.(94)

IMMUNOLOGIC PROBLEMS

In patients with lymphoma, immunosuppression has been
found even in patients with very localized disease and
of course the very treatment of this disease is immunosuppressive in itself.(95,96,97) The impairment of the immune
system in patients with lymphoma is manifested by diminution
of T-cells in HD and elevated B-cell population patients with
lymphoma.(98) The further suppression of T-cell activity
after radiotherapy can be quite prolonged.(99)

Part of the modern management of HD includes careful staging with splenectomy. Post splenectomy septicemia and meningitis can occur in as high as 10% of the children.(100,101)
Although, in the Stanford study, there was no difference in
the probability of bacterial infection with or without splenectomy, overwhelming infection occurred only in those who had
had a splenectomy and with a 1% mortality.(102,103) The
most frequent bacterial infections are sensitive to Penicillin, and prophylactic Penicillin has been advised. The use
of polyvalent pneumoccal vaccine has been widespread, although its efficacy in preventing serious illness is yet to
be established.(104,105)

By far, the most frequent viral disease is herpes zoster
varicella infection which in one series, occurred in 17% of
the HD patients and 9% of the non-Hodgkin's patients who had
their spleen in place and was significantly higher in splen-

ectomized patients.(106) Foregoing splenectomy but sub-
jecting the organ to therapeutic doses of radiation can induce splenic atrophy and the same risk of overwhelming sepsis.(107) Whether passive immunization with transfer factor
will be protective in this setting, as it has now been reported in childhood leukemia, will need to be carefully investigated.(108)

SECOND MALIGNANT NEOPLASMS

Over the years it has been well recognized that patients
with 1 primary neoplasm have a high susceptibility to a second neoplasm.(109) In studies of patients with HD and
lymphoma treated before the era of intensive chemotherapy
and/or radiation, there was a 2 to 3 fold increase in second malignant neoplasms almost entirely skin cancer.(110)
Recently Brody and Shottenfeld compared the period of 1950
to 1954, 1960 to 1964, and 1968 to 1972 at Memorial Sloan
Kettering Cancer Center (MSKCC).(111) They found a marked
increase in second malignant neoplasms in the more recent
studies, particularly in leukemia. Arseneau at the NCI was
the first to implicate the intensive radiotherapy and intensive chemotherapy used to cure patients as a significant hazard in leukemiagenesis.(112) Subsequent studies have substantiated these observations.(113,114,115) Acute non-lymphocytic leukemia occurs within the first 5 years after treatment.(116,117,118,119) Furthermore of some concern is a second undifferentiated lymphomatous neoplasm occurring after a
5 year interval which has been reported by the Stanford
group and others.(120)

An analysis of the recent experience of the CALGB in studies of advanced HD performed between 1966 & 1974 has been
done to gain insight into the risk attributable to each component of curative treatment. Protocol 6604 studied Stage
III patients with total nodal radiation, involved field radiation and/or chemotherapy. The chemotherapy consisted of
4 weeks of Vinblastine followed by 1 course of Nitrogen Mustard. Protocol 6712, 6951 and 7251 were for patients with
Stage III-B and IV HD. All but 2 induction programs contained an alkalating agent, a vincia alkaloid and Procarbazine. Approximately 25 to 30% of the patients in each of
these studies received MOPP as their induction program. The
1969 study employed maintenance therapy with Vinblastine or
Chlorambucil. The 1972 study utilized as maintenance therapy either Vinblastine alone or Vinblastine with the induction regimen repeated every 8 weeks. Fifteen hundred and
fifty-four patients were entered. One hundred and thirty
were disqualified, 97 were excluded for previous protocol
entry reasons leaving a total of 1324 evaluable cases. Eight

hundred and one patients achieved a complete remission as defined as a normalization of all initially documented disease
parameters. Systematic restaging was not required.

Only those patients whose complete remission terminated in
a second malignancy were considered. To date, there have
been 12 acute myeloid leukemias in the 801 complete responders, for a life table estimate (LTE) of 4.7%. Nine of these
leukemias occurred while the patients were in continuous,
complete remission. The median time from the entrance into
the study to the diagnosis of acute myelogenous leukemia
(AML), was 53 months with a range of 10 to 80 months. The 3
remaining patients developed AML after relapse of the HD.
The relative risk ratio (RRR) for these 9 patients was 151
which is highly significant. Life table estimates (LTE) were
4.2%. At the same time 8 other second malignancies have been
recorded while the patients were in complete remission: 2
chronic leukemias; 2 skin cancers; 1 myeloma; 1 vulva; 1 colon cancer and 1 lung cancer. The RRR was 1.3 which was not
significantly greater than expected. The LTE was 3.3%. Since
the relative risk analysis (RRA) may underestimate the expected second malignancy if the data are diluted by patients
with short follow-up time, an analysis by various minimum
number of years on study was done. This also failed to reveal any bias introduced by potential latency in the data.

There were 3 components to the treatment which these patients received: radiotherapy, induction chemotherapy and
maintenance chemotherapy. Each of these has been examined as
a hazard factor in the development of AML. Of the 801 patients in complete remission, 370 never received radiotherapy. Five of these patients developed AML for a RRR of 151
and a LTE of 5.8%. One hundred and eighty-one patients received involved field radiation, 3 of whom have developed
AML for a RRR of 250, a LTE of 5.7%. Sixty-seven patients
were treated by an extended field, one of whom has developed
AML for a RRR of 234 and a 4.5% LTE. Of the 133 patients who
received total nodal radiation none developed AML. In the 48
patients for whom it was impossible to determine exactly how
much radiation had been delivered, no AML was found. Using
the Mantel-Haenzel technique, we compared no radiotherapy to
involved field or to involved field plus extended field or to
no radiotherapy vs. any radiotherapy. The P value for all of
these was not significant.

Induction chemotherapy with MOPP or MVPP in 293 patients
resulted in 7 cases of AML for a RRR of 323 and a LTE of 10.
6%. When BCNU-OPP, CCNU-OPP; or CCNU-OPP were used on 261
patients, 1 developed AML for a RRR of 53 and a LTE of 0.5%.
When less than 4 drugs were used in 230 patients, 1 case of

AML has been seen for a RRR of 54 and a LTE of 1.5%. The
comparison of other regimens against MOPP and MVPP was highly significant with a P value of .006. This experience relates to 784 patients because of the original 801 patients,
16 received only TNI and one patient's age was unknown and
could not be used for risk analysis.

Maintenance chemotherapy with Chlorambucil appears to be a
major contributor to the development of AML. This analysis
refers to 713 patients. Eighty-eight either refused further
chemotherapy, relapsed or died prior to onset of maintenance.
There were no cases of AML in the 199 patients who received
no maintenance. One case was seen in 217 patients who received Vinblastine maintenance for a RRR of 60 and a LTE of
1.2%. Vinblastine plus reinforcement with induction chemotherapy in 139 patients was associated with 1 case of AML
for a RRR of 112 and a LTE of 1.1%. Chlorambucil plus or minus Vincristine, Prednisone in 158 patients yielded 7 cases
of AML for a RRR of 438 and a LTE of 9.1%. No maintenance
vs. Chlorambucil maintenance was significant at the P value
of .015 and non-Chlorambucil maintenance vs. Chlorambucil
maintenance had a P value of .0078.

Finally, because Chlorambucil maintenance and the inclusion
of Mechlorethamine were highly significant when considered
individually, an analysis was done matching the type of induction regimen with the type of maintenance. No case of
AML was seen in 339 patients who did not receive mustard as
part of the induction program or Chlorambucil maintenance.
On the other hand, there were 5 cases of AML in the 54 patients who received both mustard induction and Chlorambucil
maintenance for a RRR of 960 and a LTE of 21.2%. If either
of these two had been omitted, the LTE is between 2-3%. A
linear trend test was used to evaluate the association between the number of unfavorable factors present (none vs. 1,
vs. 2) and the occurrence of AML. The trend analysis of
these data had a P value of .006.

The role of radiotherapy was further examined in the Chlorambucil maintained patients adjusting for the type of induction. MOPP induction and prior radiotherapy had an extraordinarily high RRR of 1780. When no MOPP and no radiotherapy had been given to patients who were on Chlorambucil maintenance, 1 out of 59 developed AML for a RRR of 142 and a
LTE of 3.1%. The trend analysis for this comparison had a P
value of .068 which suggests that radiotherapy may add to the
risk of leukemiagenesis.

In summary, for the 801 patients in complete remission, 9
of whom developed AML, a comparison of the no radiotherapy
vs. any radiotherapy had a P value of 49, not significant.

No maintenance vs. Chlorambucil maintenance had a P value of
.015, clearly significant, and Chlorambucil maintenance vs.
non-Chlorambucil maintenance had a P value of .0078, highly
significant. Prolonged Chlorambucil maintenance appears to
be chiefly responsible for inducing a high number of cases
of AML during complete remission. Five of the 9 cases of
AML developed while in complete remission had received no
prior radiotherapy. Thus, prolonged chemotherapy in itself
is associated with the development of AML. In Chlorambucil
maintained patients, inclusion of Nitrogen Mustard in the induction regimen is associated with an appreciably increased
RRR of developing AML during CR.

Clearly, the development of a second malignant neoplasm
represents one of the most disturbing of all the late consequences of successful treatment of lymphoma. The reported
increase in skin cancer which is very successfully treated,
is not very worrisome. However there is cause for concern
for the increasing incidence of leukemia and NHL which are
extremely difficult to treat and carry a very high, and
early mortality rate. In the most recent studies, under 5%
of patients successfully treated for their lymphoma appear to
develop this problem.(121) If in an attempt to prevent the
development of a second malignant neoplasm, less intensive
treatment is delivered resulting in a 5 to 10% diminution in
survival, we have accomplished nothing.(122)

The use of alternative treatment programs must be carefully evaluated. Whether one can use less radiation either to
a diminished volume or a diminished dose alone or in combination with chemotherapy needs to be carefully assessed before changes in policy are introduced. The use of maintenance chemotherapy in HD has been shown to add nothing to
survival and has been abandoned. Alternatives to MOPP induction chemotherapeutic combinations may diminish the prospect of a second malignant neoplasm. At this time the nitrosurea combinations used in over 300 patients in the CALGB
were associated with less leukemiagenesis without the risk of
diminished efficacy in HD. Early data from Milan points in
the same direction.(123) However, it is far too soon to assume that this is the case from the 55 cases at risk in Val-
agusa's recent publication, with only 20 patients at risk 3
or more years. There is no doubt ABVD is an extremely effective induction combination and warrants careful consideration.

It is only as a consequence of the success of so many investigators over the last 20 years that we can have so many
patients surviving intensive treatment, only a small number
of whom have some troublesome problems. Many of these have

been solved by careful attention to the details of treatment, to alternate treatment programs or diminution of treatment dose or combinations. We need to be aware of the implications of treatment programs as manifested by late effects, but we can not sacrifice patients to lesser treatments just to avoid untoward consequences. Only with carefully designed, prospective, randomized, clinical trials, can we undertake to explore the questions, "is less better" or "are there better treatment combinations" and that is the challenge of the next decade.

REFERENCES

1. Moore,CV: Hodgkin's Disease. Textbook of Medicine, 11th Ed., ed.: Cecil,R. and Loeb,R., Saunders,Phila.:1963.
2. Kaplan,HS: Hodgkin's Disease. Harvard Press, 2nd Ed., Cambridge, MA, 1980.
3. Portlock,CS, Rosenberg,SA: Chemotherapy of the Non-Hodgkin's Lymphomas: The Stanford Experience. Cancer Treatment Reports,61:1040-1055,1977.
4. Wara,WM, Phillips,TL, Margolis,LW, Smith,V: Radiation Pneumonitis: A New Approach to the Derivation of Time-Dose Factors. Cancer,32:547-542,1973.
4a. C.P.C.: Case 3]-1970, Case Records of the MA General Hospital. NEJM,283:191-201,1970.
5. Lokich,JJ, Bass,H, Eberly,F, Rosenthal,D, Moloney,WC: The Pulmonary Effect of Mantle Irradiation in Patients with Hodgkin's Disease. Radiology,108:398-402,1973.
6. Evans,RF, Sagerman,RH, Ringrose,TL, Auchincloss,JH,Bowman, J: Pulmonary Function Following Mantle-Field Irradiation for Hodgkin's Disease. Radiology,111:729-731,1974.
7. Host,H, Vale,JR: Lung Function After Mantle-Field Irradiation in Hodgkin's Disease. Cancer,32:329-332,1973.
8. Libshitz,HI, Brosof,AB, Southard,ME: Radiographic Appearance of the Chest Following Extended Field Radiation Therapy for Hodgkin's Disease. Cancer,32:207-215,1973.
9. Lassvik,C, Rosengren,B, Wranne,B: Pulmonary Gas Exchange Following Irradiation of Cervical, Mediastinal, Hilar,and Axillary Nodes. Acta Radiologica:Therapy Physics Biology, 16:27-31,1977.
10. Kaplan,HS: Hodgkin's Disease. Harvard Press, 2nd Ed., Cambridge, MA, 1980, p.422.
11. Holland,JF, Frei,E: Cancer Medicine,Lea & Febiger,Phila., 1973, p.823.
12. Stewart,R, Cohn,KE, Fajardo,LF, Hancock,EW, Kaplan,HS: Radiation-Induced Heart Disease. Radiology,89:302-310,1967.
13. Cohn,KE, Stewart,JR, Fajardo,LF, Hancock,EW: Heart Disease Following Radiation. Medicine,46:281-297,1967.

14. Masland,DS, Rotz,CT, Harris,TH: Postradiation Pericarditis with Chronic Pericardial Effusion. Ann.Int.Med.,69:97-102, 1968.
15. Pierce,RH, Hafermann,MD, Kagan,AR: Changes in the Transverse Cardiac Diameter Following Mediastinal Irradiation for Hodgkin's Disease. Radiology,93:619-624,1969.
16. Ali,MK, Khalil,KG, et al: Radiation-Related Myocardial Injury: Management of Two Cases. Cancer,38:1941-1946,1976.
17. Markiewicz,W, Glatstein,E, et al: Echocardiographic Detection of Pericardial Effusion and Pericardial Thickening in Malignant Lymphoma. Radiology,123:161-164,1977.
18. Perrault,DJ, Gilbert,BW, Levy,MD, Herman,J, Adelman,AG: Long Term Effects of Upper Mantle Radiation on the Heart in Patients with Lymphoma. ASCO Abs.c-297,Proceedings,21: 349,1980.
19. Prentice,RTW: Myocardial Infarction Following Radiation. Lancet,ii:388,1965.
20. Dollinger,MR, Lavine,DM, Foye,LV: Myocardial Infarction Due to Postirradiation Fibrosis of the Coronary Arteries. JAMA,195:316-319,1966.
21. Rodgers,DL: Precocious Myocardial Infarction After Radiation Treatment for Hodgkin's Disease. Chest,70:675-677, 1976.
22. Fajardo,LF, Stewart,JR, Cohn,KE: Morphology of Radiation-Induced Heart Disease. Arch Path,86:512-519,1968.
23. McReynolds,RA, Gold,GL, Roberts,WC: Coronary Heart Disease After Mediastinal Irradiation for Hodgkin's Disease. Amer. J.Med.,60:39-45,1976.
24. Steinfeld,A, Most,A: Personal Communication.
25. Nylander,G, Pettersson,F, Swedenborg,J: Localized Arterial Occlusions in Patients Treated with Pelvic-Field Radiation for Cancer. Cancer,41:2158-2161,1978.
26. Heidenberg,WJ, Lupovitch,A, Tarr,N: "Pulseless Disease" Complicating Hodgkin's Disease. JAMA,195:488-491,1966.
27. Silverberg,GD, Britt,RH, Goffinet,DR: Radiation-Induced Carotid Artery Disease. Cancer,41:130-137,1978.
28. Weinstein,P, Greenwald,E, Grossman,J: Unusual Cardiac Reaction to Chemotherapy Following Mediastinal Irradiation in a Patient with Hodgkin's Disease. Amer.J.Med.,60:152-156,1976.
29. Bonnadonna,G, Manfardini,S: Cardiac Toxicity of Daunomycin. Lancet,1:837,1969.
30. Ingold,JA, Reed,GB, Kaplan,HS, Bagshaen,MA: Radiation Hepatitis. Amer.J.Roent.,93:200-208,1965.
31. Tefft,M, Mitus,A, Das,L, Vawter,GF, Filler,RM: Irradiation of the Liver in Children: Review of Experience in the Acute and Chronic Phases, and in the Intact Normal, and Parially Resected. Amer.J.Roent.,108:365-385,1970.

32. Glicksman,AS, Grunwald,HW: Vincristine Enhanced Hepatic Radiation Toxicity. ASCO Abs.c-114, Proceedings,20:318, 1979.

33. Malcolm,AW, Jaffe,N, Folkman,J, Cassady,JR: Bilateral Wilms' Tumor. Int.J.Rad.Onc.Biol.Phys.,6:167-174,1980.

34. Kun,LE, Camitta,BM: Hepatopathology Following Irradiation and Adriamycin. Cancer,42:81-84,1978.

35. C.P.C.: NEJM,278:1343-1349,1972.

36. Kaplan,HS: Hodgkin's Disease. Harvard Press, 2nd Ed., Cambridge, MA, 1980,p.434.

37. Danforth,DN, Javadpour,N: Total Unilateral Renal Destruction Caused by Irradiation for Hodgkin's Disease. Urology, 5:790-793,1975.

38. Churchill,DN, Hong,K, Gault,MH: Radiation Nephritis Following Combined Abdominal Radiation and Chemotherapy (Bleomycin-Vincristine). Cancer,41:2162-2164,1978.

39. Worth,PHL: Cyclophosphamide and the Bladder. Brit.Med.J., 3:182,1971.

40. Dale,GA, Smith,RB: Transitional Cell Carcinoma of the Bladder Associated with Cyclophosphamide. Urology,112:603-604,1974.

41. Wall, RL, Clausen,KP: Carcinoma of the Urinary Bladder in Patients Receiving Cyclophosphamide. NEJM,293:271-273,1975.

42. Fairchild,WV, Spence,CR, Solomon,HD, Gangai,M: The Incidence of Bladder Cancer After Cyclophosphamide Therapy. J.Urology,122:163-164,1979.

43. Royal,JE, Seeler,RA: Hemorrhagic Cystitis with MOPP Therapy, Cancer,41:1261-1264,1978.

44. Ash,P: The Influence of Radiation on Fertility in Man. Brit.J.Rad.,53:271-278,1980.

45. Lushbaugh,CC, Casarett, GW: The Effects of Gonadal Irradin in Clinical Radiation Therapy: A Review, Cancer,37:1111-1120,1976.

46. Speiser,B, Rubin,P, Casarett,GW: Aspermia Following Lower Truncal Irradiation in Hodgkin's Disease. Cancer,32:692-698,1973.

47. Hahn,EW, Feingold,S, Nisce,L: Aspermia and Recovery of Spermatogenesis in Cancer Patients Following Incidental Gonadal Irradiation During Treatment: A Progress Report. Radiology,119:223-225,1976.

48. Winstanly,TD, Peckham,MJ, Austin,DE, Murray,MAF, Jacobs, HS: Reproductive and Endocrine Function in Patients with Hodgkin's Disease: Effects of Oophoropexy and Irradiation. Brit.J.Cancer,33:226-231,1976.

49. LeFloch,O, Donaldson,SS, Kaplan,HS: Pregnancy Following Oophoropexy and Total Nodal Irradiation in Women with Hodgkin's Disease. Cancer,38:2263-2268,1976.

50. Richter,P, Calamera,JC, Morgenfeld,MC, Kierszenbaum,A, Lavieri,J, Mancini,R: Effect of Chlorambucil on Spermatogenesis in the Human with Malignant Lymphoma. Cancer,26:1026-1030,1970.
51. Sobrinho,L, Levine,R, Deconti,R: Amenorrhea in Patients with Hodgkin's Disease Treated with Antineoplastic Agents. Amer.J.Obstet.Gynec.,109:135-139,1971
52. Fairley,KF, Barrie,JU, Johnson,W: Sterility and Testicular Atrophy Related to Cyclophosphamide Therapy. Lancet,i:568-569,1972.
53. Feng,PH: Cyclophosphamide and Infertility. Lancet,i:840-841,1972.
54. Warne,GL, Fairley,KF, Hobbs,JB, Martin,FIR: Cyclophosphamide-Induced Ovarian Failure. NEJM,289:1159-1162,1973.
55. Sherins,RJ, Devita,VT: Effect of Drug Treatment for Lymphoma on Male Reproductive Capacity. Ann.Int.Med.,79:216-220,1973.
56. Asbjornsen,G, Molne,K, Klepp,O, Aakvaag,A: Testicular Function After Combination Chemotherapy for Hodgkin's sease. Scand.J.Hema.,16:66-69,1976.
57. Sherins,RJ, Olweny,CL, Ziegler,JL: Gynecomastia and Gonadal Dysfunction in Adolescent Boys Treated with Combination Chemotherapy for Hodgkin's Disease. NEJM,299:12-16, 1979.
58. Kirkland,RT, Bongiovanni,AM, Cornfeld,D, McCormick,JB, Parks,JS, Tenore,A: Gonadotropin Responses to Luteinizing-Releasing Factor in Boys Treated with Cyclophosphamide for Nephrotic Syndrome. J.Ped.,89:941-944,1976.
59. Holmes,GE, Holmes,FF: Pregnancy Outcome of Patients Treated for Hodgkin's Disease. Cancer,41:1317-1322,1978.
60. Simon,R: Statistical Methods for Evaluating Pregnancy Outcomes in Patients with Hodgkin's Disease. Cancer,45:2890-2892,1980.
61. Glatstein,E, Mchardy-Young,S, Brast,N, Eltringham,JR, Kriss,JP: Alterations in Serum Thyrotropin (TSH) and Thyroid Function Following Radiotherapy in Patients with Malignant Lymphoma. J.Clin.Endocr.,32:833-841,1971.
62. Fuks,Z, Glatstein,E, Marsa,GW, Bagshaw,MA, Kaplan,HS: Long Term Effects of External Radiation on the Pituitary and Thyroid Glands. Cancer,37:1152-1161,1976.
63. Nelson,D, Reddy,KV, O'Mara,RE, Rubin,P: Thyroid Abnormalities Following Neck Irradiation for Hodgkin's Disease. Cancer,42:2553-2562,1978.
64. Shalet,SM, Rosenstock,JD, Beardwell,CG, Pearson,D, Jones, PH: Thyroid Dysfunction Following External Irradiation to the Neck for Hodgkin's Disease in Childhood. Clinical Radiol.,28:511-515,1977.

65. Weshler,Z, Krasnokuki,D, Peshin,Y, Biran,S: Thyroid Carcinoma Induced by Irradiation for Hodgkin's Disease. Acta Rad.Onc.,17:383-386,1978.

66. Nickson,JJ, Glicksman,AS: Unpublished case.

67. Naysmith,A, Hancock,BW, Cullen,DR, Richmond,J, Wilde,CE: Pituitary Function in Patients Receiving Intermittent Cytotoxic and Coritcosteroid Therapy for Malignant Lymphoma. Lancet,1:715-717,1976.

68. Schimpff,SC, Wiernick,PH, Wiswell,J, Salvatore,P: Radiation-Related Thyroid Dysfunction in Hodgkin's Disease. ASCO Abs.c-279, Proceedings,19:376,1978.

69. Jones,A: Transient Radiation Myelopathy (with Reference to Lhermitte's Sign of Electrical Paresthesia). Brit.J.Rad., 37:727-744,1964.

70. Kaplan,HS, Stewart,JR: Complications of Intensive Megavoltage Radiotherapy for Hodgkin's Disease. Nat'l Cancer Inst Monograph,36:439-444,1973.

71. Collaborative Study: Survival and Complications of Radiotherapy Following Involved and Extended Field Therapy of Hodgkin's Disease, Stages I and II. Cancer,38:288-305,1976.

72. Marks,RD, Agarwal,SK, Constable,WC: Increased Rate of Complications as a Result of Treating Only One Prescribed Field Daily. Radiology,107:615-619,1973.

73. Rosillo-Poussin,H, Nisce,LZ, Lee,BJ: Complications of Total Nodal Irradiation of Hodgkin's Disease, Stages III and IV. Cancer,42:437-441,1978.

74. Hopfan,S, Reid,A, Simpson,L, Ager,PJ: Clinical Complications Arising from Overlapping of Adjacent Radiation Fields-Physical & Technical Consideration. Int.J.Rad.Onc. Biol.Phys.,2:801-808,1977.

75. Gagliano,RG, Costanzi,JJ: Paraplegia Following Intrathecal Methotrexate. Cancer,37:1663-1668,1976.

76. Henderson,ES: Acute Lymphoblastic Leukemia. Cancer Medicine,(Holland,JM, Frei,E), Lea & Febiger, Phila.:1973 p. 1173-1199.

77. Weiss,HD, Walker,MD, Wiernik,PH: Neurotoxicity of Commonly Used Antineoplastic Agents (Second of Two Parts). NEJM, 291:127-133,1974.

78. Perthes,G: Ueber den Einfluss der Roentgen Strahlen auf epitheliale Gerwebe, insbedondere auf das carcinoma. Arch. Klin.Chir.,71:955-1000,1903.

79. Ward,HWC: Disordered Vertebral Growth Following Irradiation. Brit.J.Rad.,38:459-464,1965.

80. Probert,JC, Parker,BR: The Effects of Radiation Therapy on Bone Growth. Radiology,114:155-162,1975.

81. Dreizen,S, Daly,TE, Drave,JB, et al: Oral Complications of Cancer Radiotherapy. Post Grad.Med.,61:85-92,1977.
82. Ihde,DC, Devita,VT: Osteonecrosis of the Femoral Head in Patients with Lymphoma Treated with Intermittent Combination Chemotherapy. Cancer,36:1585-1588,1975.
83. Sweet,DL, Roth,DG, Desser,RK, Miller,JB, Ultmann,JE: Avascular Necrosis of the Femoral Head with Combination Therapy. Ann.Int.Med.,85:67-68,1976.
84. Timothy,AR, Tucker,AK, Malpas,JS, Wright,PF, Sutcliff,SBJ: Osteonecrosis After Intensive Chemotherapy for Hodgkin's Disease. Lancet,1:154,1978.
85. Albala,NM, Steinfeld,A, Khilnani,MT: Osteonecrosis in Patients with Hodgkin's Disease Following Combined Chemotherapy. Ped.+Med.Onc.,(In Press).
86. Sykes,MP, Chu,F, Savel,H, Bonadonna,G, Mathis,H: The Effects of Varying Dosages of Irradiation Upon Sternal-Marrow Regeneration. Radiology,83:1084-1087,1964.
87. Sykes,MP, Chu,F, Gee,TS, McKenzie,S: Follow-up on the Long Term Effects of Therapeutic Irradiation on Bone Marrow. Radiology,113:179-180,1974.
88. Nelson,DF, Chaffey,JT, Hellman,S: Late Effects of X-Irradiation on the Ability of Mouse Bone Marrow to Support Hematopoiesis. Int.J.Rad.Onc.Biol.Phys.,2:39-45,1977.
89. Rubin,P, Elbadawi,NA, Thomson,RAE, Cooper,RA: Bone Marrow Regeneration from Cortex Following Segmental Fractionated Irradiation. Int.J.Rad.Onc.Biol.Phys.,2:27-38,1977.
90. Cionini,L: Bone Marrow Damage Following Total Nodal Radiation in Hodgkin's Disease Patients. Brit.J.Rad.,46:67-68, 1973.
91. Vogel,JM, Kimball,HR, Foley,HT, Wolff,SM, Perry,S: Effect of Extensive Radiotherapy on the Marrow Granulocyte Reserves of Patients with Hodgkin's Disease. Cancer,21:798-804,1968.
92. Bell,EG, Mcafee,JG, Constable,WC: Local Radiation Damage to Bone and Marrow Demonstrated by Radioisotopic Imaging. Radiology,92:1083-1088,1969.
93. Gottlieb,AJ, Bloomfield,CD, Glicksman,AS, Nissen,N, Pajak, TF: Nitrosureas in the Therapy of the Lymphomas-A Summary of the Cancer and Leukemia Group B Experience. Nitrosurea Symposium, 1980, Academic Press, NY, (In Press).
94. Kaplan,HS: Hodgkin's Disease, Harvard Press, 2nd Ed., Cambridge, MA, 1980,p.529-535.
95. Meyer,W, Leventhal,B: Late Effects of Cancer Therapy Complications of Cancer. ed. Abeloff,MD, Johns Hopkins Univ. Press, Baltimore, MD, 1979,p.397-416.

96. Leventhal,BG, Mirro,J, Yarbro,GS: Immune Reactivity to Tumor Antigens in Leukemia and Lymphoma. Sem.in Hemat., 15:157-179,1978.
97. Twomey,JJ, Rice,L: Impact of Hodgkin's Disease Upon the Immune System. Sem.in Onc.,7:114-125,1980.
98. Steele,R, Han,T: Effects of Radiochemotherapy and Splenectomy on Cellular Immunity in Long Term Survivors of Hodgkin's Disease and Non-Hodgkin's Lymphoma. Cancer,42: 133-139,1978.
99. Fuks,Z, Strober,S, Bobrove,AM, Sasuzuki,T, McMichael,A, Kaplan,HS: Long Term Effects of Radiation on T and B Lymphocytes in Peripheral Blood of Patients with Hodgkin's Disease. J.Clin.Invest.,58:803-814,1976.
100. Sutherland,RM, McCredie,JA, Inch,WR: Effect of Splenectomy and Radiotherapy on Lymphocytes in Hodgkin's Disease. Clin.Onc.,1:274-284,1975.
101. Feld,R, Bodey,GP: Infections in Patients with Malignant Lymphoma Treated with Combination Chemotherapy. Cancer, 39:1018-1025,1977.
102. Donaldson,SS, Glatstein,E, Vosti,KL: Bacterial Infections in Pediatric Hodgkin's Disease. Cancer,41:1949-1958,1978.
103. Green,DM, Stutsman,L, Blumenson,LE, Brecher,ML, Thomas, PRM, Allen,JE, Jewett,TC, Freeman,AI: The Incidence of Post-Splenectomy Sepsis and Herpes Zoster in Children and Adolescents with Hodgkin's Disease. Med.and Ped.Onc., 7:285-297,1979.
104. Siber,GR, Weitzman,SG, Aisenberg,AC, Weinstein,HJ, Schiffman,G: Impaired Antibody Response to Pneumococcal Vaccine After Treatment for Hodgkin's Disease. NEJM,299: 442-448,1978.
105. Broome,CV, Facklam,RR, Fraser,DW: Pneumococcal Disease After Pneumococcal Vaccination. NEJM,303:549-552,1980.
106. Monfardini,S, Bajetta,E, Arnold,C, Kenda,R, Bonadonna,G: Herpes Zoster-Varicella Infection in Malignant Lymphomas-Influence of Splenectomy and Intensive Treatment. Europ. J.Cancer,11:51-57,1975.
107. Dailey,MO, Coleman,CN, Kaplan,HS: Radiation-Induced Splenic Atrophy in Patients with Hodgkin's Disease and Non-Hodgkin's Lymphomas. NEJM,302:215-217,1980.
108. Steele,RW, Myers,MG, Vincent,MM: Transfer Factor for the Prevention of Varicella-Zoster Infection in Childhood Leukemia. NEJM,303:355-359,1980.
109. Warren,S, Ehrenriech,T: Multiple Primary Malignant Tumors and Susceptibility to Cancer. Cancer Res.,4:554-560,1944.

110. Berg,J: The Incidence of Multiple Primary Cancers in the Development of Further Cancer in Patients with Lymphoma, Leukemia, and Myeloma. J.Nat'l.Ca.Inst.,38:741-752,1967.
111. Brody,RS, Schottenfeld,D: Multiple Primary Cancers in Hodgkin's Disease. Sem.in Onc.,7:187-201,1980.
112. Arseneau,JC, Sponzo,RW, Levin,DL, Schnipper,LE, Bonner,H, Young,RC, Canellos,GP, Johnson,RE, Devita,VT: Non-lymphomatous Malignant Tumors Complicating Hodgkin's Disease. NEJM,287:1119-1122,1972.
113. Burns,CP, Stjernholm,RL, Kellermeyer,RW: Hodgkin's Disease Terminating in Acute Lymphosarcoma Cell Leukemia. Cancer,27:806-811,1971.
114. C.P.C.: Case 17-1974, NEJM,290:1012-1017,1974.
115. Canellos,GP, Arseneau,JC, Devita,VT, Whang-Peng,J, Johnson,REC: Second Malignancies Complicating Hodgkin's Disease in Remission. Lancet,1:947-949,1975.
116. Hutchinson,GB: Late Neoplastic Changes Following Medical Irradiation. Cancer,37:1102-1107,1976.
117. Cadman,EC, Capizzi,RL, Bertino,JR: Acute Non-lymphocytic Leukemia (A Delayed Complication of Hodgkin's Disease Therapy: Analysis of 109 Cases). Cancer,40:1280-1296,1977.
118. Coleman,CN, Williams,CJ, Flint,A, Glatstein,EJ, Rosenberg, SA, Kaplan,HS: Hematologic Neoplasia in Patients Treated for Hodgkin's Disease. NEJM,297:1249-1252,1977.
119. Kapadia,SB, Krause,JR, Ellis,LD, Pan,SF, Wald,N: Induced Acute Non-Lymphocytic Leukemia Following Long Term Chemotherapy: A Study of 20 Cases. Cancer,45:1315-1321,1980.
120. Krikorian,JG, Burke,JS, Rosenberg,SA, Kaplan,HS: Occurrence of Non-Hodgkin's Lymphoma After Therapy for Hodgkin's Disease. NEJM,300:452-458,1979.
121. Toland,DM, Coltman,CA, Moon,TE: Second Malignancies Complicating Hodgkin's Disease: The Southwest Oncology Group Experience. Cancer Clinical Trials,1:27-33,1978.
122. D'Angio,GJ, Clatworthy,HW, Evans,AE, Newton,WA, Tefft,M: Is the Risk of Morbidity and Rare Mortality Worth the Cure? Cancer,41:377-380,1978.
123. Valagussa,P, Santoro,A, Kenda,R, Bellant,FF, Franchi,F, Banfi,A, Rilke,F, Bonadonna,G: Second Malignancies in Hodgkin's Disease: A Complication of Certain Forms of Treatment. Brit.Med.J.,280:216-219,1980.

Solid Tumors 2

Germ Cell Tumors

ROBERT B. GOLBEY, M.D.

Chief, Solid Tumor Service
Department of Medicine
Memorial Sloan-Kettering Cancer Center
New York, New York

During the decade of the 1970's approximately 250 patients with advanced malignant germ cell tumors have been treated with one or more of five protocols that evolved during this period at the Memorial Sloan-Kettering Cancer Center (MSKCC). All of these patients would now be dead in the absence of effective chemotherapy. Instead 101 of these patients are alive and free of evidence of disease and have been followed long enough so that we can feel that relapse is unlikely. This is an average potential cure rate of 40% which contrasts well with the results in the 1960's when between 5 and 10% of the patients were cured. This is an encouraging increase in the number of patients who are alive and well but the increase that can be predicted for the upcoming decade of the 1980's is even greater. With the diligent application of what we know now the cure rate in the mid 1980's should approach 98%.

This optimistic prediction does not mean that all of the problems related to the treatment of these tumors have been solved, but the emphasis of the questions has shifted from how can we cure our patients to how can we best cure them. Before discussing the changes in therapy which have enabled this improvement in results it seems desirable that we understand the nature of the disease that we are treating and the importance of some of the prognostic factors that have been recognized in these tumors.

Germ cell tumors arise in the cell present in males and females which in the normal course of events gives rise to sperm and ova. They are toti-

potential in that they have the ability to differentiate into every tissue in the living body. The
tumors that are produced reflect this histologic
diversity. For a variety of embryological reasons
these cells are most commonly present in the
testicle. They are less numerous in the ovary, and
only occasionally are they found in the retroperitoneal space, in the mediastinum, and even in the
brain. Tumors arising from these cells can occur in
any of these locations. The histology of the tumors
that arise in these several sites are identical and
the responses that can be anticipated after treatment with chemotherapy are similar if one takes into
account the differences in staging and bulk of
disease at the time of initiation of therapy. The
germ cell has the capability of replicating and
differentiating. Differentiation gives rise to sperm
or to ova while replication produces more of the
primordial cells which have the capacity for
differentiation. Both of these processes are more
active in males than in females and this is one
reason that these tumors occur more frequently in
males. When the undifferentiated cell undergoes a
neoplastic change the resulting tumor in males is
seminoma while in females it is called dysgerminoma
(1). If the cell that becomes neoplastic is
somewhat more differentiated it may give rise to an
embryonal carcinoma or to an adult teratoma. After
the differentiated cell becomes neoplastic it may
retain its capability to differentiate further so
that the histology and the behavior of the tumor may
change. Embryonal carcinoma once formed may persist
as embryonal carcinoma or it may continue to
differentiate along one of two different pathways
leading either toward the development of the fetus
or to the development of the yolk sac or the
placenta. The fetal pathway provides an admixture
of teratomatous elements to the embryonal carcinoma
while the second pathway leads to choriocarcinoma or
yolk sac tumor. Mixed tumors containing clones from
more than one of these cell lines are commonly seen
(2,3). The mixture of embryonal carcinoma and a
variety of teratomatous elements has in the past
been called teratocarcinoma. It has been recognized
for some time that embryonal carcinoma and the
malignant teratomatous elements can differentiate
into histologically benign adult teratoma (4). This
occurs spontaneously as a very rare event but under

the infulence of therapy we have recognized this transition from malignant to benign with increasing frequency. The recognition of this event is important in treatment planning and in evaluation of the results of treatment. These several types of tumors are not only different under the microscope but are also different in their biological behavior. This is easiest to illustrate and is best documented in tumors arising in the testicle. Seminoma arises in the testicle and disseminates via the lymphatics which drain into the nodes in the para-aortic chain. From there they continue upward into the thoracic duct usually going to the lymph nodes in the left supraclavicular area before entering the blood stream to become hematogenously disseminated to different parts of the body. Embryonal carcinoma frequently follows this same pathway but occasionally in the testicle or in the lymph nodes blood vessel invasion occurs and early hematogenous dissemination results. Pure choriocarcinoma rarely spreads via the lymphatics and in some cases will invade the blood stream and produce distant metastases, usually in the lung, before the primary tumor in the testicle is large enough to be detected. "Teratocarcinoma", like embryonal carcinoma is capable of spreading by either route but usually it is present in the lymphatic channels where it is frequently seen as bulky and locally invasive disease in the retroperitoneal lymph nodes.

A similar spectrum can be described for sensitivity to radiation therapy (5). Seminoma is exquisitely sensitive to radiation. Choriocarcinoma is barely sensitive to radiation and the embryonal and terato-carcinomas are somewhere in between. There are also differences in sensitivity of these cell types to different chemotherapeutic agents. This was of great importance in the very early and very brief era of single agent chemotherapy and has become of lesser importance as more effective combinations which have the capability of dealing with more than one of the cell types have been developed. At the present time only pure choriocarcinoma is relatively insensitive to chemotherapy as it is presently employed. Fortunately, pure choriocarcinoma is relatively uncommon but its resistance to curative therapy is the chief reason for the projection given earlier of 98% curability

rather than 100% curability to be hoped for in the
near future. In addition to being histologically
different and biologically different these various
tumors are also chemically different (6). Choriocarcinoma produces a hormone chorionic gonadotropin
which can be measured in the blood and urine and
represents a good index of the presence and of the
activity of the tumor. Embryonal carcinoma and yolk
sac tumors produce alpha fetoprotein which similarly
is a valuable indicator of the activity of the
tumor. Since many of these tumors contain a mixture
of elements one frequently finds that both markers
are elevated. During therapy a divergence in the
response of the markers usually indicates that one
clone of the tumor is responding differently than
are the other elements. All of these tumors except
adult teratoma may produce an elevation of LDH
(lactic dehydrogenase) as a nonspecific but still
valuable indicator of the activity of the tumor (7).
When transition is seen from these malignant tumors
to adult teratoma one of the characteristic findings
is that the tumor persists but the markers decrease
to normal levels since the nonmalignant elements do
not produce any markers. This is not an absolute
differential point, however, since we have found
occasionally that a small amount of carcinoma can be
present, not producing detectable levels of marker,
and still be capable of subsequent reappearance and
metastasis. The distinction between histologically
malignant tumors can still best be made by the
pathologist after surgical removal of the nodule in
question. This fact led us to additional surgery
late in the course of the treatment of some patients
and has contributed to our improved therapeutic
results as will be demonstrated later (8,9).
    Staging initially was designed to meet the
needs of surgeons to differentiate the patients who
were potentially curable by one surgical procedure
or another from those who were not. The traditional
staging until some time in the 1970's was stage I,
II and III. Stage I being tumor confined to the
testicle, stage II being tumor present in the
retroperitoneal lymph nodes within the area that
could be encompassed by a retroperitoneal lymph node
dissection, and stage III being tumor above the
renal pedicles or metastatic to distant sites. This
staging has proven inadequate for contemporary
thinking about this disease.

The T.N.M. system has provided a useful framework in which to develop a new staging classification. Several variations are in use that are of varying degrees of complexity, but they generally agree on a few basic but essential points (10,11).

In this system "T" describes the local tumor. Major concerns are (1) whether the tumor is confined to the testicle and its appendages or not, (2) whether there is tumor in transit to the regional nodes that was not removed by orchiectomy, and (3) whether a surgical procedure has penetrated the scrotum as with a biopsy or a scrotal orchiectomy thereby opening additional pathways of lymphatic dissemination.

More immediately important than the "T" status is the "N" category describing the degree of involvement of the regional lymph nodes. Our schema defines N_1 as being microscopic involvement only, N_2 as gross involvement of lymph nodes, N_3 as large lymph nodes which have broken through their capsule, and N_4 as local invasion about the lymph node sufficient to make the mass incompletely resectable. A study which I will report to you shortly also suggested that the N_2 category should be divided into A and B with A containing grossly positive lymph nodes, fewer than five in number and with the largest node being 2 cm. or less in diameter. N_2-B includes the grossly positive nodes greater than five in number or larger than 2 cm. in diameter. This appears to be a rough dividing line between good and poor prognosis patients in whom a competent retroperitoneal lymph node dissection has been done. After a retroperitoneal lymph node dissection patients with N_1 nodes probably have as good a prognosis as do the stage I patients who could have been cured with orchiectomy alone while the N_4 lymph nodes have a prognosis that is just as poor or ironically even worse than that of the patients with distant metastases. In summary, the system consists of three stages. Stage I, tumor confined to the testicle and potentially curable by orchiectomy. Stage II-A, a few small nodes are positive and there is a high expectation of cure by retroperitoneal lymph node dissection. Stage II-B, where the hope for cure by lymph node dissection or radiation therapy decreases, and

stage III,the patients who cannot be cured by
surgery or radiation therapy alone and require
chemotherapy. At the present time the distribution
of patients when first seen is one-third stage I,
one-third stage II, and one-third stage III. There
is, of course, a difference between the cases that
are clinically staged, surgically staged and
pathologically staged after intensive review of
multiple sections of the removed tissues. As our
techniques for clinical staging have improved (12)
and as our chemotherapy for advanced disease has
improved **a** whole new series of options

have developed that may improve and simplify the
treatment of some patients. If one understands the
staging and accepts the fact that the higher the
stage the more difficult the cure, one can
understand that testicular tumors should have a
somewhat higher cure rate than the tumors that arise
in the retroperitoneum or the mediastinum or in the
ovary where by virtue of their inaccessible location
they have a greater opportunity to grow larger and
to spread further before they are detected than
does a tumor starting in the relatively exposed
testicle.
   We can now look at the treatments that have
been developed for the various histologic types and
stages of the germ cell tumors. We must divide this
discussion into Seminomas and Nonseminomatous germ
cell sections. Stage I seminoma is diagnosed and
effectively treated by orchiectomy. Since it is
impossible in most circumstances to rule out the
presence of microscopic deposits in the lymph nodes
it is the usual practice to radiate the retroperitoneal lymph nodes after orchiectomy even if the
clinical staging was I. This is good practice
because of the way that seminoma adheres to the
lymphatic pathways at dissemination and because of
its extreme sensitivity to radiation. Seminoma is
similarly curable in stage II-A by orchiectomy and
radiation therapy. In fact, 90% of all seminomas
diagnosed can be cured by orchiectomy and radiation
therapy to the retroperitoneal lymph nodes (13).
However, 10% of the patients do progress after this
treatment and require additional therapy. It seems
probable that they were the stage II-B and stage
III patients at the time of initial therapy. Many
of these seminomas are sensitive to treatment with

alkylating agents (14), however, it has recently
been realized that when a patient with seminoma
fails after therapy the metastases will frequently
present with elements other than seminoma. For this
reason we and others (15) are now treating stage
II-B and III seminomas with a chemotherapy program
identical with that used for the other germ cell
tumors. The long term results appear to have
improved but the numbers are still too small to
make any definitive conclusions.

For the nonseminomatous germ cell tumors,
optimal therapy has included orchiectomy which is
essential to the diagnosis and which will cure true
stage I patients. Because of the difficulty in
being certain by clinical means that there is not
at least microscopic involvement of the retroperitoneal nodes, it has been customary to do a
retroperitoneal lymph node dissection or to radiate
these nodes to a significantly higher dose than was
used for seminoma. We have preferred the retroperitoneal lymph node dissection because it provided a
more accurate staging for subsequent treatment
planning. A retroperitoneal lymph node dissection
is not a totally benign procedure because the
frequently unavoidable disruption of the local
nerve supply can produce functional sterility. That
is, the patient still produces active sperm in the
remaining testicle but cannot ejaculate because of
the disturbance of muscular function (16). Although
firm data is not available based on the newer
staging concepts, it seems probable that the stage
I and stage II-A patients with nonseminomatous germ
cell tumors are cured by this local therapy in up
to 85% of the cases. The more advanced degrees of
retroperitoneal lymph node involvement of stage II-
B may be cured by these local procedures in as few
as 40-50% of the cases so treated. The 15% of the
patients with stage I and stage II-A disease who
are not cured by the local procedures usually have
difficulty subsequently because of distant
metastases. In the past most of these people died
of their disease but now many can be salvaged by
the use of chemotherapy. A major impact of the past
ten years has come through the increasing efficacy
of chemotherapy in stage III disease which is by
definition disease not curable by surgery and/or
radiation therapy.

The possibility of cure of nonseminomatous

germ cell tumors with chemotherapy, even after wide
spread dissemination, has been recognized since the
late 1950's when complete responses and prolongation of disease free survival were first recognized
(17). The treatment used then was a combination of
Actinomycin D and Chlorambucil with or without
Methotrexate. This was the first effective drug
combination used. The use of this triple regimen
produced results that were better than those
achievable with any one of the drugs used alone.
Methotrexate was used because of its known activity
against gestational trophoblastic tumors (18).
Actinomycin was used because of demonstrated
activity in phase II studies. Chlorambucil was used
because of the possibility that a radiomimetic drug
would enhance the activity of the Actinomycin as
had been suggested by animal studies. The addition
of this drug did, in fact, seem to prolong the
duration of the antitumor effect achievable with
Actinomycin D alone. An effect of the Chlorambucil
that was unrecognized at the time is that it may
have helped to eliminate some of the recurrences of
seminoma that occasionally were seen after other
germ cell elements were eliminated by treatment not
containing an alkylating agent. With this
combination 50% of the patients showed some
evidence of an antitumor effect. Twenty percent had
complete disappearance of the disease for some
period but less than one in ten had prolonged
control of the disease and possible cure. This
therapy was continued for three years in most
patients before it was discontinued and the concept
that these long surviving patients with disseminated
disease might be cured did not seem real for many
years. There are, however, some survivors who were
treated with this combination now alive and well
more than twenty years later. Minor modifications
and additions of drugs to this treatment program
did not result in any improvement in response rate
or survival until the effectiveness of Vinblastine
and Bleomycin as single agents and in combination
was observed (19). This combination as originally
reported produced an overall response rate of 76%
at the cost of significant morbidity and
occasionally mortality. The activity of the
combination led us in 1972 to incorporate
Vinblastine and Bleomycin at a somewhat reduced
dosage into a combination with Actinomycin D(VAB I).

The three drugs were given as pulse doses twice in
the first week and once weekly thereafter as
tolerated. The program was well tolerated initially
but pulmonary toxicity was seen with continued
administration of Bleomycin. At this time 9 of the
68 patients (13%) treated with this combination
remain alive and well (20). This was a small but
definite improvement over the treatment employed in
the 1960's. During this period 16 of the patients
who failed this simple pulse dose regimen were
treated with a combination of Bleomycin by
continuous infusion plus a pulse dose of Cis-
Platinum. Cis-Platinum alone had recently been
described as having the capability of producing
short lived responses in patients with testicular
tumor (21) and some advantage had been described
for a continuous infusion of Bleomycin over a pulse
dose schedule (22). Sixty-eight percent, 11/16, of
these patients who had failed their primary therapy
had partial remissions on this secondary treatment
with a median duration of 2½ months. The second
protocol was designed in 1974 incorporating these
changes. In VAB II Vinblastine and Actinomycin D
were given on day 1 followed by a continuous
infusion of Bleomycin for one week and a pulse dose
of 1.2 mg/kg of Cis-Platinum on day 8. This
induction was followed by a consolidation phase
using the first three drugs weekly with substitution
of the Cis-Platinum for Actinomycin D every third
week. The induction program was repeated four months
after beginning therapy. Following this reinduction
maintenance therapy was begun with Chlorambucil
daily plus Vinblastine and Actinomycin D
intravenously every three weeks all continuing for
two to three years. Fifty patients were treated
with VAB II. All of them had measurable metastatic
disease and about half of them had previously been
treated with one or more of the drugs in the
protocol other than Cis-Platinum. The complete
response (CR) rate was 50% overall. In patients not
previously treated with drugs it was 60%. Eleven
patients (22%) remain alive and free of evidence of
disease at this time (23). While this protocol was
being studied the problem of the dose limiting
nephrotoxicity of Cis-Platinum arose. The technique
involving prehydration and mannitol induced diuresis
was developed after animal studies. This enabled a
high dose of Cis-Platinum 120 mg/M^2 (3 mg/kg) to be

administered (24). A series of patients who had
failed VAB II were treated with this "high-dose" of
Cis-Platinum. There were five PR's and one minor
remission in nine adequately treated patients all
of whom had been resistent to Cis-Platinum at doses
of 1.2 mg/kg. Nephrotoxicity was less severe and
was reversible. The remissions obtained were short
lived but encouraging since they occurred in
previous treatment failures (25). The third VAB
protocol was designed in 1975 to include high-dose
Cis-Platinum. A pulse dose of Cyclophosphamide was
also added during the induction because of its
known activity against these tumors and because of
its activity against seminoma. Several of the
patients who had failed on VAB II therapy had been
treated for an original embryonal carcinoma but had
died with disseminated seminoma. Cis-Platinum is
now known to be just as active or even more active
against seminoma than is Cyclophosphamide but this
was not known at that time. The consolidation phase
of the treatment was made less intensive by the
deletion of Bleomycin, the addition of Chlorambucil,
and by giving the intravenous drugs every three
weeks instead of weekly. Adriamycin was added to
the consolidation phase because it had been active
as a single agent in 14 of 20 patients with
testicular cancer treated in another trial. The
reinduction at about five months was retained as
was the subsequent maintenance program. This
combination was evaluated in 74 previously untreated
patients. The complete response rate was 54% with
chemotherapy alone and in 7% (5 patients) minimal
residual disease was resected before a CR was
achieved. In all five of these patients the residual
disease was histologically benign adult teratoma.
Most if not all of them would have been effectively
cured by the chemotherapy alone. The total CR rate
for chemotherapy alone and chemotherapy plus surgery
is 61%. Twenty-nine percent of these patients have
relapsed leaving 31 alive and well and free of
disease for an overall potential cure rate of 41%
(25). At about the same time that this protocol was
being studied the Indiana University group reported
on the results of treatment with a combination of
Velban, Bleomycin and Cis-Platinum. They found
another and apparently equally effective way of
delivering a higher dose of Cis-Platinum without
dose limiting nephrotoxicity. They delivered 20 mg/

M^2 daily intravenously for five consecutive days. Their reported response rate was somewhat higher than that reported here but this appeared to be more a function of staging and histology and accepted degrees of toxicity than it did of basic differences in the effectiveness of the method of administering the drugs (26). Our own experience in this and in other diseases has demonstrated clearly that the ability to induce responses is not greatly different between low dose and high dose Cis-Platinum but there is a consistent difference favoring the high dose schedule in the durability of the responses in this and in other diseases. Therefore, the comparability of the response rate between the 100 mg/M^2 in divided doses versus the 120 mg/M^2 pulse dose has not and will not be answered by the available data. Long term survival data may ultimately show some differences but they are not likely to be large. A consistent observation in our studies and in all other testicular germ cell studies is that relapses that were going to occur did so in the first 6-8 months after the onset of chemotherapy. We, therefore, designed a fourth protocol in which the induction was virtually identical to the previous protocol but a reinduction without Bleomycin was introduced at 16 weeks after the initiation of therapy followed by a full induction with Bleomycin at 32 weeks. This change did not greatly increase the complete response rate with chemotherapy alone. Forty-one previously untreated patients were evaluated. Sixty-one percent had a complete response after chemotherapy. An additional 20% were rendered free of evidence of disease by surgical removal of residual nodules. About half of these nodules were adult teratoma and others were varying mixtures of necrotic tumor and viable tumor cells. This provided a total of 81% complete responses of which 12% have relapsed. The relapse rate appeared to be the same whether the complete response was achieved by chemotherapy alone or chemotherapy plus surgery. A total of 68% of this group are alive and well and free of disease with all patients well beyond the period of anticipated relapse (27). It must be recognized, however, that increased cell kill always opens the possibility that recurrences will be seen but will be delayed beyond the anticipated period This possibility must be continually remembered but at the present

time there is no evidence that this is in fact
occurring. More time is needed to fully assess this
risk. VAB V was a protocol devised for the treatment
of very high risk previously treated patients and
it established for us the feasibility of giving a
full dose of Cis-Platinum every 28 days. This
knowledge led to the development of a sixth protocol
in which the major change is the repetition of the
full induction program once every 28 days for three
courses. If at the end of this time residual disease
is still present it is now part of the protocol to
excise the disease. We also plan to reexplore any
area where bulky disease was present prior to
therapy, as when N4 nodes were present, or there
was a large retroperitoneal or mediastinal primary
tumor. VAB VI is the protocol we are currently
using:

VAB VI

Day 1	Cyclophosphamide	600 mg/M^2 I.V.
	Vinblastine	4 mg/M^2 I.V.
	Actinomycin D	1 mg/M^2 I.V.
	Bleomycin	30 mg/M^2 I.V.
Day 1-3	Bleomycin	20 mg/M^2/day x 3 days by 24 hr. infusion
Day 4	Cis-Platinum	120 mg/M^2 I.V. c̄ hydration and mannitol diuresis

Days 1-4 repeated q 3-4 weeks x 3
Bleomycin is omitted for third course

Maintenance - given q 3 weeks for 9 months

Vinblastine	6.0 mg/M^2 I.V.
Actinomycin D	1.0 mg/M^2 I.V.

It employes the same induction as VAB III and IV
except that the dose of Bleomycin in each induction
has been reduced to a priming dose and three days
of continuous infusion. The full course is repeated
twice at monthly intervals and a third time without
Bleomycin. Occasionally a fourth course is given
without Bleomycin in patients in whom tumor
regression is incomplete but continuing. After
completion of this induction program, if necessary
and if feasible, any foci of residual tumor are
surgically resected. After resection of any viable

malignant residual tumor two additional induction
courses are administered, one without and one with
Bleomycin if the pulmonary function permits. If the
tumor is all mature teratoma or scar tissue no
further inductions are given. In either case after
the last induction maintenance therapy with
Actinomycin D and Velban is given every three weeks.
The entire period of therapy is one year. This
represents a significant decrease in the total
amount of therapy over the previous protocols which
were continued for two to three years of maintenance
therapy. A follow-up of patients treated with VAB VI
is short and conclusions must be drawn very
tentatively. However, of 25 patients adequately
treated, all of them without prior chemotherapy, 16
have achieved complete response by chemotherapy
alone. Seven had residual removal to achieve a
complete response for a total of 92%. Of this number
9% have relapsed leaving a total of 21 patients or
84% of the original group free of evidence of
disease at a median time of observation of about
1½ years. Few if any relapses are expected in this
group but only time will tell.[28] This then represents
the state of the art at our Center. The steady
improvement of results during the 1970's at MSKCC
is summarized in Table I. Variations on this theme
are producing comparable results in many other
centers most notably with the treatment plan
developed at Indiana University.

It seems clear that better results with
chemotherapy can be achieved when the tumor is small
and that results become less good as the tumor
volume increases. This fact has led to trials of
adjuvant chemotherapy in almost every type of tumor
where a partial response rate of 50% or greater can
be achieved in advanced disease with chemotherapy.
At the time when VAB I was our most effective
therapy in stage III germ cell tumors, 62 patients
with stage II disease in whom all evidence of
disease had been surgically resected were treated
with pulse doses of Velban 0.06 mg/kg, Actinomycin
0.02 mg/kg and Bleomycin 0.05 mg/kg each given
weekly x 6 followed after a two week interval by
Actinomycin D 0.02 mg/kg and Chlorambucil p.o.
0.1 mg/kg daily x 7 out of every 14 days for one
year. During the second year the interval was
increased every 21 days. Of the 62 patients treated,
9 recurred in less than 8 months, and 1 recurred at

18 months. The remaining 83% continued free of
evidence of disease. This result in stage II
patients is comparable to the result in stage I
patients with surgery alone and is significantly
better than that in stage II disease with surgery
and/or radiation therapy. Retrospectively, in this
group of 62 patients we identified a good risk and
a poor risk group. The good risk had negative tumor
markers, fewer than five lymph nodes involved and
the largest node was less than 2 cm. There were 33
patients in the good prognosis group all of whom
are free of evidence of disease with a median
follow-up exceeding two years. Of the 29 poor
prognosis patients, ten have recurred within the
two years with most of the metastases manifesting
themselves within 6-8 months after surgery. This
group, therefore, has 65% surviving free of
evidence of disease. This result in poor prognosis
patients is better than could be achieved with
surgery alone but it obviously leaves much room for
improvement. Subsequently, we treated this group of
poor risk patients which we now call stage II-B with
VAB III after it had become our best available
treatment for advanced disease. Twenty-nine patients
were treated and have been followed for a median of
24 months. All 29 remain free of disease. While we
treated this poor risk group intensively we stopped
offering adjuvant chemotherapy to stage II-A
patients on the basis that 15% of this group would
relapse but that the vast majority could then be
salvaged by the prompt utilization of our best
therapeutic program, and the majority of the group
would be spared unnecessary chemotherapy (29). This
thesis is now being tested in a nation wide cooperative study. This national study is being conducted
in two parallel parts. One utilizing the high dose
Cis-Platinum as described, while the other used the
divided dose method of administration. Despite the
very high potential cure rate in this group of
patients it remains a fact that half of these
patients or more would not have recurred even had
they not received chemotherapy. This means that one
patient in two is receiving two years of intensive
chemotherapy that he did not need. It is, therefore,
legitimate to raise the question of whether this
entire group could simply be observed until
recurrence and then treat the group who does recur
with the best available treatment with an

expectation of cure. Until recently clinical staging was sufficiently poor and the price of missing an early metastasis was so high that all of these patients after clinical staging were still treated as though they were stage II patients. Now since chemotherapy can effect cure in most of the patients who would recur the question has been raised can the initial node dissection and/or radiation therapy be omitted in patients who have been carefully staged clinically and who are stage I, with the expectation that those who subsequently relapse will be treated with chemotherapy and most will be cured. This question too is under randomized study in several centers including our own. We may be able to demonstrate that stage I patients which constitute one-third of all the patients presenting with tumors can be spared the undesirable effects of retroperitoneal lymph node dissection and/or radiation therapy, with only a small percentage of them requiring chemotherapy subsequently when and if they relapse.

This more individualized treatment is possible only in the setting where good treatment with surgery, radiation therapy and chemotherapy is available for patients in all stages of their disease. We are approaching the goal of being able to hand tailor optimal management to the individual patient on the basis of a thorough understanding of the natural history of this disease, and of the relative risks and rewards of the different modalities of treatment with a consequent effect on the use of valuable resources such as hospital time and space, and money to the betterment of the patient and the community.

In summary:

1. Chemotherapy for this disease is improving rapidly, in that, it is more effective and it is given over a shorter period of time with reduced morbidity.

2. The improvement in chemotherapy and in our ability to clinically stage the disease accurately is enabling a review of what constitutes optimal therapy for each stage of the disease.

3. Complete control of this disease is a reasonable objective for the decade of the 80's.

TABLE 1

M.S.K.C.C.

Results of Treatment 1970 - 1980

Stage 3 Germ Cell Tumors

	VAB	VAB II	VAB III	VAB IV	VAB VI
First Reported	1973	1975	1976	1979	1980
Adequate Rx #	68	50	74	41	25
Complete Response %	–	–	61%	81%	92%
chemotherapy alone	22%	50%	54%	61%	64%
chemotherapy + surg.	–	–	7%	20%	28%
Relapse after complete response	40%	52%	29%	12%	8%
# (%) Alive – Free of evidence of disease	9(13%)	12(24%)	31(41%)	28(68%)	21(84%)

REFERENCES

1. Teilum, G. Special Tumors of Ovary and Testis (ed 2). Philadelphia, Limmincott, 1976.
2. Hajdu, S.I. Pathology of Germ Cell Tumors of the Testis. Seminars in Oncology, 1979, VI(1), pp 14-25.
3. Mostofi, F.K. Pathology of Germ Cell Tumors of Testis. Cancer, 1980, 45(7) pp 1735-1754.
4. Hong, W.K., Wittes, R.E., Hajdu, S.T., et. al. The Evolution of Mature Teratoma from Malignant Testicular Tumors. Cancer, 1977, 40(6), pp 2987-2992.
5. Batata, M.A. & Unal, A. The Role of Radiation Therapy in Relation to Stage and Histology of Testicular Cancer. Seminars in Oncology, 1979, VI(1), pp 69-73.
6. Javadpour, N. The value of Biologic Markers in Diagnosis and Treatment of Testicular Cancer. Seminars in Oncology, 1979, VI(1), pp 37-47.
7. Friedman, A., Vugrin, D. & Golbey, R.B. Prognostic Significance of Serum Tumor Biomarkers (TM), Alpha-Fetoprotein (AFP), Beta Subunit of Human Chorionic Gonadotrophin (bHCG), and Lactate Dehydrogenase (LDH) in Nonseminomatous Germ Cell Tumors (NSGCT). Abstract (#C-22), AACR/ASCO Proceedings, 1980, 21, pp 323.
8. Bains, M.S., McCormack, P.M., Cvitkovic, E. et. al. Results of Combined Chemo-surgical Therapy for Pulmonary Metastases from Testicular Carcinoma. Cancer, 1978, 41(3), pp 850-853.
9. Comisarow, R. & Grabstald, H. Re-exploration for Retroperitoneal Lymph Node Metastases from Testicular Tumor. Journal of Urology, 1976, 115, pp 569-571.
10. Fraley, E.E., Lange, P.H., Williams, R.D., et. al. Staging of Early Nonseminomatous Germ Cell Testicular Cancer. Cancer, 1980, 45(7), pp 1762-1767.
11. Mostofi, F.K. Comparison of Various Clinical and Pathological Classifications of Tumors of Testes. Seminars in Oncology, 1979, VI(1), pp 26-30.
12. Barzell, W.E. & Whitmore, W.F., Jr. Clinical Significance of Biologic Markers: Memorial

Hospital Experience. Seminars in Oncology,
1979, VI(I), pp 48-52.

13. Caldwell, W.L., Kademian, M.T., Frias, Z., et
    al. The Management of Testicular Seminomas,
    1979. Cancer, 1980, 45(7), pp 1768-1774.

14. Yagoda, A. & Vugrin, D. Theoretical
    Considerations in the Treatment of Seminoma.
    Seminars in Oncology, 1979, VI(1), pp 74-81.

15. Einhorn, L.H. Chemotherapy of Metastatic
    Seminoma. In L.H. Einhorn (Ed.), Testicular
    Tumors. N.Y.:Masson Pub.Co.,1980, 151-167.

16. Whitmore, W.F., Jr. Surgical Treatment of Adult
    Germinal Testis Tumors. Seminars in Oncology,
    1979, VI(1), pp 55-68.

17. Li, M.C., Whitmore, W.F., Golbey, R.B. et al.
    Effect of Drug Therapy on Metastatic Cancer of
    the Testes. J.A.M.A., 1960, 174, pp 1291-1299.

18. Li, M.C. Chemotherapy for Gestational
    Trophoblastic Tumors. Am. J. Obstet. Gynecol.,
    1979, 135(2), pp 267-272.

19. Samuels, M.L., Holoye, P.Y. & Johnson, D.E.
    Bleomycin Combination Chemotherapy in the
    Management of Testicular Neoplasia. Cancer,
    1975, 36, pp 318-326.

20. Wittes, R.E., Yagoda, A., Silvay, O., et al.
    Chemotherapy of Germ Cell Tumors of the Testis.
    I. Induction of remissions with Vinblastine,
    Actinomycin D, and Bleomycin. Cancer, 1976,
    37, pp 637-645.

21. Higby, D.J., Wallace, H.J.,Jr., Albert D.,
    et al. Diamminodichloroplatinum in the
    Chemotherapy of Testicular Tumors. J. Urol.,
    1974, 112, pp 100-104.

22. Cvitkovic, E., Currie, V., Ochoa, M., et al.
    Continuous Intravenous Infusion of Bleomycin
    in Squamous Cancer. AACR/ASCO Proceedings,1974,
    15:179.

23. Cheng, E., Cvitkovic, E., Wittes, R. et al.
    Germ Cell Tumors (II): VAB II in Metastatic
    Testicular Cancer. Cancer, 1978, 42, pp 2162-
    2168.

24. Hayes, D.M., Cvitkovic, E., Golbey, R., et al.
    High Dose Cis-Platinum Diammine Dichloride.
    Amelioration of Renal Toxicity by Mannitol
    Diuresis. Cancer, 1977, 37, pp 1372-1381.

25. Cvitkovic, E., Hayes, D., Golbey, R. Primary
    Combination Chemotherapy (VAB III) for

Metastatic or Unresectable Germ Cell Tumors. AACR Proceedings, 1976, 17:296.

26. Einhorn, L.H. & Donohue, J.P. Cis-diammine-dichloroplatinum, Vinblastine, and Bleomycin Combination Chemotherapy in Disseminated Testicular Cancer. Ann. Intern. Med., 1977, 87, pp 293-298.

27. Vugrin, D., Cvitkovic, E., Whitmore, W.F.,Jr. et al. VAB IV Combination Chemotherapy in the Treatment of Metastatic Testis Tumors. Cancer In Press

28. Vugrin, D., Dukeman, M., Whitmore, W., et al. VAB-6: Progress in Chemotherapy of Germ Cell Tumors (GCT). AACR/ASCO Proceedings, 1980, Abstract(#C-426), 21, p 426.

29. Vugrin, D., Cvitkovic, E., Whitmore, W.F.,Jr. et al. Adjuvant Chemotherapy in Resected Nonseminomatous Germ Cell Tumors of Testis: Stages I and II. Seminars in Oncology, 1979, VI(1), pp 94-98.

Chemotherapy of Genitourinary Tumors

Alan Yagoda, M.D.

Associate Attending
Department of Medicine
Memorial Sloan-Kettering Cancer Center
New York, New York   10021

Cytotoxic chemotherapy for patients with urologic malignancies spans from marginal (adrenal, renal, prostate) and
moderate (urinary bladder, penile) efficacy to curative (testicular cancer). The significant progress in treatment of
germ cell tumors of the testis is discussed elsewhere in the
symposium; this section will delineate cytotoxic and hormonal
chemotherapy for other genitourinary tumors.

An often insurmountable, at times bewildering problem in
reviewing and collating data from numerous protocol studies
is the lack of information concerning definition and documentation of the diagnostic work-up permitting objective
assessment and re-assessment of such lesions, categories of
response, modifications in drug doses and schedules, adequacy
of trial, extent of toxicity, and more importantly, patient
selection (1,2,41,46,47,55). The paucity of "indicator"
lesions - objectively measurable, bidimensional masses -
in patients with cancer of the bladder and prostate has impeded development of Phase II disease-oriented trials (2,32,
41,46,47,55). Osseous metastases, while easily demonstrable
radiologically and on radionuclide scans, are unsatisfactory
in evaluating a > 50% (partial remission - PR -) reduction
in tumor size. Pelvic, intra-abdominal, and intravesical
lesions, particularly after irradiation, are difficult to
measure accurately even on repeated examinations under anesthesia. Evaluation of changes on intravenous pyelography or
lymphangiography are frequently too insensitive, and specific
serum biologic and biochemical markers, in contrast to their
presence in testicular cancer, are few. Potential inaccur-
acies by both physicians and patients in assessing objective
changes in "evaluable" (uni-dimensional, osseous, pelvic and

499

intra-abdominal) lesions and symptomatic parameters can be
misleading (47,55). Thus absence of similarly selected
patients and study criteria influence end-results and comparability between drug studies. Utilizing stringent response criteria (1,2,48,55) and excluding the categories of
minor remission (MR), mixed responses, and stabilization of
of disease (STAB) result in a conservative, and probably
more realistic, overall response rate. Protocol differences
in patient selection and response criteria will be discussed,
but it would be presumptive not to recognize the limitations
inherent in arbitrary decisions in the evaluation of other
investigators' data.

Adrenal Cancer

Carcinoma of the adrenal cortex is divided into functioning and non-functioning tumors, and into differentiated
and anaplastic types (16,19,58). The latter has a male pre-
dominence, shorter survival (5 vs. 19 mos.), lacks hormonal
secretion and fails to respond to mitotane (o,p'-DDD) (16).
With mitotane - a congener of the insecticide DDT approximately 30-50% of cases exhibit objective tumor regression
and improvement biochemically; steroid synthesis decreases
in 50%-86% of responders in 17 to 30 days, and tumor
masses regress in 4-10 wks. (7,13,15,18,23). Some patients
with disseminated disease given o,p'-DDD are cured with
unmaintained complete remissions (CR) persisting > 4-7 years
(7,58). Mitotane has also been called a "gloom and doom"
drug since major psychologic sequelae have been associated
with its use, particularly with high doses (7). Some investigators recommend rapid dose escalation to 10-12+ gm. Q.D.
but only 4-6 gm may be necessary for tumor control (15,23).
Exogenous steroid replacement is required with doses > 3 gm.
Q.D. After stopping o,p'-DDD, dichloroethene and acetic
acid metabolites stored in fat produce trace serum levels for
8.5-18 mos. (15,23). Although there have been no randomized
trials, adjuvant o,p'-DDD therapy has been proposed (7). Of
note, Wortsman et al. (45) have described inactivation of o,
p'-DDD's effect with spironolactone administration. Aminoglutethimide which blocks 21 hydroxylation and metapyrone
which inhibits 11 beta-hydroxylation of cortisol have also
been used to control excess steroid synthesis (34).

Studies with cytotoxic agents are limited. A recent
review (58) of 14 trials at MSKCC and 25 in the literature,
22 of which used single agents, reveals a CR for 11 mos. with
porfiromycin (21) and a PR with cisplatin (DDP) (25). Some
responses have been described with the combination of o,p'-
DDD and cytotoxic agents such as 5-fluorouracil (5-FU) and
adriamycin (ADM); such remissions could be attributed however
to the efficacy of o,p'-DDD alone (58).

Adult Kidney Cancer

Hypernephroma is a chemotherapeutically and hormonally
resistant cancer (1,2,17,49). The most extensively studied
drugs are the progestins, vinblastine (VLB) and the nitrosoureas; many other agents have been evaluated and none have
reproducible, significant, objective response rates (Table 1).
Preliminary reports in small numbers of cases often describe
high response rates but as more patients are studied rates
diminish to < 10% (10,12,49). For example, VLB's antitumor
activity in hypernephroma has been reported as >25%, yet
when MR, mixed response and STAB are excluded response rates
are < 5-10% (1,10,12,17,49). With progestins (medroxyprogesterone acetate, 1000 mg. i.m. Q.W.), Hrushesky and Murphy
(17), and Bodey (1) have observed that between 1967-1971 and
1971-1976 remissions fell from 17% (228 cases) to 2% (415
cases).

Recent disease-oriented trials find no significant antitumor effect with actinomycin D, DDP, chlorozotocin, dianhydrogalactitol, AMSA, PALA, triazinate, vindesine, and the
combinations of methyl-CCNU and VLB, medroxyprogesterone
acetate and VLB, or all three drugs (1,10-12,33,56). While
two studies report (22,40) responses (18%) with methyl-glyoxal bis-guanylhydrazone (M-GAG), another (57) has noted no
objective tumor regression in 29 cases.

Immunotherapy with immune RNA (4), vaccines, etc., has
been tried as have progestins after percutaneous intra-
arterial embolization (theoretically initiating a beneficial
immunologic reaction) prior to nephrectomy (43). While preliminary data (43) suggest positive results, lack of prospective randomized trials place both therapeutic modalities

Table 1. Selected Trials in Hypernephroma[*]

Drug		Drug	
Actinomycin D	1/89	ADM	0/31
Androgens	5/170	AMSA	0/21
Chlorozotocin (DCNU)	0/21	BLEO	0/20
Lomustine (CCNU)	4/59	CTX	7/98
Piperazenedione	0/23	DDP	0/49
Progestins	35/695	5-FU	7/90
Semustine (MeCCNU)	4/57	M-GAG	8/64
Tamoxifen	5/58	PALA	1/12
Triazinate	3/59	VLB	16-50/199+
Vindesine	0/28	+ CCNU	11/89
VP-16	1/53	DAG	0/56

[*]CR+PR in Literature + MSKCC trials/No. Entered

as well as adjuvant chemotherapy into the purely investigative area.

Bladder Cancer

During the past 5 years disease-oriented protocols in
patients with advanced transitional cell carcinoma of the
urothelial tract have defined clinically significant antitumor activity with DDP, methotrexate (MTX), and ADM (Table
2). In 1976 Yagoda et al. (51) reported an overall response
rate of 33% in 24 patients with bidimensionally measurable
metastatic disease. Updating a recent review (48) of DDP in
bladder cancer, 57 (35%) of 162 cases achieved CR+PR status -
95% confidence limits, 28-43%. Almost all responses were observed in 3-6 weeks and frequently tumor regression began in
5-14 days. Although the median remission duration was 5 mos.
(unmaintained 10-12 wks.), some persisted for > 12-48 mos. (14,
25,28,39,48).

MTX in doses of 0.5-1.0 mg/kg iv, QW, or 50-100 mg. iv
or im, Q2W has induced remissions in 28% of cases; some trials
included patients with loco-regional (T_{2-3}) disease parameters. Response occurred rapidly, 2-4 wks., and lasted 4-5 mos.
(range 2-20+) (42,48,50).

ADM 45-60-75 mg/m^2 iv, Q3W produces remission in 17% of
cases. Responses are noted in 3-9 wks. and seem to be dose-
dependent (48,53).

Other active single agents include mitomycin C (Mito C), VM-26, and possibly VLB, 5-FU and CTX (2,48). The high response rates with 5-FU and CTX used singly are based on a few cases from many drug-oriented trials which employed criteria no longer acceptable. A recent disease-oriented study with 5-FU (5) finds very limited activity. While Mito C (2, 48) and neocarcinostatin (30) appear to be active agents for intravesical lesions, the latter drug shows minimal efficacy for disseminated disease (26). Many older agents never have been evaluated in disease-oriented studies. For example, since 1960 VLB had been administered to only 16 patients with bladder cancer, 5 of whom had VLB in combination regimens; two responded (48). In a recent trial at MSKCC 7 of 22 adequately treated patients given 0.1-0.15 mg/kg iv, QW have achieved PR status.

Combination regimens are outlined in Table 2. DDP with ADM and/or CTX (54) induced remission in 40-50% of cases. Williams et al. (44) added DDP to 5-FU + ADM and reported responses in 41%. Response rates with such DDP multi-drug regimens generally fall within the 95% confidence limits of DDP used singly, and preliminary data of randomized trials of DDP vs. DDP combinations thus far have shown no statistically significant increase in response rate, complete remission, or duration of response. The addition of CTX (52) or VM-26 (29) to ADM likewise was not therapeutically synergistic. Three studies (3,6,24) have described a 40-50% rate with the combination of ADM and 5-FU - all trials included patients with loco-regional disease.

DDP was inactive against Bilharzial bladder cancer (9), and when administered intravesically or systemically was ineffective against intravesical (transitional cell carcinoma) lesions (25). In addition, some patients have shown control of disseminated (nodal, pulmonary, etc.) disease while loco-regional lesions progressed requiring surgical excision for continued remission (14,39,48). In contrast, MTX may be more effective than DDP in controlling loco-regional disease (28). Future multi-drug regimens undoubtedly will combine DDP + MTX and/or VLB.

Approximately 50-60% of patients with Stage B_2 and C lesions will die within 5 years in spite of pre-operative

Table 2.   Chemotherapy in Bladder Cancer

Drug(s)	No.	%CR+PR	Drug(s)	No.	%
DDP	162	35(28-43)	AMSA	19	11
+CTX	45	38(24-52)	BLEO	58	5
+ADM	72	42(30-53)	CTX	98+	{31}
+ADM+CTX	94	41(31-50)	5-FU	105+	{28}
+ADM+5-FU	44	41(26-55)	Mito C	42	13
MTX	151	28(21-35)	NCS	19	5
ADM	183	17(12-22)	PALA	18	0
+CTX	39	18(6-30)	VM-26	79	20
+5-FU	103	39(29-48)	VP-16	18	0
+VM-26	27	19	VLB	31	23

Data in Literature + MSKCC results. { } = small numbers of cases from many drug trials. ( ) = 95% confidence limits.

irradiation and radical cystectomy. More than 50% of such failures have tumor recur outside the pelvis. Adjuvant chemotherapy trials have been initiated in such cases, yet no current data indicates increased survival.

Penile Cancer

Squamous cell (epidermoid) carcinoma of the penis is uncommon in the United States, incidence 0.1 per 100,000, and thus, the number of disease-oriented studies has been very limited. Three drugs - DDP, MTX, and bleomycin (BLEO) - have been found to possess clinically useful anti-tumor activity. In an update of MSKCC trials (35-37) remission occurred in 3 of 10 patients given DDP, 70-120 mg/m^2 iv, Q3W, in 2 of 12 patients treated with BLEO and in 4 of 9 patients with MTX, 0.5-1.5 mg/kg iv, QW, or 250 mg/m^2 in a 2-hour infusion with citrovorum factor rescue 24 hours thereafter. Using either DDP or MTX in different doses and schedules, Merrin (25) and Frei et al. (8) have also noted response in patients with penile cancer. Tumor regression, which is frequently dramatic, is evident in 2-4 wks. and persists for 3-11+ mos. Complete remission is uncommon.

Ichikawa (20) has evaluated BLEO in penile cancer using doses of 15-30 units iv, or im, BIW-TIW to a total course of 300 mg. for 2-3 courses Q 2-3 M. Frequently, courses were also combined with irradiation, surgery, and other drugs. Local (T_1, T_2) and regional masses regressed in 39 of 59

cases. Of 113 cases in the literature (37) only 15, of whom
2 received BLEO alone, had disseminated disease. In the
MSKCC trial (37) only 2 (17%) of 12 cases with disseminated
disease responded. Thus, BLEO used singly may be of limited
value in the treatment of disseminated penile cancer.

In a comprehensive review (37) of all Phase I and II
drug and disease (epidermoid)-oriented trials published between 1960-1978, no complete or partial remissions were
described in a very limited number of cases given alanine
nitrogen mustard, CTX, 5-FU, hexamethylmelamine, hydroxybu-
sulfan, mithramycin, and MTX + cytosine arabinoside.   Of
note,   20% of 81 cases in the MSKCC series had hypercalcemia
(37).

Prostatic Cancer

Hormonal manipulation by orchiectomy or exogenous estrogen administration which modulate the hypothalamic-pituitary-
testicular axis remains the most effective form of therapy
for patients with disseminated adenocarcinoma of the prostate.
New hormonal agents include: a) steroidal antiandrogens, such
as cyproterone acetate (Androcur), b) nonsteroidal antiandrogens, such as 4'-nitro-3-trifluoromethyl isobutryanilide
(Flutamide), c) Estracyst - nor-nitrogen mustard + estradiol,
and d) prednimustine-chlorambucil + prednisolone.

The vast amount of data with hormonal manipulation can
be summarized in the following fashion: (1) No evidence indicates a survival benefit with early vs. late hormonal manipulation and therapy is best delayed until patients with disseminated disease become symptomatic. (2) Orchiectomy or
exogenous estrogens are equally effective.   (3) Increased
survival or objective tumor regression with estrogens (including Estracyst and Stilphosterol) after orchiectomy or
vice versa is uncommon; some subjective improvement may occur
for short periods of time. (4) DES in doses of 5-15 mg. is
detrimental, particularly in stage III cases because of an
increase in cardiovascular induced deaths; doses of 0.2 mg.
QD is less effective than 1 mg. and (5) DES in doses less
than 3 mg. daily does not suppress consistently serum testosterone to the levels found in castrated males; higher
doses have no additional effect.

The cardinal question remains: Does an appropriate dose

of DES (i.e. 1 mg.) or an orchiectomy prolong survival?
Some conclusions reached in the Veterans Administration Cooperative Urologic Research Group (VACURG) studies have been
misinterpreted. The limitations and qualifications were
clearly stated - results "pertain only to the initial treatment to which patients were assigned", some patients with
advanced disease "clearly do benefit" from DES, and many
patients "were not held indefinitely on the treatment originally assigned". In fact, more than 75% of protocol changes occurred in the placebo group. In the second VACURG study
patients with stage III disease given placebo had at 12 and
24 mos. a higher survival rate than those patients given DES
while in stage IV patients some benefit was noted with 1 mg.
The VACURG study proved that no overall increase in survival
was discerned when hormones were administered prophyllactic-
ally or therapeutically. The question of the effectiveness of
hormonal manipulation in increasing survival was not answered.

During the past 5 years there has been a resurgent interest in the use of cytotoxic chemotherapy for disseminated
prostatic cancer. Classic definitions of response employed
in Phase II disease-oriented trials have been expanded with
the use of the term "objective" response (32). Objective
response indicates that stabilization of disease is to be
considered a significant response since such patients have
a longer survival compared to nonresponders (progressors).
Since the natural history of prostatic cancer is variable,
the time interval from recognition of hormone failure to
initiation of cytotoxic chemotherapy becomes important. In
patients with slow growing disease, the "lead time", that is,
the time from diagnosis to cytotoxic drugs or from hormonal
failure to protocol, has been shortened, and in certain subsets of patients (i.e. slow growing disease) survival after
initiation of cytotoxic chemotherapy may appear to be prolonged. Many investigators use the National Prostatic Cancer Project response criteria, however, the inadequacies and
difficulties in evaluating response in this tumor are evidenced by the plethora of systems employed.

Single agents and combination regimens have been reported to induce "objective response" in 14 to 53% of cases
(Table 3) (2,32,28,41). However, when STAB is excluded

Table 3. Selected Chemotherapy Trials in Prostate Cancer

Drug	n	% Response	Drug	n	% Response
ADM	83	13*(30)	CTX	139	3 (28)
AMSA	19	0 (0)	+5-FU	41	2 (10)
CCNU	30	13 (33)	+ADM	92	12 (39)
DDP	91	22 (30)	+5-FU+ADM	21	0 (57)
DTIC	64	3 (22)	+5-FU+MTX	20	15 (35)
5-FU	74	7 (26)	Estracyst	265	7-15(51-83)
NCS	19	0 (0)	Stereocyst	71	1 (21)
MeCCNU		– (30)	Matulane	44	0 (29)
CTX ——125		– (35)	Streptozotocin	35	0 (29)
Hydrea		– (15)	Stereo + Estra	75	8 (28)
VCR – ~70+		– (18)	MTX+VCR+5-FU +	25	24 (72)
+Estra		– (27)	Melphalan+Pred		

* = "objective regression", CR+PR.

( ) = "objective response", CR+PR+ stabilization of disease.

remissions decrease < 10-20% (41,55). CTX, 5-FU, ADM and ADM containing regimens, and possibly DDP have exhibited some efficacy. The effectiveness of multi-drug regimens or adjuvant programs still require confirmation in prospective, randomized trials.

References:

1. Bodey GP: Current status of chemotherapy in metastatic renal cancer. In Johnson DE, Samuels ML (Eds): Cancer of the Genitourinary Tract. Raven Press, New York, 1979, pp 67-76.
2. Carter SK: Chemotherapy and genitourinary oncology. Cancer Treat Rev 5:85-93, 1978.
3. Cross RJ, Glashan RW, Humphrey CS et al: Treatment of advanced bladder cancer with adriamycin and 5-fluorouracil. Br J Urol 48:609-615, 1976.
4. DeKernion JB, Ramming KP: The therapy of renal adenocarcinoma with immune RNA. Invest Urol 17:378-381, 1980.
5. Duchek M, Edsmyr F, Naeslund I: 5-Fluorouracil in the treatment of recurrent cancer of the urinary bladder. In Pavone-Macaluso M, Smith H, Edsmyr F (Eds): Bladder Tumors and Other Topics in Urological Oncology. Plenum Press, New York, 1980, pp 381-385.

6. EORTC: The treatment of advanced carcinoma of the bladder with a combination of adriamycin and 5-fluorouracil. Eur Urol 3:276-278, 1977.

7. Exelby PR: Adrenal cortical carcinoma in a child. Clin Bull 5:26-31, 1975.

8. Frei E, Blum RH, Pitman SW, et al: High dose methotrexate with leucovorin rescue. Amer J Med 68:370-376, 1980.

9. Gad-el-Mawla N, Chevlen E, Hamza R, et al: Phase II trial of cis-dichlorodiammineplatinum (II) in cancer of the Bilharzial bladder. Cancer Treat Rep 63:1577-1578, 1979.

10. Hahn RG, Tempkin NR, Savlov ED, et al: Phase II study of vinblastine, methyl CCNU and medroxyprogesterone in advanced renal cell cancer. Cancer Treat Rep 62:1093-1095, 1978.

11. Hahn RG, Bauer M, Wolter J, et al: Phase II study of single agent therapy with megesterol acetate, VP-16-213, cyclophosphamide, and dianhydrogalactitol in advanced renal cell cancer. Cancer Treat Rep 63:513-515, 1979.

12. Hahn RG, Berg CB, Davis T: Phase II trial of vinblastine-CCNU, triazinate, and actinomycin D in advanced renal cell cancer. Cancer Treat Rep (in press).

13. Helson L, Wollner N, Murphy ML, et al: Metastatic adrenal cortical carcinoma. Clin Chem 17:1191-1193, 1971.

14. Herr H: Diamminedichloride platinum II in the treatment of advanced bladder cancer. J Urol 123:953-855, 1980.

15. Hogan TF, Citrin DL, Johnson BM, et al: o,p'-DDD (Mitotane) therapy of adrenal cortical carcinoma. Cancer 42:2177-2181, 1978.

16. Hogan TF, Gilchrist KW, Westring DW, et al: A clinical and pathological study of adrenocortical carcinoma. Cancer 45: 2880-2883, 1980.

17. Hurshesky, WJ, Murphy GP: Current status of the therapy of advanced renal carcinoma. J Surg Oncol 9:277-288, 1977.

18. Hutter AM, Kayhoe DE: Adrenal cortical carcinoma - Results of treatment with o,p'-DDD in 138 patients. Am J Med 41:581-592, 1966.

19. Huvos AG, Hadju SI, Basfield RD, et al: Adrenal cortical carcinoma - Cliniopathologic study of 34 cases. Cancer 25: 353-261, 1970.

20. Ichikawa T: Chemotherapy of penis cancer. In Grundmann E, Vahlensieck W (Eds): Tumors of the male genital system. Springer Verlag, Berlin, 1977, pp 140-156.

21. Izbicki R, Al-Sarraf M, Reed ML, et al: Further clinical trials with porfiromycin. Cancer Chemother Rep 56:615-624, 1972.

22. Knight WA, Livingston RB, Fabian C, et al: Phase I-II trial of methyl-GAG. Cancer Treat Rep 63:1933-1937, 1979.

23. Lupitz J, Freeman L, Okun R: Mitotane use in inoperable adrenal cortical carcinoma. JAMA 223:1109-1112, 1973.

24. Martinos, Samal B, Al-Sarraf M: Phase II study of 5-fluorouracil and adriamycin in transitional cell carcinoma of the urinary tract. Cancer Treat Rep 64:161-163, 1980.

25. Merrin CE: Treatment of genitourinary tumors with cis-dichlorodiammineplatinum (II): Can Tr Rep 63:1579-158, 1979.

26. Natale RB, Yagoda A, Watson RC, et al: Phase II trial of neocarcinostatin in patients with prostatic and bladder cancer. Cancer 45:2836-2842, 1980.

27. Nissen NI, Pajak TF, Leone LA, et al: Clinical trial of VP 16-213 (NSC 14150) i.v. twice weekly in advanced neoplastic disease. Cancer 45:232-235, 1980.

28. Oliver RTC: The place of chemotherapy in the treatment of patients with invasive carcinoma of the bladder. In Pavone-Macaluso M, Smith PH, Edsmyr F (Eds): Bladder Tumors and Other Topics in Urological Oncology. Plenum Press, New York, 1980, pp 381-385.

29. Rodriguez LH, Johnson DE, Holoye PY, et al: Combination VM-26 and adriamycin for metastatic transitional cell carcinoma. Cancer Treat Rep. 61:87-88, 1977.

30. Sakamoto S, Ogata J. Ikegami K, et al: Chemotherapy for bladder cancer with neocarcinostatin: Eur J Can 22: 103-112, 1980.

31. Samuels ML: CISCA combination chemotherapy. In Johnson DE, Samuels ML (Eds): 2nd Annual Conference on Cancer of the Genitourinary Tract. Raven Press, New York, 1979, pp 97-106.

32. Schmidt JD: Chemotherapy of hormone-resistant Stage D prostatic cancer. J Urol 123:797-805, 1980.

33. Schneider RJ, Woodcock TM, Yagoda A: Phase II trial of 4'-(9-acridinylamino)methanesulfon-m-anisidide (AMSA) in patients with metastatic hypernephroma. Can Tr Rep 64:183-185, 1980.

34. Schteingart DE, Cask R, Conn JW: Aminoglutethimide and metastatic adrenal cancer. JAMA 198:143-146, 1966.

35. Sklaroff RB, Yagoda A: Cis-diamminedichloride platinum II in the treatment of penile cancer. Cancer 44:1563-1565, 1979.

36. Sklaroff RB, Yagoda A: Methotrexate in the treatment of penile carcinoma. Cancer 45:2214-2216, 1980.

37. Sklaroff RB, Yagoda A: Chemotherapy of penile cancer. In Spiers AS (Ed): Chemotherapy and Urological Malignancy. Springer Verlag, Berlin (in press).

38. Smith PH: Medical management of prostatic cancer. Eur Urol 6:65-68, 1980.

39. Soloway MS: Cis-diamminedichloroplatinum (II) (DDP) in advanced bladder cancer. J Urol 120:716-719, 1978.

40. Todd RF, Garnick MR, Canellos GP: Chemotherapy of advanced renal adenocarcinoma with methyl-glyoxal bis-guanylhydrazone. Proc Am Assoc Cancer Res 21:340, 1980.

41. Torti FM, Carter SK: The chemotherapy of prostatic adenocarcinoma. Ann Intern Med 92:681-689, 1980.

42. Turner AG, Hendry WF, William GB, et al: The treatment of advanced bladder cancer with methotrexate. Br J Urol 49:673-678, 1977.

43. Wallace S, Chuang V, Green B, et al: Diagnostic radiology in renal carcinoma. In Johnson DE, Samuels ML (Eds): Cancer of the Genitourinary Tract. Raven Press, New York, 1979, pp 33-45.

44. Williams SD, Einhorn LH, Donohue JP: Cis-platinum combination chemotherapy of bladder cancer. Cancer Clin Trials Cancer Chemotherapy 2:355-358, 1979.

45. Wortsman J, Soler NG: Mitotane-spironolactone antagonism in Cushing's syndrome. JAMA 238:2527-2528, 1977.

46. Yagoda A: Non-hormonal cytotoxic agents in the treatment of prostatic adenocarcinoma. Cancer 38:388-394, 1973.

47. Yagoda A: Future implications of phase II chemotherapy trials in ninety-five patients with measurable advanced bladder cancer. Cancer Res 37:2275-2280, 1977.

48. Yagoda A: Chemotherapy of metastatic bladder cancer. Cancer 45: 1879-1888, 1980.

49. Yagoda A. Macchia RJ: Antineoplastic chemotherapy of genitourinary cancer. In Nealon TF (Ed): Management of the Patient with Cancer. Saunders, Philadelphia, 1976, pp 601-632.

50. Yagoda A, Watson RC, Whitmore WF: Phase II trial of methotrexate in bladder cancer. Proc Am Assoc Cancer Res 21:427, 1980.

51. Yagoda A, Watson RC, Gonzalez-Vitale JC, et al: Cis-dichloro-diammineplatinum (II) in advanced bladder cancer. Cancer Treat Rep 60:917-923, 1976.

52. Yagoda A, Watson RC, Grabstald H, et al: Adriamycin and cyclophosphamide in advanced bladder cancer. Cancer Treat Rep 61:97-99, 1977.

53. Yagoda A, Watson RC, Whitmore WF, et al: Adriamycin in

advanced urinary tract cancer. Cancer 39:279-285, 1977.

54. Yagoda A, Watson RC, Kemeny N, et al: Diamminedichloride platinum II and cyclophosphamide in the treatment of advanced urothelial cancer. Cancer 41:2121-2130, 1978.

55. Yagoda A, Watson RC, Natale RB, et al: A critical analysis of response criteria in patients with prostatic cancer treated with cis-diamminedichloride platinum II. Cancer 44: 1553-1562, 1979.

56. Yagoda A, Watson RC, Blumenreich R, et al: Phase II trials in urothelial tumors with AMSA and PALA. Proc Amer Assoc Cancer Res 21:427, 1980.

57. Zeffren J, Yagoda A, Watson RC, et al: Phase II trial of methyl-glyoxal bis-guanylhydrazone in advanced renal cancer. Cancer Treat Rep (in press).

58. Zeffren J, Yagoda A: Chemotherapy of adrenal cortical carcinoma. In Spiers AS (Ed): Chemotherapy and Urological Malignancy. Springer Verlag, Berlin (in press).

Cancers of The Stomach,
Pancreas and Large Bowel

PHILIP S. SCHEIN

Professor of Medicine & Pharmacology
Georgetown University School of Medicine
Vincent T. Lombardi Cancer Researrch Center
Washington, D.C.   20007 USA

FREDERICK P. SMITH

Assistant Professor of Medicine
Georgetown University School of Medicine

PAUL V. WOOLLEY, III
Associate Professor of Medicine & Pharmacology
Georgetown University School of Medicine

JOHN NEEFE
Assistant Professor of Medicine
Georgetown University School of Medicine

PATRICK J. BYRNE
Instructor in Medicine
Georgetown University School of Medicine
Vincent T. Lombardi Cancer Research Center
Washington, D.C.   20007 USA

INTRODUCTION

Malignant disease of the gastrointestinal tract has
in the past been the leading cause of cancer death in the
United States, although it has recently been surpassed in
frequency by cancers of the lung due to the rising
incidence of these tumors in smoking women. Nevertheless

despite the importance of gastrointestinal cancer as an
international health problem, only in the past six years
has there been adequate effort to define the role of
non-surgical therapies. These tumors have been perceived
as resistant to cytotoxic drugs and to radiation therapy
and this preconception, coupled with difficulties in each
diagnoses have dampened the enthusiasm of clinical
investigations. Because of the renewed interest in these
important cancer there exists a new and growing base of
therapeutic information which defines the importance of
combination chemotherapy and combined modality treatment.
This review of the three major organ sites must be regarded
as only a progress report, but it will serve to emphasize
that more can be accomplished than had previously been considered possible and that continued intensive research is
essential.

GASTRIC CANCER

        Gastric cancer is the most responsive of the gastro-
intestinal adenocarcinomas to chemotherapy (1). While only
a few drugs have been adequately evaluated, response rates
ranging from 10% to 25% have been established for 5-fluoro-
uracil (5-FU), doxorubicin (Adriamycin), mitomycin-C and
the chloroethyl nitrosoureas BCNU and methyl CCNU (2).
Single agent therapy, however, produces responses of brief
duration and there is little impact on patient survival.
The most important recent development in the chemotherapy
of advanced gastric cancer is the demonstration that
adriamycin containing drug combinations produce a significant increase in therapeutic activity over single agents.

COMBINATION CHEMOTHERAPY IN ADVANCED DISEASE

        The drug regimens that have been used for metastatic
gastric carcinoma have all employed 5-FU in combination
with either nitrosoureas, adriamycin and/or mitomycin.
Kovach et al (3) have reported the results of a randomized
trial comparing 5-FU or BCNU as single agents, or in
combination. The regimen of 5-FU plus BCNU produced a
higher response rate (41%) than either 5-FU or BCNU used
alone (29% and 17% respectively). Survival for patients
treated with BCNU alone was inferior to that of the other
two treatment groups, and was essentially identical to an
untreated historical control. Superior survival with the
combination was observed at 18 months of follow-up with 25%
alive versus 10% with the single drugs. A subsequent study

from the Eastern Cooperative Oncology Group (ECOG) reported that the combination of 5-FU and methyl-CCNU was superior in both response rate and survival to methyl-CCNU alone (4); in addition, the latter drug produced only an 8% response rate in this trial, compared to 40% with the combination.

Based upon these data the ECOG undertook a three-arm, randomized study, which compared the former regimen of 5-FU and methyl-CCNU with a combination of 5-FU and mitomycin or adriamycin as a single agent. Patients treated with 5-FU plus mitomycin-C achieved a response rate of 32% whereas 5-FU and methyl-CCNU produced objective responses in 24%, lower than that previously recorded by this same group. This modest response rate for the latter combination has been confirmed in a trial conducted by the Gastrointestinal Tumor Study Group (5). In patients who had not received prior chemotherapy, a 22% response rate was obtained with adriamycin.

Buroker et al (6) have reported results of the Southwest Oncology Group's randomized trial comparing 5-FU given in a continuous 96 hour infusion with either intra-venous mitomycin-C or oral methyl-CCNU. Responses were seen in only six of 43 (14%) patients treated with the former combination, compared to 5 of 54 (9%) treated with the 5-FU plus methyl-CCNU.

Ota et al in Japan (7) and DeJager et al from the Memorial Sloan Kettering Cancer Center (8) have conducted trials with the combination of 5-FU, mitomycin-C and cytosine arabinoside (FMC). In the former trial, a 55% response rate was reported. The GITSG undertook a compara-tive study of a similar combination versus Adriamycin alone and the combination of 5-FU, Adriamycin and methyl-CCNU (FAMe) (9). The FMC regimen employed in this study produced a disappointing 17% response rate in patients with no prior chemotherapy, but the authors note that the dose schedule was different from that employed in the Japanese and MSKCC Studies. The activity of single agent Adriamycin for gastric cancer was confirmed with objective responses recorded in 24% of patients with advanced measurable tumor. FAMe produced objective responses in 47% of pre-viously untreated cases. Furthermore, patients treated with FAMe had statistically better survival and a longer time to disease progression than did those treated with FMC or with Adriamycin alone.

In 1974 the Division of Medical Oncology at the Vincent T. Lombardi Cancer Research Center initiated a Phase II trial of a combination of the three most active

drugs for gastric cancer, 5-fluorouracil, Adriamycin and
mitomycin-C (FAM). In this regimen, 5-FU 600 mg/m^2 was
administered i.v. on weeks 1,2,5 and 6, Adriamycin
30mg/m^2 i.v. on weeks 1 and 5, and mitomycin-C 10mg/m^2
i.v. week 1 only. This schedule for mitomycin-C was chosen
in recognition of the delayed and cumulative bone marrow
toxicity of this agent, and the cycle was repeated every 2
months. A response rate of 43% was recorded in 62 patients
with advanced measurable disease (10). Responders evidenced a median survival of 12.5 months compared to 3.5
months for non-responders, a statistically significant
improvement. FAM was well tolerated with mild to moderate
myelosuppression as the main dose-limiting toxicity.
Bitran et al have presented confirmatory data employing a
slightly modified FAM regimen and achieving a 55% response
rate with significant survival benefit for responders
(11). The activity of FAM has further been substantiated
by a randomized study performed by the Southwest Oncology
Group (SWOG) which compared the FAM regimen to a sequential
schedule of the same three drugs (12). A total of 123
patients with advanced metastatic disease were evaluated.
Responses were recorded in 44% of those treated with the
original FAM regimen compared to 27% of those treated
sequentially with the same three drugs (13). For advanced
gastric cancer, FAM has become the standard of comparison
for advanced stages of disease. Phase III comparative
protocols with FAM are now in progress in several cooperative groups, and this regimen is now being evaluated as a
surgical adjuvant therapy.

At the Vincent T. Lombardi Center, we have recently
initiated a Phase II trial of a new combination of
5-fluorouracil, adriamycin and cis-diamminedichloroplatinum (FAP). The inclusion of cis-platin is based upon
the findings of LaCave et al who report objective tumor
regression in 5 of 19 patients with advanced gastric cancer
who had previously been treated with multiagent therapy
(14). In addition, Magill et al. had obtained responses in
3 of 12 patients with gastric cancer treated with cisplatin and anhydro-ara-5-fluorocytidine (15). Lastly,
there are suggestions of synergy between adriamycin and
cis-platin in both in vitro and in vivo studies (16).

In summary, the introduction of Adriamycin into
combination with 5-FU for gastric cancer has resulted in a
tangible improvement in patient response. This is
supported by the results achieved with the FAM program, as
well as with FAMe and the combination of 5-FU, adriamycin
and BCNU (FAB) which produced a 52% response rate in a

recently reported Phase II trial (17).

LOCALLY UNRESECTABLE GASTRIC CANCER

This stage of gastric cancer encompasses those cases in which local tumor extension into a lymph nodes or adjacent organs precludes complete en bloc surgical resection. In practical therapeutic terms, the residual cancer can be encompassed within a moderate sized radiation port. Falkson et al. (18) studied the combined use of radiation therapy and 5-FU for patients with locally unresectable gastric cancer. They reported an objective improvement in 55% of patients, treated with the combination, while none were improved with radiation alone, and only 17% responded to 5-FU. Subsequently, the Mayo Clinic reported a controlled trial of combined modality therapy for patients with locally unresectable gastric cancer (19). All patients received a radiation dose of 3500-4000 rads. By random selection, half of the patients received 5-FU at a daily dose of 15mg/kg for 3 days. The median survival of patients treated with the combination was approximately 7 months versus 5 months for irradiation alone. There was, however, a significant increase in mean survival of the radiation/5-FU group compared to radiation alone (13.0 vs 5.9 months respectively), with 3 patients (12%) alive at 5 years.

The Gastrointestinal Tumor Study Group has subsequently undertaken a randomized trial to compare the value of chemotherapy alone to combined radiation and chemotherapy for locally advanced gastric cancer (20). One group received intravenous 5-FU, 325mg/m^2 on days 1-5 and 375mg/m^2 on days 36-40 combined with methyl-CCNU, 150 mg, orally on day 1, all repeated in 10 week cycles. The combined modality group received irradiation in 2 courses of 2500 rad, each given over 3 weeks and separated by a 2 week rest period. This was accompanied by intravenous 5-FU, 500mg/m^2 for the first 3 days of each radiation course. The latter group was then placed on maintenance chemotherapy with the same 5-FU plus methyl-CCNU regimen. The initial analysis of this demonstrated improved survival and patient tolerance for the chemotherapy alone group. In a recent update of this study, median survival for the chemotherapy alone group remains favorable - 70 weeks compared to 36 weeks for the combined modality group (20). The difference is accounted for by an increase in early toxicity and hematologic and nutritional complications, as well as tumor-related deaths in the combined modality

group. Interestingly, approximately 20% of two arms of the
survival curves have now crossed, and demonstrate a long
term survival advantage for patietns who received combined
modality. In contrast, patients who received chemotherapy
alone have shown a continuing probablity for tumor relapse
of their disease. In addition, palliative resection of the
primary tumor improves the survival results with both forms
of postoperative treatment. This result can be improved by
reducing the toxicity of upper abdominal radiation therapy,
more careful attention to nutrition and the use of a more
effective form of chemotherapy.

ADJUVANT THERAPY OF GASTRIC CANCER

        The value of adjuvant chemotherapy in high-risk
surgically resected patients remains to be demonstrated.
The few published studies have consisted largely of
short-term single-agent therapy with Thiotepa (a drug
without known efficacy for this tumor), mitomycin-C or
5-fluorodeoxoyuridine (21-23). Nakajima, et al have
reported a possible benefit to a short course of
combination chemotherapy with 5-FU, mitomycin-C and
cytosine arabinoside followed by oral 5-FU or Ftorafur,
when compared to a control group (24). Disease free
survival at 36 months was 71% and 61% respectively for the
treated groups compared to 58% for the controls. There was
no statistical analysis provided. The GITSG and the ECOG
are presently evaluating a randomized trial of 5-FU plus
methyl-CCNU compared to control in the adjuvant setting of
gastric cancer. With the demonstration of improved
efficacy of the Adriamycin containing regimens, such as
FAM, in advanced gastric cancer, these combinations are now
being evaluated in randomized trials by the CALGB and the
SWOG as adjuvant therapy for patients with gastric cancer
who remain at high risk for relapse because of serosal or
lymph node involvement. It must be emphasized the response
rate and duration now being achieved with combination
chemotherapy for advanced gastric cancer are equivalent to
that in metastatic breast cancer, where such treatment in
the adjuvant setting made an apparent impending impact on
survival.

PANCREATIC CANCER

        In the past few years, several extensive reviews of
the chemotherapy of pancreatic cancer have stressed the
need for renewed interest in systematic investigation of

therapy for this disease and in particular the evaluation of newly developed anticancer agents (25,26). The incidence of this malignancy has been rising over the past four decades, and it now ranges as the fourth most common cause of cancer death in the United States. Less than 10-15% of patients are resectable for "cure"; and even with "curative" surgery less than 4% of resected cases survive 5 years. Consequently chemotherapy or combined-modality therapy will of necessity play an important role in attempt to improve the care of these patients. There are very few single chemotherapeutic agents that have been studied, 5-FU has been the most extensively investigated agent in all gastrointestinal malignancies and pancreatic cancer presents no exception. Although response rates recorded with the use of this agent vary, a 20% figure is most frequently encountered (86). Other agents with limited effectiveness include adriamycin, streptozotocin and mitomycin-C with response rates varying from 10-20% (26). In the chloroethylnitrosoureas, BCNU and methyl-CCNU have negligible activity (26). Despite the limited number of agents for the design of drug combinations, several regimens have been evaluated.

Kovach et al in a randomized study compared 5-FU by continuous infusion with BCNU alone and with the combination of 5-FU plus BCNU (27). Eighty-two patients with advanced pancreatic carcinoma were randomized to one of these three treatment regimens; sixteen percent of the patients treated with 5-FU alone evidenced an objective response, but 0 of 21 cases responded to BCNU alone. Nevertheless, it was found that 10 of 30 patients treated with the combination achieved an objective response. However, there was no survival benefit when patients treated with the combination were compared with either of the single agent groups. Lokich and Skarin administered 5-FU and BCNU in combination (28). They obtained 27% objective responses, and responding patients had a longer median survival than non-responders.

Buroker and colleagues studied two regimens of 5-FU administered by continuous intravenous infusion (29), with either mitomycin-C or methyl-CCNU. One hundred and forty-four patients with advanced measurable pancreatic carcinoma were randomized. The combination of 5-FU and mitomycin-C produced a response rate of 30%, which was statistically superior to the 17% response rate observed with the nitrosourea combination.

The three drugs with the highest reported single agent activity are: streptozotocin, 5-FU, and

mitomycin-C. The Vincent T. Lombardi Cancer Research
Center of Georgetown University developed a combination of
these three drugs (SMF) which was used in the treatment of
23 consecutive patients with advanced measurable pancreatic
cancer (30). Forty-three percent of the patients demonstrated an objective response and one patient with biopsy
proven hepatic metastases achieved a complete remission for
more than four years from initiation of SMF therapy. The
median survival of all cases was 6 months, but responders
achieved a median survival of 10 months, while non-
responders survived only 3 months. The majority of
patients in this study were of good performance status,
that is, asymptomatic or symptomatic but ambulatory. Only
three of 23 patients were bedridden greater than 50% of the
time. The good performance status of the patients in this
trial stands in contrast to most other treatment series
which have included patients that were near bedridden or
jaundiced from hepatic metastases.

The activity of the SMF regimen at the Vincent T.
Lombardi Cancer Research Center have been confirmed (31).
At the Cleveland Clinic, Aberhalden et al had described a
series of 16 patients treated with a similiar regimen; 5-FU
was given as a loading course, $500mg/m^2$/day IV x 5;
streptozotocin was given $300mg/m^2$/day IV x 5; and
mitomycin-C was given $10mg/m^2$ IV on day 1. The cycle was
repeated every eight weeks. An objective response was
recorded and 31% of the patients treated, and the three
drug combination was superior to the two drug combination
of 5-FU and streptozotocin.

Following the demonstration that Adriamycin had
independent activity for advanced pancreatic cancer (32),
the Vincent T. Lombardi Cancer Research Center initiated a
study of the FAM regimen in this disease (33). This
combination had previously been evaluated in advanced
gastric cancer, with a response rate of 43% (20). Thirty-
nine patients with pancreatic cancer have been treated with
this regimen; twenty-seven of the patients were evaluable
for response. Ten of the 27 (37%) achieved a partial
response with a median survival of 12 months compared to 3
months in non-responders ($p<0.01$).

Bitran, et al, have since confirmed the activity of
analogous FAM regimen (11). Six of 15 patients with
pancreatic cancer obtained partial tumor regression with a
median survival in responders in excess of 13 months. The
FAM regimen is currently being further evaluated in Phase
III trials by the Cancer and Acute Leukemia Group B (CALGB)
and GITSG.

The Cleveland Clinic have reported on 18 patients with localized and disseminated pancreatic cancer who were treated with the FAM regimen, to which streptozotocin was added (34). Six responses (33%) and three cases with disease stablization (17%) were recorded.

LOCALLY ADVANCED DISEASE

Combined modality therapy of locally advanced pancreatic cancer has been the standard form of therapy for this stage of disease since the demonstration by Moertel and Childs that the addition of 5-fluorouracil to 3500-4500 rads of split course regional radiation could result in improved patient survival (35).

A subsequent report by Haslam et al suggested that a higher dose of regional irradiation, 6000 rads, by split course was more effective. However, many of the patients in this study had also received chemotherapy (36).

The Gastrointestinal Tumor Study Group has substantiated the benefit of combined modality therapy in a randomized study comparing 5-FU plus 4000 rad or 6000 rad to 6000 rad administered alone (37). One hundred and six patients with higtologically confirmed carcinoma of the pancreas have been evaluated in this three arm study. Radiation was delivered in 2000 rad courses given over two-week periods separated by two-weeks rest intervals. In the two groups receiving 5-fluorouracil, 500mg/m^2 IV was given on the first three days of each 2000 rad course. Both 4000 rad + 5-FU and 6000 rad + 5-FU produced a significantly longer survival than 6000 rad alone. Survivals were 36 weeks, 40 weeks and 20 weeks respectively. Thus the combined modality approach of 5-FU plus irradiation must now be the standard of comparison in this stage of pancreatic cancer. However, relatively few patients survive as long as two years, and local control remains an important problem. With the encouraging albeit results of combination chemotherapy in advanced disease, it would appear warranted to conduct comparative trials of such therapy alone, as well as in combined modality treatment for locally advanced disease.

The combination of 5-FU and fast neutron therapy has been evaluated at the Vincent T. Lombardi Cancer Research Center in cooperation with the Mid-Atlantic Neutron Association Therapy (38). Nineteen patients with locally advanced pancreatic carcinoma were treated with 1716 rads of 15 MEV neutrons with and without 5-FU. The intent of this study was to exploit the theoretic advantages of

neutrons, viz. their higher radiobiologic effectiveness and
linear energy transfer and the lower oxygen enhancement
ratio. The median survival of all patients was 6 months
and is less than that reported with 5-fluorouracil and
conventional photon irradiation. Gastrointestinal toxicity
was considerable, hemorrhagic gastritis in 5 patients,
colitis in 2, and 1 patient developed radiation myelitis.
With this toxicity and lack of therapeutic advantage of
neutron we caution any enthusiasm for this treatment
modality in the management of locally advanced pancreatic
cancer.

There is now considerable interest in the use of
interstitial radiation therapy, and in particular with
Iodine - 125 because of its physical characteristics. This
isotope decreases the level of exposure to hospital
personnel and also permits a sharp limit of the high-dose
volume of the absorbed radiation to within the implanted
volume. This allows for the safe delivery of external beam
radiation therapy to the tumor bed and regional lymph
nodes. Shipley et al, have conducted a pilot study to
evaluate the efficacy of intraoperative Iodine-125 implantation in combination with postoperative external beam
radiation therapy (4000-4500 rad) (39). The projected
median survival was 11 months, with 4 of the 12 patients
still surviving at the time of this report. While local
control was improved, distant metastases remain on important problem emphasizing the need for systemic chemotherapy.

Intraoperative electron beam irradiation is
undergoing an evaluation in the joint Howard
University-Georgetown University Cancer Center Program, as
well as at the Massachusetts General Hospital. This
approach allows for the single delivery of 1000-3000 rads
of electrons to a carefully design field which prevents
injury to the bowel. An electron energy can be chosen
which allows for penetration into the tumor, while sparing
the spinal cord and major blood vessels, this technique is
best performed in specialized centers will have a linear
accelerator in an operating room, is at the Howard
University Medical Center in Washington, D.C.

Adjuvant Therapy

There is no information available on the surgical
adjuvant management of the relatively few patients with
pancreatic cancer who had undergone a resection with
curative intent. The majority of these patients are at

great risks for recurrence when one considers a four
percent five year survival.

COLORECTAL CANCER

Colorectal cancer represents the second leading
cause of death in both males and females. One hundred and
twelve thousand new cases of colorectal cancer were diagnosed in 1979, and approximately one-half of this group
will die from disseminated disease. While early diagnosis
and surgical management remain the most important factor
for improving these statistics, there remains an important
need to develop an effective postoperative therapy for the
Dukes B_2 and C cases.

ADVANCED DISEASE

5-Fluorouracil has been the most extensively studied
antineoplastic agent in colorectal cancer with responses
recorded in approximately 20% of cases. Intravenous 5-FU
has been demonstrated to be superior to oral 5-FU, hepatic
artery infusions has failed to produce a significant
increased response or survival compared to intravenous
therapy for patients with hepatic metastases (40).
The value of combination chemotherapy for advanced
colorectal cancer remains to be established. Moertel and
co-workers reported the results of a controlled clinical
trial in which the combination of 5-FU, methyl-CCNU and
vincristine was compared to 5-FU as a single agent (41).
The combination produced a 43.5% response rate compared to
5-FU alone at 19%; however, there was no survival benefit.
Subsequent trials of 5-FU plus methyl-CCNU with and without
vincristine combinations, unfortunately, have failed to
uphold the initial encouraging activity of this multiagent
therapy in colorectal cancer (42-45).
Kemeny, et al at the Memorial-Sloan Kettering Cancer
Center attempted to improve patient tolerance to he 5-FU,
methyl-CCNU, vincristine combination (MOF) by administering
the nitrosourea in a daily schedule (i.e. 30 mg/m^2/day
p.o. x5) and compared this to the conventional regimen of
single nitrosourea dosage (45). The response rates of the
two schedules were identical and disappointing, 11-12%. Of
note, however, was the finding that the daily times five
schedule of methyl-CCNU was better tolerated with reduced
nausea and vomiting.

These investigators have now reported the results of adding streptozotocin, a naturally occurring methylnitrosourea, to the latter MOF schedule (46). 5-FU was administered at a dose of 300 mg/m^2 i.v. daily x5; vincristine at a dose of 1 mg i.v. every 5 weeks; methyl-CCNU 30 mg/m^2/day x5 orally and streptozotocin 500 mg/m^2 i.v. weekly, MOF-streptozotocin. The criteria for objective partial tumor regression were strict and included a 50% of greater decrease in the sum of three distinct measurements of the liver span. Minor responses were a less than 50% but greater than 25% reduction in the above measurements. Of 54 patients treated, 33% achieved an objective response, and 25% a minor response. The MOF-streptozotocin regimen has now been compared to MOF in a prospectively randomized controlled trial at the same institution with further demonstration of the superiority of MOF-streptozotocin regimen. Confirmatory studies are in progress by the GITSG.

Adjuvant Treatment

Large bowel cancer has been one of the most extensively invstigated malignancies in regard to therapy; however relatively little progress has been made as is reflected in the rather static survival statistics over the past 3-4 decades. It is for this reason that a major emphasis in clinical research has been directed toward surgical adjuvant therapy, an approach which was first evaluated in the late 1950's.

This experience in the treatment of colorectal cancer has resulted in an appreciation of some of the major prognostic variables which serve to identify patients at high risk for relapse (47). A heavy emphasis has been given to the Dukes' classification which correlated the degree of penetration of he colonic wall and involvement of lymph nodes with ultimate survival prospects. This classification system has undergone a series of adaptions and at the present time the Astler-Coller modification is the most widely accepted. Patients with tumor that has invaded through the muscularis and serosa, or spread to lymph nodes have a relatively poor prognosis, with an approximate 10-50% 5-year survival after surgical resection with curative intent. While experience differs from center to center, this population with B$_2$ and C disease represent a substantial proportion of all cases of colorectal cancer, in the range of 70-80%. The number of involved lymph nodes as well as their location relative to the primary tumor also has significance for survival. Recently, several studies have shown that the pre-operative CEA concentration functions as an independent prognostic variable that complements the Dukes' classification; patients with a CEA greater than 5ng/ml demonstrate an inverse relationship between the elevated level of this plasma tumor marker and the time to tumor recurrence (48).

Despite an enormous effort extending over a 20-year period it can be safely stated that surgical adjuvant chemotherapy has failed to make a significant impact on survival for this high risk group of patients. This experience stands in direct contrast with the gains that have been recently achieved in breast cancer for patients with nodal metastases. The first controlled clinical trials in colorectal cancer involved the use of an alkylating agent, Thio-Tepa. In these studies, initiated in 1957 the Veterans Administration Surgical Adjuvant Group, resected patients received either chemotherapy or placebo. In the original protocol Thio-Tepa, 0.2mg/kg, was administered intraperitoneally and intravenously in the operating room, followed by two additional doses on the first and second post-operative days. Because of suspected increased postoperative mortality in treated cases, the intraoperative intravenous dose was discontinued. Between 1957 and 1961, 1,064 patients who underwent curative resection was entered onto the program. The overall results favored the placebo group which had a 57% 5-year survival compared to 50% for thio-Tepa treatment. An independent study, with similar results, was reported by the University Hospitals group.

Following the identification of the fluorinated pyrimidines, 5-FU and FUdR, as a class of agents capable of producing objective regressions in advanced disease, attention was directed toward the use of these drugs in the surgical adjuvant setting (49,50). An initial controlled trial using 5-fluorodeoxyuridine given at time of operation and in the immediate post-operative period in a manner similar to the Thio-Tepa study similarly failed to produce an improvement in 5-year survival.

The next trials in colon cancer undertaken by the Veterans' Administration Surgical Adjuvant Group employed 5-FU, but delayed drug administration until two weeks following operation. Patients were randomized to receive chemotherapy consisting of 5-FU, 12 mg/kg, for 4 consecutive days with single repeat course in 7 weeks, or no further therapy. At 5 years of followup the survival of the 308 patients in the curative resection group was 59%

for those receiving 5-FU compared to 49% in controls. This
difference was not statistically significant. Similarly
small non-significant improvements in survival were noted
in the patients who had undergone only palliative resections.
    The second controlled trial with 5-FU conducted by
the Veterans Group was designed to study the efficacy of
prolonged intermittent courses of chemotherapy. In this
study patients with colorectal cancer who were considered
to have a poor prognosis based upon a histologic review of
the resected specimen were randomized to receive 5-FU or no
further treatment. 5-FU was administered at a dose of 12
mg/kg i.v. for 4 successive days. The first course was
given two weeks following operation and repeated at 6-8
weeks intervals until the 19th postoperative month, or 12
courses. Between 1969-1973 522 patients who had undergone
a curative resection were entered into the trial. The
results of this study have recently been analyzed. They
demonstrate no significant improvement in 5-year survival
with 5-FU treatment, 49% versus 44% for the control group.
In addition, 163 patients had resection with proven
residual disease were also randomized. Survival at 18
months was 38% in the treated group compared to 26% in
controls - again not a statistically significant
difference.
    It has been demonstrated that optimal response rates
for 5-FU in colorectal cancer require that a moderate
degree of myelosuppressive toxicity be produced. One of
the criticisms of the VA prolonged intermitent therapy
study was that over 75% of the patients failed to develop
leukopenia during the 19 months of treatment.
    A somewhat more intensive trial of 5-FU adjuvant
chemotherapy has been conducted by the Central Oncology
Group (51). Patients undergoing curative or palliative
resection were randomized to receive 5-FU chemotherapy or
no further treatment until relapse. 5-FU was administered
intravenously using a dose-schedule of 12 mg/kg daily for 4
days followed by 6 mg/kg on alternate days for 4 additional
doses. Following a 7-14 day rest, weekly maintenance
chemotherapy 12 mg/kg was continued for one year. In
contrast to the VA study, 60% of patients developed some
degree of leukopenia. A total of 372 patients had been
entered on this study, of which 81% were acceptable for
analysis, including 92 patients with Dukes' B, and 97
patients with Dukes' C colorectal cancer who had undergone
surgical resections with curative intent. A significant
increase in disease-free interval was demonstrated for

patients with Dukes' C cancer treated with 5-FU who demonstrated a median relapse free interval of 24 months versus 16 months control. However, there was no significant improvement in survival when compared to control.

The prognostic importance of drug induced leukopenia was also analyzed. The disease-free interval is significantly longer for patients in whom the white blood cell count dropped below 4,000, but this made no impact on survival.

Taylor, et al have recently reported their follow-up on a trial of adjuvant continuous infusion of 5-fluoro-uracil by umbilical vein catheter (52). Patients were randomized to receive either 5-FU, 1,000 mg/day by umbilical vein catheter (53). Patients were randomized to receive either 5-FU, 1,000 mg/day by umbilical vein infusion along with 5,000 units of heparin for 7 days, or no additional postoperative therapy. Dukes' stages B and C as well as A lesions were included and appeared to be evenly distributed between the two groups. Most patients received liver scans and none had intraoperative evidence of metastases to the liver. Ninety patients (47 control, 43 perfusion) are currently evaluable with a mean follow-up of 25 months. Twenty-three of 47 patients have died in the control group compared to 7/43 in the perfusion group. The control group had 5 patients with liver metastases only, 8 with liver metastases plus other sites and 7 with local recurrence only, whereas the perfusion group had one patient, one patient and 4 patients in the treated group (p=0.01). Patients with Dukes' C lesions benefited most: 17 in the control group have died compared to 5 in the treatment arm. Five patients developed transient granulo-cytopenia ($<$ 3,500) and 3 patients thrombocytopenia ($<$ 60,000), which returned to normal after completion of infusion. There was one death from sepsis in the treated group. There was also transient elevation of liver function tests seen in both. This is an ongoing study and further followup will be necessary to confirm the results. Local control has not been as effective and the addition of peripheral systemic 5-FU for maintenance needs to be studied.

In summary, the use of peripheral intravenous single agent 5-FU in the adjuvant setting of colon cancer cannot be defended, and new approaches are required. In 1975 the Gastrointestinal Tumor Study Group (GITSG) initiated a prospective controlled trial comparing 5-FU + meCCNU + MER, and a control group for patients with Dukes' B_2 + C colon

cancer. A total of 566 eligible patients were randomized
by August, 1979 when the study was closed to accession.
The recurrence rates as of September, 1980 are unexpec-
tantly low, 10% of Dukes' B_2, 29% of C,and 50% of C_2,
for an overall recurrence of only 25%. There is no
significant difference in recurrence between any of the
four treatment options, including surgery alone. The
survival statistics closely parallel recurrences, with no
significant difference between treatment groups. The
relatively low recurrence and survival from surgery alone
compared to NCI-ACS statistics, emphasized the continued
need for carefully controlled randomized trials, which
include a non-treatment control group.
        In summary, adjuvant chemotherapy of resected colon
cancer remains to be demonstrated to be of significant
benefit.

Rectal Cancer

        Rectal cancer requires some special consideration
the potential role of radiation therapy. There is little
question that rectal cancer is sensitive to radiation
therapy. Effective symptomatic palliation and objective
regression locally unresectable and recurrent disease can
be effected in nearly 80% of patients. However, almost 10%
of such cases achieve long-term benefit. As with chemotherapy, there is reason to believe that radiation therapy
might be maximally effective in the surgical adjuvant
setting, with a patient with minimal residual disease.
        Gunderson and Socci have reported a valuable
analysis of areas of failure found at reoperation following
curative resection for rectal cancer (53). Of 75 patients
with Dukes' B_2 and C, 52 were found to have recurrent
tumor. Distant metastasis as a sole expression of relapse
was an uncommon finding and was demonstrated in only 7% of
cases. However, local failure and regional lymph node
metastases occurred frequently, as the only site of failure
in approximately 48% of cases and as a component in a 92%.
This pattern of failure was predictable based upon
anatomical factors, specifically the direct extension of
the tumor to contiguous tissues and organs, and lymphatic
drainage patterns: the upper rectum drains to lymph nodes
which follow the superior hemorrhoidal and inferior
mesenteric arteries. The latter vessel inserts into the
aorta at about the level of L2. The lower rectum drains
inferiorly to the internal iliac nodes.

The importance of this study is the demonstration
that a high percentage of surgical failures in rectal
cancer occur in an anatomic distribution that is readily
encompassed in a pre- or postoperative radiation port.

The rationale for preoperative radiation therapy has
been discussed by Higgins and Kligerman, who have been the
strongest proponents for this approach. The largest single
experience with preoperative radiation as a surgical
adjuvant for rectal cancer has been reported by Memorial
Hospital. Between 1937 and 1951 1,276 cases including 396
Dukes' C were treated preoperatively at dose levels of
1,500-2,000 rads. In a non-randomized comparison 37% who
received radiation therapy were alive at 5 years compared
to 27% for a non-irradiated group (54).

A subsequent randomized study performed at the same
institution failed to demonstrate any survival benefit with
radiation (55). In addition, it can be seen that in both
studies radiation therapy did not alter the relative
incidence of Dukes' C cases, a claim that is now being made
in several other studies.

In 1964 the VA Surgical Adjuvant Group initiated a
randomized controlled trial of 2,000 rads preoperative
radiation to a pelvic port followed by surgery. A total of
700 patients were entered into the study (56,57). There
was no difference in the operability or resectable rate in
the treated and control groups. For the 453 patients in
whom a "curative" resection was possible the 5-year
survival was 49% for treated versus 39% for controls. The
difference was not statistically different. The data were
also analyzed for the type of operation performed: 414
patients under an abdominoperineal resection. The 5-year
survival for radiation treatment was 41% which was significantly different from the 38% for controls. However,
when this group is broken down to curative resection (no
gross evidence of residual disease, or Dukes' C cases), the
result is no longer statistically valid. In addition,
there was no observed difference in survival when resection
other than the abdominoperineal approach were employed,
for higher lesions above the peritoneal reflection. The
five year survival of 39% was identical for the treated and
the control groups.

The VA study did find a reduction in involved lymph
nodes in resection in patients who received preoperative
radiation therapy - 28% Dukes' C versus 41% in the control
group. Similar data have been reported by Kligerman using
a dose of 4,500 rads in 5 weeks comparing the expected
incidence of Dukes' C cases previously found at Yale-New

Haven Hospital, and at the University of Oregon using 5,000
rads in using retrospective controls.

In 1975, the GITSG initiated a four arm controlled
randomized trial in postoperative rectal carcinomas of
stages B_2 and C. The three treatment arms were a)
radiation therapy 4,000 rads alone; b) chemotherapy with
5-FU and MeCCNU for 18 months; c) radiaton therapy with
5-FU sensitization followed by 5-FU and MeCCNU. These were
compared to the use of surgery alone. As of September
1980, 189 patients have been analyzed and there have been
70 recurrence (37%). An inferior arm of this program was
identified in February 1980 with a 52% recurrence; this was
found to be surgery alone. In contrast, all three forms of
postoperative treatment have reduced numbers of relapses of
39%, 32% and 21%, differences which are statistically
superior. This study was uncoded in September of 1980.
While none of the three forms of postoperative treatment
can be classified as the best based upon statistical
analysis, a 21% overall recurrence with a 3% local/regional
relapse was recorded with the combination of pelvic
irradiation and combination chemotherapy. This result with
the combined modality therapy represents an important new
advance in the management of this common solid tumor.

SUMMARY

        Cancer of the stomach is the most responsive tumor
to drug treatment, and recently developed regimens of
combination chemotherapy employing Adriamycin have made a
tangible improvement in patient response. In addition to
the identification of new drugs for gastric cancer and the
development of combinations, the emphasis for chemotherapy
in the 1980's must be the completion of surgical adjuvant
trials with FAM and other programs. For locally unresectable gastric cancer, combined modality therapy appears to
carry the best prospect for long term disease-free
survival, after a palliative resection of the primay tumor
when technically possible. A reduction of toxicity from
upper abdomen irradiaton and the use of more effective
combination chemotherapy should result in an improvement in
the 20% four-year disease-free survival now being achieved.
        The problem of pancreatic cancer remain more
difficult. The poor survival, even after curative surgery,
and the increasing incidence demand that more effective
forms of chemotherapy and radiation therapy be defined.
The most important need is the identification of new
anticancer agents with specific activity for this tumor.

This will allow for the development of more effective drug combinations. While the empirical Phase II clinical trial in patients with measurable disease remains the standard and accepted approach for drug evaluation, it is hoped that the development of a simple _in_ _vitro_ stem cell assay will in the future allow for prospective treatment selection.

Local control remains a important problem for the locally unresectable stage of the pancreas, even after the administration of 6000 rads of external photon irradiation, or the equivalent dose of fast neutrons, with 5-FU. The early results with interstitial irradiation, where local doses of 16,000 rads can be delivered, appear promising. Ultimately, these measures must be combined with chemotherapy for control of microscopic distant metastases.

The chemotherapy of advanced colorectal cancer has made little progress since the introduction of 5-FU into clinial trial some 25 years ago. There is a continued need to test newly developed anticancer agents in Phase II trials. The newly reported results of postoperative treatment of resected rectal cancer suggest that our current therapies are not biologically inert, and that a significant reduction in tumor recurrence can be achieved. This is important new data considered of overall importance, and previous refractoriness of this tumor.

Lastly, we must now recognize that each of these important tumors of the gastrointestinal tract are distinctly different, not only in regard to possible etiologic factors and methods for diagnosis, but also in the form of therapy that must be separately defined based on site and stage. This poses an important challenge for the clinical investigator, and let us hope that we are equal to the task.

REFERENCES

1. Moertel, C.G.: Carcinoma Of The Stomach. In: Cancer Therapy; Prognostic Factors And Criteria Of Response To Therapy, Chapter 3, p.229. Ed. M.J. Staquet. Raven Press, New York, (1975).

2. Woolley, P.V., Macdonald, J.S., Schein, P.S.: Chemotherapy Of Malignancies Of The Gastrointestinal Tract. Progr. Gastroenterol., 3:671, (1977).

3. Kovach, J.S., Moertel, C.G., Schutt, A.J., Hahn, R.G., Reitemeier, R.J.: A Controlled Study Of Combined 1,3-bis-(2-chloroethyl)-1-nitrosourea And 5-Fluorouracil Therapy For Advanced Gastric And Pancreatic Cancer. Cancer, 33:563, (1974).

4. Moertel, C.G., Mittelman, J.A., Bakemeier, R.F., Engstrom, P., Hanley, J.: Sequential And Combination Chemotherapy Of Advanced Gastric Cancer. Cancer, 38:678, (1976).

5. Moertel, C.G., Lavin, R.T.: Phase II-III Chemotherapy Studies In Advanced Gastric Cancer. Cancer Treatment Report, 63:1963, (1979).

6. Buroker, T., Kim, P.N., Groppe, C., McCracken, J., O'Bryan, R., Pannettiere, F., Costanzi, J., Bottomley, R., King, G.W., Bonnet, J., Thigpen, T., Whitecare, J., Hass, C., Vaitkevicivus, V.K., Hoogstraten, B., Heilbrun, L.: 5-FU Infusion With Mitomycin-C vs. 5-FU Infusion With Methyl-CCNU In The Treatment Of Advanced Upper Gastrointestinal Cancer. A Southwest Oncology Group Study. Cancer, 44:1215, (1979).

7. Ota, K., Kurita, S., Nishimura, M., Ogawa, M., Kamei, Y., Imai, K., Ariyoshi, Y., Kataoka, K., Murakami, M.O., A. Hoshino, A., Amo, H., Kato, T.: Combination Therapy With Mitomycin-C, 5-Fluorouracil And Cytosine Arabinoside For Advanced Cancer In Man. Cancer Chemotherapy Rept. 56:373, (1972).

8. DeJager, R.L., Magill, C.B., Golbey, R.B., Krakoff, I.H.: Combination Arabinoside In Gastrointestinal Cancer. Cancer Treat. Rept. 60:1973, (1976).

9. The Gastrointestinal Tumor Study Group: Phase II-III Chemotherapy Study In Advanced Gastric Cancer. Cancer Treat. Rept. 63:1971, (1979).

10. Macdonald, J.S., Schein, P.S., Woolley, P.V., Boiron, M., Gisselbrecht, C., Brunet, R., Lagarde, C.: 5-Fluorouracil, Mitomycin-C and Adriamycin (FAM) Combination Chemotherapy For Advanced Gastric Cancer. Ann. Int. Med. (In Press).

11. Bitran, J.D., Desser, R.K., Kozloff, M.F., Billings, A.A., Shapiro, C.M.: Treatment Of Metastatic Pancreatic and Gastric Adenocarcinoma With 5-Fluorouracil, Adriamycin, And Mitomycin-C (FAM). Cancer Treat. Rep. 63:2049, (1979).

12. Panettiere, F., Heilbrun, L.: Comparison of Two Different Combinations Of Adriamycin, Mitomycin-C And 5-FU In The Management Of Gastric Carcinoma. A SWOG Study. Proc. Amer. Soc. Clin. Oncol. 20, No. C-102, (1979).

13. Panettiere, F.: Personal Communication. Manuscript In Preparation.

14. Brugolaris: Personal Communication.

15. Magill, G.B., Golbey, R.B., And Burchenal, J.H.: Combined Anhydro-ara-5-fluorocytidine (AAFC) And Cis-platinum Diamminodichloride (PDD) Therapy. Proc. Am. Soc. Clin. Onc. 19:353, (1978).

16. Bonomi, P.D., Slayton, R.F., And Walter, J: Phase II Trial Of Adriamycin And Cis-dichlorodiammineplatinum (II) In Squamous Cell, Ovarian And Testicular Carcinoma. Cancer Treat Rep. 62:1211-1213, (1978).

17. Levi, J.A., Dalley, D.M., Aroney, R.S.: Improved Combination Chemotherapy In Advanced Gastric Cancer. British Med. J., 2:1471, (1979).

18. Falkson, G., And Falkson, H.C.: Fluorouracil And Radiotherapy In gastrointestinal Cancer. Lancet 2:1252-1253, (1969).

19. Moertel, C.G., Childs, D.S., Reitemeier, R., Colby, M.Y., And Holbrook, M.A.: Combined 5-Fluorouracil And Supervoltage Radiation Therapy Of Locally Unresectable Gastrointestinal Cancer. Lancet, 2:865, (1969).

20. Schein, P.S., Novak, J: For The Gastrointestinal Study Group: Combined Modality Therapy (XRT - Chemo) Versus Chemotherapy Alone For Locally Unresectable Gastric Cancer. Proc. Amer. Soc. Clin. Oncol. 21, (1980).

21. VASAG - Veteran's Administration Cooperative Surgical Adjuvant Study Group Use Of Thiotepa As An Adjuvant To Surgical Management Of Carcinoma Of The Stomach. Cancer 18:291, (1965).

22. Hattori, T., Ito, I., Katsvr, H., Hirata, K., Iizuka, T., Abe, K.: Results Of Combined Treatment In Patients With Cancer Of The Stomach: Palliative Gastrectomy, Large Dose Mitomycin-C, And Bone Marrow Transplantation Gann, 57:441, (1966).

534   Philip S. Schein et al.

23. Serlin, O., Wolhoff, J.S., Amadeo, J.M., Keehn, R.J.:
Use of 5-Fluorodeoxyuridine (FUDR) As An Adjuvant To
Surgical Management Of Carcinoma Of The Stomach.
Cancer, 24:223, (1969).
24. Nakajuma, T., Ota, H., Takagi, K., Kajitani, T.:
Combination Of Multi-Drug Therapy (i.v.) And Long-term
Oral Chemotherapy As An Adjuvant To Surgery For Gastric
Cancer. J. Jpn. Soc. Cancer Ther., 15th Congr. 226,
(1977).
25. Macdonald, J.S., Widerlite, L., And Schein, P.S.:
Current Diagnosis/And,Management Of Pancreatic
Carcinoma. J. Nat. Cancer Inst. 56:1093, (1976).
26. Smith, F.P., and Schein, P.S.: Chemotherapy Of
Pancreatic Cancer Seminars in Oncology, 6:368, (1979).
27. Kovach, J.S., Moertel, C.G., Schutt, A.J., Hahn, R.G.,
Reitermeier, R.J.: A Controlled Study Of Combined
1,3-Bis(2-chloroethyl)-1-Nitrosoureas And
5-Fluorouracil Therapy For Advanced Gastric And
Pancreatic Cancer. Cancer 33:563-567, (1974).
28. Lokich, J.J., Skarin, A.T.: Combination Therapy With
5-Fluorouracil (5-FU) And 1,3-Bis(2-chlorethyl)-1-
nitrosourea (BCNU) For Disseminated Gastrointestinal
Carcinoma. Cancer Chemother. Rep. 56:653-657, 1972.
29. Buroker, T., Kim, P.N., Heilbrun, L., et al.: 5-FU
Infusion With Mitomycin-C (MMC) vs 5-FU Infusion With
Methyl CCNU (Me) In The Treatment Of Advanced Upper
Gastrointestinal Cancer. Proc. ASCO 19:310, (1978).
30. Wiggans, G., Woolley, P.V., Macdonald, J.S., et al.:
Phase II Trial of Streptozotocin, Mitomycin-C And
5-Fluorouracil (SMF) In The Treatment Of Advanced
Pancreatic Cancer. Cancer 41:387-391, (1978).
31. Aberhalden, R.T., Bukowski, R.M., Groppe, C.W., et al.:
Streptozotocin (STZ) And 5-Fluorouracil (5-FU) With And
Without Mitomycin-C (Mito) In The Treatment Of Pan-
creatic Adenocarcinoma. Proc. ASCO 18:301, (1977).
32. Schein, P.S.: For The Gastrointestinal Tumor Study
Group: A Randomized Phase II Clinical Trial Of
Adriamycin, Methotrexate And Actinomycin-D In Advanced
Measurable Pancreatic Carcinoma. Cancer, 42, (1978).
33. Smith, F.P., Macdonald, J.S., Woolley, P.V., Hoth, D.,
Smythe, T., Lichtenfeld, L., Levin, B., And Schein,
P.S.: Phase II Evaluation Of FAM, 5-Fluorouracil,
Adriamycin And Mitomycin-C, In Advanced Pancreatic
Cancer. Cancer (In Press).

34. Schacter, L., Bukowski, R.M., Hewlett, J.S., Gropper, C., Weick, J., And Reimer, R.: Combination Chemotherapy With 5-Fluorouracil, Adriamycin, Mitomycin-C And Streptozotocin Of Pancreatic Cancer. Proc. Amer. Soc. Clin. Oncol., 21:420, (1979).

35. Moertel, C.G., Childs, D.S., Reitemeier, R.J., et al.: Combined 5-Fluorouracil And Supervoltage Radiation Therapy Of Locally Unresectable Gastrointestinal Cancer. Lancet 2:865-867, (1969).

36. Haslam, J.B., Cavanaugh, P.J., Stroup, S.L.: Radiation Therapy In the Treatment Of Irresectable Adenocarcinoma Of The Pancreas. Cancer 32:1341-1345, (1973).

37. Gastrointestinal Tumor Study Group. A Multi-institutional Comparative Trial Of Radiation Therapy Alone And In Combination With 5-Fluorouracil For Locally Unresectable Pancreatic Carcinoma. Ann. Surg. 189:205, (1979).

38. Smith, F.P., Woolley, P.V., Rogers, C., Ornitz, R., And Schein, P.S.: Fast Neutron Therapy For Locally Advanced Pancreatic Carcinoma (LAP). Proc. Am. Soc. Clin. Onc. 21:367, (1980).

39. Shipley, W.U., Nardi, G.L., Cohen, A.M., And Ling, C.C.: Iodine-125 Implant And External Beam Irradiation In Patients With Localized Pancreatic Carcinoma Cancer. 45:709-714, (1980).

40. Grage, T.B., Shingleton, W.W., Jubert, A.V., Elias, E.G., Aust, J.B., And Moss, S.E.: Results Of A Prospective Randomized Study Of Hepatic Artery Infusion With 5-Fluorouracil vs Intravenous 5-Fluorouracil In Patients With Hepatic Metastases From Colorectal Cancer. A Central Oncology Group Study (CO6 7032). In Frontiers Of Gastrointestinal Research; Gastrointestinal Cancer. ed. P. Rosen, S. Edelman, T. Gilat, S. Karger; Basel pp. 116-129 (1979).

41. Moertel, C.G.: Chemotherapy Of Gastrointestinal Cancer. N. Engl. J. Med. 288:1049, (1978).

42. Baker, L.H., Talley, R.W., Matter, R., Legane, D.E., Ruffner, B.W., Jones, S.E., Morrison, F.E., Stephens, R.L., Gehan, Z.A., Vaitkevicuis, J.K.:   Phase III Comparison Of The Treatment Of Advanced Gastrointestinal Cancer With Bolus Weekly 5-FU vs. Methyl-CCNU Plus Bolus Weekly 5-FU: A Southwest Oncology Study. Cancer: 38:1-7, (1976).

43. Lokich, J.J., Skarin, A.T., Mayer, R.J. And Frei, E.: Lack Of Effectiveness Of Combined 5-Fluorouracil And Methyl-CCNU Therapy In Advanced Colorecal Cancer. Cancer 40:2792-2796, (1977).

44. Engstrom, P., MacIntyre, J., Douglas, H., And Carbone,
    P.: Combination Chemotherapy Of Advanced Colon
    Cancer. Proc. Am. Soc. Clin. Oncology 19:384, (1978).
45. Kemeny, N., Yagoda, A., Braun, D., Jr., And Golbey,
    R.: A Randomized Study Of Two Different Schedules Of
    Methyl-CCNU, 5-FU, And Vincristine For Metastatic
    Colorectal Carcinoma. Cancer 43:78, (1979).
46. Kemeny, N., Yagoda, A., Golbey, R.: Methyl-CCNU
    (meCCNU), 5-Fluorouracil (5-FU), Vincristine And
    Streptozotocin (MOF. Strep) For Metastatic Colorectal
    Carcinoma. Proc. Amer. Soc. Clin. Oncol. (1980).
47. Hoth, D.F., And Petrucci, P.E.: Natural History And
    Staging Of Colon Cancer. Sem. Oncology 3:331-336,
    (1976).
48. Wanebo, H.J., Rao, B., Pinsky, C.M., Hoffman, R.G.,
    Stearns, M., Schwartz, M., And Oettgen, H.F.:
    Preoperative Carcinoembryonic Antigen Level As A
    Prognostic Indicator In Colorectal Cancer. N. Engl.
    Med. J. 299:448-451, (1978).
49. Woolley, P.V., Higgins, G.A., And Schein, P.S.:
    Ongoing Trials In The Surgical Adjuvant Managment Of
    Colorectal Cancer. Recent Results In Cancer Res.,
    Vol. 68:231-235, (1979).
50. Higgins, G.A. (Jr.), Humphrey, E., Jules, G.L., LeVeen,
    H.H., McCaughan, J., and Keehn, R.J.: Adjuvant
    Chemotherapy In The Surgical Treatment Of Large Bowel
    Cancer. Cancer 38:1461-1467, (1976).
51. Grage, T.B., Metter, G.E., And Correll, G.W.: Adjuvant
    Chemotherapy With 5-Fluorouracil After Surgical
    Resection Of Colorectal Carcinoma. Am. J. Surg.
    133:298-305, (1977).
52. Taylor, I., Rowling, J., And West, C.: Adjuvant
    Cytotoxic Liver Perfusion For Colorectal Cancer. The
    British Journal of Surgery, Vol. 66: No. 12, Dec., pg.
    833-837, (1979).
53. Gunderson, L.L. And Sosin, H.: Areas Of Failure Found
    At Reoperation (Second Or Symptomatic Look) Following
    "Curative Surgery" For Adenocarcinoma Of The Rectum.
    Cancer 34:1279, (1974).
54. Quan, S.H.: Preoperative Radiation For Carcinoma Of
    The Rectum. N.Y. State J. Med., 66:2243, (1966).
55. Stearns, M.W., Deddish;, M.R., Quan;, S.H., And
    Learning, R.H.: Preoperative Roentgen Therapy For
    Cancer Of The Rectum And Rectosigmoid. Surg. Gynecol.
    Obstet., 138:584, (1975).

56. Higgins, G.A., Conn, J.H., Jordan, P.H., Humphrey,
E.W., Roswit, B., And Keehn, R.J.: Preoperative
Radiotherapy For Colorectal Cancer. Ann. Surg.
181:624-631, (1975).
57. Roswit, B., Higgins, G.A., And Keehn, R.J.:
Preoperative Irradiation For Carcinoma Of The Rectum
And Rectosigmoid Colon: Report Of A National Veterans
Administration Randomized Study. Cancer 35:1597,
(1975).

LUNG CANCER

A. PHILIPPE CHAHINIAN, M.D.,F.A.C.P.

Associate Professor
Department of Neoplastic Diseases
Mount Sinai School of Medicine
City University of New York
New York, New York 10029

Nothing in cancer epidemiology has been more tragic than
the increase in mortality from lung cancer over the past four
decades. In 1912, 374 cases of lung cancer were collected by
Adler from the world literature. In 1980, the death toll from
lung cancer in the United States is expected, for the first
time to exceed 100,000 (75,000 men and 26,000 women.)[12] Compared to 1970, this represents an increase of 50% in men and 260%
in women. Lung cancer is by far the leading cause of mortality
from cancer. The steadily widening gap in mortality between
lung cancer and other cancers is likely to continue in the
future. Reputedly a cancer of the male, its incidence in
females is increasing even more rapidly. Lung cancer now ranks
second in cancer mortality in women, behind breast. If the
present trend persists, however, it will also become number one
in women by the mid 80's. Whereas smoking is by far the most
important causative agent, the incidence of lung cancer among
nonsmokers is also increasing.

In contrast the overall prognosis of lung cancer has not significantly improved in the past decades. The one-year survival
remains below 30%, and the five year survival below 10%. Treatment is still based on surgery for localized disease, and radiotherapy for locoregional disease. There is a biologic asymptote
for these modalities, since they are both local therapies,where-
as lung cancer is with some exceptions, a systemic disease.
Surgery can no longer become more curative. The impact of conventional radiotherapy on survival is low. In a major trial
conducted by the Veterans Administration, 554 patients with
localized but inoperable lung cancer were randomized between
radiotherapy alone (4,000 to 6,000 rads in 4 to 6 weeks)versus
placebo. The median survival of the radiotherapy group was 142
days, versus 112 days for the placebo group. One-year survival
was 18% and 14% respectively.

539

It appears therefore, that the only hope to improve present cure rates is the development of more effective systemic therapies. In the past decade such therapies have already transformed the prognosis of at least one cell type of lung cancer: the small cell ("oat-cell") anaplastic lung cancer.

ACHIEVEMENTS: SMALL CELL ANAPLASTIC CARCINOMA

Representing about 20% of all primary lung cancers,[11] small cell anaplastic carcinoma of the lung (SCCL) has unique biologic features. Its cell of origin is most likely the 'K-cell' (Kulchitsky-like), previously called 'clear cell' by Feyrter.[5] The presence of cytoplasmic neurosecretory type granules detected by electron microscopy in K cells and SCCL can explain the high frequency of paraneoplastic syndromes and ectopic hormone production. It also suggests a relationship between SCCL, carcinoid tumors, and the APUD system. The cellular kinetics of SCCL are characterized by the highest labeling index among all primary lung tumors,[13] with a short tumor doubling time[6] and a high metastatic potential,including bone marrow and central nervous system. Only 4 to 7% of patients with SCCL have intrathoracic involvement only at autopsy.[3] Untreated SCCL carries the poorest prognosis of all primary lung cancers,with a median survival of 14 weeks for limited and 6 weeks for extensive SCCL(defined by spread beyond the supraclavicular lymph nodes). It is only an apparent paradox that SCCL, the most malignant tumor of the lung, has now become the most responsive to chemotherapy, which can take advantage of its peculiar cellular kinetics to achieve greater efficacy. During the past decade, the median survival in SCCL has increased 5 to 6-fold. This is largely attributable to combination chemotherapy,which has been developed and improved step by step following a logical scheme. An increasing fraction of these patients(10% for limited and 1% for extensive SCCL) remain in prolonged complete remission over 2 years, raising the hope for cure.[9] SCCL has become treatable, and potentially curable.

Two randomized trials conducted in the late 60's proved the efficacy of chemotherapy, and gave an impetus to further studies.[5] The Veterans Administration compared placebo versus cyclophosphamide (CYC) in 144 patients with extensive SCCL. Median survival was 6 weeks and 16 weeks, respectively. In 41 patients with limited SCCL, radiotherapy alone was compared to radiotherapy plus CYC at the Ontario Cancer Foundation. Median survival was 21 weeks and 42 weeks respectively. CYC was therefore an active agent both for limited and extensive SCCL. It is now established that a number of single agents are active in SCCL, with response rates between 15 to 47%. They include CYC, mechlorethamine, methotrexate, adriamycin, vincristine, and procarbazine. More recently, agents with similar activity have

TABLE I. Small Cell Lung Cancer Chemotherapy Trials

INSTITUTION Regimens*	No. Pts.	Response rates % CR	PR	CR+PR	Median Survival (weeks)	1 year Survival
ECOG						
CYC vs	112	3	19	22	17	<15%
CYC + CCNU	106	12	31	43	20	<20%
	80% exten.	p=.02		p=.002	p=.07	
NCI-VA						
CYC+MTX vs	24	–	–	38	23	8%
CCM (low)	30	–	–	56	32	6%
	100% exten.			N.S.	N.S.	
FINSEN,DK.						
CCM vs	52	–	–	75	25	9%
CCM + VCR	53	–	–	78	33	28%
				N.S.	p<.01	
NCI-VA						
CCM (low) vs	9	0	45	45	20	11%
CCM (high)	23	30	66	96	42	30%
	84% exten.			p<.05		
CALGB #7283						
CYC (2 gm/m²) vs	12	8	0	8	16	–
CYC+MTX vs	40	10	13	23	18	–
CYC+MTX+ VCR vs	25	12	12	24	21	–
CYC+HDMTX+ VCR	33	9	27	36	23	–
	100% exten.			N.S.	N.S.	

* CYC= cyclophosphamide, MTX= methotrexate, HDMTX= high dose
  methotrexate with citrovorum rescue, VCR= vincristine.
  CCM= CYC+CCNU+MTX (low or high dose).

been identified, including VP16-213, hexamethylmelamine and
vindesine. VP16-213 is presently a major new agent in SCCL.[3]
It has been thoroughly evaluated in more than 200 patients,
with a mean response rate of 44%, mostly in previously treated
patients. The complete response rate to single agents, however,
is low and varies between 0 to 7%. Since complete response is
a prerequisite for cure,many drug combinations have been evaluated in the past ten years in order to improve these figures.
Table 1 summarizes such stepwise attempts before the inclusion
of adriamycin. The addition of CCNU and/or methotrexate to
CYC did not generally improve survival,although response rates
were higher. These trials showed, however, that high dose
chemotherapy (CCM high) can achieve higher response rates and
survival. The addition of vincristine appeared beneficial in

TABLE 2: Effect of Chest Irradiation in Extensive SCCL.
Randomized Trials

INSTITUTION Regimens*		No. Pts.	CR%	PR%	Median Survival (Months)	%Chest Relapse
STANFORD						
POCC	vs	12	42	50	11	58%
POCC + RT		13	38	31	9	62%
(3000 rads x 2 wks, involved site after 2 or 3 cycles)						
SYDNEY, Australia						
CAV	vs	35	20	54	9	23%
CAV + RT		13	-	-	9.5	15%
(4000 rads x 3 wks, after response)						
CALGB #7782 (coded)						
CCV/AV	vs		10	24	7	-
MACC	vs	178+	to	to	to	-
MACC + RT			14**	33**	8	-
(3000 rads x 12 days, after 2 cycles)						

*POCC= procarbazine, vincristine, CYC, CCNU. CAV= CYC, ADR,
vincristine. CCV/AV= CYC, CCNU, vincristine, alternating with
ADR, vincristine. MACC= MTX. ADR. CYC, CCNU. RT= radiotherapy
to chest. **Preliminary results.

one trial, but not in the other. The Cancer and Leukemia Group
B (CALGB) study also showed that maintenance chemotherapy after
complete response was beneficial in terms of survival. In subsequent trials, adriamycin (ADR)has generally been included in
combination chemotherapy. Although the precise impact of this
agent is difficult to evaluate,there has been a steady increase
in response rates to chemotherapy in the past decade. Complete
response rates to combination chemotherapy alone went from an
average of 6% between 1973 to 1975, to 10% in 1976 and 22% in
1977 (cumulative data on 1004 patients).[5]
    Subsequent attempts to improve these results may derive from
the concept of alternating non-cross resistant combinations.
The NCI-VA group piloted a combination of vincristine, adriamycin and procarbazine (VAP) in 17 patients who progressed on
CCM. There were 4 complete responders (24%) and 6 partial
responders (35%). Lack of cross-resistance between CCM and VAP
led to the use of this alternating combination as a first line
therapy,in order to increase complete response rates and therefore long-term survival. Sixty-one patients (69% extensive)
received CCM at high dose, followed by VAP after 6 weeks.
Addition of VAP increased the complete response rate from 30%

TABLE 3: Effect of Chest Irradiation in Limited SCCL.
Randomized Trials

INSTITUTION Regimens*	No. Pts.	CR%	PR%	Median Survival (Months)	%Chest Relapse
FINSEN, DK.					
CCMV vs	69	92		14	47%
CCMV + RT	65	87		11	32%
(4000 rads split,				p<0.01	
wk 7 & 11)					
INDIANA					
CAV vs	16	50	25	11.5	37%
CAV + RT	14	71	29	13	36%
(3500 rads split,					
wk 3 & 5)					
SYDNEY, Australia					
CAV vs	57	21	56	15.5	41%
CAV + RT	21	–	–	17	14%
(4000 rads x 4 wks,					
after response)					
NCI-VA					
CCM/VAP vs	14	46	–	too early	
CCM/VAP + RT	14	77	–		
(4000 rads x 3 wks,					
wk 1)					
* See Tables 1 & 2.					

to 48%. (42% to 74% in limited disease and 24 to 36% in extensive disease). Toxicity was high with 3 treatment related deaths,and requirement for platelet transfusions in 23 patients. Patients were also randomized to receive VP16 and ifosfamide, without demonstrable benefit. Overall 1 year survival was 45%, and median survival 43 weeks. These figures are not much different from those reported for CCM alone by the same investigators (Table 1). Analysis of survival is difficult, however, since 46 patients were also randomized to receive immunotherapy with Thymosin Fraction V (low dose or high dose)or not. A subsequent report on these 46 patients revealed that the only long-term survivors (over 18 months)were in the high-dose thymosin group. Therefore, randomized trials are necessary to confirm the validity of non-cross resistant alternating combinations. The current CALGB protocols 7781 and 7782 address that question in both limited and extensive SCCL. Patients are randomized between a straight combination (MACC: methotrexate, adriamycin, CYC and CCNU) versus a combination of CYC,CCNU and vincristine alternating with adriamycin and vincristine (CCV/AV). The studies are still coded, but preliminary results show no significant difference in response rates and survival.

The role of radiotherapy remains controversial in SCCL.
Despite excellent responses to chemotherapy which remains the
cornerstone of treatment in this disseminated neoplasm, intrathoracic relapses in the primary tumor and mediastinal nodes
are frequent. Therefore, chemotherapy and radiotherapy to the
chest have been combined in a large number of trials. The most
intensive one was conducted at the NCI, with various schedules
of radiotherapy combined with vincristine,adriamycin and cyclophosphamide. Among 50 patients, complete response rate was 66%,
partial response 8%,but toxicity was formidable with 20% treatment related deaths. There was no major benefit in survival for
21 patients with extensive SCCL (median = 10.5 months),but the
calculated median survival for patients with limited SCCL exceeded 2 years,with 36% projected disease-free survival. Maintenance was not given in that trial. Intrathoracic recurrence
was observed in 13/18 complete responders at relapse. Other
less intensive chemotherapy-radiotherapy programs have been
evaluated. There appears to be no benefit in terms of survival
when radiotherapy is added to chemotherapy in patients with extensive SCCL. (Table 2). In limited SCCL, cumulative data from
the literature comparing combined radiotherapy and chemotherapy
versus chemotherapy alone suggest a slight increase in complete
response rates for the former (48% versus 28%),but no apparent
benefit in survival (median = 11.9 months and 10.3 months respectively).[10]   It is of importance that about 30 to 50% of
irradiated patients relapse within the chest. Randomized trials
have been conducted (Table 3). Although the incidence of intrathoracic relapse is slightly lower in irradiated patients,there
is no apparent benefit in survival. In one trial there was, in
fact,a detrimental effect of added radiotherapy for survival.

An important area where radiotherapy has been effective is
the prevention of brain metastases,a sanctuary site for chemotherapy. Randomized trials conducted by the major cooperative
groups (CALGB, ECOG, SWOG) have demonstrated a significant
decrease in brain metastases in patients who received prophylactic brain irradiation(5% versus 22%). Survival, however, was
not influenced, probably because patients relapsed elsewhere.
The effect of nitrosoureas(CCNU) suggest some activity in this
area, at least at high dose(100 mg/m^2), but await confirmation
by controlled trials.

Chemotherapy with or without immunotherapy has also been
evaluated in randomized trials. C. parvum has been beneficial
for survival but not for response in the original trial in
France. Such effect has not been confirmed at UCLA and Mount
Sinai. BCG,MER-BCG,and levamisole have not been beneficial so
far. Thymosin fraction V given at two dose levels versus chemotherapy alone in a total of 46 patients at the NCI-VA hospital
has increased survival at high-dose only. Confirmation by a
larger trial is necessary.

CHALLENGES: CELL TYPES OTHER THAN SMALL CELL

Often grouped as "nonsmall cell" lung cancer,(nonSCCL)these
types include essentially squamous cell carcinoma (SQC),adeno-
carcinoma (ADC) and large cell anaplastic carcinoma (LCC). The
most frequent used to be SQC,but recently it has been replaced
by ADC in several centers in the United States. This is important because the frequency of extrathoracic metastasis is higher
in ADC than SQC.[7] These cell types are more refractory to
chemotherapy than SCCL. Six major single agents have shown some
activity, including CYC, mechlorethamine, methotrexate, (MTX)
hexamethylmelamine, adriamycin (ADR) and CCNU.[3] Overall range
of response is very wide,and this can be explained by varying
criteria of response. When standard criteria(CR, PR) are used,
response rates to most active single agents are usually not
higher than 10 to 15%(Table 4).[4] In contrast to SCCL,no single
agent has yet been shown to increase survival in these types.
Three major randomized trials have compared CYC alone versus
combinations. In ECOG, CYC alone was compared to CYC + CCNU.
In 162 patients with ADC, response rates were 13% and 12% respectively,and median survival 16 weeks and 26 weeks (p=0.07).
At M.D. Anderson, CYC alone was compared to 'COMB' (CYC, vincristine, methylCCNU, bleomycin) in 47 patients with SQC.
Response rates were 4% and 5% and median survival 14 weeks and
11 weeks, respectively. The only trial with a significant
result was conducted by the Veterans Administration where CYC+
ADR doubled the survival of patients with SQC (but not ADC or
LCC)compared to CYC alone (24 weeks versus 12 weeks, p<0.001).
In the same trial,no benefit over CYC was noted with CYC+CCNU
or ADR + CCNU. In almost all trials comparing other single
agents vs combinations,no clear difference was demonstrated for
survival. Many combinations have been piloted with encouraging response rates (over 30%). The one year survival, however,
is often below 10%.[8] One major problem remains the reproducibility of these results. Table 5 shows that, with the exception of MTX,subsequent trials yielded lower response rates than
initial trials. It must be remembered that lung cancer is a
heterogeneous disease, and that many factors besides cell type
affect prognosis, including performance status, prior therapy,
site of metastases, etc. Lack of stratification by prognostic
factors may thus at least partly explain these differences.
Different doses and schedules of some drugs can also influence
results. As an example, the MACC combination (MTX, ADR, CYC,
CCNU) was originally piloted at Mount Sinai with a response
rate of 44% in 68 patients with nonSCCL and an overall one year
survival of 25%.[2] As seen in Table 5, response rate dropped to
12% in ECOG. Several differences between both studies are

TABLE 4:   MAJOR SINGLE AGENTS.   Response Rates
(No. of Patients) According to Criteria of Response,
All Cell Types Lung Cancer.*

DRUG	OVERALL RANGE OF RESPONSE	NONSTANDARD CRITERIA	STANDARD CRITERIA (CR & PR)
Cyclophosphamide	0-63%	37%(182)	16%(396)
Mechlorethamine	0-68%	26%(247)	6%(145)
Methotrexate	3-43%	30%(79)	11%(291)
Adriamycin	0-50%	22%(41)	14%(358)
CCNU	0-41%	36%(50)	8%(216)
* Modified from Ref. 4.			

noteworthy. The ECOG trial was a large multi-institutional one,
where about 20 centers contributed to include 43 patients,where-
as the original trial was based on a single institution. Distribution of cell types was different with 63% SQC in ECOG vs
32% at Mount Sinai. Changes in weight and performance status
were included in criteria of response in ECOG. High dose MACC
was given to all ECOG patients,and there was no requirement for
nadir counts,contrary to earlier recommendations from the Mount
Sinai group. Therefore toxicity became prohibitive in ECOG,
leading to early discontinuation of the trial. Activity of MACC,
however,has been reported by others using a low-dose schedule,
or a modified schedule given on day 1 and 8(ASCO 1980). Another
combination,CAMP (CYC, ADR, MTX, procarbazine),added to radiotherapy in some patients,has produced results similar to MACC,
but awaits confirmation. The fact is that there is presently no
accepted standard regimen of chemotherapy in nonSCCL. To further confuse the issue,conflicting results from prospective randomized trials have been reported.[3] Combinations of alkylating
agents and nitrosoureas have been most popular in view of results obtained in Lewis lung tumor in mice. In patients with
nonSCCL however,the addition of CCNU to CYC or mechlorethamine
did not increase response rates or survival. The addition of
CCNU to CYC and MTX,however,improved response and survival in
ADC. One might therefore speculate that there is a synergistic
action between CCNU and MTX. In another trial,however,the addition of MTX to a nitrosourea(methylCCNU)and vincristine did not
improve response or survival over methylCCNU and vincristine.
   There is an urgent need for more effective agents. Table 6
summarizes cumulative results obtained with 20 new drugs in
lung cancer.[3] Only a few of them,including Baker's antifolate,
ifosfamide and vindesine have shown some activity. Cisplatin is
presently undergoing Phase II trials, and preliminary results
indicate an objective response rate of 14% (4/29)in previously

TABLE 5: REPRODUCIBILITY OF RESULTS IN LUNG CANCER
% OBJECTIVE RESPONSE (NO. OF PATIENTS)

DRUG(S)*	CELL TYPE	INITIAL TRIAL	SUBSEQUENT TRIAL
MTX .6mg/kg IM BiW	All	6%(31) RPMI	21%(48)ECOG
CCM	Adeno	38%(28)NCI-VA	14%(56)WP-L
CAP	Nonsmall	39%(41)Mayo	27%(120)Toronto
COMB	Squamous	33%(33)MD Anderson	5%(20)MDAnderson
BACON	Squamous	45%(38)MD Anderson	21%(116) SWOG
PACCO	Squamous	87%(15)RPMI	25%(12)Wisconsin
CCM/VAP	Small	94%(61)NCI-VA	39%(18)Montefiore
MACC	Nonsmall	44%(68)Mt.Sinai	12%(43) ECOG

*CAP: CYC+ADR+Cisplatin. BACON: Bleomycin+ADR+CCNU+vincristine
+Nitrogen mustard. PACCO: cisplatin+ADR+CYC+CCNU+vincristine.

untreated patients. The combination of vindesine with two dose
levels of cisplatin piloted at Memorial Sloan-Kettering has produced a 39 to 50% objective response rate in 59 patients. Duration of response was longer for the high dose cisplatin group.

Immunotherapy combined with chemotherapy has also been evaluated in advanced nonSCCL. Although immunotherapy is most effective in case of minimal tumor burden, the paucity of active
drugs and the results in some experimental systems justify such
attempts. Several randomized trials versus chemotherapy alone
have been conducted.[3] The addition of C. parvum to chemotherapy
significantly increased survival but not response rates in the
original trial in France and also at Roswell Park. A minor and
nonsignificant effect was reported at E. Lansing and UCLA. BCG
and MER-BCG were not beneficial at UCLA and Roswell Park respectively. At Mount Sinai an ongoing randomized trial is comparing
MACC alone vs MACC + C. parvum vs MACC + levamisole. Interim
analysis on 101 patients,all cell types,revealed no differences
in overall response rates and survival. Analysis by cell type,
however, showed a benefit for survival in patients with LCC
receiving C. parvum or LMS. Numbers are still small,but these
results cast doubt on the validity of lumping different cell
types in a"nonsmall cell"category without stratification. Human
leukocyte interferon has,so far,provided no objective response
in 9 patients with nonSCCL at Memorial Sloan-Kettering (AACR
1980).

Adjuvant therapy after surgical resection of Stage I and Stage
II disease can be evaluated only by prospective randomized
trials with an untreated control arm. In this setting,no program of adjuvant chemotherapy has been convincingly beneficial
in nonSCCL. All trials,however,used single agents or combinations which are not,or would not,be effective in advanced lung

A. Philippe Chahinian

TABLE 6:   INVESTIGATIONAL AGENTS IN LUNG CANCER
No. responses/no. of pts. - Cumulative results

DRUG	ALL TYPES	Non-small	SQC	ADC	LCC
ACNU		0/23	0/10	0/13	
5-Azacytidine	7/45				
Baker's Antifolate			0/6	4/31	
Chlorozotocin		2/30	1/11	1/18	0/1
DDMP			0/5		
Dianhydrogalactitol		8/83	6/46	0/20	2/17
Dibromodulcitol		10/51	9/39	1/12	
Dichloromethotrexate	2/22				
Emetine		3/27	1/15	1/11	1/1
ICRF-159		4/43	1/15	2/20	1/8
Ifosfamide		14/38	11/28	0/4	3/6
Maytansine		3/42	1/12	1/17	1/13
MTX Hi-dose & CF		8/34	2/5	2/9	2/4
Methyl-GAG			1/6		
Neocarzinostatin	1/15				
Pyrazofurin		0/24	0/14	0/10	
Rubidazone			0/16		
Sarcolysin		0/17	0/14	0/2	0/1
Streptonigrin	1/ 7				
Vindesine	13/51	10/44	3/13	6/28	1/3

cancer. Adjuvant immunotherapy is theoretically seductive in this situation. Intrapleural BCG(IP-BCG)has been pioneered at Albany,N.Y. as a mean of local and systemic immunotherapy and production of an experimental empyema. Following resection, patients are randomized to receive INH only or INH and IP-BCG, 10^7 viable units once(Tice strain).[14]   There is presently a significant advantage for the BCG group in terms of recurrence rate and survival in 58 patients with Stage I disease only. The National Lung Cancer Study Group is conducting a similar trial with no significant difference to date in recurrence rate among 383 patients with Stage I disease. The Seattle group is randomizing patients between placebo only,IP-BCG,or IP-BCG + levamisole. Recurrence rates are respectively 36%, 27% and 51%,in 134 patients with no significant differences at this time.   At Nottingham, no significant benefit was seen for IP-BCG versus controls in 50 patients with Stage I disease. That particular trial,however,used a different source of BCG (Glaxo) and less febrile reactions were noted than with the Tice strain. Definitive results of ongoing trials will be soon available.   In one European trial,levamisole at a fixed dose reduced hematogeneous metastases after surgery. This effect was found retrospectively in patients weighing less than 70 kg.

There are presently several other immunotherapy protocols
using intradermal BCG, intratumoral BCG, allogeneic soluble
tumor antigens, complete Freund's adjuvant, intrapleural
C. parvum, etc. Results are too preliminary at this time.

PROSPECTS

1. In SCCL, the potential for curability should sustain intensive efforts in three directions. (i) Systemic Therapy.
The search for new active agents has already been successful
(VP16-213) and should continue. Noncross resistant alternating regimens need prospective evaluation. The concept of late
intensification also deserves testing. Duration of treatment
and need for maintenance should be more precisely defined. New
supportive techniques are of potential importance including
bone marrow protection (autologous transplantation,lithium),
prevention of leukopenic sepsis and of nutritional disorders.
Nonchemotherapeutic systemic treatments such as immunotherapy,
anticoagulation, are of interest because of lack of additive
toxicity with chemotherapy. (ii) Local control. Relapse in
the area of bulky disease, (primary site and mediastinum)re-
mains a major problem. New techniques of radiotherapy, such
as high linear energy transfer particles and radiosensitizers
should be piloted. Half-body or total body irradiation techniques are under study. Hyperthermia could potentiate the
effect of chemotherapy or radiotherapy. Finally, surgery deserves investigation whenever it is or becomes technically
feasible. (iii) Sanctuary sites. Prophylactic brain irradiation should be considered in good risk patients (limited disease). Leptomeningeal metastases may become a rising problem
in the future. The role of intrathecal or systemic therapies
such as nitrosoureas and high-dose methotrexate,will require
prospective evaluation.
 Many of these approaches are being tested now, and rapid
developments are expected.
2. In the other cell types, the frustrating lack of effective
agents requires a different approach. (i) Experimental
screening. Presently Lewis lung tumor in mice is the only
experimental system where new drugs are routinely tested. It
has been a poor predictor for the selection of drugs active
in human lung cancer. There are 14 different types of spontaneous or induced lung tumors in mice, three in rats and one
in hamsters. It is time to use them. More direct information can also be obtained from human tumors transplanted in
immunodepressed mice, or grown in vitro by tumor stem cell
assays. (ii) Clinical Trials. Each new agent should be
clinically tested in advanced lung cancer. In addition,
Phase II and III trials of new agents and new combinations

should be intensively and rapidly conducted.   (iii) <u>Adjuvant</u>
<u>Trials</u>. The present situation should not deter physicians
from referring patients for adjuvant trials.   Even a slight
increase in cure rate can have a great impact.
3. Finally,it is a paradox that the most lethal cancer is also the most preventable. Any policy aimed at long-term control cannot be successful without a campaign against smoking.

REFERENCES*

1. Broder LE, Cohen MH, Selawry OS:Treatment of bronchogenic
   carcinoma.II. Small cell. Cancer Treat Rev.4:219-260,1977.
2. Chahinian AP, Mandel EM, Holland, JF, et al:MACC (Methotrexate, adriamycin, cyclophosphamide and CCNU)in advanced
   lung cancer.   Cancer 43:1590-1597, 1979.
3. Chahinian AP, Hansen HH: Chemotherapy of lung cancer.
   New York, Bristol-Myers Co. Int. Div., 1980.
4. Cohen MH, Perevodchikova NI:Single agent chemotherapy of
   lung cancer.   In ref. 9, pp 343-374.
5. Greco FA, Einhorn LH (eds): Small cell lung cancer.
   Semin Oncol 5:233-340, 1978.
6. Harris CC (ed): Pathogenesis and Therapy of Lung Cancer.
   New York, Marcel Dekker, 1978.
7. Israel LI, Chahinian AP (eds):Lung Cancer. Natural History, Prognosis and Therapy. New York, Academic Press,1976.
8. Livingston RB: Combination chemotherapy of bronchogenic
   carcinoma. I.Non-oat cell. Cancer Treat Rev 4:153-165,1977.
9. Muggia FM, Rozencweig M (eds): Lung Cancer. Progress in
   Therapeutic Research.   New York, Raven Press, 1979.
10. Salazar OM, Creech RH: "The state of the art" toward de-
    fining the role of radiation therapy in the management of
    small cell bronchogenic carcinoma.   Int J Radiat Oncol
    Biol Phys 6:1103-1117, 1980.
11. Selawry OS, Hansen HH: Lung cancer, in Holland JF,
    Frei III E (eds): Cancer Medicine. Philadelphia, Lea
    & Febiger, 1973, pp 1473-1518.
12. Silverberg E: Cancer statistics 1980. CA30:23-38, 1980.
13. Straus MJ (ed): Lung Cancer. Clinical Diagnosis and
    Treatment. New York, Grune & Stratton, 1977.
14. Terry WD, Windhorst D (eds): Immunotherapy of Cancer. Pre-
    sent Status of Trials in Man. New York,Raven Press,1978.

*Limited to general bibliography. Specific references can
be obtained upon request to author.

Head and Neck Cancer

ROBERT E. WITTES, M.D.

Associate Attending Physician
Solid Tumor Service, Department of Medicine
Memorial Sloan-Kettering Cancer Center
New York, New York

Etiology and Prevention

Although only about 6% of all cancer in the United States
arises in the head and neck area, these tumors have an
importance in medicine which belies their modest relative
incidence. Involving as they most often do the epithelium
of the upper aerodigestive tract, they usually interfere
with nutrition, communication, and appearance in ways that
cannot easily be concealed. Therapy for established disease
must often be radical and may itself leave both psychological
and physical sequelae. Treatment is frequently protracted
and expensive, with significant economic implications for
patients and society.

The epidermoid cancers of the upper aerodigestive tract
(hereafter, simply head and neck cancer) are, in principle,
far easier to prevent primarily than to cure.Epidemiologic
studies have long suggested the important etiologic role
of tobacco usage. As with lung cancer, there appears to be
a dose-effect relationship, at least at certain sites (44).
Moreover, concomitant alcohol abuse appears to augment
greatly the effect of tobacco at any given level of tobacco
usage (34), such that the two agents appear to be acting
synergistically. The striking effects of tobacco are not
limited to cigarettes, since cigar and pipe users also are
at increased risk, both in the oral cavity and the larynx.
Nor, for that matter, is smoking itself necessary; in areas
of the world where tobacco is incorporated into quids of
various types, or chewed alone, the incidence of oral cancers
is clearly increased in users compared with non-users. The
magnitude of this effect is such that in India, where such
habits are common, head and neck cancer is a major cause of
cancer-related morbidity and mortality. Admittedly, since
the quids often have many ingredients, tobacco may not be
the only culprit. Whether the substitution of low-tar
cigarettes for the standard variety will have a substantial

impact upon the incidence of any of the tobacco-related
cancers in Western society won't be known for many years.
Meanwhile efforts to educate the population must be
broadened and expanded into a national priority, especially
in the younger age groups, where peer pressure to conform
sets lifetime patterns of behavior.

Not all epithelial head and neck cancer shows such a
strong effect of tobacco. Nasopharynx cancer (NPC), rather
rare in the U.S,is common among southern Chinese. The
original observations linking NPC to measurable circulating
anti-EB virus antibody has led to expanded efforts to
define the relationship between the EB virus and NPC in
humans (see a full discussion elsewhere in this Symposium).
Epidemiologic studies have also suggested that other factors
such as diet and possibly genetic predisposition may play a
role in increasing the susceptibility of certain segments
of the population (17,26). In short, it is likely that
many of the head and neck cancers will prove to have
multifactorial etiologies and that a fuller understanding of
the process of carcinogenesis, based upon further work in
epidemiology, molecular biology, and immunology, will suggest
reasonable strategies for primary prevention. As our
experience with tobacco demonstrates, however, the design of
strategies which are both scientifically based and socially
acceptable will be no small task.

Diagnosis

The relationship between late stage at diagnosis and a poor
prognosis has been apparent for many years. It is therefore
reasonable to suppose that earlier diagnosis would lead to
at least some reduction in the morbidity and mortality from
head and neck cancer. One might also expect that symptoms
in such vital areas of the body would cause rapid self-
referral to physicians or dentists but in fact a very
sizable proportion of the patient population presents with
advanced disease and has lived with symptoms for some time
before seeking consultation (6,28). The problem of patient
delay is, of course, not unique to head and neck cancer
and may improve somewhat as general pessimism about cancer
disappears. Nevertheless, it is probably still true that
therapy for these neoplasms is more frightening than for
most, and at least the alcoholic segment of the patient
population at high risk for the development of head and
neck cancer is not noted for seeking medical consultation
at the first sign or symptom of disease.

Clinical experience also suggests that suboptimal
handling by physicians is an occasional cause of delay in
diagnosis. It is ironic that physicians trained in the

minutiae of cardiac and neurological physical diagnosis are often incompetent to perform a simple mirror examination of the larynx or a digital examination of the base of the tongue. Patients presenting with a lump in the neck and a sore throat are still sometimes given penicillin and a six-month return appointment. Although there is no evidence that such practice is a quantitatively important cause of death from advanced disease, lack of physician awareness or ability is still a suitable target for continuing medical education.

Treatment

During the past decade some attitudes toward therapy have shifted significantly and new directions have opened. These include: (a) a wider acceptance of the efficacy of combined surgery and irradiation in enhancing locoregional control rates; (b) new developments in radiation therapy which may improve the effectiveness of this modality against advanced disease; (c) a vast increase in interest by medical oncologists and a corresponding upsurge in the number of disease-oriented clinical chemotherapy trials in advanced disease, with the incorporation of chemotherapy into various combined modality approaches to therapy.

(a) Surgery + radiation therapy. As many have noted (12,29) these two types of therapy are complementary rather than competing. Each tends to be effective where the other is most prone to fail. Surgery rids the patient of bulky tumor with unparalleled efficacy but, despite meticulous surgical technique, often leaves behind unrecognized deposits of tumor which may cause recurrence. Conversely, radiotherapy is often strikingly successful in sterilizing subclinical foci of locoregional disease but usually gives unsatisfactory control rates when used as primary therapy for massive tumor. Over the past two decades or so, radiation and surgery have been used together in a great number of different combinations, depending upon the primary site, the distribution of tumor, and the preferences of the clinicians. The sequencing of the two treatments, the time-dose fractionation, total dose, and ports of the radiotherapy, and the scope of the surgery have all been important variables that often differ widely from study to study. In addition, very few investigators have employed a prospective, randomized design but have resorted instead to the use of either historical controls treated with one modality alone, or else a control group which may be more or less contemporaneous but chosen by a technique other than random assignment. Even the randomized trials may suffer from small sample sizes (24).

Despite these apparent difficulties, it is difficult to avoid the conclusion that, at least for some sites, combined therapy results in enhanced locoregional control rates over treatment with surgery or radiotherapy alone (5,12,14,20,29). We must recall, however, that not all trials showing improved local control rates with combined therapy show a corresponding advantage in survival (5,13,25,29). In some instances, such as with cancers of the hypopharynx, as local control rates have risen with combined therapy, the rate of appearance of distant metastases has increased as well (13,25). Moreover, head and neck cancer patients are notoriously fragile and may die from unrelated causes even if anticancer treatment is successful; while such deaths are not attributable to either the cancer or its treatment, they reduce the number of patients available for analysis of treatment-related effects late in the course of the trial. The propensity of these patients to develop subsequent new primary cancers, even after cure of the first, has a similar effect.

In any case, current data suggests benefit from combined treatment in selected circumstances. In addition to increased locoregional control rates, many have used the effectiveness of radiotherapy as a tool to allow a scaling down of the scope of surgery (14,20,27,29). Though no controlled trials exist, it certainly seems that at selected primary sites and in the neck, aggressive radiotherapy can permit the performance of less radical operations without compromising the patient's chances of cure.

More work is necessary to define the optimum combinations of surgery and radiotherapy in the various head and neck cancers; for all the reasons stated above, this is a most complex task. Moreover, reliable data, convincing to the medical community at large, will not be forthcoming unless adequate methodology is employed for the very difficult and time-consuming clinical trials that are necessary. In this respect the current efforts of the Radiation Therapy Oncology Group (RTOG) are exemplary.

(b) Advances in radiotherapy. The total radiation dose achievable in the clinic is most often limited by normal tissue tolerance. Techniques have been developed and refined whereby tumors can be implanted with radioactive materials, insuring over time a very high radiation dose to the tumor with relative sparing of the surrounding normal tissues. Local control rates in expert hands are good (36) and the technique appears very promising as salvage therapy for persistant but still localized disease (38).

Because hypoxic conditions in the interior of large tumors

may be of major importance in determining resistance to radiation-induced killing (15), much effort is being directed towards the development of techniques which increase the sensitivity of hypoxic cells to radiation. Treatment with accelerated particles (neutrons and pions) and the use of hypoxic cell sensitizers with irradiation are currently under active scrutiny for the treatment of head and neck cancer. The results of the randomized trial at the Hammersmith Hospital (7,8) comparing neutrons with photons in the treatment has suggested an advantage for neutrons, but systematic differences in the handling of the patient groups, as well as the suboptimal beam character-istics, primitive techniques of immobilization, and limited field sizes of the Hammersmith cyclotron make definitive conclusions impossible. Cooperative trials are currently in progress at several centers in the U.S. (33) in which treatment with neutrons and with a mixed beam of neutrons and photons are compared with photons alone. Because of the formidable costs involved in setting up facilities of this kind, the clinical trials will have to show a sub-stantial advantage for treatment with neutrons to create enthusiasm for wide adoption of the technique.

Trials with pions (23) are in a less advanced state, in part because only one pion generator has been in use in the U.S. for any length of time. Results of a small pilot study in head and neck cancer at the Los Alamos Meson Physics Facility and the University of New Mexico have been suf-ficiently encouraging to warrant expansion of the trial into a randomized comparison with more standard radiotherapy.

A vastly cheaper, more easily applicable solution to the problems of hypoxic cells might be provided by chemical sensitizers such as misonidazole (10), a congener of the commonly used trichomonacide metronidazole. Dosage schedules have been developed which minimize the vexing problem of both central and peripheral neurotoxicity and this compound is currently in a Phase III randomized trial in the RTOG for patients with advanced head and neck cancer.

As is equally true of the chemotherapy + radiotherapy approach discussed below, even if early results appear promising, the new developments in radiotherapy will not be fully evaluable for many years. Only when sufficient time has elapsed for the complete assessment of both long-term disease-free survival rates and the evolution of any chronic toxicities will a definitive judgment be possible.

(c) Increased activity in clinical chemotherapy. This area has been recently reviewed in detail (41,42). In common with most of the solid tumors, head and neck cancer

has seen an impressive increase in the sheer number of
disease-oriented trials of new drugs and drug combinations.
Although the mere quantity of studies in progress and
published during the past decade is not an automatic guaran-
tee of progress, there is surely reason for optimism.
Several drugs show significant activity in head and neck
cancer patients when they are used singly; the activity of
methotrexate, cisplatin, and bleomycin have been defined
most clearly, but 5-FU, cyclophosphamide, doxorubicin,
hydroxyurea, and vinblastine also appear potentially useful,
though more precise activity data would be desirable. The
short duration of remissions with single agent treatment
and the notable effects of combination chemotherapy in
other solid tumors have led to many attempts at defining
useful combinations of drugs in head and neck cancer.
Combinations of cisplatin and bleomycin (32,19), cisplatin +
methotrexate + bleomycin (11,21), cyclophosphamide + methotrexate + 5-FU + bleomycin (18), and other regimens (31)
have been reported to have very significant antitumor
effects, with remission rates in excess of 40-50%. From
nearly all these trials, it seems clear that previously
untreated tumors are more sensitive to chemotherapy than
those which have survived previous therapy with radiation
and/or surgery.

The activity of chemotherapy in previously untreated
patients, coupled with the well-known difficulties with
locoregional control in very advanced head and neck cancer
and the appreciable incidence of distant metastases in
this group of patients, has motivated a large number of
pilot studies within the past 2-3 years in which chemotherapy has been used as initial treatment prior to the
local modalities. Regimens have included cisplatin (43),
methotrexate (22), and many combinations of these and other
drugs (11,19,21,31,32). Experience with this approach has
yielded high regression rates with a variety of combinations
(70-90%CR+PR). Moreover the sequential use of chemotherapy
followed by radiotherapy and/or surgery appears not to
result in an increase in complications from the local treatment (19,32,43). Occasionally, resected specimens show no
obviously viable tumor by histological criteria, but more
commonly there is ample evidence of residual tumor on
microscopic examination, even when clinical evidence of
regression has been very impressive. The ultimate effects
of initial chemotherapy on relapse-free interval, survival,
relapse patterns, and incidence of second malignancies are
totally unknown at this time. Happily, there is general
awareness in the community of physicians, surgeons, and

radiotherapists who treat head and neck cancer that such questions will only be answered by large-scale randomized trials, and several are currently in progress, both in the U.S. and the U.K..

Since many commonly used cytotoxic agents may function as radiosensitizers both in cell culture systems and in vivo, many clinical trials have explored the simultaneous delivery of chemotherapy and radiotherapy. As usual, the large majority of such trials are not randomized comparisons and rely heavily on historical controls. Evidence from controlled trials of the superiority of combined chemotherapy + radiotherapy over radiation alone is not persuasive, although positive trials, at least for some subsets of patients, have been reported for both 5-FU (3) and bleomycin (37). Combinations of drugs have also been examined with simultaneous radiotherapy. Although unrandomized, the trial of Clifford with vincristine, methotrexate, bleomycin, and radiotherapy has suggested a possible advantage to combination therapy over radiation alone (9). It is obvious however, from nearly all studies of simultaneous treatment that patient tolerance to the therapy is frequently poor, and that the local toxicities of radiotherapy may be significantly augmented by the simultaneous use of chemotherapy. A very real question exists, therefore, concerning the presence or absence of any selectivity in the action of the radiosensitizer; if the drug is simply sensitizing normal cells to the same degree as the tumor cells, it is unlikely that any net therapeutic gain will result. Multi-institutional trials are in progress in the U.K. to test the efficacy of Clifford's regimen; the Northern California Oncology Group is examining the use of bleomycin with radiation.

No discussion of therapeutic alternatives in head and neck cancer would be complete without mentioning the potential for effective immunotherapy. Studies on populations of patients with these diseases have established a very significant incidence (30-50%) of failure to mount a delayed hypersensitivity response to skin test antigens (4,16) as well as of defects in in vitro T cell function(40). This apparent defect in cell-mediated immunity appears even in patients with tumors localized to the primary site and probably cannot be totally explained by the confounding variables of malnutrition, alcoholism, or tobacco use, although this issue has not been entirely settled. Moreover, early-stage patients who fail to react to DNCB have inferior survivorship compared to those whose delayed hypersensitivity is not impaired (16). Non-specific immunostimulation has been used as an adjunct to chemotherapy in several studies of patients

with advanced disease, with unimpressive results to date.
A randomized, controlled, double-blind trial of levamisole
(2), given after local control is achieved with standard
treatment, is currently in progress at the Memorial Sloan-
Kettering Cancer Center (39). Until the completion of this
and of other controlled trials, it seems fair to conclude
that no immunotherapy is of established value as an adjuvant
in the treatment of head and neck cancer.

Conclusions

The decade ahead will be a period of further progress in
therapy-related research. A major problem will be the
optimum sequencing of the various modalities to obtain the
maximum benefit from each without sacrificing the efficacy
of the others. Most of the multimodality studies now in
progress using chemotherapy employ drugs as initial treatment for a brief time period. It is not at all obvious that
this is the best approach. On the other hand, the use of
chemotherapy only after conclusion of surgery and/or radiation would usually mean waiting many weeks to permit healing
from any ablative and reconstructive procedures and the sub-
sidence of significant radiation reactions. Since experiments in animal models show the importance of starting postoperative chemotherapy as early as possible after surgery,
long delays may well prejudice the chances of success. In
addition, common clinical experience suggests that a protracted period of adjuvant chemotherapy may be psychologically unacceptable to a significant fraction of this patient
population, which tends to be tired and impatient to resume
a normal life after a stressful period of surgery and radiotherapy.

In many respects, perhaps the most important achievement
of the past 10 years has been the formation of a real commitment to prospective multimodality trials in head and neck
cancer by oncologists in surgery, radiation and medicine.
It would be a disaster if a shortage of supporting funds
from governmental and private sources were to stunt the
growth of clinical trials in this area just when they seem
to hold so much promise. The National Cancer Institute, by
the formation of the Head and Neck Cancer Contracts Program,
has indicated a commitment to support and coordinate therapeutic efforts. The coordination is as important as the
support. Dr. Simon Kramer has estimated that no more than
600-1000 patients with advanced, previously untreated epidermoid head and neck cancer are likely to find their way
into prospective clinical trials each year in the U.S.A..
Close coordination is therefore highly desirable if needless
duplication of effort is to be avoided.

References

(1)   Al-Sarraf, M., Amer, MH, Vaisham-Payan, G, et al.: A
      multidisciplinary therapeutic approach for advanced
      previously untreated epidermoid cancer of the head and
      neck: preliminary report. Int. J. Rad. Oncol Biol.
      Phys. 5:1421-1423 (1979).

(2)   Amery, WK, Spreafico, F, Rojas, AF, et al: Adjuvant
      treatment with levamisole in cancer. A review of experi-
      mental and clinical data. Cancer Treat. Rev. 4:167-195
      (1977).

(3)   Ansfield, FJ, Ramirez, G, Davis, HL, et al.: Treatment
      of advanced cancer of the head and neck. Cancer 25:78-
      82 (1970).

(4)   Browder, JP, Chretien, PB: Immune reactivity in head
      and neck squamous carcinoma and relevance to the design
      of immunotherapy trials. Sem. Oncol. 4:431-440 (1977).

(5)   Cachin, Y, Eschwege, F: Combination of radiotherapy and
      surgery in the treatment of head and neck cancers.
      Cancer Treat. Rev. 2:177-192 (1975).

(6)   Cady, B, Catlin, D: Epidermoid carcinoma of the gum: a
      20 year survey. Cancer 23:551-569 (1969).

(7)   Catterall, M: The treatment of cancer of the head and
      neck: fast neutrons-the way ahead? Sem.Oncol. 4:407-
      412 (1977).

(8)   Catterall, M, Bewley, DK, Southerland, I: Second report
      on results of a randomized clinical trial of fast
      neutrons compared with X or gamma rays in the treatment
      of advanced tumors of the head and neck. Brit. Med. J.
      1:1642 (1977).

(9)   Clifford, P., O'Connor, AD, Durden-Smith, J, et al.:
      Synchronous multiple drug chemotherapy and radiotherapy
      for advanced (Stage III and IV) squamous carcinoma of
      the head and neck. Antibiot. Chemother. 24:60-72 (1978).

(10) Dische, S, Saunders, MI, Flockhart, IR, et al.: Misoni-
      dazole-a drug for trial in radiotherapy and oncology.
      Int. J. Rad. Oncol. Biol. Phys. 5:851-860 (1979).

(11) Elias, EG, Chretien, P, Monnard, E, et al.: Chemotherapy
      prior to local therapy in advanced squamous cell carci-
      noma of the head and neck. Cancer 43:1025-1031 (1979).

(12) Fletcher, GH: Place of irradiation in the management of

head and neck cancers. Sem. Oncol. 4:375-386 (1977).

(13) Fletcher, GH: Textbook of Radiotherapy, 2nd Ed., 1973, Philadelphia, Lea & Febiger, p.284..

(14) Fletcher, GH, Jesse, RH: The place of irradiation in the management of the primary lesion in head and neck cancers. Cancer 39:862-867 (1977).

(15) Fowler, JF : Developments in radiotherapy other than heavy particle beams. Int. J. Rad. Oncol. Biol, Phys. 3:351-358 (1977).

(16) Hilal, EY, Wanebo, HJ, Pinsky, CM, et al.: Immunologic evaluation and prognosis in patients with head and neck cancer. Am. J. Surg. 134:469-473 (1977).

(17) Ho, JHC: An epidemiologic and clinical study of naso-pharyngeal carcinoma. Int. J. Rad. Oncol. Biol. Phys. 4:181-198 (1978).

(18) Holoye, PY, Byers, RM, Gard, DA, et al.: Combination chemotherapy of head and neck cancer. Cancer 42:1661-1669 (1978).

(19) Hong, WK, Shapshay, SM, Bhutani, R, et al.: Induction chemotherapy in advanced squamous head and neck carci-noma with high-dose cis-platinum and bleomycin infusion. Cancer 44:19-25 (1979).

(20) Jesse, RH, Fletcher, GH: Treatment of the neck in patients with squamous cell carcinoma of the head and neck. Cancer 39:868-872 (1977).

(21) Kaplan, BH, Vogl, SE, Chiuten, D, et al.: Chemotherapy of advanced cancer of the head and neck with metho-trexate, bleomycin, and cis-diamminedichloroplatinum in combination. Proc. Am. Soc. Clin. Oncol. 20:384 (1979).

(22) Kirkwood, J, Miller, D, Pitman, S, et al.: Initial high-dose methotrexate-leucovorin in advanced squamous cell carcinoma of the head and neck. Proc. Am. Soc. Clin. Oncol. 19:398 (1978).

(23) Kligerman, MM, Knapp, EA, Peterson, DF; Biomedical pro-gram leading to therapeutic trials of pion radiation at Los Alamos. Cancer 36:1675-1680 (1975).

(24) Levitt, SH, Beachley, MC, Zinberg, Y, et al.: Combina-tion of preoperative irradiation and surgery in the treatment of cancer of the oropharynx, hypopharynx, and larynx. Cancer 27:759-770 (1971).

(25) Lord, JJ, Briant, TD, Rider, WD, Bryce DP: A comparison of pre-operative and primary radiotherapy in the treat-ment of carcinoma of the hypopharynx. Br. J. Radiol. 46:175-179 (1973).

(26) Miller, D: The etiology of nasopharyngeal cancer and its management. Otolaryngol. Clinics North Amer.

13:467-476 (1980).

(27) Million, RR: Elective neck irradiation for T_xN_0 squamous carcinoma of the oral tongue and floor of mouth. Cancer 34:149-155 (1974).

(28) O'Brien, PH, Catlin, D: Cancer of the cheek (mucosa). Cancer 18:1392-1398 (1965).

(29) Perez, CA, Marks, J, Powers, WE: Preoperative irradiation in head and neck cancer. Sem. Oncol. 4:387-398 (1977).

(30) Pitman, SW, Kowal, CD, Papac, RJ, Bertino, JR: Sequential methotrexate-5 fluorouracil: a highly active drug combination in advanced squamous cell carcinoma of the head and neck. Proc. Am. Soc. Clin. Oncol. 21:473 (1980).

(31) Price, LA, Hill, BT, Dalley, VM, et al.: Improved results in combination chemotherapy of head and neck cancer using a kinetically-based approach: a randomized study with and without adriamycin. Oncology 35:26-28(1978).

(32) Randolph, VL, Vallejo, A, Spiro, RH, et al.: Combination therapy of advanced head and neck cancer: induction of remissions with diamminedichloroplatinum (II), bleomycin, and radiation therapy. Cancer 41:460-467 (1978).

(33) Rogers, CC, Hussey, DH, Parker, RA: The future neutron therapy clinical trials in the United States. Int. J. Rad. Oncol. Biol. Phys. 3:263-270 (1977).

(34) Rothman, K, Keller, A: The effect of joint exposure to alcohol and tobacco on risk of cancer of mouth and pharynx. J. Chron. Dis. 25:711-716 (1972).

(35) Seagren, S, Byfield, J, Nahum, A, Bone, R: Concurrent cyclophosphamide, bleomycin, and ionizing radiation in advanced squamous cell carcinoma of the head and neck. Proc. Am. Soc. Clin. Oncol. 20:324 (1979).

(36) Seydel, HG: Interstitial implantation in head and neck cancer. Sem. Oncol. 4:399-406 (1977).

(37) Shanta, V, Krishnamurthi, S: The combined therapy of oral cancer. GANN Monograph on Cancer Res. 19:159-170 (1976).

(38) Syed, A: Management of extensive residual cancer with interstitial iridium implant, in Hilaris, B (ed): Afterloading, 20 years of experience, New York, Memorial Sloan-Kettering Cancer Center, 1975.

(39) Wanebo, HJ, Hilal, EY, Pinsky, CM, et al.: Randomized trial of levamisole in patients with squamous cancer of the head and neck: a preliminary report. Cancer Treat. Rep. 62:1663-1669 (1978).

(40) Wanebo, HJ, Jun, MY, Strong, EW, et al.: T cell deficiency in patients with squamous cell cancer of the head and neck. Am. J. Surg. 130:445-451 (1975).

(41) Wittes, RE: Chemotherapy of head and neck cancer. Otolaryngol. Clinics North Amer. 13:515-520 (1980).

(42) Wittes, RE : Combination chemotherapy of head and neck cancer in the United States. Recent Results in Cancer Res., in press.

(43) Wittes, RE, Heller, K, Randolph, V, et al.: Cis-diamminedichloroplatinum (II)-based chemotherapy as initial treatment in advanced head and neck cancer. Cancer Treat. Rep. 63:1533-1538 (1979).

(44) Wynder, EL, Mabuchi, K, Hoffmann, D: Tobacco, in Schottenfeld, D (ed): Cancer Epidemiology and Prevention, Springfield, Illinois, 1975, pp. 102-125.

Chemotherapy of Gigacytomas: The Treatment
and Curability of "Solid" Tumors with Drugs.

JAMES F. HOLLAND, M.D.

Professor and Chairman
Department of Neoplastic Diseases
Mount Sinai Medical Center
New York, N.Y. 10029

I do not like and have never liked the ambiguous and in-
correct term, solid tumors. I am not one who advocates
calling certain diseases by a negative nomenclature such
as non-lymphocytic leukemia, or non-Hodgkin's lymphoma to
describe diseases for which there have been perfectly adequate alternative names for nearly a century.
  Solid tumors are not solid. There may be extensive necrosis, cavitation, hemorrhage, edema and other serous and
cellular infiltrates that belie the solidity of solid tumors. I propose instead to consider the chemotherapy of
gigacytomas. Since this is a new term, its derivation is
of importance. In this taxonomy, a tumor with a thousand
cells is a kilocytoma, a tumor with a million cells is a
megacytoma, and a tumor with a billion cells, which is
approximately 1 milliliter in volume is a gigacytoma. If
these cells are spread around in small islands, rather than
the coalescent tumor of gigacytoma, the term is gigacytosis. The Greek numerical units focus our attention on the
very phenomena that Skipper and Schabel have taught us
over the last 16 years that have been so critical to the
progress of chemotherapy. We are dealing with specific
numbers of tumor cells in kinetic situations that are dy-
namic. One can even deal with big "solid" tumors, which
are generically gigacytomas. The Greeks had a word for it:
Dekagigacytoma for a ten billion cell tumor, hectogigacy-
toma for 100 billion (approximately 100 grams) and for that
tumor of 10^{12}, approximating a kilogram, teracytoma. And
lastly, for a leukemic patient with a trillion cells, 10^{12},
the applicable term would be leukemic teracytosis (Table I).

TABLE I
Characteristics And Names Of "Solid" Tumors

Cells	Exponent	Volume ml.	Name
1,000	10^3	.000001	Kilocytoma
1,000,000	10^6	.001	Megacytoma
1,000,000,000	10^9	1.0	Gigacytoma
10,000,000,000	10^{10}	10.0	Dekagigacytoma
100,000,000,000	10^{11}	100.	Hectogigacytoma
1,000,000,000,000	10^{12}	1000.	Teracytoma

We tend to think of leukemic patients with so many thousands of cells per cu. mm. of blood, or so many billions of cells per liter. For purposes of the therapy of cancer, I suggest that it would be well to calculate the total body burden, despite the necessarily imprecise assumptions. It has been pointed out in the experimental circumstance that one can give or take a log order or two without changing the principles of the extrapolation in any important way. Just because teracytosis exists does not mean that diseases are incurable. The progression of survival curves for all acute lymphocytic leukemias from the Cancer and Leukemia Group B, contains patients whose mean body burdens at onset of treatment have been calculated to be very close to a trillion cells (15), Fig. 1. Gigacytosis, one billion cells spread around the body, is almost impossible to demonstrate microscopically. Acute lymphocytic leukemia is generically a gigacytosis (tens or hundreds of billions) and often a teracytosis, for which there is an increasing cure rate.

It is possible to separate cancers in terms of the chemotherapeutic effect on them into curable, subcurable, and precurable cancer (Table 2). The curable cancers, by my definition, are those in which 50% or more of the cancers can be cured by chemotherapy alone. The cancers subcurable by chemotherapy are those wherein chemotherapy augments the cure rate appreciably, but by less than 50%. The precurable cancers are not incurable by chemotherapy, but the chemotherapeutic contribution to cure is still uncommon.

Among the curable cancers, one can cure gigacytomas and even teracytosis, often involving primary and metastatic tumor. In the subcurable cancers we are usually limited to micrometastatic cancer or megacytosis as the curative target. In precurable cancer, since we are not in the stage where we reproducibly can effect cure, results depend on

FIGURE I

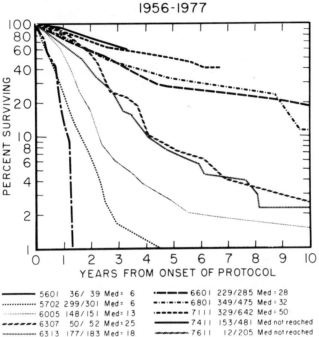

CANCER AND LEUKEMIA GROUP B
Survival of acute lymphocytic leukemia in
children under 20
1956-1977

——— 5601 36/ 39 Med= 6	•———— 6601 229/285 Med = 28	
·············· 5702 299/301 Med= 6	—·—·—·• 6801 349/475 Med = 32	
············· 6005 148/151 Med= 13	■—■——■ 7111 329/642 Med = 50	
✦✦✦✦✦ 6307 50/ 52 Med=25	——— 7411 153/481 Med not reached	
············· 6313 177/183 Med= 18	✧✧✧✧ 7611 12/205 Med not reached	

the size and the nature of the neoplasm. In curable cancer,
local and regional assistance from surgery and radiotherapy
may be helpful. In subcurable cancer local assistance is
essential, and in the precurable cancers it is still insufficient. Chemotherapeutically curable cancers are curable by single drug treatments, such as methotrexate, or
cyclophosphamide, or by combinations. In the subcurable
cancers it is uncommon that a single agent be sufficient.
Combination chemotherapy is usually superior. In the precurable cancers, most of the chemotherapeutic treatments
have not been adequately or appropriately tried. What
chemotherapy has been attempted has often been in patients
with very large tumors, hectogigacytomas and teracytomas,
often extensively pretreated with other ineffective approaches. Studies have rarely been conducted under circumstances where one could anticipate curability.

TABLE 2
Classification Of Tumors By Chemotherapeutic Effect
1980

	Curable	Subcurable	Precurable
Curability:	>50%	<50%	Uncommon
Effects On:	Metastatic	Micrometastatic	Either
Susceptible Tumors:	Gigacytomas	Megacytosis	
Local Assistance:	Helpful	Essential	Insufficient
Drugs:	Single or combination	Combination	Mostly untried
Monitoring:	Biochemical, anatomic	Usually ineffective	Absent or ineffective

Another characteristic of the curable tumors is that they are usually easy to monitor, either by biochemical techniques or by anatomic circumstance. The correlation of human chorionic gonadotropin titer with gestational choriocarcinoma, for example, has made it easy to treat seemingly healthy women in remission with continuing intensive drug therapy to attain disease eradication. The patterns of growth and metastasis of curable tumors make it relatively easy to stage them and to know their extent and disposition with some confidence. Monitoring techniques in the subcurable tumors are usually ineffective. A major contribution can be made among the subcurable cancers, moving them more assuredly into the curable area, by dicovery of effective monitoring techniques that would allow closure of the feedback loop, knowing when tumor is present or not, and thus knowing when treatment is necessary or not. In the precurable tumors, monitoring techniques of biochemical nature or anatomical staging are either absent or ineffective.

It is relevant to inquire how the therapies that have been discovered for the three categories of cancer were found. For the curable cancers, by and large, it has been by revelation. Serendipity has played a part. The first use of methotrexate in choriocarcinoma was serendipitous. But the people plowing that garden could see a flower growing rather than a weed, and paid attention. Li continued the methotrexate treatment which Condit had given to the first patient with choriocarcinoma as a pharmacologic trial, not a therapeutic effort, because the titer of HCG had dropped (16). Burkitt treated children in Uganda with "a

handful of pills" and saw total permanent regressions. None
of the curative treatments, including the MOPP treatment in
Hodgkin's disease nor the initial studies that made major
differences in acute lymphocytic leukemia were executed as
a controlled trial. The findings were such a dramatic departure from the expected background of cancer medicine
that the recognition was a revelation. For subsequent improvements upon curative regimens for cancer, however, controlled trials have produced the most significant benefits.

In the subcurable cancers, often there has been a major
deviation from usual expectation. Not of the same miraculous splendor perhaps as is true of the curable cancers,
but nonetheless striking. An example of this is Cooper's
first recognition of the activity of vincristine, prednisone, cyclophosphamide, methotrexate and fluorouracil, the
VPCMF, or Cooper regimen for women with metastatic breast
cancer. It was logically formulated in his head, and properly tested in women with metastatic cancer where it was found
to be dramatically active, a major departure (6). Unfortunately, it was never reported in a full paper. Cooper then
undertook to study his regimen in women at such high risk,
with 4 or more metastatic axillary lymph nodes, that 85% were
doomed to relapse within 10 years as has been shown by Fisher
(11). The Cooper regimen given for only 9 months was also
dramatically active in this adjuvant setting. Since it was
not a prospectively randomized study, background comparisons
with 21,000 American women who were at better initial prognosis are valuable to illustrate the major deviation from expectation (7), Fig. 2. Subsequently a controlled trial of
this has been undertaken in the Cancer and Leukemia Group B,
superintended by Dr. Douglas Tormey. We have demonstrated
that the 5 drug Cooper regimen given adjuvantly at the time
of surgery for women with 4 nodes or more is significantly
superior (P=.01) to CMF, the 3 drugs which are derivative of
the original Cooper regimen (20). The CALGB data for CMF are
superimposable upon the Bonadonna data for CMF. Since there
is a significant difference of CMFVP from our own CMF data,
and the CMF data from CALGB intertwine with the Milan CMF
data, we submit that CMFVP is a better treatment for women
with 4 nodes or more (Fig. 3). From Bonadonna's controlled
experiment, the contribution of radical mastectomy alone to
disease-free survival can be estimated as 30% at 4 years (2).
The Milan CMF data and the CALGB CMF data confirm each other
in adding approximately 20% to relapse-free survival. The
CMFVP program adds another 20%, and thus approaches the
arbitrary 50% definition that would move it into the curative
classification. Further time is required to reach the final
plateaus of cure expectancy. The more curable the tumor and

FIGURE 2

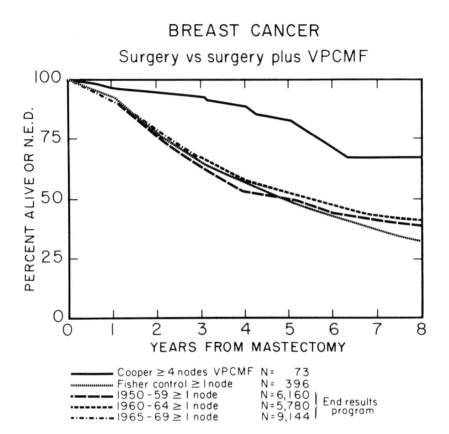

BREAST CANCER
Surgery vs surgery plus VPCMF

Legend	N=
Cooper ≥ 4 nodes VPCMF	73
Fisher control ≥ 1 node	396
1950 - 59 ≥ 1 node	6,160
1960 - 64 ≥ 1 node	5,780
1965 - 69 ≥ 1 node	9,144

End results program

the more curative the regimen, the earlier the plateau will begin.

It is my interpretation of the information that Veronesi and coworkers have gathered, presented in this symposium by Bonadonna, that the surgical component of breast cancer therapy may indeed shrink as the chemotherapeutic component becomes more effective.

The precurable neoplasms so far have shown minor deviations from expectation in single arm studies or in controlled trials.

Subcurative chemotherapies (as well as curative therapies) are associated with failure or relapse. It is necessary to determine why relapses occur, because if they did not, from the apparent initial effectiveness of the treatment we might attain curative treatments. One reason pa-

FIGURE 3

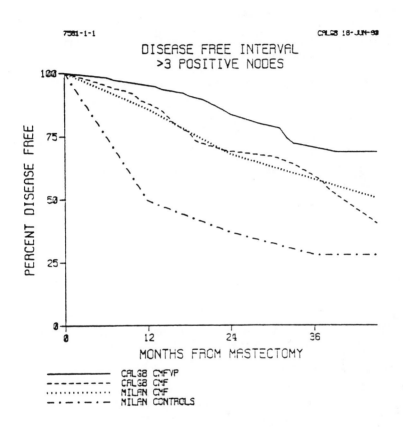

7581-1-1   CALGB 18-JUN-80

DISEASE FREE INTERVAL
>3 POSITIVE NODES

Legend:

- CALGB CMFVP
- CALGB CMF
- MILAN CMF
- MILAN CONTROLS

tients relapse is that chemotherapy exceeds normal tissue tolerance. Myocardial degeneration from an anthracycline antibiotic is an example. We have learned how to prevent this by restricting cumulative doses, but dose restriction may be deleterious insofar as it jeopardizes killing the tumor (Table 3).

Kinetic resistance is difficult for the individual phy-

TABLE 3
Relapse On Primary Resistance Causes Of Chemotherapy
1980

Curative	Subcurative	Precurative
	Exceeding normal tissue tolerance	Ineffective drugs
	Kinetic resistance	Ineffective use of drug schedules
	Clonal selection	Combinations
	Biochemical resistance	Drug transport
	Immunologic factors Treatment related Tumor related	Tumor kinetics
	Patient-Physician exhaustion	

sician to recognize before it is too late. It is nonetheless common. Norton has emphasized that Gompertzian tumor kinetics make novel alterations in dose schedule appropriate (17). A mathematical model of the effect of chemotherapy studied in the adjuvant surgical program of the Cooper regimen is shown (Fig. 4). An induction treatment course of CMFVP for 6 weeks was administered and then maintenance treatments 2 weeks on, 2 weeks off sequentially during the first year. Decreases in drug dose are arbitrarily factored in, since drug toxicity is frequent and such drug adjustments lead to less drug being administered than was prescribed. Bonadonna has cited drug reduction as having major impact on the results of CMF treatment (2). A new program we have been exploring is also shown in which an identical induction course is followed by 6 weeks recovery, and then another full induction course is administered seriatim. The same dose adjustments that may be necessary as one pursues these treatments have been modelled in. Norton assumed Gompertzian growth of a gigacytoma, and the growth characteristics are identical in the two examples (18). With the same drugs, the same schema for dose alterations, and the same assumptions of tumor growth and tumor regression, one regimen could lead to relapse and the other to eradication.

FIGURE 4

INFLUENCE OF DIFFERENT PLANS OF CHEMOTHERAPY ON REGRESSION OF A SMALL GOMPERTZIAN TUMOR

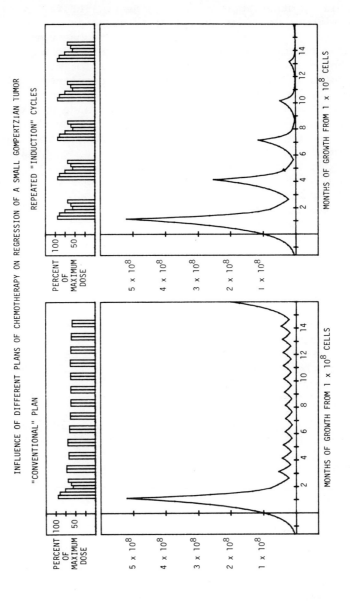

Thus kinetic resistance can lead to relapse, possibly avoidable by other appropriate regimens. The failing regimen in the model does not always fail, since it is the successful 5-drug program which we have shown to be superior to the 3-drug regimen in women with 4 or more metastatic nodes in the course of breast cancer (20). Pilot studies on the repeated induction regimen have been completed, and it will be put to test in an adjuvant surgical program by the CALGB.

In addition to normal tissue tolerance and kinetic resistance, clonal selection in the tumor by killing off sensitive cell lines is possible. Clonal lines within tumors can be readily recognized in malignant melanoma, for example, where different cutaneous metastases may be densely pigmented or amelanotic. Some nodules appear to be mixtures of two clones. If different amounts of tyrosinase can occur in isolated metastases of melanoma, it is apparent that the other biochemical properties in sublines of tumor cells might be similarly different in other ways, including drug metabolism. Biochemical resistance can also develop adaptively in tumor cells, but may not be as important for human cancer using the present techniques of chemotherapy as the attainment of host tolerance, kinetic resistance, or clonal selection.

Other factors which can compromise the effectiveness of subcurative chemotherapy are immunologic factors related to the treatment, and immunologic factors related to the tumor. Such phenomena as depletion of killer cells, the appearance of blocking factors, and induced appearance of suppressor cells are all relevant and have been described (1).

One of the most critical reasons for the failure of subcurative chemotherapy to succeed is patient-physician exhaustion. Determination to continue with the treatment is essential. Patients who leave the therapeutic program are failures of the regimen. Such patients could constitute a significant proportion of failures of some future regimen that might be curative. Maintenance of intensive dosing, avoidance of toxicity, nonadherence to prescribed regimens, and loss to followup (which usually means the patient has voted with his feet) all relate to curative chemotherapy.

It is now appropriate to question why cancers remain in the precurable category. It is not that they may not be curable. The first and obvious answer that many would put forth is that there are ineffective drugs. Yet many of the drugs that we know to be effective in other cancers have not been convincingly tested in this group of tumors. The ineffective use of drugs can be illustrated in the classic research of Goldin showing the extraordinary effect of intermittency of methotrexate dosing on early L1210 leukemia, (megacytosis) and the inactivity of this drug at the same doses and schedules in the late tumor (gigacytosis) (13). In the early tumor modifications of schedule can alter therapeutic effectiveness. In the advanced tumor it doesn't matter what schedule is used. The opportunity to apply a curative approach may be lost with an ineffective schedule and precluded altogether by the consequences of a massive tumor.

Drug transport in many precurable tumors has not been studied. Drugs may not gain entry to or remain within the tumor to accomplish their effect. Tumor kinetics of the neoplasms that are among the chemotherapeutically precurable cancers is quite different from the kinetics of those in the curable category, with a smaller proliferating pool and much greater differentiation. It is also possible that repair enzymes are substantially more active in the more differentiated cells thereby retrieving genetic and biochemical abnormalities resultant from drug interaction with macromolecules that are unrepaired and lethal in primitive curable tumors.

As a summary aspect of cancers classified by chemotherapeutic sensitivity, curable tumors are undifferentiated and very close to the stem cell of the tissue involved (Table 4). They have a very short G_1, a rapid cell cycle, and cure is moderately independent of tumor size. Even grossly metastatic tumors are responsive. The subcurable tumors are generally more differentiated. The G_1 period of these tumors is probably shortened by the local assistance treatments. The tumor size is critical. Data have been referred to herein (7)(20)(2) that a substantial proportion of high risk

---

TABLE 4
Classification Of Tumors By Chemotherapeutic Effect
1980

	Curable	Subcurable	Precurable
Morphology:	Undifferentiated	Differentiated	Differentiated
G_1 in cell cycle	Short	Shortened	Long
Size:	Moderately independent	Critical	Critical

breast cancer patients can be rendered disease-free by intensive chemotherapy assisted by local removal. These patients
are women with metastatic breast cancer, clinically inapparent, but nonetheless metastatic, probably as megacytosis.
For patients who present with clinically manifest metastatic
breast cancer, gigacytomas, it's an extreme rarity with the
drugs and strategies we use today to attain cure. Kilocy-
tomas and megacytomas may be eradicable when gigacytomas
are not.

The precurable tumors are, by and large, highly differentiated tumors. It seems likely that the tumor stem cell
is also quite differentiated rather than just a commitment
for post mitotic cells to mature. Their G_1 is long. Their
growth may be slow, but it is inexorable, and size is undoubtedly critical for any approach to chemotherapeutic
curability.

The chemotherapies of gigacytomas and gigacytoses as of
1980 can be arranged by their effectiveness (Table 5).
Choriocarcinoma was cured in 1956, and is, comparatively,
relatively size independent and responds to single drugs.
The pre-T cell (common antigen) acute lymphocytic leukemia,
those cells that are more immature than T-cell leukemias,
was reproducibly curable by about 1963. Burkitt's tumor is
influenced by stage (cellular number and host factors) but is
curable with single drugs. Hodgkin's disease is chemotherapeutically curable with the 4 drug combination that DeVita
and coworkers introduced at the beginning of '66. Acute
promyelocytic leukemia, found curable by Bernard and colleagues requires not just proper diagnosis and proper anthracycline chemotherapy, but proper host supportive therapy
with heparin and thrombocytes. This is a highly fatal neoplasm transformed into a curable tumor by an appropriate
comprehensive approach. Large follicular center cell lymph-

TABLE 5
Curative Chemotherapy Of Gigacytomas
And Gigacytoses - 1980

Choriocarcinoma 1956
Wilms' tumor 1960
Pre-T cell acute lymphocytic leukemia 1963
Burkitt's tumor 1965
Hodgkin's disease 1966
Acute promyelocytic leukemia 1974
Large follicular center cell
    (diffuse histiocytic) lymphoma 1975
Embryonal carcinoma of testis 1977

oma, particularly with indented nuclei, which is a subset of what has been termed diffuse histiocytic lymphoma was curable by 1975, and embryonal carcinoma of the testes by 1976. The concept is surfacing that the less differentiated forms of Hodgkin's disease, lymphocyte depletion and mixed cellularity, are more susceptible to chemotherapy than is nodular sclerosis Hodgkin's disease (9). It is widely recognized that the more differentiated lymphoid neoplasms are not nearly so curable as Burkitt's tumor and the large follicular center cell lymphomas. Golbey has observed that if embryonal carcinoma of the testis matures in the tumor to show teratomatous elements, the cure rate is lower (12). The tumors curable by chemotherapy are undifferentiated, primitive, rapidly growing cells with short G_1 periods and a proportionately longer time in the S phase.

The subcurative chemotherapies of gigacytomas and gigacytoses apply to T-cell acute lymphocytic leukemia, wherein dramatically rapid responses occur, but tumor killing is incomplete, most remissions are not sustained, and relapse occurs (Table 6). Nonetheless an appreciable percentage attains a prolonged disease-free state consistent with cure. Acute myelocytic leukemia is in the early stage of curative treatment, and thus is subcurative. A progressive march has been in process over a ten year period in the data of the Cancer and Leukemia Group B, based on 2,500 patients with acute myelocytic leukemia (Fig. 5). The tails of the curves have begun to break on semilog plotting indicating the low percentage of patients (now up to 20%) who are departing from the expected behavior and who remain disease-free. It is therefore reasonable to recognize that cure is in progress in acute myelocytic leukemia.

Small cell carcinoma of the lung is one subset of the dreadful epidemic of lung cancer that could be preventable

---

TABLE 6
Subcurative Chemotherapy Of Gigacytomas
And Gigacytosis - 1980

T cell acute lymphocytic leukemia
Acute myelocytic leukemia
Small cell carcinoma of lung
Squamous cell carcinoma of upper
    aerodigestive tract
Adenocarcinoma of ovary
Adenocarcinoma of breast
Osteosarcoma
Ewing's sarcoma
Embryonal rhabdomyosarcoma

FIGURE 5

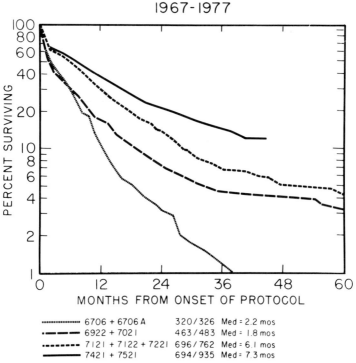

CANCER AND LEUKEMIA GROUP B
Survival of acute myelocytic leukemia
1967-1977

▪▪▪▪▪▪▪▪▪▪▪ 6706 + 6706A	320/326	Med = 2.2 mos
▪—▪— 6922 + 7021	463/483	Med = 1.8 mos
▪▪▪▪▪▪▪▪ 7121 + 7122 + 7221	696/762	Med = 6.1 mos
—— 7421 + 7521	694/935	Med = 7.3 mos

with effective social and regulatory posture concerning
cigarette smoking. A proportion of patients with small cell
carcinoma of the lung are long term disease-free survivors
if there is no evidence of disseminated metastasis at the
onset of treatment with chemotherapy and radiotherapy.
    Squamous cell carcinoma of the upper aerodigestive tract
is now showing major response to several chemotherapeutic
regimens containing cisplatin, bleomycin, vinblastine or
methotrexate. Here the timing is critical, since chemotherapy after surgical and radiation failures also fails.
Carcinoma treated first with intensive short-term chemotherapy usually regresses at least partially promptly, and
some have even not been detectable on the pathological specimen a few weeks later at the time of surgery. Chemotherapy is being used to attempt avoidance of disfiguring
surgery by Clifford and colleagues who have observed patients

with T-3 and T-4 head and neck cancers treated with chemotherapy and radiotherapy without surgery, whose disease-
free survival at 5 years projects to 48%. This is substantially better than standard treatment (5).

Adenocarcinoma of the ovary is chemotherapeutically subcurable. In an interim analysis at Mount Sinai, 41 patients from 88 who had received cisplatin in combination,
primarily in our adriamycin-platinum combination, were
clinically free of disease at the end of one year. They
were thus subjected to a second laparotomy. Nine had gross
tumor that wasn't detectable externally, 15 had only microscopic tumor on extensive biopsy procedure, and 17 had no
evidence of disease. Sixteen of these women were living
without recurrence of tumor with observations extending to
48 months. Ovarian cancer is chemotherapeutically subcurable, and both surgery and chemotherapy are essential
aspects of the overall treatment strategy.

Adenocarcinoma of the breast is an example, par excellence, of a disease subcurable by chemotherapy.

Metastatic osteosarcoma masses, even deka- and hectogigacytomas, may regress temporarily from adriamycin or methotrexate. These two agents are effective as single drug
treatments, and are the prime factors in combination drug
regimens that have been effective in prolonging disease-free
survival in association with amputation. Combination regimens have also caused nearly total histological regression
of a substantial proportion of primary osteosarcomas, allowing conservative limb salvage surgery, and together with
postoperative chemotherapy, a high proportion of disease-
free survivors (8). Some observers believe the results
might be attributable to improved surgery alone and that the
need for certainty requires an untreated control population
(10). There is an extremely steep dose response curve for
the treatment of osteosarcoma (and probably for most cancers). In studies of the CALGB, when physicians or patients
do not adhere to the protocol (which makes allowance for
dose adjustments at specific thresholds of toxic phenomena)
pulmonary metastases appear and the results are demonstrably
inferior. This demonstrates that the tumors are still viru-
lent, if not eradicated. For patients who receive the intensive treatment stipulated as 30 mg/m^2 x 3 days for 6
courses over a period of 6 months for a total of 540 mg/m^2
of adriamycin (with adjustments as necessary according to
protocol) the disease-free survival is impressive (Fig. 6).
A few small tumors had 50% disease-free survival. Patients
whose tumors were 5 to 10 cm. in diameter, however, the
disease-free survival is 90%. This is not consistent with

FIGURE 6

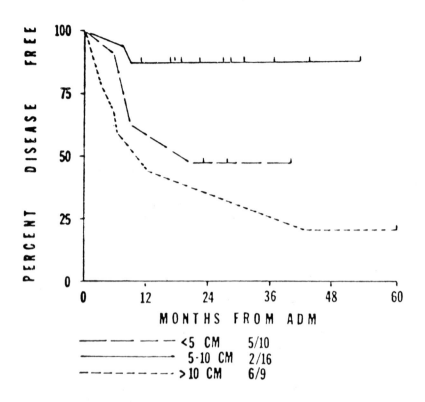

— — — — <5 CM	5/10
—————— 5-10 CM	2/16
— — — — — >10 CM	6/9

surgery alone for this disease. Those who have huge tumors do poorly. The large tumor probably correlates with poly-megacytosis in the disseminated micrometastases which thus prevents chemotherapeutic cure. The chemotherapeutic contribution to cures of Ewing's sarcoma and embryonal rhabdomyosarcoma are presented elsewhere in this symposium (14).

The cancers that are not ordinarily cured with chemotherapy are precurable (Table 7). They are not incurable, however, since some credible studies report suggestive but statistically insignificant trends of improvement over local and regional treatment alone. Carcinoma of the lung is a nearly preventable disease. We appear to be totally ineffective at a political level. The oncologist is being asked to rescue patients from the consequences of vested inaction in health politics, while the patient is being permitted suicidal slow puffing. It is a medical and political disgrace. With imaginative progressive taxation based on cigarette tar content, a penny a milligram, inhalational carcinogenesis can be diminished.

TABLE 7
Precurative Chemotherapy Of Gigacytomas
And Gigacytoses - 1980

Carcinoma Of Lung
squamous cell
adenocarcinoma
large cell anaplastic

Carcinomas Of
esophagus, stomach,
pancreas, liver,
biliary tract, colon

Carcinoma Of
endometrium, cervix

Carcinoma Of
kidney, bladder,
prostate

Carcinoma Of
thyroid

Gliomas

Melanomas

Carcinoids

Chronic Myelocytic Leukemia

Chronic Lymphocytic Leukemia

Multiple Myeloma

The gastrointestinal tract is in the stage of precurative chemotherapy. Adriamycin containing regimens are active in advanced gastric cancer. Reorganization to study these regimens in the state of megacytosis rather than on gigacytomas has been undertaken (19). Small improvements in the response to drugs or to radiotherapy and drugs has also been seen for pancreatic cancer, allowing a sensible program moving by small steps to continue toward the target. Elsewhere in this symposium Schein gives evidence that progress is being made toward converting precurable carcinoma of the rectum to a subcurable classification (19). Carcinoma of the anus is a rare tumor but there too, tumor eradication

appears to be attainable with chemotherapeutic and radiotherapeutic and surgical methods which were not achieved
previously with surgical and radiotherapeutic methods alone
(3).

We are still in the precurative chemotherapy of gigacytomas and gigacytoses of endometrial carcinoma, probably for
a very different reason than in cancers of the gastrointestinal tract. Endometrial carcinoma is so well cared for by
the conventional techniques of surgery and radiotherapy that
only a small percentage of patients relapse. Because of
this, because there is no monitoring technique to tell which
patient will relapse, we are usually precluded from undertaking what would seem to be chemotherapy at the optimal
time in the stage of megacytosis, and are obliged to wait
until a clinically manifest gigacytoma reappears indicating
relapse. Nonetheless endometrial carcinoma appears to be a
sensitive neoplasm even as a gigacytoma and I believe that
it will move into the subcurative stage quickly (4).

In the urinary tract, despite evidence of chemotherapeutic activity on prostatic carcinoma, we certainly are in
the precurative phase. Similarly, bladder carcinoma is responsive to chemotherapy, but reproducible cures have not
been observed (21).

The most persuasively remote from cure are those cancers
with the most differentiated cells. It is as if tumors that
show anatomic and functional maturation have tumor stem
cells which alrady have many metabolic commitments to differentiation. The chemotherapeutic sensitivity of such
tumor stem cells is probably substantially less than that of
the stem cell in tumors with little maturation. Chronic
myelocytic leukemia, chronic lymphocytic leukemia and multiple myeloma are neoplasms containing the most differentiated cells of the hematopoietic system. Cures have been
extremely rare in these diseases. Prolonged apparent
disease-free intervals in a few patients with myeloma may
be a consequence of slow doubling time of a tumor that regressed under therapy rather than truly having disappeared.

In addition to the therapeutic approaches that are being
tested in an attempt to effect maturation of the cancer
cells into their normal counterpart, one viable strategy
would seem to be to organize therapeutic approaches to block
maturation of cells so that the dividing stem cells were
less mature, less committed to differentiation, and perhaps
more chemotherapeutically susceptible. One way to accomplish this, apparently, is by bulk reduction of tumor. This
may be the significance of surgery and of radiotherapy as
local treatments allowing for chemotherapeutic successes in

the adjuvant setting. It then becomes realistic to ask which is the adjuvant therapy, or are they coequal partners?

The tumors that are in the precurative category constitute two thirds of human cancer in western societies. I believe however, that we are much closer than readily apparent to transferring some of these cancers to the subcurable category. This requires surgical and radiotherapeutic control of major tumor masses. It raises the question whether we will ever find curative therapies for clinically massively disseminated neoplasms such as melanoma or metastatic carcinoma of the kidney using the techniques we currently know. I believe it will take a much more organized strategy of exploratory treatment of patients in the postoperative period, when the tumor may be, because of bulk reduction, somewhat more susceptible to our chemotherapeutic ministrations. Such research will require a long term systematic plan, because it will require control patients who do not receive the chemotherapy to know what has been accomplished in treating the biology of the unseen. A reasonable start could be made examining the therapies that are known to be of value in other cancers when treated as megacytoses, despite the fact that the same drugs may have been shown of no value in the advanced differentiated cancers when tested against gigacytomas, or more usually, teracytoses. To this end, the emerging technology of the study of human cancer cells in vitro for their therapeutic responsiveness should provide a basis for accelerating the shift from the precurable towards subcurable cancer, and a diminution in the two thirds of patients who are currently not susceptible of cure by chemotherapy. Revelations may come unexpectedly for some of the cancers, but slow stepwise progress seems much more likely.

It has been only 33 years since the recognition of aminopterin as a drug able to induce temporary remissions of acute lymphocytic leukemia. I believe that the next 33 years, or probably much less, with attention to the concepts and strategies emerging, will be even more fruitful.

References

1) Bast Jr., R.C.: Effects of Cancers and Their Treatment
   on Host Immunity. In J.F. Holland and E. Frei, III (eds.)
   Cancer Medicine. Philadelphia, Pa. Lea & Febiger, (In
   Press) 1981.
2) Bonadonna, G., Valagussa, P., Rossi, A., Tancini, G.,
   Bajetta, E., Marchini, S. and Veronesi, U.: In S.E.
   Jones and S.E. Salmon (eds.), Adjuvant Therapy of
   Cancer II. New York: Grune and Stratton, 1979, 227-235.
3) Bruckner, H.W., Spigelman, M.K., Mandel, E., Cohen, C.J.,
   Deppe, G., Turell, R. and Schiavone, R.: Carcinoma of
   the Anus Treated with a Combination of Radiotherapy and
   Chemotherapy. Cancer Treatment Reports 1979, 63:395.
4) Bruckner, H.W. and Deppe, C.: Combination Chemotherapy
   of Advanced Endometrial Adenocarcinoma with Adriamycin,
   Cyclophosphamide, 5-fluorouracil and Medroxyprogesterone
   Acetate. Obstet. & Gynec. 1977, 50:10.
5) Clifford, P.: Personal Communication 1980.
6) Cooper, R.G.: Combination Chemotherapy in Hormone
   Resistant Breast Cancer. Proc. Am. Assoc. Cancer
   Res. 1967, 10:15.
7) Cooper, R.G., Holland, J.F. and Glidewell, O.: Adjuvant
   Chemotherapy of Breast Cancer. Cancer 1979, 44:693-696.
8) Cortes, E.P., Holland, J.F. and Glidewell, O.: Adjuvant
   Therapy of Operable Primary Osteosarcoma - Cancer and
   Leukemia Group B Experience. In G. Bonadonna, G. Mathe
   and S.E. Salmon (eds.) Recent Results in Cancer Research
   68, Springer-Verlag Berlin Heidelberg 1979, 16-24.
9) DeVita, V.T., Glatstein, E.J., Yount, R.C., Hubbard, S.M.,
   Simon, R.M., Ziegler, J.L. and Wiernik, P.H.: Changing
   Concepts: The Lymphomas. In S.E. Jones and S.E. Salmon
   (eds.), Adjuvant Therapy of Cancer II. New York: Grune
   and Stratton, 1979, 173-190.
10) Edmonson, J.H. and Green, S.J.: Methotrexate as Adjuvant
    Treatment for Primary Osteosarcoma. New England J. Med.
    1980, 303:642-643.
11) Fisher, B., Slack, N., Katrych, D. and Wolmark, N.: Ten
    Year Followup Results: Patients with carcinoma of the
    breast in a cooperative clinical trial elevating surgical
    adjuvant chemotherapy. Surg. Gynec. Obstet. 1975,
    140:528-534.

12) Goldberg, R.B.: Germ Cell Tumors. Cancer; Achievements, Prospects and Challenges for the 1980s. New York, Grune and Stratton, 1981.

13) Goldin, A., Venditti, J.M., Humphreys, S.R. and Mantel, N.: Modification of Treatment Schedules in the Management of Advanced Mouse Leukemia with Amethopterin. J. Nat. Cancer Inst. 1956, 17:203-212.

14) Hammond, D.: Pediatric Overview. Cancer: Achievements, Prospects and Challenges for the 1980s. Grune and Stratton, 1981.

15) Holland, J.F.: The Acute Leukemias. In P.B. Beeson and W. McDermott (eds.) Textbook of Medicine 15th edition. W. B. Saunders Co., 1979, 1813-1821.

16) Li, M.C., Hertz, R. and Spencer, D.B.: Effect of Methotrexate Therapy upon Choriocarcinoma and Chorioadenoma. Proc. Soc. Exp. Biol. (N.Y.) 93:361-366, 1956.

17) Norton, L., Simon, R.: New Thoughts on the Relationship of Tumor Growth Characteristics to Sensitivity to Treatment. Methods in Cancer Research 1979, 27:53-90.

18) Norton, L.: Unpublished data.

19) Schein, P.S.: G.I. Tumors. Cancer: Achievements, Prospects and Challenges for the 1980s. New York, Grune & Stratton, 1981.

20) Weiss, R.B., Tormey, D.C., Holland, J.F., Weinberg, V.E., Lesnick, G., Perloff, M., Falkson, G. and Glidewell, O.: A Randomized Trial of Postoperative 5-Drug Vs. 3-Drug Chemotherapy After Mastectomy: A Cancer and Leukemia Group B Study. Recent Results in Cancer Research. Springer-Verlag Berlin Heidelberg New York 1980.

21) Yagoda, A.S.: GU Tumors. Cancer: Achievements, Prospects and Challenges for the 1980s. New York, Grune & Stratton, 1981.

Chemotherapy

Development of Coordinated Cancer
Chemotherapy in Western Europe

H.J. TAGNON
*Emeritus Professor of Medicine and Oncology, University of
Brussels Medical School,
Former Chief of Clinical Investigation, Institut Jules
Bordet, Brussels,
Past President, E.O.R.T.C.*

OMAR C. YODER, PH.D.
Division of Cancer Treatment
National Cancer Institute

By 1962 a group of clinical and laboratory scientists
from the countries of Western continental Europe, later
joined by representatives from Great Britain, had decided
to make a concerted effort and pool resources in order to
develop a program of cancer chemotherapy of an international
West-European scope. The justification for this decision
was firstly the relative underdevelopment of chemotherapy
research in Europe as compared with the United States,
secondly the lack of response of national foundations or
governments to the challenge represented by this underdevelopment. An important factor of the success of the
group was their initial enthusiasm and the unanimous agreement among the representatives of these neighbour countries
on the long term objective to be won : this was clearly
expressed as the pooling of research resources in the
laboratory as well as in the hospital in order to increase
the efficiency of the European participation in cancer
therapeutic research and create the conditions for active
participation and collaboration with the United States and
other advanced countries' programs of research. Thus was
created the European Organization for Research on Treatment
of Cancer, or E.O.R.T.C. (1). This was from the beginning
and still is a non governmental organization grouping the
different scientific disciplines contributing to the
progress and development of cancer therapeutic research.
The founder members are listed on the inside front cover of
the European Journal of Cancer.

FIGURE 1
Map of Cities with Participating Centers

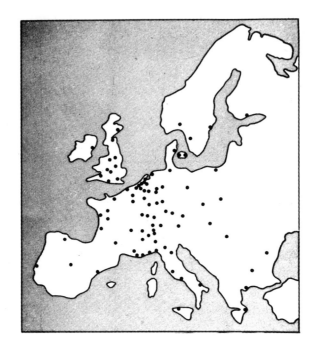

EORTC has a Council which plans and supervises the
activities within the organization. The Administrative
Board prepares the meetings of the Council and handles the
daily work involved with administrative and financial
matters. Within the EORTC clinical and laboratory research
is carried out by some 27 clinical and preclinical cooperative project groups, and working parties.

Membership

Members of Council are elected for a period of 3 years
after which they can be considered for re-election according
to the same procedure as in the case of new members. The
chairmen of cooperative groups and project groups are
elected Council members for the tenure of their respective
chairmanship. Membership to clinical cooperative group is,
in essence, open to every interested clinician. A new
member is elected by the group for two years. Election to
active membership will depend on his/her contribution to the
group's work during the two year period. Research Project
Groups are open for scientists wishing to participate in the
respective research programme.

Statutes

The statutes approved by the general assembly of the
organization have been deposited according to the Belgian
law, and EORTC has been recognized as an "International
Association with Scientific Aims" by Decree no. 3344
published in the Belgian Gazette (Moniteur Belge) of 11th
July 1963, page 1229. The same statutes form the basis for
the registration of EORTC with the Court of Ulm as
"eingetragener Verein". Statutes regulating the work in the
clinical cooperative groups have been adopted by the Council
and the groups in 1971 and bylaws were adopted in 1979.

Meetings

The Council meets 2 to 4 times, the Administrative Board
4 to 6 times a year in the various European institutes
associated with EORTC to discuss scientific as well as
administrative matters. At regular intervals it reviews the
results of the drug screening programmes and those of the
clinical cooperative groups and the research project groups.
Project groups meet as often as their activity requires.
An annual plenary meeting is organized in June for all
members of suborganizations of EORTC on one or more subjects

related to the treatment of cancer.

Therefore the EORTC is not a scientific society in the
usual meaning of the word : it is an association of workers
who get together on projects lending themselves to collaborative approaches. It does not pretend to monopolize cancer
research in Europe. There are of course a large number of
laboratories and hospitals which carry out outstanding
research outside of the EORTC. Similarly it does not wish
to supplant national programs of research in progress in the
different countries grouped in the EORTC. However, the EORTC
over the years has become a well established and well
recognized institution in Europe, having attracted a high
proportion of the best oncologists and the most important
cancer centers of the continent.

Therapeutic cancer research in the EORTC is conceived in
its broadest meaning from organic chemistry through biology,
genetic, pharmacology, etc. to the ultimate of therapeutic
research which is the controlled clinical trial and the
application of new acquisitions to the practice of medicine.

Later in 1970 the initiation of the inspiring cancer
program in the United States had a profound repercussion in
the EORTC membership and provided added intellectual stimulation and psychological support for the pursuance of our plan
which became more and more ambitious with successive
presidents and the availability of new resources.

In short EORTC assigns itself the task of promoting
actively in the field collaborative research bringing together scientists from the participating countries and
endeavoring to associate laboratory workers and clinicians
around the same table and in collaborative projects for
better efficiency improvement and broadening of the thinking
process and acceleration of the transit from theoretical
results to practical application. Success has been achieved
in what some observers have called a spectacular way in two
main areas : firstly the screening of new compounds and
experimental pharmacology ; secondly the setting up of
cooperative clinical and preclinical groups, assisted and
monitored by a strongly structured Data Center. We will
first discuss the Data Center and the cooperative groups
gravitating around it.

THE EORTC DATA CENTER

There were as of the end of last year 72 clinical studies
being monitored by the Data Center, from 13 countries, 255
institutions with the participation of over 1500 clinicians.
This important participation of physicians from cancer
centers and general hospitals represents a type of postgraduate medical education in oncology which has proved to
be very effective and much superior to other forms of postgraduate education as for instance formal courses or lectures.
The Data Center of the EORTC is composed of a Director who
is physician and biostatistician, 3 statisticians, 3 computer
analysts and programmers, 8 data managers and 4 medical
secretaries (Table 1). The Data Center has today 6500 to
7000 patients on study with 1000 new patients being
registered each year. Obviously much clinical therapeutic
research is carried out outside of the EORTC and without
the assistance of the EORTC Data Center. This is as it
should be.   Nevertheless the number of study groups
requesting the assistance of the EORTC Data Center is increasing every year and the saturation point has now been
reached. This is perhaps a sign that centralized offices
are a more efficient and also economical system of data
evaluation than small individual units for each hospital.
The question of the right size of such a centralized office
remains open and should be subject to evaluation from time
to time. Indeed one can visualize a not too distant future
with several centralized Data Centers in different geographic
areas of Europe. There are already some in the making at
present. However the formation of an efficient, professional
type Data Center requires a number of years and it is perhaps
fortunate that the pionneer action of the EORTC Data Center
has rendered it capable of assisting and helping in many
ways the new developing Centers : one of the important
factors of success is to gain the confidence of the participating clinicians as we have learned over the years and
this takes time.
    Therapeutic protocols are designed by each cooperative
clinical group with the assistance of our statistical staff.
There is always a statistician present at each group meeting
to assist the clinicians in the stratification of patients,
evaluation of old and new therapies, determination of sample
size and duration of the trial. Discussion and elaboration
of the protocol is the responsibility of the clinical group.
However after completion each protocol is submitted to a
Protocol Review Committee which makes an evaluation from a

TABLE 1
Composition of Data Center

Maurice M. STAQUET	Director and Coordinator for Clinical Cooperative Groups
Richard SYLVESTER	Assistant Director
Stefan SUCIU	Statistician
Otilia DALESIO	Statistician
Martine VAN GLABBEKE	Computer Analyst
Marc BUYSE	Computer Analyst
Jean-Paul HATUNGIMANA	Computer Analyst
Georgette RENARD	Chief Data Manager
Marleen DE PAUW	Data Manager
Jennifer McCREANNEY	Data Manager
Gabriel SOLBU	Data Manager
Nicole DUEZ	Data Manager
Nicole ROTMENSZ	Data Manager
Denis THOMAS	Data Manager
Anne KIRKPATRICK	Data Manager
Dominique EECKHOUDT	General Secretary
Julie TYRRELL	Secretary
Anne-Marie STIFT	Secretary
Dolores DE BEL	Secretary

scientific as well as an ethical viewpoint. A completed
protocol is an important document, comprising 14 different
items, and going into every detail of the project (Table 2).
Once the protocol has been finalized, a set of forms and
procedures is designed by the Data Center for the approval
of the group clinicians. There is a registration form, an
on study form, a flow sheet, a summary form and a progress
report form. Some groups require additional specialized
forms. The clinical cooperative groups carry out randomized
and non randomized studies. In general, the EORTC groups
have favored the randomized studies as opposed to studies
using historical controls although the choice is left to the
individual groups. For randomized trials, a random log must
be created before patients can be entered on study. The log
is usually designed in such a way that treatments are
balanced between patients from participating institutions
and also balanced in regard to important prognostic variables or strata as specified in the protocol. Such a log is
created by a standard computer program which allows for the
particular features of an individual study. Randomizations
are usually made by institutions telephoning the data
managers' office at the Data Center, but can be made also
by telex, telegram or letter. The first step in registering
a patient for a particular study is for the data manager to
check with the caller that the patient satisfies the eligibility criteria specified in the protocol. Once this preliminary check is made, the name of the patients is entered on
the next space in the random log under the appropriate
institution and stratum. The treatment assigned is then read
from the random log and given to the caller. At this stage
a "registration form" is completed by the data manager.
The physician in charge of the patient then completes an "on
study form" which contains basic patient information such as
previous history, description of the disease and the treatment group assigned by randomization, and send it to the
Data Center normally within one week of registration. The
on-study form serves as a second check on whether the patient
is eligible to enter the study and whether the correct
treatment is being given. Once a registration has been
completed, the patient is on study and information is
collected periodically on treatment forms and flow sheets.
These forms are returned periodically to the Data Center and
indicate whether the protocol is well followed. A summary
form is sent when a patient goes off study. However the
most important function of the Data Center is to review all
patient forms that are received for drug toxicity, ambi-
guities, completeness and protocol violations.

TABLE 2
Content of Protocol

1. Background and introduction

2. Purpose of the study

3. Selection of patients

4. Design of the study, including a scheme

5. Pretreatment studies

6. Therapeutic regimens

7. Toxicity

8. Follow up and duration of the study

9. Criteria of evaluation

10. Registration and randomization of patients

11. Submission of forms

12. Statistical considerations

13. Administrative responsibilities

14. References

Appendices : Performance status scale, TNM classifications.

The data are processed in the Center to be added to the computer file after careful verification for accuracy by the data manager and the computer itself.

Cooperative groups meet at least twice a year for progress reports and quality control of the results.

The Data Center uses two large and powerful C.D.C. (Control Data Corporation) computers for storing the large quantity of data. They are necessary because of the complexity of the statistical techniques required to analyze the data. Access to the computer files can be made by several techniques not to be detailed here, but preserving professional secrecy.

At the end of the study, eligibility of patients for evaluation and inclusion in the final analysis is made by the Data Center in collaboration with the responsible clinicians. The final statistical analysis preceeding publication of the results is also carried out in the Center. Publication is under an authorship decided by each cooperative trial group. The Data Center does not publish results of the studies it monitors.

The activity of the cooperative groups working in collaboration with the Data Center is probably best described by the bibliography of the published work by these cooperative groups. This bibliography is listed each year in a book entitled : "Current Research of the EORTC Cooperative Groups" which can be obtained from the Data Center in Brussels and is available in most medical libraries. As of today and for the last 6 years, over one hundred such studies have been published.

To conclude for the Data Center presentation, this is a type of central organization with several years experience in serving a large number of cooperative clinical groups in their controlled studies of new or old forms of treatment of cancer. This experience seems to indicate that centralization of data is a desirable form of giving high quality statistical and methodological assistance to a large number of teams of physicians engaged in clinical investigation. This assistance is given freely and experience has shown that over the years it has served a powerful binding force to bring together physicians of diverse trainings, nationalities and languages into working groups who define their own protocol and accept responsibility for respecting the terms of their protocol. Probably no better method has been available so far to render more uniform, at the highest level of quality of care delivered to patients in all the participating countries. The educational value of the association of large number of physicians in discussion groups with a

diversity of opinions and personalities has had enormous
educational value for the medical profession at large.

THE COOPERATIVE CLINICAL GROUPS AND THE CONTROLLED CLINICAL TRIALS

General Consideration

In recent years, the number of clinical trials undertaken
by the EORTC clinical groups has increased importantly. The
clinical groups organize themselves elect their President and
Secretary and meet two to three times a year. They write
their own protocol, revise it several times to make it
acceptable to the Protocol Review Committee. Financial
support in the form of EORTC grants for secretarial help and
some travel is given by the Administrative Board of EORTC on
recommendation of the Protocol Review Committee. This
support is still very limited.

There are currently 20 groups actively engaged in clinical
cooperative work. There were at the end of last year 101
clinical studies in progress of which 72 were monitored by
the Data Center whose activities were described in Chapter 2.

Not all working groups are clinical cooperative groups.
There are really three types of association that are encouraged by the EORTC. A club is a very informal group who meet
to discuss a particular area of interest which could be
either clinical or in the basic sciences. A project group
is the precursor of the cooperative group. Project groups
may start in one country and if they are doing well they will
attract participants from other countries and develop into
a multinational cooperative group. Most cooperative groups
conduct their business in English. Groups that are unable
or unwilling to do so usually remain at the national level
and do not develop into EORTC groups.

Most cooperative groups are disease oriented, breast
cancer or lung cancer for instance. However there are also
groups emphasizing treatment modalities, for instance the
radiochemotherapy group. Each group is expected to prepare
a critical review of their work each year for presentation
at their meeting. The cooperative groups once accepted by
EORTC receive the support of the Data Center.

The EORTC is made of diverse personalities and must deal
tactfully rather than in an authoritarian mode across
national boundaries, different philosophical orientations
and various language barriers, the latter in part solved by
the adoption of English as the common language. Despite
these difficulties, it has been estimated by a group of

foreign observers that it is doing a "truly impressive job
of developing an increasingly well disciplined quality
oriented cooperative cancer clinical trials program in
Europe". This is due in great part to the organization of
the Data Center and the increasing pride each institution
and participant derives from being identified with EORTC.

The cost of participation is assumed almost completely
by the participating institutions. Individuals take the
responsibility of securing support for their travels,
secretarial work and investigator's time. The care of the
patients, including the cost of drugs, hospitalisation,
nursing and laboratory work is entirely supported by the
national health service of each country and this represents
a tremendous local contribution to the program of clinical
trials in Europe amounting to approximately 10 million
dollars a year.

The importance of the EORTC activity in clinical medicine
comes from the fact that a multinational agency for supporting research that could represent in Europe what the N.C.I.
is doing for cooperative trials involving different states
or regions in the U.S. has never existed. Support for
research is strictly national. Therefore EORTC had to move
and develop its program despite this financial handicap and
this was encouraged by a grant from the N.C.I. to the Data
Center which made it possible to initiate the coordination
and evaluation indispensable for the constitution of the
groups. This grant which is being gradually phased out in the
presence of increasing contributions from European sources,
has had an immense enabling influence on the overall progress
toward high quality cooperative clinical research, the
results of which are made fully available to the medical
profession of the U.S. All this inaugurates extension of
the multinational collaborative research on cancer and the
establishment of international standards for reporting,
thereby facilitating comparison and epidemiological studies.

The Protocol Review Committee is becoming more and more
exacting in its requirements for approval of a protocol and
approval of a protocol is necessary to make it an EORTC
protocol. This is due to the increasing sophistication of
the members of the committee, the accelerated introduction
of a second generation type of young oncologists with good
training and high standards of evaluation in the Committee
and the growing number of proposed protocol creating a
competitive situation calling for selectivity and elimination of the unfit.

A list of the cooperative groups and other associations of
the EORTC is given in Table 3, together with the chairmen
and secretaries : these change every 2 to 4 years. The two
Task Forces listed in this Table are temporary organizations established for specific purposes such as confronting
past results from different sources and proposing multidisciplinary programs for the future.

It is impossible to list here all the publications by the
cooperative groups of the EORTC. At this point, it should
be repeated that the EORTC is far from monopolizing clinical
therapeutic research and controlled trials in Europe.
There are numerous excellent studies emanating from hospitals,
members or non members of EORTC who work without the assistance of our Data Center. In general, as said before, the
number of institutions requesting the Data Center's assistance is increasing steadily and we have a tendency, perhaps
unjustified, to trust our independent data analysis and
evaluation more than others when they are carried out by
isolated statisticians responding to the clinician. These
publications amount to over 100, counting only the collaborative trials work to the exclusion of numerous clinical
investigations arising more or less directly from the
clinical trials.

It may be interesting to review briefly the results of
one of the cooperative groups, the breast cancer group, as
an example of one of the interaction of American and European
cancer research. The first cooperative group carrying out
controlled trials in Europe originated in 1958 under the
stimulation of Albert Segaloff, George Escher and the late
Isidore Ravdin. This trial confirmed on a larger scale the
essentially equivalent therapeutic effectiveness of Δtesto-
lactone as compared to testosterone propionate. It definitely fixed the rate of response of a mean population of
advanced breast cancer in postmenopausal women at 14% and
showed also that nothing whatsoever was gained by combining
the two hormonal compounds each of which given alone carried
the same rate of remissions (3). Later, the same group
showed that estramustine, in a phase I trial, accomplished
the same rate of remission as the estrogen component of the
molecule given alone (4). The same group demonstrated the
limited effectiveness of one of a new class of compounds :
chrysenex in advanced breast cancer but this compound,
despite its interest, did not gain acceptance because of
difficulties of formulation and gastrointestinal intolerance
(5). The same group pionneered the adrenalectomy in
Europe and accumulated a large series of successful results
at a time when other institutions had hardly begun. (6)

TABLE 3-1
List of Cooperative Groups (with Chairmen and Secretaries) — 1980.

Group	Chairman	Secretary
Screening and Pharmacology	F. SPREAFICO	P. LELIEVELD
Clinical Screening	P. CAPPELAERE	M. HAYAT
Leukemia and Hematosarcoma	C. HAANEN	M. HAYAT
Bronchial Carcinoma	O. MONOD	A. DEPIERRE
Breast Cancer	A. ENGELSMAN	W.H. MATTHEIEM
G.I. Tract Cancer	J. LOYGUE	A. GERARD
Thyroid Cancer	P. DOR	J. COLON
Genito-Urinary Tract Cancer	P. PAVONE-MACALUSO	P.H. SMITH
Melanoma	E. MACHER	F.J. LEJEUNE
Radiotherapy / Chemotherapy	M. HAYAT	E. VAN DER SCHUEREN
Radiotherapy	E. VAN DER SCHUEREN	J.C. HORIOT
Head and Neck	Y. CACHIN	A. JORTAY
Brain Tumors	L. CALLIAUW	J. HILDEBRAND
Early Clinical Trials	H.H. HANSEN	M. HANSEN
Cancer of the Ovary	J.P. WOLFF	A. MASKENS
Soft Tissue and Bone Sarcoma	G. BONADONNA	H.M. PINEDO
		A.T. VAN OOSTEROM

TABLE 3-2
EORTC Project Groups

Group	Chairman	Secretary
Gnotobiotic	D. VAN DER WAAIJ	P.J. HEIDT
Antimicrobial Therapy	J. KLASTERSKY	H. GAYA
Metastases	K. HELLMANN	
Tumor Invasion	P. STRAULI	A. HAGENBEEK
High Let Therapy	W. DUNCAN	J.J. BATTERMANN
Pharmacokinetics and Metabolism	J.F. SMYTH	H.M. PINEDO

With the advent of chemotherapy and polychemotherapy, the
EORTC breast group kept in front of the advances in the field
and carried out original clinical studies on the estrogen
receptors as applied to the clinic.

There are not two classes of mammary cancers in respect
to estrogen receptors but instead a continuous spectrum from
low to high receptors carrying breast cancers. This concept
was introduced when the group discovered that over 80% of
all specimens received from the operating room revealed the
presence of variable amounts of receptors (7,8). All or
practically all tumours contain some cells with estrogen
receptors, although many do not have enough of these cells
to make them responders in the clinical sense (50% regression) to hormonal manipulation. Therefore, hormonal treatment would appear to be always useful in conjunction with
cytotoxic chemotherapy : this is why the EORTC breast group
added tamoxifen to the CMF from the very beginning of its
chemotherapy program and it appears now that a controlled
trial has confirmed the value of this combined therapy and
the validity of the concept (9).

Numerous other studies have been conducted or are being
conducted by the EORTC breast group, including negative ones
with prolactine inhibitors, bromocryptin, L-dopa and also
studies on the primary treatment. There have been several
symposiums and workshops initiated by this group and
published in the form of books or supplements to cancer
journals.

This short review of the activities of one of the cooperative groups of EORTC shows the definitely sizable contribution of these EORTC activities to our common problem. All
this work is carried out in close collaboration with the U.S.
oncologists. In the more than 12 monographs published by
the EORTC in the last 10 years, over one half of the contributions emanate from the U.S. : these monographs represent
the meetings and workshops organized in Europe under the
sponsorship of EORTC to get together the active representatives of cancer research in the world.

There are cooperative groups carrying out preclinical
research. For instance, there is a screening and pharmacology cooperative group with laboratories and representatives
in Brussels, Leiden, Milano and Villejuif (Paris). This
group maintains a close contact with pharmacologists in
universities and industry on one side and with the clinical
groups on the other side.

THE "LIAISON OFFICE" OF THE NCI-EORTC

This office is intimately connected with the procurement
of drugs from the European continent. In recent years,
there has been an increasing number of active anticancer
drugs originating in Europe. Cyclophosphamide and its
numerous derivatives originated in Germany, and several
anthracyclines in Italy and France. A recent article in
"Cancer Chemotherapy and Pharmacology" lists the major
European drugs contributed to the pharmacopeia up to 1978
(10).

For a number of years the collaborative office has been
established in Brussels as an initiative of the Brussels
office of the EORTC to which the NCI responded and is well
known by the scientific community in cancer research in
Europe and accepted as the intermediary link between the two
scientific communities, Western Europe and North America.
In this respect, it is fulfilling an irreplaceable function
which is that of bringing together some of the best minds of
the two continents and creating the contacts between individuals having common interests and who otherwise might never
be able to exchange ideas and methods. The office is also
fulfilling the important function of an observation center
where European scientific news and events are gathered and
communicated to all interested parties in the U.S.
Conversely, this has now become the office to which Europeans
turn to obtain first hand information on scientific life,
activities and developments in the United States.

The "liaison" function of the office has been mostly useful in the broad field of experimental and clinical pharmacology, clinical trials, exchange of professional personnel
(physicians, nurses, biologists) as well as the organization
of workshops and symposia jointly with American and European
participation.

The prospection of European pharmaceutical and chemical
industry in Europe and the evaluation of its potentialities
for cancer research is a most remarkable achievement which
has never been successfully attempted before and by itself
would amply justify the continuation of the collaborative
program.

Since this is a cost sharing contract it may be difficult
to enumerate all the additional benefits which have or will
likely result from this collaboration between the NCI and the
EORTC through the Institut Jules Bordet. Although the support given by the NCI to this projet is modest compared to
the effort now coming from Europe, the U.S. participation
continues to be essential.

Organizational Background

The liaison office is established at EORTC headquarters based at the Institute Jules Bordet which include :

a) the office of the Division of Therapeutic Research
b) the coordinating center for the EORTC cooperative groups
c) the Data Center which handles and collects data on clinical trials from Europe
d) many of the Secretaries and/or Chairmen of the cooperative groups
e) the EORTC Foundation, legally registered as a non-profit organization under Belgian law, provides financial support from European sources to the EORTC.

The editorial staff of the European Journal of Cancer is located at the Institut J. Bordet. The EORTC Monograph series, published by Raven Press, New York is also edited here.

New Drugs

Compounds with antitumor activity

Table 4 represents a breakdown of the various countries which have supplied compounds to the NCI Drug Development Program. It should be pointed out that approximately 18% of all the compounds selected for tumor panel testing by the NCI originate from Europe. A majority of these compounds came through the NCI effort in Brussels and originate in the EORTC countries. An additional 40 substances with confirmed activity are now under review to determine possible selection for tumor panel testing. It is anticipated that a significant number of these will be selected for further development. The input from the European program represents a rather large contribution given the fact that a very small percentage of the Drug Development Program is allocated for the activities in Europe (less than 1%). The Institut Jules Bordet has the facilities to test new compounds coming from European sources. Since the European firms have the possibility of submitting their compounds for testing in Brussels, they are encouraged to actively participate in the synthesis of new structures. Several firms not involved in the cancer field until recently have now appropriated substantial support for synthetic program as a result of their collaboration with this Office.

TABLE 4
List of Countries

PANEL COMPOUNDS

FROM EUROPE		FROM OTHER COUNTRIES	
West Germany	65	Japan	82
England	55	Australia	10
France	14	USSR	8
The Netherlands	14	Canada	3
Denmark	10	Israel	3
Belgium	9	New Zealand	3
Italy	9	India	2
Ireland	2	Brazil	1
Sub total E.E.C.	178	Iran	1
Other European countries		Taiwan	1
Sub total	30		
TOTAL	208	TOTAL	114
= 18%		= 9%	

TOTAL COMPOUNDS IN PANEL AT N.C.I., FEB. 28, 1980 = 1200.

Compounds of clinical interest

Several new compounds are currently being pursued toward clinical trial. One of particular interest, now in phase I study is NSC 296934 which was supplied by a firm in Germany. This compound was discovered approximately two years ago in Brussels and has undergone all the necessary preclinical toxicology in Europe without any direct cost to the NCI program. A sulfate derivative of platinum : NSC 311065 will also be tested in clinical trial in the very near future. Thioproline (Norgamem) is currently in phase II clinical trial in the EORTC.

The Institut Jules Bordet in collaboration with the EORTC and the NCI will expand the drug development program for phase I and phase II clinical trials. New drugs will be tested in Europe without major expense to the participating institution since most of the patient care as well as the consulting physicians' and nurses' salaries are covered by the individual social security systems. The only major expense is the administration costs and the data evaluation. In view of resource considerations at N.C.I., quite frequently a choice has to be made to select only one new drug for further development out of a series of possible candidates, the active collaboration with the EORTC makes it possible to develop in Europe analogues of such compounds in parallel with the NCI. Such a program can be carried out without any financial burden on the NCI program. Taking this approach, NCI can substantially increase the number of new drugs evaluated in the clinic at no additional cost to the taxpayer.

As of now (summer 1980) 3 original compounds are undergoing trials within the EORTC testing grounds :

1) α 1,3,5 triglycidyl-s-triazine trione (α TGT : NSC 296 934) : this compound from Germany was screened at Institut J. Bordet and is now in a concerted phase I study in Brussels, Geneva and Amsterdam.

2) 2-formylpyridine thiosemicarbazone zinc sulfate (NSC 294721) or picazone, obtained from Italy was studied in phase I in Brussels but so far toxicity has prevented introduction in clinical trials.

3) cis-dichloro 1,1 (aminomethyl) cyclohexane platinum (II) (NSC 269608) developed in Brussels, has been formulated in the form of sulfate to increase solubility. It reverts to chloride immediately after parenteral injection. The chloride salt is the active form. This compound is undergoing clinical trials.

These are just examples of compounds developed under the European program and showing promising clinical activity.

PUBLICATIONS

Collaborative and scientific work is often reported in the European Journal of Cancer. In addition, an EORTC Newsletter is published with information on Council and cooperative group activities and other news on general interest. Two book series are regularly edited by EORTC. The EORTC Monograph Series (Raven Press, New York) edited by M. Staquet deals with topics selected from symposia and EORTC Cancer Chemotherapy Annual Series (Excerpta Medica, Amsterdam), edited by H. Pinedo which reports on recent advances in drug therapy.

It should be noted that US research is the second most important contributor to the European Journal of Cancer and this is another manifestation of the close relationship between European and American cancer research (11).

SOURCES AND EVOLUTION OF FINANCIAL SUPPORT

As said before, the cost of the care of patients, including hospitalization, remuneration of physicians and medical personnel, drugs and in general all types of treatment, all this is supported by the social security system of each individual participating country. A low estimate of the cost of every one patient in clinical trials sums up to 1500 $ With 6500 to 7000 patients per year, the European contribution to the project amounts to approximatey 10 million $ per year. This is of course normal and represents the cost of the care of the nationals of European countries. The budget of the EORTC as presented every year does not mention this item because paying for patients care is not the responsibility of EORTC since it is fully assumed by the social security systems. The responsibility of EORTC is to budget expenses for which there is no provision from the individual nations. This is represented by the Data Center (salaries and office equipment), the Newsletter, grants to the clinical groups, etc. The budget as defined here was 730.000 $ last year of which 256.000 $ were contributed by the EORTC European Foundation, 140.000 $ by the scientific division of the European Economic Community and 237.000 $ by a grant from the NCI. The yearly support from Europe proper jumped from 130.000 $ in 1975 to 1.400.000 $ in 1978.

If the EORTC program took off to reach an international dimension, it is to be credited to the initial grant of the NCI. This grant was entirely destined to the support of the coordinating activities between participating countries and no part of it was ever spent on care of patients. However, this coordination was and still is the essence of the mission of the EORTC and we will always be grateful to the U.S. to have understood this long before the Europeans did. But the lesson has now been learned. Under the preceding presidency of the EORTC, the acknowledgment of EORTC as a continental research association with European financial support supplementing the national financing of patient's care got off to a good start with the help of the newly created EORTC Foundation. Also negotiations with the Commission of the European Community came finally to a conclusion and the first contract between EORTC and EEC was signed in 1979. As all these initiatives come to fruition we can now look forward with confidence to a continued fertile association with the U.S. cancer research and maintain an intellectual partnership with shared financial responsibility.

REFERENCES

1. Tagnon H.J. : Recent Achievements in Cancer Cooperation and Data Treatment. In "Cancer Centers",Cancer Campaign, Vol. 3, E. Grundmann and J.W. Cole Edit., Gustave Fischer Verlag, Stuttgart, New York, 1979.
2. Groupe Européen du Cancer du Sein (H.J. Tagnon : coordinateur) : Le traitement hormonal du cancer du sein en phase avancée. Rev. franç. Etud. clin. biol. 7, 1067, 1962.
3. Groupe Européen du Cancer du Sein (H.J. Tagnon : coordinateur) : Le traitement hormonal du cancer du sein en phase avancée. Comparaison entre le proponiate de testostérone et la combinaison propionate de testostérone-delta-1-testolactone. Rev. franç. Etud. clin. biol. 9, 88, 1964.
4. Groupe Européen du Cancer du Sein : Essai clinique du phénol bis (2-chloroéthyl) carbamate d'oestradiol dans le cancer mammaire en phase avancée. Europ. J. Cancer, 5, 1, 1969.
5. Groupe Européen du Cancer du Sein : Induction par le 6-aminochrysène de rémission du cancer du sein en phase avancée chez la femme. Europ. J. Cancer, 3, 75, 1967.
6. H.J. Tagnon, A. Coune, J.C. Heuson and M. Van Rymenant : Problems in the treatment of disseminated cancer of the breast : selection of patients for hormone treatment. In New Trends in the Treatment of Cancer (Edited by L. Manuila, S. Moles, P. Rentchnick) p. 126, Springer-Verlag, Berlin, 1967.

7. Tagnon H.J. : Antioestrogens in treatment of breast cancer. Cancer, 39, 2959, 1977.
8. Leclercq G., Heuson J.C., Deboel M.C. and Mattheiem W.H. : Oestrogen receptors in breast cancer : a changing concept. Brit. Med. J. 1, 185, 1975.
9. Heuson J.C., Engelsman E., Blonk Van der Wijst J. et al. : Comparative trial of nafoxidine and ethinyloestradiol in advanced breast cancer. An EORTC study. Brit. Med. J. 1, 711, 1975.
10. Mathé G. and van Putten L.M. : New cancer chemotherapy drugs in Europe. Cancer Chemother. Pharmacol. 1, 5, 1978.
11. Tagnon H.J. : A message from the Editor. Europ. J. Cancer 16, 6, June 1980.

Addendum

. List of Presidents with years of tenure :

1962	G. MATHE
1966	S. GARATTINI
1969	D. VAN BEKKUM
1975	H. TAGNON
1979	L.G. LAJTHA

. List of Treasurers with years of tenure :

1962	P. LOUSTALOT
1967	H. TAGNON
1975	L.M. van PUTTEN

Pitfalls in the
Interpretation of the
Chemotherapy Literature

STEPHEN K. CARTER

Director
Northern California Cancer Program
Palo Alto, California

The chemotherapy literature is vast and ever growing. A
practicing oncologist is faced with an onslaught of speciality
journals as well as an increase in oncology papers in the
general medical journals. There exists a new bewildering array
of regimens which are reported as active and choosing between
them can be a difficult task. This task is complicated by the
lack of comparability which is found in the literature. This
lack of comparability makes abstract reading a dangerous
procedure for therapeutic decision making. Therapeutic decision
making requires a careful reading of a clinical experiment
with close scrutiny of the methods section.

As far back as 1969 Moertel [14] highlighted, in dramatic
fashion, the lack of comparability in the literature concerning
the use of 5-Fluorouracil in the therapy of advanced large
bowel cancer. He outlined a series of journal reports all of
which administered the drug on the standard loading course
approach. The response rates in those papers ranged from a
low of 8% to a high of 85%! Unfortunately, this is not an
isolated occurance.

The comparability factors which exist in clinical trials
are very extensive and are outlined in Table I. They begin
with the patient selection factors, followed by the
pre-therapeutic work that is done for the patient and the
staging definition. After staging, there is the treatment
prescription for the patient, and the delivery of therapy with
the variety of factors that go into it (such as, dose level,
schedule, duration, titration to toxicity) which is an essential
element in the equation. Then there is criteria of response,
adequacy of follow-up, and data reporting techniques, including
defining the numerator, which is the criteria response, and
defining the denominator.

The performance status is one of the most important patient selection variables which affect prognosis and response for cancer chemotherapy studies in advanced diseases. The performance status is an evaluation of how well a given patient can function in a normal life situation. A variety of scales have been developed to try to quantify the performance status which is in essence a subjective determination. The most commonly utilized scale is one developed by Dr. David Karnofsky at Memorial Hospital and named for him. It starts from ten, which is the best performance status, fully functional, and goes down to one in which the patient is nearly moribond and clearly non-ambulatory. In every advanced solid tumor situation situation in which it has been evaluated, the performance status is an important prognostic indicator of survival length and response to active drug treatment. In bronchogenic carcinoma it may be the most potent variable of all and should be a stratification variable in every comparative clinical trial in advanced disease patients.[11] In an idealized trial, if drug "A" gives a median survival of 20 weeks, and drug "B" gives us a median survival of 4 weeks, then impression could be that drug "A" is clearly superior to drug "B". If the data show, however, that all patients treated with drug "A" had a Karnofsky performance status of 8 to 10, and all the patients treated with drug "B" had a Karnofsky status of 1 to 4, then what is being seen are not differences in drug effect, but a difference due to inbalances of patient selection factor in the trial. It is essential in analyzing a clinical trial for decision making to be aware of the important prognostic variables for response for the disease being treated.

The potential heterogeneity in selection factors that patients with a given kind of cancer bring to a clinical trial is one of the major reasons for the utilization of randomization techniques to attempt to assure comparability. Besides randomization, clinicians and statisticians like to use stratification so that one separates out subsets of patients that have particular prognostic groupings so as to ensure comparability with randomization.

It is the purpose of this paper to highlight examples of the comparability problems in the literature on the chemotherapy of advanced breast cancer.

The chemotherapy of advanced breast cancer in the decade of the 1970's was predominantly combination chemotherapy. It began with the abstract publications in 1969 of a regimen involving cyclophosphamide (C), Methotrexate (M), 5-Fluorouracil (F), Vincristine (V) and Prednisone (P) by Cooper.[4]

Table I
Comparability Factors in Clinical Trials

I. Patient selection factors
II. Pre-therapeutic work-up
III. Staging definition
IV. Delivery of therapy
    a. dose level
    b. schedule
    c. duration
    d. titration to toxicity
V. Criteria of response
    a. objective regression
    b. survival
VI. Adequacy of follow-up
VII. Data reporting techniques
    a. defining numerator
    b. defining denominator

This abstract is of such historical importance, and is so short, it is reproduced in its entirety below:

COMBINATION CHEMOTHERAPY IN HORMONE RESISTANT BREAST CANCER. Richard G. Cooper, Buffalo Medical Group, Buffalo, N.Y.

Sixty unselected patients with far advanced disease were treated with vincristine, 35 mcgm./kg., I.V. weekly, cyclophosphamide, 2.5 mgm./kg., p.o. daily, prednisone, 0.75 mgm./kg., p.o. daily, 5-Fluorouracil, 12 mgm./kg., I.V. daily for 4 doses and 5-Fluorouracil, 500 mgm. with 25 to 50 mgm. Methotrexate, I.V. weekly for an 8-week induction phase. Therapy was reduced for maintenance. Patients were categorized by site of major recurrence. Complete remission was noted in 8 of 9 with lung lesions, 19 of 22 with liver metastases, 14 of 16 with bone recurrence, 7 of 8 with brain metastases and 5 of 5 with massive skin recurrence. Toxicity was manifest by alopecia in 67%, marked leukopenia in 45% and G.I. symptoms in 10%. Two drug related deaths occured. Complete remission lasted an average of 10 months and was unrelated to age or prior hormonal control.

It is worth noting that the CMFVP regimen published in
abstract form in 1969 was never followed by a paper in the
literature giving details as to patient selection factors,
response criteria, etc. Despite the fact that earlier in the
1960's Greenspan[7] had reported response rates of higher
than 80% with a similar type regimen, this CMFVP combination
of Cooper became a focal point for the great mass of
chemotherapy clinical research in the early 1970's.

A near deluge of confirmatory studies with CMFVP following
the abstract subsequently appeared in the literature with
widely varying results. The 90% complete response rate
reported initially by Cooper could not be confirmed. The
overall response rates in 8 series ranged from 20% to 70%
with an overall cumulative response rate of 47% in 529
patients.[3] The confirmatory studies were followed by a
vast numer of exploratory type studies which attempted to
dissect or modulate the CMFVP regimen. This involved studies
of CMFV, CMFP, CMF and CFP, as well as other regimens
attempting to drop out one or more of the five original drugs.
Other studies attempted schedule modifications such as giving
the drugs on an intermittent rather than a continuous schedule.
Out of all this CMF, on an intermittent schedule, evolved as
the most commonly used modification of the orignial continuous
CMFVP. Again a wide range of response rates were reported
with these regimens.[3]

In the early to mid seventies Adriamycin's [A] activity
became known and a great degree of clinical research focused
on combinations involving this compound. The most commonly
used combination has become Cyclophosphamide + Adriamycin +
5-Fluorouracil. This regimen has been called "FAC" or "CAF"
or "AFC" depending upon the group using it. As with other
combinations,the range of response rates has varied widely
(Table II).

In analyzing the differing results with CMFVP or FAC in
the literature, four major factors can be seen as playing a
role in the lack of comparability. These include the therapy
itself, the prognostic variables within the patient populations,
the criteria of response and the data reporting technique.

Variables In The Therapy Itself

A difficulty often encountered in the literature, is that
confirmatory studies are often not in truth what they set
out to be. Instead of reproducing the combination, they set
out to confirm that many protocols change the regimen as to
dose and/or schedule of one or more of the drugs in the
regimen. Table II details the dose schedules for the four
different papers studying the combination of Adriamycin, 5-FU

TABLE II

Adriamycin, Cyclophosphamide
And 5-FU In
Breast Cancer (6-9)

Regimen Group	Adriamycin	5-FU	Cyclophos- phamide	Cycle Interval	No. of Pts.	No. Resp.	% Resp.
M.D. Anderson "FAC" (9)	50 D1	500 D1.8	500 D1	3 wks.	44	32	73
SWOG "AFC" (17)	40 D1	400 D1.8	400 D1	3 wks.	105	52	49
NCI "CAF" (2)	30 D1.8	500 D1.8	100 D1-14	4 wks.	38	31	82
SEG "CAF" (15)	50 D1	500 D1	500 D1	3 wks.	59	38	64

Cycle Dose In mg/m^2

611

and Cyclophosphamide. It is obvious that these studies are not
comparing exactly the same regimens. While the drugs are
the same, the schedules and dose levels differ significantly.

Prognostic Variables

In the decade of the 1960's, when hormonal therapy dominated
the treatment of advanced breast cancer, three prognostic
variables were considered paramount in terms of objective
response. These were sites of dominant lesion (local-regional,
osseous, or visceral), disease-free interval after surgery
and menopausal status. In the decade of the 1970's, these
have been replaced to a significant degree by new prognostic
variables such as performance status, prior therapy and most
recently estrogen receptor status. Swenerton et al [16]
studied 619 patients treated at M.D. Anderson, mostly with
the FAC combination, retrospectively to identify those host,
tumor, or treatment characteristics that might be of prognostic
importance for response and survival. They found that
pre-treatment weight loss, poor performance status (Table III)
and abnormal biochemical and hematological values were of
adverse prognostic significance. There was a trend for
patients with bone involvement to have a better survival
than patients with other metastatic sites. Shorter survival
times were observed among patients exposed to extensive
prior radiotherapy and those who failed to respond to prior
hormonal treatment.

Creech et al [5] in their studies of CMF with or without
the addition of Adriamycin (CAMF) divided patients into good
or poor risk category. Good risk was defined as ambulatory,
minimally symptomatic and no life threatening visceral
metastatic disease. Regardless of whether the patients in
this study were classified as responding, stable disease, or
progressing, the good risk patients had a longer median

TABLE III
Impact of Performance Status on Patients
Treated with FAC Regimen

Data of Swenerton et al
Cancer Res. 39:1522,1979

Performance Status	No. of Patients	No. Resp.	% Resp.	(wks) Median Survival
1	196	140	71	123
2	359	232	65	90
3,4	64	25	39	42

survival than did the poor risk patients. This is equally true for the stable and progressing patients as is shown for CMF in Table IV.

Manni et al [12] have demonstrated that prior response to hormonal therapy is of positive prognostic significance for patients treated with CMFVP. In their series, they treated 110 patients with CMFVP of which 97 were evaluable and 62 responding for a response rate of 56% to 64% depending on the denominator chosen. These patients were analyzed by prior endocrine therapy (Table V). Responders to endocrine therapy had a 74% response rate and a median survival of 53 months in comparison to a 50% response rate and 13.5 month median survival for these with no previous endocrine therapy.

Tumor Response

A critical variable in data analysis is the definition of tumor response. In advanced disease, criteria of response are not uniform and a wide variety of definitions exist. Many groups report some "responses" that are are less than the 50% shrinkage which most investigators define as the minimal shrinkage required for partial response. Most groups measure a lesion in two perpendicular diameters and take the product of these two measurements.

In the chemotherapy of breast cancer today, most of the objective responses observed are less than complete. Because of this, it is of critical importance to define a "partial response." Defining a partial response is an area of great complexity, despite the fact that > 50% shrinkage of measurable lesions is now an accepted generality.

TABLE IV
Impact of Patient Risk Status
on Patient Survival with
CMF in Breast Cancer

Data of Creech et al
Cancer 43:51, 1979

Patient Risk Status	No. of Patients	Median Survival in Months by Response Category		
		Response	Stable	Progression
Good Risk*	18	24	12	19+
Poor Risk	21	17	7	3
Total	39	19	12	3

*Ambulatory, minimally symptomatic, no life threatening visceral metastatic disease.

What is difficult to elucidate in breast cancer patients
is how a partial response is defined with multiple lesions. As
can be seen in Table VI, there are four general possibilities
for defining a partial response with multiple lesions utilizing
the 50% shrinkage criterion. These are distinctly not
comparable and can lead to differing partial response rates
with the same clinical material.   An example is shown in Table
VII, where the measurements of three lesions are shown. These
lesions measure 10 x 10, 3 x 3, and 4 x 4. If eight weeks
later the 10 x 10 lesion has shrunk to 2 x 2 and the other two
lesions have remained stable, is this a partial response? If a
50% decrease in the sum of the products of all measurements of
lesions is used as the criterion, this is a partial response
as the sum of the products has declined from 125 to 29. On the
other hand, if shrinkage of all lesions, or even half the
lesions, is the criterion then this is not a partial response.
If eight weeks later, the two smaller lesions have disappeared
but the large lesion has remained unchanged then the situation
reverses.   On the basis of the sum of products this is not
a partial response, but using the criterion of shrinkage of
more than half the lesions it is. In both cases, the strict
criterion of all lesions shrinking would exclude a partial
response definition. In both cases, the liberal definition
of only one lesion having to shrink would report a partial
response. It should therefore be required that partial
response criteria go into greater detail as to how a partial
response is defined in the face of multiple lesions.

Attempts have been made to develop response criteria
for advanced breast cancer studies.[1,8] Major investigators
and funding agencies should come together and agree on the
utilization of these criteria or some acceptable modification.
Once this is accomplished, the editors of major journals
should develop baseline criteria of what should be included
in the literature reporting of a study. If general criteria
becomes widely accepted then methodology sections can be
shortened by just stating these criteria, with reference to
an appropriate publication. What should no longer be accepted
is the anarchy of a free enterprise approach to data reporting
in the oncologic literature.

TABLE V
Response to Treatment
with CMFVP in Advanced
Breast Cancer Correlated with
Previous Therapy

Data of Manni et al
Cancer Treatment Reports
64:111, 1980

Prior Treatment Category	No. of Patients	% CR&PR	Median Duration of Remission (mos)	Median Survival (mos)
Responders to Endocrine Therapy	27	74	11	53*
Failures to Endocrine Therapy	39	64	9	23
No Previous Endocrine Therapy	26	50	5	13.5

Total Response Rate in
Evaluable Patients 64%

*P < 0.0005

TABLE VI
Possibilities for Defining Partial Response
with 50% Shrnkage when Multiple Lesions Exist

1. All lesions must shrink by 50% (product of perpendicular measurements)
2. More than half the lesions must shrink by 50%, while others remain stable.
3. Only one lesion must shrink by 50%, while others remain stable.
4. 50% decrease in sum of products of all lesions.

Other Variables
1. Duration
2. Bone lesions
3. Liver enlargement
4. CNS lesions
5. Pleural effusions
6. Lymphangitic pulmonary metastasis

Unfortunately, the measuring of lumps and bumps and the measuring of x-ray shadows with calipers and rulers is not as precise a science as might be thought. This difficulty is illuminated by a study reported by Moertel and Hanley.[13] An experiment was performed with balls of varying sizes placed under foam rubber. The balls were placed under the foam rubber and investigators of the Eastern Cooperative Oncology Group came in and were asked to measure the size of the "lesion" with their calipers. Their measurements were put on a flow sheet as if they were performing a clinical study. Sixty-four of these investigators measured the same "lesion" twice without being aware of it. What was observed was that 19% of the time the difference was greater than a 25% shrinkage, in 8% of the observations the difference was greater than a 50% shrinkage which is the classic definition of objective response (Table VIII). This indicates that there exists a background noise of investigator variability in measurement. Utilization of less stringent criteria (> 25% shrinkage) should be avoided because then the background noise of investigator variability in measurement begins to approach 20% which is considered meaningfull activity for some tumors. In the same series when two different investigators measured the same mass the variability was even greater. (Table IX)

Data Reporting Techniques

All trials have a patient flow which relates to how the data will be reported (Table X). All trials begin with patients who are considered for the trial. Out of this group comes the number actually found to be eligible for the trial. Only a subset of those found eligible will actually be entered in the trial. After the patients are entered into the trial, there will be a percentage of patients deemed unevaluable for a variety of reasons. There is no comparability between various groups and studies as to what the criteria

TABLE VIII
Measuring Error in Objective Response Determination
Moertel and Hanley
Cancer 38:388, 1976

No. of Repeat Same Investigator Evaluations	No. of Investigators Who Reported Objective Response	
	> 25% Shrinkage	> 50% Shrinkage
64	12 (18.8%)	5 (7.8%)

TABLE VII

Idealized Situation with Three Lesions and Selected Shrinkage 8 Weeks Later

	Lesion Measurement				Is this a "PR"			
	1	2	3	Sum of the Products	50% Shrinkage in Sum of Products	All Lesions Shrink 50%	Half the Lesions Shrink 50%	One Lesion Shrink 50%
Base Line	10x10	3x3	4x4	125	—	—	—	—
8 wks Later Example 1	2x2	3x3	4x4	29	Yes	No	No	Yes
8 wks Later Example 2	10x10	0x0	0x0	100	No	No	Yes	Yes

for evaluability will be. Another subset of patients are
those deemed adequately treated by whatever criteria may be
used by the study group.

A response rate consists of a numerator and a denominator.
The denominator can be chosen from number of patients entered,
evaluable or adequately treated. Depending upon which
denominator is chosen, the response rate can vary. This
variation in response rate can be significant if there is a
large difference between the number of patients entered and
the number evaluable within a study.

A black box in any literature report of a study is the
gap that may exist between the number of patients considered
for a study and those actually entered within a given
institution. If this gap is a wide one, the study becomes
an experience in a highly selected group of patients. The
study may therefore not fully apply to the full range of
patients, with the particular tumor and stage under study,
seen in general oncologic practice. This could be solved by
having registries set up within institutions to detail
eligible patients who do not become entered on a study and
the reasons why. Unfortunately, clinical research support
for such registries rarely receives a high priority.

Davis et al[6] have taken a population of breast cancer
patients treated by the Central Oncology Group (COG) and has
re-analyzed them using the response criteria of four other
groups, including the Eastern Cooperative Oncology Group
(ECOG), Southwest Oncology Group (SWOG) and Southeastern
Cooperative Groug (SEG). Response rates were tabulated
using four different denominators:

1. Total entered minus ineligible patients.
2. Total entered minus ineligible and cancelled patients.
3. Total entered minus ineligible, cancelled,
    unevaluable and early withdrawals due to drug toxicity
    and early deaths.
4. Total evaluable patients as defined by each groups
    criteria.

Using the fourth denominator above (total evaluable as
defined by each group) the denominators broke down as follows,
with the numbers in parenthesis being the first denominator
(total minus ineligible patients):

1.	COG	88	(106)
2.	ECOG	91	(109)
3.	SWOG	92	(110)
4.	SEG	93	(111)

TABLE IX
Erroneously Declared Objective Responses When Two
Different Investigaotors Measure Tumor Which Has
Remained the Same Size

No. of Different Investigator Pairings	No. of Pairings Who Report Objective Responses > 25% Shrinkage	> 50% Shrinkage
		Moertel and Hanley Cancer 38:388, 1976
1920	497 (24.9%)	130 (6.8%)

Progression	
> 25% Growth	> 50% Growth
604 (31.5%)	342 (17.8%)

TABLE X
Patient Flow in Clinical Trials

Patients Potentially Available for the Study

Patients Considered for the Study

Patients Eligible for the Study

Patients Entered in the Study

Patients Evaluable in the Study

Patients Adequately Treated in the Study

Patients with Adequate Follow-Up

Using the different groups criteria for response, the following number of "responses," in this identical group of patients, broke down as follows:

1. COG 46
2. ECOG 43
3. SWOG 42
4. SEG 35

When the above numerators are put together with the four potential denominators the response rates range from 32% to 59% (Table XI). The differences in response rates within a group between the four denominators range from a low of 6% (SEG) to a high of 9% (COG). The range of response rates between groups at a given denominator ranged from a high of 15% (denominator 3) to a low of 11% (denominator 1). The 27% difference between the highest and lowest response rate calculated can explain a good deal about the variability that exists within the literature.

An example of the problem of interpretation, especially if only abstracts are read, can be seen in a recent paper by Hug et al.[10] The abstract is given in its entirety as follows:

A phase II trial of Peptichemio (PTC) was conducted on 56 patients with advanced breast cancer that had been resistant to treatment with cyclophosphamide. The overall response rate was 32%, with one complete remission, seven partial remissions, and ten instances of improved disease status. Soft tissue and bone

TABLE XI
Comparative Response Rates
With An Identical Group of Patients
Utilizing Criteria of Four Cooperative Groups [6]

No. of Responses	COG 46	ECOG 43	SWOG 42	SEG 35
Denominator 1	106(43)	109(38)	110(39)	111(32)
Denominator 2	102(45)	105(41)	106(40)	107(33)
Denominator 3	83(55)	85(51)	86(49)	87(40)
Denominator 4	88(52)	91(47)	92(46)	93(38)

Percent response in parenthesis

Denominator
1. Total minus ineligible.
2. Total minus ineligible, cancelled.
3. Total minus ineligible cancelled, unevaluable early withdrawal due to drug toxicity, early deaths.
4. Total evaluable patients as defined by each group's criteria.

lesions were the primary sites of response. The
median duration of response was 11 weeks, with a
range of 6 - 30 weeks. Major toxicities were
myelosuppression affecting predominantly the platelets
and sclerosing phlebitis. Myelosuppression was
cumulative and thrombocytopenic bleeding was a
likely contributing factor in the death of 2 patients.
This trial showed that PTC is another alkylating
agent with definite activity in the treatment of
breast cancer. More importantly, it showed that
cross-resistance with cyclophosphamide does not exist,
at least in breast carcinoma.

This abstract states that the response rate for this
alkylating agent is 32% in patients prior treated with
cyclophosphamide and that cross-resistance does not exist.
How was the 32% derived? A reading of the paper shows
that 60 patients were treated and 56 considered evaluable.
There were 8 complete and partial responses and 10 patients
"improved." The response rate of 32% is obtained by adding
the improved patients into the numerator to make 18 over a
denominator of 56. A conservative approach might be a
numerator of 8 and a denominator of 60 for a response rate of
13% which might lead to a different interpretation. The
abstract is correct given the definitions used to determine
response. A practicing oncologist who did not read the paper
in its entirety would miss the more traditional conservative
approach to determining response which might change the
therapeutic decision making reaction.

Sumary
Reading the vast, and ever expanding oncology literature
is a difficult task due to a lack of comparability in data
reporting techniques and definitions of response. Reading
abstracts only is dangerous for therapeutic decision making.
Without standardization of data reports it is "Caveat Emptor"

REFERENCES

1. Breast Cancer Task Force Treatment Committee, National
   Cancer Institute: Breast cancer: Suggested protocol
   guidelines for combination chemotherapy trials and for
   combined modality trials. Publication No. (NIH) 77-1192.
   Washington, D.C.; United States Department of HEW 1977.
2. Bull JM, Tormey DC, Li SH, Carbone PP, Falkson GF, Blom J,
   Perlin E and Simon R: A Randomized Trial of Adriamycin

vs Methotrexate in Combination Drug Therapy. Cancer 41: 1649-1657, 1976.

3. Carter SK: Intergration of Chemotherapy into Combined Modality Treatment of Solid Tumors VII-Adenocarcinoma of the Breast. Cancer Treatment Reviews 3:141-174, 1976.

4. Cooper RG: Combination Chemotherapy and Hormone Resistant Breast Cancer. Proc Am Assoc Cancer Res 10:15, 1969.

5. Creech RH, Catalano RB, Harris DT, Engstrom PF and Grotzinger PJ: Low Dose Chemotherapy of Metastatic Breast Cancer with Cyclophosphamide, Adriamycin, Methotrexate, 5-Fluorouracil (CAMF) vs Sequential Cyclophosphamide, Methotrexate, 5-Fluorouracil (CMF) and Adriamycin. Cancer 43:51-59, 1979.

6. Davis HL, Multhauf P, Klotz J: Comparisons of Cooperative Group Evaluation Criteria For Multiple Drug Breast Cancer Therapy. Cancer Treat Rep, in press.

7. Greenspan E: Regression of Metastatic Hepatomegaly from Mammal Carcinoma-Cytotoxic Combination with 5-FU. NY State J Med 64:2442-2449, 1964.

8. Hayward JL, Carbone PP, Heuson JG, et al: Assesment of Response to Therapy in Advanced Breast Cancer. Cancer 39: 1289-1294, 1977.

9. Hortobagyi GN, Gutterman JU, Blumenschein GR, et al: Combination Chemotherapy of Metastatic Breast Cancer with 5-Fluorouracil, Adriamycin, Cyclophosphamide and BCG. Cancer 43:1225-1233, 1979.

10. Hug V, Hortobagyi GN, Buzdar AU, Blumenschein GR, Grose W, Burgess MA and Bodey GP: A Phase II Study of Peptichemio in Advanced Breast Cancer. Cancer 45: 2524-2528, 1980.

11. Lagakos SW: Prognostic Factors for Survival Time in Inoperable Lung Cancer, in Strauss M (ed): Lung Cancer: Clinical Diagnosis and Treatment. New York, Grune and Stratton, 1977, pp 271-280

12. Manni A, Trujillo JE and Pearson OH: Sequential Uses of Endocrine Therapy and Chemotherapy for Metastatic Breast Cancer-Effects on Survival. Cancer Treat Rep 64:111-116, 1980.

13. Moertel C and Hanley JA: The Effect of Measuring Error on the Results of Therapeutic Trials in Advanced Cancer. Cancer 38:388-394, 1976.

14. Moertel CG and Reitemeier OJ: Advanced Gastrointestinal Cancer/Clinical Management and Chemotherapy. New York, Heeber Medical Division of Harper and Row, 1969, p 74

15. Smalley RV, Carpenter J. Bartolucci A, Vogel C and Kauss S: A Comparison of Cyclophosphamide, Adriamycin, 5-Fluorouracil (CAF) and Cyclophosphamide, Methotrexate, 5-Fluorouracil, Vincrinstine, Prednisone (CMFVP) in patients with Metastatic Breast Cancer. Cancer 40:625-632, 1977.
16. Swenerton KD, Legha SS, Smith T, Hortobagyi GN, Gehan EA, Yap HY, Gutterman JU and Blumenschein GR: Prognostic Factors in Metastatic Breast Cancer Treated with Combination Chemotherapy. Cancer Res 39:1552-1562, 1979.
17. Tranum B, Hoogstraaten B, Kennedy A, Vaughn CB, Samal B, Thigpen J, Rivkin S, Smith F, Polmen RL, Constanzi J, Tucker WG, Wilson H and Maloney T: Adriamycin in Combination for the Treatment of Breast Cancer-A Southwest Oncology Group Study. Cancer 41:2078-2083, 1978.

Bone Marrow Transplantation

Bone Marrow Transplantation

E. DONNALL THOMAS

Professor & Head, Division of Oncology
Department of Medicine
University of Washington School of Medicine
Fred Hutchinson Cancer Research Center
Seattle, Washington

At the end of the 1960s there was a revival in interest in the possibility of utilizing bone marrow transplantation in the treatment of patients with leukemia based on more effective antileukemic agents, increased knowledge of human histocompatibility typing and better supportive care of the patient without marrow function by platelet and granulocyte transfusions, more effective antibacterial agents and improved isolation techniques.[25] During the following 5 to 7 years most marrow donors were siblings who were HLA identical with the patient and these transplants carried out by the Seattle Marrow Transplant Team will be reviewed first.

HLA IDENTICAL SIBLING TRANSPLANTS FOR PATIENTS IN LEUKEMIC RELAPSE

For obvious ethical reasons the initial studies were carried out in leukemic patients who had relapsed after failure of the best available chemotherapeutic regimens. Because of advanced illness, these patients were poor candidates and their subsequent survival was very poor. Figure 1 shows the Kaplan-Meier product-limit estimates of percentage surviving of the first 110 patients transplanted in Seattle.[21] The first 10 patients were prepared with 1000

This investigation was supported by Grant Numbers CA 18029 and CA 15704, awarded by the National Cancer Institute, DHHS. Dr. Thomas is a recipient of a Research Career Award AI 02425 from the National Institute of Allergy and Infectious Diseases. Address Reprint Requests to E. Donnall Thomas, Fred Hutchinson Cancer Research Center, Division of Oncology, 1124 Columbia Street, Seattle, Washington 98104.

rad total body irradiation (TBI) and the next 100 were given
cyclophosphamide (CY), 60 mg/kg x 2, a few days before the
TBI. Based on studies in the canine model, all patients
were given a regimen of methotrexate in the first 100 days
after grafting in an effort to prevent graft-versus-host
disease (GVHD). No other antileukemic treatment was given.

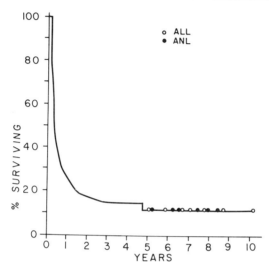

There was a high initial mortality due to advanced illness, infection and complications of GVHD. Leukemic relapse
was common during the first year after grafting and uncommon
thereafter. The latest relapse occurred 27 months after
grafting. Twelve patients are alive and in remission after
5 to 10 years. Although the overall survival was poor, the
long-term survivors are unique since no other therapeutic
approach has produced such long-term survivors in leukemic
patients who have relapsed. The flat disease-free survival
curve indicates[23] that these patients are cured of their
disease. The fact that some patients in end stage relapse
can be cured is most encouraging.

     Some of our patients received additional antileukemic
therapy before CY and TBI without an improvement in survival. Dr. Robert Gale has recently reviewed the experience
of the transplant centers throughout the world and has
described a long-term survival rate of approximately 10% for
patients transplanted in relapse after a variety of
different preparative regimens.[11] His review indicates that
efforts to prevent the subsequent recurrence of leukemia by
more aggressive chemoradiotherapy before transplantation
have, in general, been unsuccessful probably due to increased toxicity of these regimens.

HLA IDENTICAL SIBLING TRANSPLANTS FOR PATIENTS
WITH ACUTE LYMPHOBLASTIC LEUKEMIA (ALL) IN REMISSION

Encouraged by the few long-term survivors described
above, we initiated marrow transplantation earlier in the
course of the disease. Although many patients with ALL can
be cured by chemotherapy alone, the prognosis is generally
poor once relapse has occurred. Acccordingly, we decided to
undertake marrow grafting for patients in second or subsequent remission. Figure 2 provides an update of the Kaplan-
Meier plot of survival of the first 22 patients transplanted
in remission and, for comparison, a concurrent series of 26
patients transplanted in relapse.[24] Although there are long-
term survivors in both groups, survival is clearly greater
for patients transplanted in remission (p = 0.01). For comparison, most chemotherapy regimens for patients with ALL in
second remission give a median survival of approximately 6
months and less than 10% are alive at 2 years. The
principal cause of death is leukemia.

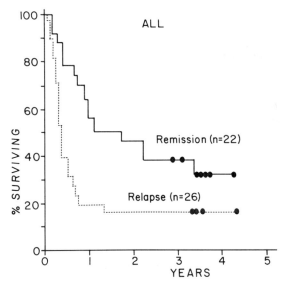

For patients with ALL transplanted in second remission,
recurrence of leukemia has continued to be a major problem.
For example, 12 of the 22 patients cited above died of
recurrent leukemia. These recurrences, in host type cells,
indicate that the chemoradiotherapy regimen failed to
eradicate the leukemic cell population.

HLA IDENTICAL SIBLING TRANSPLANTS FOR PATIENTS WITH
ACUTE NONLYMPHOBLASTIC LEUKEMIA (ANL) IN FIRST REMISSION

Virtually all chemotherapy regimens for patients with ANL
have resulted in a median survival, for those who achieve a
remission, of less than 2 years. Accordingly, it seemed
ethically acceptable to initiate a trial of marrow transplantation for these patients in first remission. Figure 3
provides an update of the survival curve of the first 19
such patients transplanted in Seattle.[22] More than half the
patients are living in remission, and the median duration of
the first remission will not be less than 34 months. Fifty-
eight such patients have now been transplanted in Seattle,
including 18 who received a fractionated irradiation regimen, and a Kaplan-Meier plot of their survival is shown in
Figure 4. The majority of the deaths have been associated
with GVHD and opportunistic infections during the period of
lack of immunologic competence post-grafting. Two other
transplant centers have recently reported the results of
transplantation for patients with ANL in first remission.[1,18] Through the courtesy of Dr. Ray Powles and Dr.
Karl Blume an update of the survival of their patients is
also shown in Figure 4.

In contrast to patients with ALL in second remission, recurrent leukemia has, so far, not been a major problem for
patients with ANL transplanted in first remission. For
example, only 3 of the 58 Seattle patients have suffered a
relapse. The apparent ability to eradicate the leukemic
cell population in patients with ANL but not in ALL is unexplained. It may be related to the nature of the diseases.
However, it may be that patients with ALL might be cured
more readily if transplanted in first remission.

IDENTICAL TWIN TRANSPLANTS FOR PATIENTS WITH
ACUTE LEUKEMIA IN RELAPSE

The patient with leukemia who has a normal identical twin
provides an opportunity to study the effects of "supralethal" chemoradiotherapy with restoration of marrow function by the syngeneic graft without the associated problems
of GVHD. In Seattle, 34 such transplants (18 ALL, 16 ANL)
had been[9] performed by July 1978 after preparation with CY
and TBI. Recurrence of leukemia (13 ALL, 10 ANL) was the
principal cause of death. However, 8 of these patients (3
ALL, 5 ANL) remain in complete remission without any maintenance chemotherapy at 29 to 103 months (median, 80) after
transplant. A Kaplan-Meier plot of survival for these 34

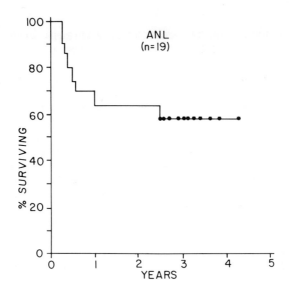

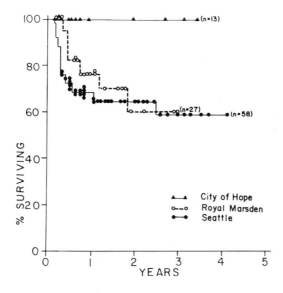

patients shows the long-term survivors to be far out on a plateau indicating cure of the disease. Since these patients were not given methotrexate after grafting and since an antileukemic effect of GVHD could not have been operative, it appears that the preparative regimen of CY and TBI was effective in eradicating the disease in some patients.

MARROW TRANSPLANTATION IN PATIENTS WITH
CHRONIC MYELOGENOUS LEUKEMIA

Patients with chronic myelogenous leukemia in blast crisis are known to have a poor probability of response to all reported chemotherapeutic regimens, and the duration of response is usually limited to a few months. Marrow transplantation in these patients has been difficult, and the early mortality rate, as for other patients transplanted in relapse described above, has been high. Nevertheless, 1 of 6 recipients of an identical twin transplant is living in remission 52 months after grafting and 3 of 24 recipients of HLA identical sibling marrow are living in remission after 30 to 60 months. Although the fraction of long-term survivors is low, these patients illustrate the feasibility of cure in patients with this otherwise disastrous disease.

In an effort to undertake marrow grafting in the presumably more favorable chronic phase of chronic myelogenous leukemia we have transplanted $_8$4 patients with identical twins to serve as marrow donors. All 4 are living after 36 to 54 months. One patient had the reappearance of the Philadelphia chromosome 30 months after marrow grafting, but the other 3 do not have the Philadelphia chromosome that was present in the patients but not the donors before grafting. An additional 8 such patients have now been transplanted. One died of pneumonia in the post-grafting period and the other 7 are well without evidence of the Philadelphia chromosome.

GVHD

Despite the use of an HLA identical sibling as the marrow donor and the administration of methotrexate as an immunosuppressive drug in the immediate post-grafting period, acute GVHD continues to be a major problem in the first 3 months after grafting. Acute GVHD shows a wide clinical spectrum ranging from a mild skin rash to severe involvement of the skin, gut and liver with an associated profound immunodeficiency and susceptibility to opportunistic infections. In Seattle, the incidence of severe acute GVHD has decreased significantly from approximately 49% of the patients before 1977 to 26% since then and, for the patients who get GVHD, the mortality rate has decreased from 55% to 32%. The reason for these decreases has not been identified.

Efforts to treat established GVHD with corticosteroids and/or horse antithymocyte globulin have been only partially successful, and efforts to avoid GVHD by the prophylactic use of horse antithymocyte globulin have been unsuccessful.

Chronic GVHD, a new syndrome, has been observed in about one-fourth of the long-term survivors. It is characterized by dyspigmentation and scleroderma-like lesions of the skin, oral and ocular sicca and, occasionally, by involvement of the esophagus, the gut or the liver. In its advanced form contractures may develop and bacterial infections and weight loss are common. Recently, early and prolonged treatment of chronic GVHD with corticosteroids and azathioprine has been successful in approximately 80% of the patients.

The accompanying article by Dr. Rainer Storb gives details regarding GVHD and the immunologic status of the transplant recipient.

GRAFT-VERSUS-LEUKEMIA

Although GVHD is usually considered an undesirable complication of allogeneic marrow grafting, a recent analysis has shown that the recurrence rate of leukemia is less in those patients having severe GVHD as compared to those with no GVHD.[26] These observations suggest that graft-versus-host disease may be of therapeutic value in preventing the recurrence of leukemia but, unfortunately, appropriate methods for the initiation of GVHD and its subsequent control are not yet available.

OPPORTUNISTIC INFECTIONS

In the 2 to 4 week period of granulocytopenia following the marrow graft, bacterial infections, particularly by gram negative organisms, are likely to occur. With current antibacterial therapy, isolation techniques and granulocyte transfusions, bacterial infections have accounted for less than 10% of the deaths on our marrow transplant ward. During the period of profound immunological depression, roughly the first 100 days after grafting, viral, fungal and protozoan infections constitute a grave threat.[15] Fungal infections account for a great deal of morbidity and about 15% of the deaths despite the use of amphotericin. Newer antifungal agents are presently being studied. The use of prophylactic trimethoprim-sulfamethoxazole has largely eliminated the 10% of deaths that had been due to Pneumocystis carinii. After day 100 the incidence of infections decreases but vigilance must be maintained, particularly for varicella-zoster infections and bacteremic pneumococcal infections. Interstitial pneumonia continues to be a major cause of morbidity and mortality, particularly in the first 100 days after grafting.[16] A recent tabulation shows the following incidence of interstitial pneumonia: allogeneic transplant for leukemia in relapse, 104/216 (48%) with 65% case fatality; allogeneic transplant for ANL in first remission 26/63 (41%) with 54% case fatality; syngeneic transplant 17/100 (17%) with 41% case fatality. About half of the pneumonias are associated with cytomegalovirus infection. Efforts to treat cytomegalovirus associated interstitial pneumonia with adenine arabinoside or interferon have been unsuccessful and avoidance of these pneumonias by adenine arabinoside prophylaxis has also been unsuccessful. A few of the interstitial pneumonias have been due to other agents, such as varicella-zoster virus, but no candidate pathogen has been identified for most of them. These "idiopathic" pneumonias may be due to agents that have not been identified despite intensive studies. The irradiation exposure may play a role in all of the interstitial pneumonias whether or not a pathogen is identified.

RECURRENCE OF LEUKEMIA

Leukemia that recurs after marrow grafting has, as expected, usually involved cells of host type. An analysis of 128 such recurrences in the patients transplanted in Seattle showed that 64 either had no genetic marker or insufficient material was available for analysis. However, 64 patients were shown by cytogenetic studies to have recurrence in host type cells. Presumably, these recurrences are due to leukemic clones that survived the preparative regimen and proliferated resulting in the relapse.

However, recurrent leukemia in two patients in the Seattle series and two patients reported by other transplant groups has been shown to be in donor type cells.[7,10,12,20] Several hypotheses have been invoked to explain these recurrences in donor cells: 1) leukemia might be a disorder of a control mechanism so that a normal cell might take on the growth characteristics of a leukemic cell, 2) a somatic cell hybridization followed by a diploidization might have resulted in a leukemic cell having a donor sex chromosome, 3) chronic allogeneic stimulation of donor lymphoid cells might have resulted in a malignant transformation, 4) there might be a leukemogenic virus in the host, perhaps induced by the TBI, which effected the malignant transformation.

Despite extensive study there is as yet no evidence for the existence of any of these mechanisms.

Recent laboratory studies have shown that viral or non-viral transforming genes can be transferred to and expressed in certain types of recipient cells following transfection with free chromatin and/or DNA.[5] These studies offer an alternate possibility that cellular genes responsible for malignant transformation may have been transferred into donor type cells. The two Seattle patients with recurrence in donor type cells had ALL in advanced relapse and they were prepared with 1000 rad TBI. Cellular genes released from the large mass of leukemic cells undergoing rapid disintegration after this preparative regimen may have brought about this type of transfection phenomenon. Further study of the phenomenon of recurrence in donor type cells should provide insight into the nature of the origin of the leukemia.

DIRECTIONS OF CURRENT RESEARCH

Many research activities are underway in several transplant centers designed to improve the clinical results described above. In addition, a great deal of work in animal systems and in the laboratory is in progress in an effort to provide a better understanding of the complex problems of transplantation biology as related to leukemia. Some of these areas of research are the following:

Antileukemic Therapy Before Grafting

Damage to the patient's normal bone marrow is the most common limiting factor in the aggressive use of antileukemic therapy. In theory, marrow transplantation would permit the use of any potent antileukemic drug with or without TBI in an effort to achieve a maximum leukemic cell kill without regard to associated marrow toxicity. The Johns Hopkins Team is studying high dose busulfan before grafting[19] and the MD Anderson Team is investigating the use of piperazine-dione.[6] Newer agents, such as AMSA, may prove useful in this context.

Fractionated Irradiation

In theory, fractionation of irradiation might result in a desirable antileukemic cell kill while sparing normal

tissues such as the gut and the lung. For two years the
Seattle Team has been conducting a randomized study of 1000
rad in one exposure compared to 200 rad per day for 6 days
for patients with ANL in first remission. Thirty-six
patients have been entered, but it is too early to evaluate
the results. At Johns Hopkins a study,[14] now modified, involving 300 rad on each of 4 days with shielding of the lung
on the third day is underway. In an effort to reduce the
recurrence rate for patients with ALL transplanted in
relapse, the Seattle Team is conducting a study of 225 rad
per day for 7 days. The regimen is quite well tolerated,
but it is too early to evaluate the antileukemic effect.
The Memorial-Sloan Kettering Team has reported preliminary
data on a regimen of fractionated irradiation totaling 1320
rad in a 3 day period.[13] It appears that a large number of
patients will have to be entered on these studies in order
to assess the antileukemic effect and the tolerance of
normal tissues.

Interferon

The Seattle Team has initiated a randomized study of the
administration of interferon in the post-grafting period for
patients with ALL in second remission. The objectives are
to determine the role of interferon in preventing cytomegalovirus associated pneumonia and to evaluate the possible antileukemic effect of interferon, especially at a time when the
body burden of leukemic cells is known to be minimal.

Cyclosporin A

Cyclosporin A is a new immunosuppressive agent with many
unusual properties but without significant marrow toxicity.
The Royal Marsden Team[17] has published preliminary data concerning the use of this agent for the prevention and/or the
treatment of GVHD and studies are also underway in Paris,
Baltimore, Basel and Seattle. As with any new agent, much
work must be done before the toxic properties and optimal
application of cyclosporin A can be defined.

Monoclonal Antibodies

Monoclonal antibodies produced by hybridized cells offer
exciting possibilities for the in vitro treatment of marrow
in order to inactive T cells or T cell subsets thought to

cause GVHD, for treatment or prevention of GVHD when administered after marrow grafting and for the antileukemic
effect of antibodies directed toward leukemia associated
antigens. The accompanying article by Dr. John Hansen
describes these possibilities in detail.

The Use of Mismatched Donors

Several marrow transplant teams have carried out marrow
grafts using donors who are not HLA identical with the recipient. In Seattle, there are now a number of long-term
survivors and, in general, the outcome of these mismatched
grafts appears to be more a function of the problems associated with the underlying disease rather than with the
degree of tissue compatibility.[3] The accompanying article
by Dr. Bo Dupont provides an overview of these studies.

SELECTION OF THE RECIPIENT

As indicated in the sections above, most marrow grafts
for patients with ALL have been carried out following the
first relapse. Experience with the chemotherapy of ALL has
led to the identification of patients with a poor prognosis
who may be, therefore, candidates for a marrow transplant.
Several transplant centers are carrying out marrow transplants for patients with poor prognosis ALL during first
remission.

In theory, any responsive tumor might be treated with
high dose chemoradiotherapy and a subsequent marrow graft.
Tumors currently being studied include certain non-Hodgkin's
lymphomas and small cell carcinoma of the lung. Any
inherited disorder of the bone marrow might be corrected by
destruction of the abnormal marrow and its replacement with
a marrow graft. For example, the Boston Team has utilized
this approach for patients with disorders of leukocyte
function[2] and the Minnesota Team for patients with
osteopetrosis.[4]

OVERVIEW

The replacement of any diseased organ by transplantation
is an admission of failure. It would obviously be better to
have a specific treatment for the disease or, best of all,
to prevent the disease in the first place. The long range
goal of medical science is to accomplish these ends. A

realistic appraisal is that it will take decades of research at all levels ranging from the molecular to the bedside before we have the knowledge necessary to accomplish these ends. In the meantime, the treatment of leukemia with marrow grafting is saving the lives of an ever increasing number of patients with an otherwise fatal disease while providing basic information in immunology and the patho-biology of leukemia.

REFERENCES

1. Blume KG, Beutler E, Bross KJ, Chillar RK, Ellington OB, Fahey JL, Farbstein MJ, Forman SJ, Schmidt GM, Scott EP, Spruce WE, Turner MA, Wolf JL: Bone-marrow ablation and allogeneic marrow transplantation in acute leukemia. N Engl J Med 302:1041-1046, 1980.
2. Camitta BM, Quesenberry PJ, Parkman R, Boxer LA, Stossel TP, Cassady JR, Rappeport JM, Nathan DG: Bone marrow transplantation for an infant with neutrophil dysfunction. Exp Hematol 5:109-116, 1977.
3. Clift RA, Hansen JA, Thomas ED for the Seattle Marrow Transplant Team: The role of HLA in marrow transplantation. Transplant Proc (in press)
4. Coccia PF, Krivit W, Cervenka J, Clawson C, Kersey JH, Kim TH, Nesbit ME, Ramsay NKC, Warkentin PI, Teitelbaum SL, Kahn AJ, Brown DM: Successful bone-marrow transplantation for infantile malignant osteopetrosis. N Engl J Med 302:701-708, 1980.
5. Copeland NG, Zelenetz AD, Cooper GM: Transformation of NIH/3T3 mouse cells by DNA of Rous sarcoma virus. Cell 17:993-1002, 1979.
6. Dicke KA, Zander A, Spitzer G, Verma DS, Peters L, Vellekoop L, McCredie KB, Hester J: Autologous bone-marrow transplantation in relapsed adult acute leukaemia. Lancet 1:514-517, 1979.
7. Elfenbein GJ, Brogaonkar DS, Bias WB, Burns WH, Saral R, Sensenbrenner LL, Tutschka PJ, Zaczek BS, Zander AR, Epstein RB, Rowley JD, Santos GW: Cytogenetic evidence for recurrence of acute myelogenous leukemia after allogeneic bone marrow transplantation in donor hemato-poietic cells. Blood 52:627-636, 1978.
8. Fefer A, Cheever MA, Thomas ED, Boyd C, Ramberg R, Glücksberg H, Buckner CD, Storb R: Disappearance of Ph^1-positive cells in four patients with chronic granu-locytic leukemia after chemotherapy, irradiation and marrow transplantation from an identical twin. N Engl J Med 300:333-337, 1979.

9. Fefer A, Cheever MA, Thomas ED, et al.: Personal communication.

10. Fialkow PJ, Thomas ED, Bryant JI, Neiman PE: Leukaemic transformation of engrafted human marrow cells in vivo. Lancet 1:251-255, 1971.

11. Gale RP: Clinical trials of bone marrow transplantation in leukemia. Transplant Proc (in press).

12. Goh KO, Klemperer MR: In vivo leukemic transformation: Cytogenetic evidence of in vivo leukemic transformation of engrafted marrow cells. Am J Hematol 2:283-290, 1977.

13. Kim JH, Chu FC, Grossbard E, Hopfan S, Simpson L, Shank B, Reid A, Finegan DM, O'Reilly RJ: A new radiation dose fractionation schedule of total body irradiation (TBI) in bone marrow transplantation for refractory leukemia. Proc Am Soc Clin Oncol 21:p 436, C-464, 1980 (abstract)

14. Lichter AS, Tutschka PJ, Wharam MD, Elfenbein GJ, Sensenbrenner LL, Saral R, Kaizer H, Santos GW, Order SE: The use of fractionated radiotherapy as preparation for allogeneic bone marrow transplantation. Transplant Proc 11:1492-1494, 1979.

15. Meyers JD, Thomas ED: Infection complicating bone marrow transplantation, in Young LS, Rubin RH (eds): Clinical Approach to Infection in the Immunocompromised Host. New York, Plenum Press (in press).

16. Neiman PE, Meyers JD, Medeiros E, McDougall JK, Thomas ED: Interstitial pneumonia following marrow transplantation for leukemia and aplastic anemia, in Gale RP, Fox CF (eds): Biology of Bone Marrow Transplantation. New York, Academic Press (in press).

17. Powles RL, Clink HM, Spence D, Morgenstern G, Watson JG, Selby PJ, Woods M, Barrett A, Jameson B, Sloane J, Lawler SD, Kay HEM, Lawson D, McElwain TJ, Alexander P: Cyclosporin A to prevent graft-versus-host disease in man after allogeneic bone-marrow transplantation. Lancet 1:327-329, 1980.

18. Powles RL, Morgenstern G, Clink HM, Hedley D, Bandini G, Lumley H, Watson JG, Lawson D, Spence D, Barrett A, Jameson B, Lawler S, Kay HEM, McElwain TJ: The place of bone-marrow transplantation in acute myelogenous leukaemia. Lancet 1:1047-1050, 1980.

19. Santos GW, Sensenbrenner LL, Anderson PN, Burke PJ, Klein DL, Slavin RE, Schacter B, Borgaonkar DS: HL-A-identical marrow transplants in aplastic anemia, acute leukemia, and lymphosarcoma employing cyclophosphamide. Transplant Proc 8:607-610, 1976.

20. Thomas ED, Bryant JI, Buckner CD, Clift RA, Fefer A,

Johnson FL, Neiman P, Ramberg RE, Storb R: Leukaemic transformation of engrafted human marrow cells in vivo. Lancet 1:1310-1313, 1972.

21. Thomas ED, Buckner CD, Banaji M, Clift RA, Fefer A, Flournoy N, Goodell BW, Hickman RO, Lerner KG, Neiman PE, Sale GE, Sanders JE, Singer J, Stevens M, Storb R, Weiden PL: One hundred patients with acute leukemia treated by chemotherapy, total body irradiation, and allogeneic marrow transplantation. Blood 49:511-533, 1977.

22. Thomas ED, Buckner CD, Clift RA, Fefer A, Johnson FL, Neiman PE, Sale GE, Sanders JE, Singer JW, Shulman H, Storb R, Weiden PL: Marrow transplantation for acute nonlymphoblastic leukemia in first remission. N Engl J Med 301:597-599, 1979.

23. Thomas ED, Flournoy N, Buckner CD, Clift RA, Fefer A, Neiman PE, Storb R: Cure of leukemia by marrow transplantation. Leukemia Research 1:67-70, 1977.

24. Thomas ED, Sanders JE, Flournoy N, Johnson FL, Buckner CD, Clift RA, Fefer A, Goodell BW, Storb R, Weiden PL: Marrow transplantation for patients with acute lymphoblastic leukemia in remission. Blood 54:468-476, 1979.

25. Thomas ED, Storb R, Clift RA, Fefer A, Johnson FL, Neiman PE, Lerner KG, Glucksberg H, Buckner CD: Bone-marrow transplantation. N Engl J Med 292:832-843, 895-902, 1975.

26. Weiden PL, Flournoy N, Sanders JE, Sullivan KM, Thomas ED: Antileukemic effect of graft-versus-host disease contributes to improved survival after allogeneic marrow transplantation. Transplant Proc (in press)

Graft-Versus-Host Disease, Immunologic Reconstitution and Graft-Host Tolerance in Marrow Graft Recipients

RAINER STORB

Professor of Medicine, Division of Oncology

KERRY ATKINSON

Assistant Professor of Medicine, Division of Oncology

LAWRENCE G. LUM

Assistant Professor of Pediatrics, Division of Oncology

KEITH M. SULLIVAN

Assistant Professor of Medicine, Division of Oncology

MANG-SO TSOI

Research Associate Professor of Medicine, Division of Oncology

PAUL L. WEIDEN

Associate Professor of Medicine, Division of Oncology

ROBERT P. WITHERSPOON

Assistant Professor of Medicine, Division of Oncology

University of Washington School of Medicine
Fred Hutchinson Cancer Research Center
Seattle, Washington

This investigation was supported by Grant Numbers CA 18221, CA 18029, CA 15704, and CA 18047, awarded by the National Cancer Institute, DHHS, and CH 137 awarded by the American Cancer Society. K.M.S. is supported in part by a Junior Faculty Clinical Fellowship from the American Cancer Society.

Over the past decade syngeneic and allogeneic marrow transplants have been used with increasing success for the treatment of severe aplastic anemia and acute leukemia.[15] These
studies have involved ablation of the host's hematopoietic
and immunologic system by high doses of chemotherapeutic
agents either given alone or in combination with total body
irradiation. Many patients have become long-term survivors
with neither recurrence of their original disease nor with
occurrence of graft-versus-host disease (GVHD). Others,
however, have died from recurrent disease or, more frequently, from complications related to the transplant.
Further improvement of clinical marrow grafting results
hinges upon progress and better understanding in (1) prevention and treatment of GVHD, (2) recovery of immunologic
reactivity in marrow graft recipients, and (3) elucidation
of mechanisms of stable graft-host tolerance and of GVHD.
The present report summarizes some of the studies in these
areas.

                          ACUTE GVHD

    GVHD describes the clinical and pathological syndrome
which results from the reaction of immunologically competent
donor lymphocytes against histocompatibility antigens of the
host.[3] Both, an acute and chronic form of GVHD are
recognized. The manifestations of acute GVHD are limited to
the skin, liver, intestinal tract and lymphoid system.
    The prevention and treatment of acute GVHD in man remains
problematic. Although many other approaches have been
explored in experimental animals, based on studies in random
bred dogs almost every transplant center has employed post-
grafting methotrexate.[13,15] The prophylactic administration
of horse antithymocyte globulin in addition to methotrexate
failed[19] to decrease the incidence or severity of acute
GVHD. More recently Powles et al.[9] have used cyclosporin
A to prevent GVHD with encouraging preliminary results.
Recent interest has also focused on in vitro manipulations
of marrow in attempts at eliminating immunocompetent cells
while retaining hemopoietic cells.[1]
    Treatment of established acute GVHD has proven to be
frustrating. In a recent study, we demonstrated that either
corticosteroids or antithymocyte globulin resulted in an
apparent decrease in severity of acute GVHD, but many patients died and one-fourth went on to develop chronic GVHD.
    One encouraging note is a curious decrease in the in-
cidence, severity and fatality of acute GVHD over the last 5
years among patients transplanted in Seattle and perhaps in

other transplant centers as well. The cause(s) of this may be due to earlier transplantation, improvements in supportive care, especially therapeutic and prophylactic parenteral nutrition, and perhaps a refinement in the diagnostic criteria for and, thus, earlier treatment of GVHD.

CHRONIC GVHD

In the last 5 years chronic GVHD has been recognized as a major problem of allogeneic marrow grafting, affecting[4,5,12] approximately 30% of patients surviving 180 days. Increasing patient age and presence of acute GVHD are associated with a greater chance of developing chronic GVHD.

Clinically chronic GVHD resembles autoimmune diseases. It occurs 100-300 days after transplant, may persist for years and affects more target organs than acute GVHD. Initial lesions include malar erythema, mottled dyspigmentation, papulosquamous eruptions and desquamation. In untreated patients dermal induration, ulceration, wasting, scleroderma and joint contracture are the rule. Liver function is frequently abnormal and biopsies show severe cholestasis and/or hepatocellular injury.[12] Ocular and oral sicca and oral mucositis, ulceration and striae are common. Less frequently, esophagitis, polymyositis, enteritis and serositis have been observed. Antinuclear, antimitochondrial and antismooth muscle antibodies, rheumatoid factor, direct Coombs' reactivity and eosinophilia are also detected.

Some patients with limited disease of skin and liver have a favorable course without treatment.[12] In contrast, extensive chronic GVHD involves multiple organs and, without treatment, most patients either died or had major disabilities. Mortality was often the result of recurrent bacterial infections[1] while morbidity resulted from wasting, sicca and joint contractures.

We have treated 21 patients with a combination of prednisone and either procarbazine, cyclophosphamide or azathioprine and 16 (76%) survived more than 2 years after transplant with Karnofsky scores $\geq$70%.[14] Light microscopic and direct immunofluorescence examination of skin and oral biopsies or findings of keroconjunctivitis sicca can predict subsequent development of chronic GVHD. Early detection allows immunosuppressive therapy before clinical deterioration or disability. However, treatment is often prolonged and its long-term hazards are currently unknown.

GRAFT-VERSUS-TUMOR EFFECT

Confirmation of the existence of a graft-versus-leukemia effect in human recipients of allogeneic marrow transplants has recently been obtained.[21] The relative rate of leukemia relapse among allogeneic recipients with moderate to severe acute GVHD was 2.5 times less than among recipients with no or only mild acute GVHD or syngeneic recipients. For patients transplanted between 1970 and 1977, however, the decreased rate of leukemia relapse did not result in increased survival because of an increased risk of dying from nonleukemic causes.

Patients transplanted during 1977 and 1978, however, had a lower incidence and fatality rate of acute GVHD. Nevertheless, the antileukemic effect associated with GVHD did not change, i.e. the probability of being in remission 2 years after transplantation was higher among patients with GVHD compared to those without. The net effect of these trends on <u>survival</u> of patients with acute nonlymphoblastic leukemia in remission or relapse or acute nonlymphoblastic leukemia in relapse at the time of transplantation was as follows: survival was better for patients with grade II-IV acute GVHD (50% at 2 years) than for those with no or grade I acute GVHD (25% at 2 years).[20] Future studies may attempt to manipulate GVHD and exploit its apparent antileukemic effect. It should be noted that leukemic relapse is rare in patients with acute nonlymphoblastic leukemia transplanted in remission regardless of presence or absence of GVHD.

IMMUNOLOGIC RECONSTITUTION AFTER MARROW GRAFTING

We have previously reported an evaluation of immunologic reactivity in 56 patients who had survived for 1-6 years after allogeneic marrow grafting for aplastic anemia or hematologic malignancy.[8] Other investigators have reported similar studies.[reviewed in 8] More recently, we completed a study of 153 patients with allogeneic and 48 patients with syngeneic marrow grafts which allowed us to evaluate more accurately the influence of various factors on the tempo and magnitude of immunologic recovery after marrow grafting.

Some general conclusions can be drawn from those studies. Firstly, all patients regardless of whether they were recipients of syngeneic or allogeneic grafts, regardless of underlying disease or whether they had GVHD or not, had pronounced impairment of all immunologic parameters studied during the first 4-5 months post-grafting.

Secondly, recipients of syngeneic grafts and recipients

of allogeneic grafts, who had either no or only transient GVHD, showed subsequently uneventful recovery of immunologic function. This indicates that the major determinants of the pace of immunologic recovery after syngeneic and allogeneic marrow grafting are the speed with which the lymphoid tissues are repopulated by mature donor cells.

Thirdly, patients with chronic GVHD, treated or untreated, remain immunologically crippled. They show no skin test responsiveness to neoantigens, poor antibody titers to both T-dependent and independent antigens and inability to switch from IgM to IgG antibody after repeated challenge. Consequently, they are plagued by recurrent gram positive bacterial infections, usually pneumococcal.[7]

Fourthly, despite the poor immune reactivity in vivo early after grafting, many in vitro parameters of immunity (responses in mixed leukocyte culture and to mitogens, recovery of cells with various surface markers etc.) rapidly returned to the normal range. This was also true for cytotoxic effector cells mediating natural killing, antibody-dependent and lectin-dependent cellular cytotoxicity which returned to normal within 30 days of grafting.[6] Furthermore, there were no significant associations between in vitro cytotoxic activity and infections, GVHD and recurrence of leukemia. These data suggest that most tests and lymphocyte markers used to date are not clinically relevant after marrow grafting and point out the need for new in vitro approaches.

Fifthly, a promising in vitro approach appears to be the study of in vitro antibody secretion by patient lymphocytes[10] using polyclonal activator systems.[10] A recent study revealed the following aberrations in patients with chronic GVHD: a) failure of B cells to secrete Ig in the presence of normal helper T cell activity, b) lack of helper T cell activity, and c) presence of T cells capable of suppressing normal Ig synthesis by normal T and B cells. As a rule, long-term healthy patients lacked B and T cell defects and none showed evidence for suppressor cells.

Finally, these data have some relevance for the management of marrow graft recipients. Early after grafting, there is a need for extreme vigilance with regard to prevention of infection in all patients. Whether this period of profound immunologic deficiency can be abbreviated by the use of thymosin or thymic transplants is uncertain at present. Long-term survivors without GVHD can lead perfectly normal lives without infection while continued protection with antibiotics or perhaps hyperimmune serum is necessary in patients with chronic GVHD. Knowledge of the immune status will be a guide for attempts at vaccinations against pathogens.

IN VITRO STUDIES OF GVHD AND GRAFT-HOST TOLERANCE

Antihost immune reactivity and suppressor cell activity were examined to understand the mechanisms of acute and chronic GVHD and graft-host tolerance after marrow grafting from HLA identical sibling donors. Similar studies were performed in dogs given marrow grafts from DLA nonidentical littermate donors. The following findings were obtained.

I. Dermo-Epidermal IgM Deposits

The presence of cutaneous Ig was investigated in 88 human chimeras.[18] Minimal amounts of IgM were found at the dermo-epidermal junction in 11% of healthy individuals and patients before grafting and in 39% of patients with acute GVHD, but more extensive deposits were present in 86% of patients with chronic GVHD. Chimeras who never had GVHD or had recovered from it and those with syngeneic grafts showed findings not different from those in healthy individuals. These observations raised the possibility that humoral immunity was involved in the development of chronic GVHD.

II. Cellular Immunity to Host Antigens

A. Mixed Leukocyte Response (MLR) in Human Chimeras

Lymphocytes (of donor origin) from 34 human chimeras were tested for MLR to host lymphocytes cryopreserved before grafting.[19] Lymphocytes from 14 of 22 long-term chimeras with chronic GVHD showed MLR to host lymphocytes manifested as high stimulation indices compared to lymphocytes from only 1 of 12 long-term chimeras without GVHD. The results are consistent with in vivo sensitization of donor lymphocytes to non-HLA host antigens in patients with chronic GVHD.

B. Lymphocytotoxicity to Host Fibroblasts

Lymphocytes from 63 human chimeras were tested for toxicity to host fibroblasts (unpublished data) using a ^{51}Cr cytotoxic assay. Cells from 13 long-term stable chimeras lacked cytotoxicity against host skin fibroblasts; in contrast, cells from 4 of 12 long-term chimeras with chronic GVHD, 2 of 20 short-term patients without acute GVHD and 9 of 18 short-term patients with acute GVHD had anti-host cytotoxicity. Statistical analysis showed a significant difference in results between long-term patients with and without chronic GVHD and between short-term patients with and without acute GVHD. These data suggest an involvement of cell-mediated cytotoxicity in human acute and chronic GVHD.

C. MLR to Host Lymphocytes in Canine Chimeras

The MLR to host lymphocytes was examined in 16 canine chimeras transplanted from DLA nonidentical mixed leukocyte culture (MLC) reactive littermates.[2] These chimeras uniformly showed MLC reactivity to cryopreserved host lymphocytes during episodes of both acute GVHD (10 of 10 dogs) and chronic GVHD (6 of 6 dogs). During the periods of clinical good health intervening between episodes of acute and chronic GVHD, however, this reactivity was absent or greatly diminished, while reactivity to third party lymphocytes remained intact. These findings indicate that anti-host reactivity was present during acute and chronic GVHD.

III. Suppressor Cell Activities

A. "Nonspecific" Suppressor Cells in Human Chimeras

Mononuclear cells from 107 chimeras were tested for their ability to suppress the MLR of marrow donors to unrelated alloantigens in MLC.[16] Cells from only 1 of 32 long-term patients without chronic GVHD showed suppression, compared to cells from 21 of 40 patients with chronic GVHD (p $<$ 0.001). It is tempting to speculate that suppressor cells are involved in the severe immunodeficiency of patients with chronic GVHD.

B. "Specific" Suppressor Cells in 35 Human Chimeras

An active cellular suppressor mechanism in long-term stable human chimeras was sought by testing their lymphocytes for ability to inhibit donor MLR to trinitrophenyl-modified (TNP-) host lymphocytes stored before transplantation.[17] and unpublished data We also tested the effect of chimera lymphocytes on donor MLR to unmodified unrelated stimulating cells ("nonspecific" suppression). The results showed that most stable chimeras without GVHD had circulating suppressor cells that "specifically" inhibited donor MLR to TNP-host cells but not to TNP-donor, TNP-unrelated or unmodified unrelated lymphocytes. In comparison, most chimeras with active chronic GVHD lacked suppressor cells that inhibited donor MLR to TNP-host while at the same time showing cells that inhibited donor MLR to unmodified unrelated lymphocytes. These results suggest that stable chimerism in man is maintained by "specific" suppressor cells.

C. Stable Graft-Host Tolerance in Canine Chimeras

Four dogs transplanted from DLA incompatible MLC reactive littermate donors became long-term survivors without GVHD.[2] All 4 showed absence or marked diminution of MLC reactivity to host lymphocytes while demonstrating normal reactivity to third party cells. We were unable to demonstrate cells in the blood of these chimeras suppressive of the positive donor response. We were also unable to demonstrate chimera lymphocytes cytotoxic to host cells in cell-mediated lympholysis. We propose that newly generated lymphoid cells capable of reacting with host antigen are inactivated by a suppressor mechanism in the central lymphoid tissues. The reason for the apparent differences in mechanism of stable graft-host tolerance between human and canine chimeras remains unclear but may be related to the difference in the degree of histoincompatibility in the two systems examined.

In summary, anti-host immune reactivity has been demonstrated in human and canine chimeras with acute and chronic GVHD after marrow grafting. Long-term stable chimeras and short-term chimeras without GVHD in general lacked in vitro evidence of an anti-host response. In humans long-term survivors without GVHD transplanted from HLA identical donors, "specific" suppressor cells inhibiting donor MLR to TNP-host lymphocytes were observed suggesting that an active cellular suppressor mechanism is responsible for graft-host tolerance. Suppressor cells could not be demonstrated in long-term stable canine chimeras transplanted from DLA non-identical donors. In humans, the lack of "specific" suppressor cells, the presence of "nonspecific" suppressor activity, and the presence of anti-host immune reactivity appear to be the characteristics of chronic GVHD.

REFERENCES

1. Atkinson K, Storb R, Prentice RL, Weiden PL, Wither-spoon RP, Sullivan K, Noel D, Thomas ED: Analysis of late infections in 89 long-term survivors of bone marrow transplantation. Blood 53: 720-731, 1979.
2. Atkinson K, Storb R, Weiden PL, Deeg HJ, Gerhard-Miller L, Thomas ED: In vitro tests correlating with presence or absence of graft-vs-host disease in DLA nonidentical canine radiation chimeras: Evidence that clonal abortion maintains stable graft-host tolerance. J Immunol 124:1808-1814, 1980.
3. Billingham RE: The biology of graft-versus-host reactions. Harvey Lectures 62:21-78, 1966.
4. Graze PR, Gale RP: Chronic graft versus host disease: A syndrome of disordered immunity. Am J Med 66:611-620, 1979.
5. Lawley TJ, Peck GL, Moutsopoulos HM, Gratwohl AA, Deisseroth AB: Scleroderma, Sjögren-like syndrome, and chronic graft-versus-host disease. Ann Intern Med 87:707-709, 1977.
6. Livnat S, Seigneuret M, Storb R, Prentice RL: Analysis of cytotoxic effector cell function in patients with leukemia or aplastic anemia before and after marrow transplantation. J Immunol 124:481-490, 1980.
7. Lum LG, Seigneuret MC, Storb R, Witherspoon RP, Thomas ED: T and B-cell deficiencies in patients with chronic graft-versus-host disease after HLA identical marrow transplantation. Transplant Proc (in press).
8. Noel DR, Witherspoon RP, Storb R, Atkinson K, Doney K, Mickelson EM, Ochs HD, Warren RP, Weiden PL, Thomas ED: Does graft-versus-host disease influence the tempo of immunologic recovery after allogeneic human marrow transplantation? An observation on 56 long-term sur-vivors. Blood 51:1087-1105, 1978.
9. Powles RL, Barrett AJ, Clink H, Kay HEM, Sloane J, McElwain TJ: Cyclosporin A for the treatment of graft-versus-host disease in man. Lancet 2:1327-1331, 1978.
10. Ringden O, Witherspoon RP, Storb R, Ekelund E, Thomas ED: Increased in vitro B-cell IgG secretion during acute graft-versus-host disease and infection. Observa-tion in 50 human marrow transplant recipients. Blood 55:179-186, 1980.
11. Rodt H, Netzel B, Kolb HJ, Janka G, Rieder J, Belohradsky B, Haas RJ, Thierfelder S: Antibody treat-ment of marrow grafts in vitro, in Baum SJ, Ledney GD (eds): Experimental Hematology Today. New York, Springer Verlag (in press).

12. Shulman HM, Sullivan KM, Weiden PL, McDonald GB, Striker GE, Sale GE, Hackman R, Tsoi MS, Storb R, Thomas ED: Chronic graft-versus-host syndrome in man: A clinicopathological study of 20 long-term Seattle patients. Am J Med 69:204-217, 1980.

13. Storb R, Epstein RB, Graham TC, Thomas ED: Methotrexate regimens for control of graft-versus-host disease in dogs with allogeneic marrow grafts. Transplantation 9:240-246, 1970.

14. Sullivan KM, Shulman HM, Storb R, Weiden PL, Witherspoon RP, McDonald GB, Schubert MM, Atkinson K, Thomas ED: Chronic graft-versus-host disease in 52 patients: Adverse natural course and successful treatment with combination immunosuppression. Blood (in press).

15. Thomas ED, Storb R, Clift RA, Fefer A, Johnson FL, Neiman PE, Lerner KG, Glucksberg H, Buckner CD: Bone-marrow transplantation. N Engl J Med 292:832-843, 895-902, 1975.

16. Tsoi MS, Storb R, Dobbs S, Kopecky KJ, Santos E, Weiden PL, Thomas ED: Nonspecific suppressor cells in patients with chronic graft-vs-host disease after marrow grafting. J Immunol 123:1970-1976, 1979.

17. Tsoi MS, Storb R, Dobbs S, Santos E, Thomas ED: Specific suppressor cells and immune response to host antigens in long-term human allogeneic marrow recipients: Implications for the mechanism of graft-host tolerance and chronic graft-versus-host disease. Transplant Proc (in press)

18. Tsoi MS, Storb R, Jones E, Weiden PL, Shulman H, Witherspoon R, Atkinson K, Thomas ED: Deposition of IgM and complement at the dermo-epidermal junction in acute and chronic cutaneous graft-vs-host disease in man. J Immunol 120:1485-1492, 1978.

19. Weiden PL, Doney K, Storb R, Thomas ED: Antihuman thymocyte globulin for prophylaxis of graft-versus-host disease. A randomized trial in patients with leukemia treated with HLA-identical sibling marrow grafts. Transplantation 27:227-230, 1979.

20. Weiden PL, Flournoy N, Sanders JE, Sullivan KM, Thomas ED: Antileukemic effect of graft-versus-host disease contributes to improved survival after allogeneic marrow transplantation. Transplant Proc (in press).

21. Weiden PL, Flournoy N, Thomas ED, Prentice R, Fefer A, Buckner CD, Storb R: Antileukemic effect of graft-versus-host disease in human recipients of allogeneic-marrow grafts. N Engl J Med 300:1068-1073, 1979.

The Use of Separated Allogeneic Hematopoietic Precursors to Circumvent Graft vs. Host Disease Following Marrow Transplantation

RICHARD J. O'REILLY, M.D.

Director, Marrow Transplantation Program
Memorial Sloan-Kettering Cancer Center

YAIR REISNER, Ph.D., NEENA KAPOOR, M.D.

Memorial Sloan-Kettering Cancer Center
1275 York Avenue
New York, New York 10021

In the last twelve years, marrow transplantation has emerged as the treatment of choice for lethal congenital immunedeficiencies[14], aplastic anemia[3] and possibly certain forms of leukemia [39]. However, application of this approach is largely limited to the 30 or 40% of patients who have an HLA-identical sibling, since transplants of marrow from HLA-haploidentical or fully allogeneic donors have, once engrafted, regularly induced lethal graft vs. host disease [14]. Although we and others have demonstrated that transplants from related or even unrelated donors who are HLA phenotypically identical or haploidentical and mismatched for a restricted number of HLA determinants on the other haplotype may produce full and durable hematopoietic and lymphoid reconstitution without[4] lethal[11] GvHD[22,74], identification of such donors is currently possible for no more than 5-10% of cases [9]. Thus, for over 50% of patients with lethal blood diseases for which a transplant might be curative, this approach cannot be used, for want of an appropriate donor.

In the past decade, studies in murine models have established that graft vs. host disease is initiated by thymic derived T lymphocytes [43] and more importantly, that selective removal of the T lymphocytes capable of initiating this response allows for transplantation across major histocompatibility barriers with subsequent development of stable chimeras without lethal graft vs. host disease [41,43]. In Table 1, are listed 6 techniques which have been developed in murine models

This investigation was supported by National Institutes of Health Grants:CA23766,CA08748,CA19267,CA17404;by the Charles A. Dana Foundation,Robert J. Kleberg,Jr. and Helen C. Kleberg, Foundation,Arthur Vining Davis Foundation, Judith Harris

TABLE 1

Techniques for Depleting Alloreactive
T Lymphocytes from Hematopoietic Tissue Grafts

1. Density gradient techniques
2. In vitro "suicide" techniques
3. Preincubation or fractionation with antibody
4. Fractionation with lectins
5. In vitro culture of hematopoietic cells
6. Fetal liver transplants

for depleting alloreactive T lymphocytes from marrow or other
hematopoietic tissues for the purposes of transplanting across
histocompatibility barriers without risk of lethal graft vs.
host disease. In this review, we will briefly examine the
biological basis for each technique, the in vitro and in vivo
evidence derived from animal experimentation supporting its
use, and, where available, the accumulated experience in
clinical marrow transplantation.

The use of density gradient techniques was initially
proposed by Dicke et al. [7] and was based on the concept that
early hematopoietic precursors were of lighter density than
alloreactive T lymphocytes permitting their separation by
differential centrifugation in continuous or discontinuous
albumin density gradients. Accumulated results using these
techniques have failed to demonstrate a clear differential in
buoyant density between early hematopoietic precursors and
alloreactive T lymphocytes, particularly activated T lymphocytes. While results of transplants in animals suggest that
survival may be prolonged following transplants of precursor
rich populations [7] , graft vs host disease has been seen
in the majority of cases. Clinical experience with this
approach is largely limited to transplants in children for
severe combined immunedeficiency [8]   . To date, there is no
evidence that the use of density gradient techniques to remove alloreactive T cells will abrogate the GvH potential of
a fully allogeneic or HLA haploidentical separated marrow
graft.

The in vitro "suicide" techniques, initially developed
by Zoschke and Bach [46] and by Rich et al. [31], is based on
differential uptake of a pulse of toxic DNA precursors such
as bromodeoxyuridine or highly labelled [3]H Thymidine, by
alloreactive T lymphocytes of donor origin induced to proliferate in response to host alloantigenic determinants in

Selig Memorial Fund, The Sherman Fairchild Foundation-New
Frontiers, International Paper Company Foundatioh, The Jeanne
and Robert Rimsky Cellular Engineering Fund, The New Hope
Chapter, Siegfried and Josephine Bieber Foundation.

in vitro mixed lymphocyte culture. This results in a selective depletion of T lymphocytes specifically responsive to the host, preserving lymphocytes with other specificities. This technique has been utilized in inbred mouse models of marrow transplantation, where it was found that tritiated thymidine pulsed, host antigen-stimulated, donor marrow cells could be selectively depleted of host specific T lymphocytes. Subsequent transplantation of the treated marrow led to stable chimerism without GvHD.[31] As shown in Table 2, four attempts to extend this technique to man have not been successful. Two patients succumbed to infection before the graft could be evaluated.[35,28] One patient achieved limited engraftment with minimal GvHD but remained immunodeficient and died of infection;[30] one patient died with GvHD and a viral infection.[28] The GvHD noted in the last case may have been caused by allostimulated T lymphocytes not immediately induced into a proliferative cycle. A more inclusive method for insuring depletion of allospecific T lymphocytes was devised by Romano et al.[34] and is based on the observation that allostimulated T lymphocytes are selectively susceptible to lytic infection by vesicular stomatitis virus whether or not they are induced to proliferate. Transplants of histoincompatible marrow treated with this virus after exposure to host cells, results in stable chimerism without GvHD. While this system presents a particularly effective system for depletion of allospecific T cells, the requirement of preincubation with virus makes it unlikely that this technique will be extended to man.

A third technique involves pretreatment of an allogeneic bone marrow or spleen cell graft with an antiserum specific for T lymphocytes. This technique was initially introduced by von Boehmer, Sprent and Nabholz[41], who pretreated parental strain marrow or spleen cells with an anti-serum specific for the theta antigen characteristic of T lymphocytes prior to injection into F$_1$ hybrid mice, and achieved in long-lived stable chimeras with full hematologic vigor and without detectable GvHD. In subsequent work, in the rat model by Muller Rucholz[19], and in murine models by Onoe et al.[21] and Krown et al.[16], it has been shown that this technique is also effective in preventing GvHD in fully allogeneic crosses. Kolb et al.[15] have recently used this approach for marrow transplants in outbred dogs. Results have been encouraging but less consistent with frequent graft failures, possibly due to the relatively poor specificity of heteroantisera raised against dog T lymphocytes. Clinical experience with HLA-mismatched marrow grafts pretreated with either heteroantisera

TABLE 2

*Clinical Experience With Histoincompatible Marrow Grafts
Following T Lymphocyte Depletion*

Patients	Disease	Pre-BMT Treatment	Method of T Cell Depletion	Outcome	Source
2	SCID	None	Marrow T cell suicide by exposure to BUDR and light	1 early infectious death, 1 GvHD viral disease	Parkman et al.
2	SCID	None	Marrow T cell suicide by HOT 3H Thymidine pulse	1 limited engraftment, min. GvHD, persist. immunodef.; 1 no engraftment, early infectious death	Sieber et al. Salmon et al.
2	SCID	None	Heterologous ATG pre-treatment	2 early infec. deaths	Niethammer Park et al.
1	SCID	None	Monoclonal Anti-OKT3 Pre-treatment	Early infect. death	Parkman et al.
1	Leukemia	CTX,TBI	Monoclonal Anti-OKT3 Pre-treatment	Early infect. death	Parkman et al.

or monoclonal antibodies raised against thymis derived lymphocytes is extremely limited (Table 2), and unevaluable since
the patients treated died of infections before engraftment
was achieved. [20,27,28]

Another technique developed by Reisner et al. [32] involves
separation of T lymphocytes from other hematopoietic precursors in the bone marrow by differential adsorption to plant
lectins, such as soybean agglutinin or peanut agglutinin.
These lectins bind to specific sugar moieties in the surface
glycoproteins of the cell wall. The sugars present in the
glycoprotein thus define the cell's affinity for each lectin.
In initial experiments, Reisner et al.[32] demonstrated that soybean agglutinin and peanut agglutinin bound to early hematopoietic precursors but failed to bind to T lymphocytes in
marrow or spleen. Marrow fractions agglutinated by these
lectins were highly enriched for hematopoietic precursors but
void of functional T cells demonstrable by transformation
responses against allogeneic cells or the mitogen PHA. Transplantation of marrow or spleen cells agglutinated by soybean
agglutinin and peanut agglutinin resulted in stable long-term
chimeras without evidence of GvHD. More recently, Reisner
et al. [33], have compared mouse, monkey and human bone marrow
for the reactivity of their T lymphocytes and hematopoietic
precursors with the different plant lectin. In contrast to
the mouse, it was found that both human and primate (Cynomologus monkey) hematopoietic precursors fail to agglutinate
with soybean agglutinin, whereas their T lymphocytes bind to
soybean agglutinin and are largely eliminated by this agglutination step. By combining an initial differential sedimentation of T lymphocytes forming spontaneous rosettes with
sheep red cells and a secondary removal of residual T cells
by agglutination with soybean agglutinin, one is left with a
cell fraction highly enriched for hematopoietic precursors
but totally void of reactivity in mixed lymphocyte culture,
in allospecific cell mediated lympholysis assays, or in
transformation responses to the mitogen PHA. The content of
early myeloid cells in this T cell depleted population accounts for over 25% of the myeloid cells in unfractionated
marrow, yet the total number of cells represents less than
25% of the monoclonal cells in the unseparated marrow fraction. Recently, we have used marrow precursor-rich fractions
for transplantation into fully allogeneic Cynomologus monkeys
which were pretreated with lethal irradiation and Cyclophosphamide. Hematopoietic reconstitution has been rapid. Pathologic examination of the tissues of these animals has failed
to demonstrate any evidence of GvHD. Thus, this technique,

now extended to a preclinical primate model which has strong
analogies to man, may soon be applicable to the human situation.

Recently, Dexter and Moore[5] developed techniques for
sustained in vitro culture of hematopoietic precursors with
potential for differentiation along any of the hematopoietic
lines. Transplantation of hematopoietic precursors derived
from long term in vitro culture across major H2 barriers in
the mouse has also produced full, stable hematopoietic
chimeras without GvHD[6]. Critical to the success of this
approach is the fact that T lymphocytes capable of inducing
GvHD die off during the period of prolonged culture. Modifications of this technique such as the addition of cortisone
to the culture have promoted rapid elimination of T lymphocyte populations. There are now indications that approaches
of this type can also be applied to the culture of human bone
marrow. As methods for propagation of human bone marrow
cells become available, this technique may be applied to
marrow transplantation in instances where an HLA identical
or compatible donor is not available.

The last approach which will be discussed, was initially
developed in the mouse in 1958 by Uphoff et al.[40] This technique involves transplantation of hematopoietic precursors
derived from the fetal liver at a stage of gestation antedating development of the thymus. Transplantation of these
very immature cells into lethally irradiated H2 incompatible
recipients has been shown to be effective in producing long
term chimeras without GvHD. This early technique was early
applied to clinical transplantation. Studies of the ontogeny
of the immune system in man indicated that the fetal liver is
the major site of hematopoiesis from approximately the 8th to
the 18th week of fetal gestation . It was also shown that
lymphoid infiltration of the thymus begins between the 12th
and 14th week of fetal gestation[2] at which time functionally mature T lymphocytes are demonstrable in the thymus by
their responses to mitogens[18,37] and their capacity to induce
a local GvHD in xenogeneic recipients[1]. The first evidence that fetal liver transplants could be successful in
reconstituting immune function without GvH, was presented by
Keightly et al.[13] This patient, who developed significant
evidence of both T and B cell immunity, ultimately died of a
nephritis 13 months after transplantation. A rather dramatic example of the potential of fetal liver transplants is
illustrated by a patient transplanted on our service in 1975.
Prior to engraftment of the fetal liver cells, this patient
suffered from a disseminated Mycobacterium avium infection
and was totally void of evidence of immunologic reactivity.
The patient exhibited no evidence of granulomatous responses

to the Mycobacterium prior to engraftment. However, with engraftment of fetal liver derived lymphoid precursors demonstrable by HLA typing of peripheral blood lymphocytes, and
thereafter the development of T cell function, shown by transformation responses to mitogens, antigens and allogeneic
cells, the patient rapidly developed the capacity to react to
the Mycobacterium avium generating a marked granulomous response in affected tissues and ultimately eradicating this
infection. This patient, who continues chimeric with normal
T and B cell function, provided by a lymphoid system which,
by HLA typing, is totally distinct from his own, recently
overcame a primary varicella infection with little evidence
to suggest immunedeficiency. At no time has he developed
any clinical or pathological evidence of GvHD. [25,26]
    In reviewing the world's experience (Table 3), it is
clear that GvHD is either absent or mild in recipients of
fetal liver transplants. Indeed, there has been only one
death ascribed to GvHD following a fetal liver transplant.
This patient received, concurrently, a thymus from a 16 week
gestational aged fetus and would therefore have been expected
to develop GvHD. However, this experience also illustrates
the major problems which may be anticipated when fully allogeneic cells are used for the purposes of transplantation.

TABLE 3

Fetal Tissue Transplants In SCID

Type of Donor

	Graft vs Host Disease		
	No.	o-1+	2-y+
HLA-identical sibling marrow	25	80%	20%
Non-sibling HLA-D compatible marrow	10	30%	70%
Fully allogeneic fetal liver and thymus	12	83%	17%

TABLE 4

Summary of Fetal Liver Transplants
For Severe Combined Immunodeficiency

Total number of treated patients	68
Patients unevaluable due to early infectious deaths	16
Patients with evaluable transplants	52
Failure of engraftment	33(51)**
Sustained engraftment with chimerism	19
Reconstitution of T lymphocyte function only	8
Reconstitution of T and B cell function	7
Reconstitution of B lymphocyte function only	1
Long term survival with reconstitution	6(11%)

First, as can be seen in Table 4, the incidence of engraftment of these cells is extraordinarily low; even in a
population of individuals who have no evidence of classical
immunity. It would be anticipated that the incidence of engraftment would be even more restricted in patients with
aplasia or leukemia who have been sensitized to allogeneic
donors by virtue of prior transfusion. Secondly, the immune
reconstitution attending successful engraftment of fetal
liver cells is rarely complete. The studies of Zinkernagel
and Doherty[44] suggested that the major histocompatibility region may serve to promote interaction between cooperative
cells both in interpretation of an antigenic challenge and
also in the genesis of effector responses such as production
of antibody by B cell in cooperating with helper T cells and
in virus-specific T cell cytotoxic responses. Such cooperation did not occur when the T cells did not share H2 determinants with the B cells or with virus-infected target cells.
The studies of our own group demonstrated that the majority
of patients with combined immunedeficiency treated with
either marrow or fetal tissue transplants, achieve engraftment of donor T lymphocytes but rarely achieve engraftment of
donor B cells[26] . We have also observed that in instances
in which the T and B cell are derived from fully HLA-dispa-
rate donors, cooperation between donor T and host B cells,
as evidence by antibody production, is minimal. A failure of

** Number of grafts

effective interactions due to genetic disparity between the donor T lymphocyte and host cooperating cell has been observed in certain fully allogeneic radiation chimeric mice,[4,5] and might serve to explain the low incidence of survival and effective immunologic reconstitution in human recipients of fetal tissue grafts. The recent studies of Onoe et al.[21] and Katz et al.[12] however, suggest the possibility that through certain manipulations of the host, early lymphoid precursor cells of donor type may be induced to develop within the host thymic environment and thereby be educated to recognize the host as self. As a consequence of such adaptive differentiation, allogeneic donor T cell precursors are able to cooperate appropriately with host tissues in the development of an effective immune response.

From the above, it is clear that transplantation of fully allogeneic hematopoietic precursors depleted of T lymphocytes can be effective in reconstituting hematopoietic function and, in certain instances, the immune system without evidence of lethal GvHD. Experience with fully allogeneic grafts of fetal tissues and T cell-depleted bone marrow, both in mouse and in man, suggests that engraftment will be markedly more difficult to achieve when such grafts are used and further, that the immune reconstitution achieved may be limited. Many of the difficulties attending the use of fully allogeneic hematopoietic tissues, however, may be obviated through the use of haploidentical donors since sharing of HLA specificities may not only reduce the incidence of graft rejection but also promote effective lymphoid cooperation with the host in the development of an immune response.

If it were possible to transplant histoincompatible hematopoietic cells without risk of lethal GvHD, what advantages might be accrued to the human host? First, it is clear that such transplants, if successful, would extend the application of marrow transplantation to the majority of patients who are currently lacking histocompatible donors thereby markedly enhancing the usefulness of marrow transplantation for the treatment of lethal hematopoietic diseases. It is also clear that if such manipulations are effective in abrogating or eliminating the GvHD potential of a marrow graft, the acute morbidity and mortality associated with marrow transplants even from histocompatible siblings, would be markedly reduced.

A second advantage to the recipient may attend the introduction of lymphoid precursors of a different genetic background. In individuals transplanted for neoplastic disease, such grafts might potentiate immune responses against malignant cells (graft vs. leukemia). Indeed, the recent studies

of Weiden at al.[42] in patients transplanted for acute lymphoblastic leukemia suggest that individuals developing GvHD are
at lower risk for developing late relapse in the post transplant period. Such graft vs. leukemic response is well-known
in mice models of transplantation. However, in the horse it
is often difficult to differentiate the anti-leukemic effect
from the reaction of the donor lymphoid system against alloantigens of the host. However, there are some systems, particularly transplantation models in germ-free animals, which
would suggest that a distinction between GvHD and graft vs.
leukemia can be made.[30] Further evidence for such a distinction is presented in the results of transplants between animals resistant and susceptible to a specific pathogen or
tumor, transplants which may confer resistance to a specific
exogenous pathogen to genetically susceptible animals. Examples of this phenomenon are provided by work of Galelli et
al.[10] which demonstrated that immunization with LPS of genetically susceptible mice chimeric with bone marrow derived
from genetically resistant mice, confers on those animals a
degree of resistance to subsequent challenge with Klebsiella
pneumoniae comparable to that of the genetically resistant
donor strain. Similarly, the work of Lopez et al.[17] examining resistance to HSV virus, demonstrates that genetically
susceptible mice who have been lethally irradiated and transplanted with bone marrow from (C57 black 6 x AJ)F1 mice which
are genetically resistant, are rendered resistant to subsequent challenge with HSV   . More recently, the studies of
Tanaka et al. , have extended this type of manipulation to
the study of genetic resistance to malignancies [38] . Thus,
AKR mice which have been lethally irradiated and transplanted
from genetically resistant B6, D10 mouse donors have a low
incidence of spontaneous leukemia, a finding which sharply
contrasts with the high incidence of leukemia in untreated
AKR mice or AKR mice transplanted with syngeneic bone marrow.
     In summary, experimental work in murine models has led
to a definition of those cells responsible for initiating
GvHD and to the development of a number of techniques for depleting those cells from the bone marrow graft which permit
transplants of marrow across major histocompatibility
barriers. Many of these techniques will soon be applicable
to human marrow transplantation. Such techniques should
markedly reduce morbidity and mortality attributable to GvHD
which currently limits the success of HLA-identical marrow
transplants in patients with acutely, lethal blood disorders,
and prohibit the use of this approach in other disorders such
as sickle cell anemia and thalassemia. Such techniques
should also permit marrow transplants in patients lacking an

HLA histocompatible donor. Ultimately, such techniques may allow us to explore the true potential of a genetically disparate immune and hematopoietic system in enhancing the host's resistance to neoplasia.

REFERENCES

1. Asantila, T., Sorvari, T., Hirvonen,T.,Tolvanen,P.: Xenogeneic reactivity of human fetal lymphocytes. J. Immunol. 111:948-987, 1973.
2. August, C.S., Berkel, A.J. et al.:Onset of lymphocyte function in the developing human fetus. Ped.Res.5:539,1971.
3. Camitta, B. M., Thomas, E.D., et al.:Severe aplastic anemia: A prospective study of the effect of early marrow transplantation on acute mortality. Blood 48:63-70,1976.
4. Clift, R. A., Hanse, J.A., et al.:Marrow transplantation from donors other than HLA-identical siblings. Transplan. 28:235-242, 1979.
5. Dexter, T.M., Moore, M.A.S.,Sheridan,A.P.C.: Maintenance of hemopoietic stem cells and production of differentiated progeny in allogeneic and semiallogeneic bone marrow chimeras in vitro. J. Exp. Med. 145:1612, 1977.
6. Dexter, T. M., Spooncer, E.: Loss of immunoreactivity in long term bone marrow culture. Nature 275:135-136, 1979.
7. Dicke, K.A., Triderte,G., van Bekkum, D.W.: The selective elimination of immunologically competent cells from bone marrow and lymphocyte cell mixtures. Transplant.8:422,1969.
8. Dicke, K.A., van der Waaij,D., van Bekkum,D.W.: The use of stem cell grafts in combined immune deficiencies. Birth Defects:Original Article Series. 11:391-396,1975.
9. Dupont. B.: HLA factors and bone marrow grafting (elsewhere in this volume)

10.Galelli, A., LeGarree,Y. et al.: Transfer by bone marrow cells of increased natural resistance to Klebsiella pneumoniae induced by lipopolysaccharide in genetically deficient C3H/He mice. Infec. and Immun. 23:232-238,1979.
11.Hansen, J.A., Clift,R.A. et al.: Transplantation of marrow from an unrelated donor to a patient with acute leukemia. N. Engl.J. Med. 303:565-567, 1980.
12.Katz,D.H.,Katz,L.R. et al.:Adaptive differentiation of murine lymphocytes II. J. Exp. Med. 149:1360-1370, 1979.
13.Keightley,R.G., Lawton,A.R. et al.:Successful fetal liver transplantation in a child with severe combined immunodeficiency. Lancet 2:850-853, 1975.

14. Kenny,A.B., Hitzig,W.G.: Bone marrow transplantation
for severe combined immunodeficiency disease.Eur.J.Ped.
131:155-177,1979.
15. Kolb,H.J.,Rieder,I. et al.:Antilymphocytic antibodies and
marrow transplantation VI. Graft vs. host tolerance in
DLA-incompatible dogs after in vitro treatment of bone
marrow with absorbed anti-thymocyte globulin.Transpl.27:
242-245,1979.
16. Krown,S.,Coico,R.et al:Immune function in fully allogeneic
mouse bone marrow chimeras. Clin. Immunol.Immunopath.
In Press.
17. Lopez,C.:Immunological nature of genetic resistance of
mice to Herpes simplex virus Type 1 infection. In: Onco-
genesis and Herpesviruses III.(G.de The,W.Henle,F.Rapp,ed)
1978. W.H.O. Lyon, France, pp. 775-782.
18. Lowenberg, B.: Fetal liver transplantation. Radiobiol.
Inst., Rijswijk, Netherlands, 1975.
19. Muller-Ruchholtz, W., Wotlge, W.U., Muller-Hermelink,H.K.
Bone marrow transplantation in rats across strong histocompatibility barriers by selective elimination of
lymphoid cells in donor marrow. Transpl.Proc.8:537,1976.
20. Niethammer, D., Goldman,S.F., et al:Bone marrow transplantation for severe combined immunodeficiency with the HLA-
A incompatible but MLC-identical mother as donor. Transpl.
Proc. 8:623, 1976.
21. Onoe, K., Fernandez, G., Good, R.A.:Humoral and cell-
mediated immune responses in fully allogeneic bone marrow
chimera in mice. J. Exp. Med. 151:115-132, 1980.
22. O'Reilly, R.J.,Pahwa, R., et al: Successful transplantation of marrow from an HLA-A,B,D mismatched heterozygous
sibling donor into an HLA-D homozygous patient with
aplastic anemia. Transp.Proc. 10:957-961, 1978.
23. O'Reilly, R.J.,Kapoor,N. et al: Reconstitution of immunologic function in a patient with severe combined immunodeficiency following transplantation of marrow from an
HLA-A,B,C, non-identical but MLC compatible paternal donor.
Transpl. Proc. 11:1934-1937, 1979.
24. O'Reilly, R. J., Dupont,B. et al: Reconstitution in severe
combined immunodeficiency by transplantation of marrow
from an unrelated donor. N. Engl. J. Med. 297:1311-1318,
1977.
25. O'Reilly,R.J., Pahwa,R., et al.:Transplantation of foetal
liver and thymus in patients with severe combined immunodeficiency. In: The Immune System. Function and Therapy
of Dysfunction(G.Doria,A.Eshisol,eds.)Acad. Press 1980,
pp. 241-253.

26. O'Reilly, R.J., Kapoor, N. et al.: Fetal tissue transplants for severe combined immunodeficiency. Proc. Symp. on Primary Immunodeficiencies. Royaumont, France, 1980. Elsevier/North Holland. In Press.

27. Park, B. H., Biggar, W.D., Govo,R.A.:Transplantation of imcompatible bone marrow in infants with severe combined immunodeficiency disease. Birth Defects: Original Article Series. 11:380-384, 1975.

28. Parkman, R., Gelfand, E.W.,Rosen,F.S.:Attempted immunologic reconstitution of patients with combined immune deficiency syndrome with bone marrow transplantation from histocompatible donors. Birth Defects:Original Article Series. 11:417-420, 1975.

29. Parkman, R. : Personal Communication.

30. Pollard, M., Truitt, R. L.: Allogeneic bone marrow chimerism in germ free mice. I. Prevention of spontaneous leukemia in AKR mice.Proc.Soc.Exp.Biol.Med.144:659-665,1973.

31. Rich, R. R., Kilpatrick, C. H.,Smith,T.K.:Simultaneous suppression of responses to allogeneic tissues in vitro and in vivo. Cell.Immunol. 5:190, 1972.

32. Reisner, Y., Itzicovitch,L. et al.:Hematopoietic stem cell transplant using mouse bone marrow and spleen cells fractionated by lectins.Proc.Nat.Acad.Sci.75:2933-2936,1978.

33. Reisner, Y., Kapoor,N.,et al: Allogeneic bone marrow transplantation using stem cells fractionated by lectins.III In vitro analysis of human and monkey bone marrow cells fractionated by sheep red blood cells and soybean agglutinin. Lancet. Submitted.

34. Romano,T.J., Nowakowski,M. et al.: Selective viral immunosuppression of the graft versus host reaction. J.Exp.Med. 145:666-675, 1977.

35. Salmon, S.E.,Smith,B.A. et al:Modification of donor lymphocytes for transplantation in lymphopenic immunological deficiency. Lanct 2:149,1970.

36. Sieber,O.F.,Fulginiti,V.A. et al:Immunological reconstitution in severe combined immunodeficiency disease with transplantation from a non-compatible donor. Clin.Res. 22:230,1974.

37. Stites,D.P.,Carr,M.C.,Fudenberg,H.H.:Ontogency of cellular immunity in the human fetus. Cell.Immunol.11:257,1974.

38. Tanaka, T., Obata, Y. et al.:Prevention of leukemia in lethally irradiated AKR mice by CBA/H marrow transplantation. Proc. Am. Assoc.Cancer Res. 20:114,1979.

39. Thomas, E.D.,Buckner,D.D. et al:Marrow transplantation for acute nonlymphoblastic leukemia in first remission. N. Engl.J. Med. 301:597-599, 1979.

40. Uphoff, D.: Preclusion of secondary phase of irradiation syndrome by inoculation of fetal hematopoietic tissue following lethal total-body X-irradiation. J.Nat.Cancer Inst. 20:625-632,1958.
41. von Boehmer, H., Sprent,J., Nabholz, M.: Tolerance to histocompatibility determinants in tetraparental bone marrow chimeras. J.Exp. Med. 141:322, 1975.
42. Weiden, P.L., Fluorney,N. et al.:Anti-leukemic effect of graft vs. host disease in human recipients of allogeneic marrow grafts. N. Engl.J. Med.300:1068-1073, 1979.
43. Yunis, E.J., Good, R. A. et al: Protection of lethally irradiated mice by spleen cells from neonatally thymecto-mized mice. Proc.Natl. Acad. Sci. 71:2544, 1974.
44. Zinkernagel,R.M., Doherty,P.C.: MHC-restricted cytotoxic T cells:Studies in the biological role of polymorphic major transplantation antigens, determining T cell re-striction specificity, function and responsiveness. Adv. Immunol. 27:42, 1979.
45. Zinkernagel, R.M., Althage, A.,et al: On the immunocompe-tence of H-2 incompatible irradiation bone marrow chimeras. J. Immunol. 124:2356-2365, 1980.
46. Zoschke, D.C., Bach,F.H.: Specificity of allogeneic cell recongition by human lymphocytes in vitro. Science 172:1350-1352, 1971.

Monoclonal Antibodies and Marrow Transplantation

John A. Hansen

Associate Professor, Division of Oncology,
Department of Medicine, University of Washington
Puget Sound Blood Center
Fred Hutchinson Cancer Research Center
Seattle, Washington

and

Paul J. Martin

Associate in Medical Oncology
Fred Hutchinson Cancer Research Center
University of Washington
Seattle, Washington

The potential value of serotherapy in the treatment of malignant disease and in clinical transplantation has long been appreciated. For this purpose, antisera to human cell-surface antigens have been produced by heteroimmunizations in multiple species. This type of approach, however, has generally failed to yield antibody sources of sufficient specificity, titer and supply. These limitations can now be overcome by the techniques introduced by Kohler and Milstein (1) for the generation and selection of hybrid cells that secrete monoclonal antibodies. Hybrid cell lines have already been used to obtain antibodies against human tumor associated antigens (2-7) and lymphoid-hematopoietic differentiation antigens, including human Ia-like antigen (8-12), T cell (12-23) and thymus antigens (24-26), monocyte antigen (27), and common-ALL antigen (28).

This work has been supported by Grant Number HL 17265 awarded by the National Heart Lung Blood Institute and by Grant Numbers CA 29548 and CA 18029 awarded by the National Cancer Institute. Address Reprint Requests to: John A. Hansen, Fred Hutchinson Cancer Research Center, 1124 Columbia Street, Seattle, Washington 98104.

As discussed elsewhere in this symposium (29-30), marrow transplantation can be a definitive form of therapy for immune deficiency, bone marrow failure, and for leukemia. Despite recent successes, a number of formidable obstacles remain, including graft versus host disease (GVHD), graft rejection, recurrent leukemia, and opportunistic infections. Overcoming these obstacles could become feasible with the advent of monoclonal antibodies (see Table 1).

Table 1.   Potential Uses of Monoclonal Antibodies in

Clinical Marrow Transplantation

I.   Treatment of Bone Marrow Cells in vitro

for removal of residual leukemia cells from patient's marrow prior to autologous transplantation

for prevention of graft-versus-host disease by removal of donor T cells prior to allogeneic transplantation.

II.   Treatment of the Marrow Graft Recipient

for immunosuppression pre-transplantation

for anti-leukemia therapy

for therapy of graft-versus-host disease

for prevention or therapy of viral infections

PREVENTION OF GVHD

Serious GVHD remains a major problem in marrow transplantation even when HLA-identical sibling donors are used. In rodent models, experimental evidence indicates that the primary responder and effector cells responsible for acute GVHD are T cells. Thus, acute GVHD can be induced when tissues containing immunologically mature T cells are transferred to a genetically disparate and immunologically deficient recipient (33-34). Immature T cells, however, obtained from fetal tissues or from spleens of newborn mice do not cause GVHD (35-37). Of special relevance to clinical marrow transplantation are experiments in mice and rats in which antisera were used to remove mature T cells from donor marrow (38-43). Following this treatment, donor stem cells can differentiate in allogeneic recipients into fully mature cells, including functionally normal lymphocytes that are specifically tolerant to the histocompatibility antigens of the recipient.

In humans, donor marrow is collected by performing multiple marrow aspirations. Invariably a considerable amount of peripheral blood is obtained as well, so that the marrow graft contains not only stem cells, but also a large number of peripheral lymphocytes. If mature T cells could be eliminated from the donor marrow, GVHD might be prevented. Clinical adaptation of the experimental approaches successful in rodent models requires consideration of several questions: 1) Which monoclonal anti-T cell antibody would be most suitable? 2) What are the optimal conditions for effecting T cell lysis in vitro? and 3) Are there circumstances in which some T cells might be necessary for "helping" engraftment of stem cells?

The animal experiments that were successful in preventing GVHD by pretreatment of marrow cells made use of anti-T cell sera (highly absorbed anti-lymphocyte sera or antitheta serum) that reacted with all mature T cells. For initial clinical trials in man, it might therefore be most prudent to select monoclonal antibodies that similarly recognize all mature T cells, since it is not known whether any single functionally distinct T cell subset is responsible for induction of GVHD. The monoclonal antibodies thus far described that appear to meet this requirement, the so-called "pan-T cell" antibodies, are listed in Table 2. Final selection of the most appropriate reagent for clinical trial should be based on in vitro studies demonstrating abrogation of T cell function following treatment with antibody and complement (15).

Table 2. Cell-Surface Antigens on Mature T cells

Cell Surface Antigen	Distribution of Antigen Peripheral blood T cells	Thymocytes	Molecular Characteristics of Antigen	References
9.6	>99%	>99%	Single chain; 50,000 - 55,000	Kamoun et al., 1980
10.2	84-92%	>99%	Multimeric complex; 67,000 and 65,000	Martin et al., 1980
Leu1	80-95%	>99%	Multimeric complex; 67,000 and 65,000	Engelman and Levy, 1980 Wang et al., 1980
Leu5	>99%	>99%	Single chain; 45,000 - 50,000	Howard et al., 1980
T101	>99%	>99%	Multimeric complex; 67,000 and 65,000	Royston et al., 1980
OKT1	>99%	10%		Reinherz et al., 1979a
OKT3	>99%	10%		Kung et al., 1979 Reinherz et al., 1979b

In the experimental model, T cell depletion can be accomplished simply by pretreating marrow in vitro with a specific T cell antiserum followed by infusion of the treated cells into the recipient. Elimination of T cells presumably occurs in vivo by fixation of complement, by opsonization and phagocytosis, or by the activity of K cells in antibody-dependent cell-mediated cytotoxicity (ADCC). There is no data available regarding the efficacy of these cell lysis mechanisms in vivo in humans. An alternative method for removing T cells is treatment of antibody-coated cells in vitro with complement. We have begun screening pools of rabbit serum in order to identify a complement source with optimal specific lytic activity against T cells and minimal nonspecific toxicity against human hematopoietic cells. For this purpose, we test each batch of complement for toxicity against the erythroid burst forming unit (BFU-E), a relatively immature committed precursor cell assayed in vitro by culture of peripheral blood or bone marrow mononuclear cells in plasma clots with erythropoietin.

Although it is unlikely that there is an absolute requirement for T cell interactions during stem cell proliferation and differentiation in vivo, it can be shown that T cells enhance hematopoiesis in vitro (44-46). Moreover, there is a suggestion from the canine model and from the marrow grafting experience in patients with aplastic anemia that T cells and possibly certain other accessory cells may help to overcome the phenomenon of allograft resistance (47-48). Failure of engraftment is usually not a problem in patients with leukemia, probably because the vigorous cytotoxic therapy (high dose cyclophosphamide and total body irradiation) used before transplantation results in adequate immunosuppression.

Treatment of Established GVHD

Treatment of acute GVHD has been attempted using corticosteroids and/or antithymocyte globulin (ATG) with equivocal results (29-30). Prophylactic treatment with horse ATG early after transplantation has not been effective in preventing acute GVHD (49). In recent years, chronic GVHD has become a significant clinical problem as well. A monoclonal antibody specific for cytotoxic cells might control GVHD without the broad lympholytic effects of currently used ATG preparations.

Pretransplant Immunosuppressive Therapy
for Patients with Aplastic Anemia

The major limiation to successful marrow transplantation in patients with aplastic anemia has been graft rejection (48). Even when the marrow donor is an HLA identical sibling, 30-40% of aplastic patients who received transfusions before transplantation reject their marrow grafts. The risk of graft rejection is higher for transfused patients than for untransfused patients. In this setting, alloantigen - stimulated T cells probably play a role in the rejection mechanism. Combined immunosuppressive regimens which incorporate ATG have been reported successful in overcoming graft rejection (50). Toxic complications of other regimens have been severe (48).

Adjunct Leukemia Therapy and Allogeneic
Marrow Transplantation

In the treatment of leukemia, marrow transplantation from an HLA identical sibling donor appears to be of greatest therapeutic value when performed for patients with acute nonlymphocytic leukemia in remission (51). Relapse of leukemia after marrow transplantation unfortunately persists as a major problem for patients with acute lymphocytic leukemia (ALL) (52). Several approaches for overcoming ALL relapse have been suggested and are discussed in the accompanying article by Dr. E. Donnall Thomas (29).

Experimental models for treatment of murine leukemia using monoclonal antibodies have been recently described (53-54) and application of similar methods for treatment of human leukemia and lymphoma has already been attempted (55-56). Tumor associated differentiation antigens restricted in distribution to the hematopoietic system but not present on stem cells are candidates as target determinants for adjunct antileukemic serotherapy during marrow transplantation. Leukemic patients in remission carry a minimum body burden of leukemic cells (estimated at less than 10^9 cells). An infusion of monoclonal antibodies throughout the period of cytoreduction prior to marrow transplantation might be effective in helping to achieve complete erradication of the malignant clone. If several monoclonal antibodies recognizing two or more tumor associated antigens could be administered in combination, the probability of a lytic "hit" would be increased, and the effect of cell surface modulation might be diminished. The phenomenon of modulation is well described for the murine Tla system (57) and has recently been observed clinically (56).

Removal in vitro of Leukemic Cells from Patient's Marrow Prior to Autologous Marrow Transplantation

Details of autologous marrow transplantation are dis-cussed in an accompanying manuscript by Dr. George Santos (31). Briefly, leukemia patients without marrow donors might benefit from ablative cytotoxic therapy if reconstitution with normal marrow stem cells were possible. A number of cell separation procedures, including serotherapy have been attempted (58). Monoclonal antibodies that recognize dis-tinct lymphoid and myeloid differentiation might offer new methods for eliminating leukemic cells or the lineage (12-19) from which they emerge. Monoclonal antibodies specific for T cell antigens (12-19), thymus-associated antigens (24-26), myeloid-monocyte antigens (27), B cell chronic lymphocytic leukemia antigens (13,19,22,23), the common acute lymphocytic leukemia antigen (28) and the lymphoma-associated antigen (7) potentially each have a role for in vitro treatment of leukemic marrow

Prevention or Treatment of Virus Infections

As discussed in the accompanying paper by Dr. E. Donnall Thomas (29), interstitial pneumonia remains a major cause of morbidity and mortality during the first 100 days after marrow transplantation, affecting approximately 50% of pa-tients grafted for leukemia, with nearly two-thirds of cases being fatal. Cytomegalovirus (CMV) alone accounts for roughly one half of cases. The high incidence of CMV infec-tion early after transplantation is likely related in part to the severely immunosuppressed condition of the patients dur-ing this period. The availability of monoclonal antibodies specific for viral associated antigens might offer new means of providing protection against CMV infection during the time of greatest risk. Recent reports of the successful produc-tion of hybrid clones that synthesize human antibodies sug-gest exciting new prospects for the treatment of opportun-istic infections in immunosuppressed hosts (59-60).

Summary

The frequent and severe complications that accomapny allogeneic marrow transplantation persist as a challenge to our ingenuity. If techniques for effective prevention or treatment of these complications were available, then marrow transplantation could find wider application in the therapy of both malignant and non-malignant diseases. It appears certain that monoclonal antibodies will provide new avenues of approach towards solving many of these problems in the coming decade.

REFERENCES

1. Kohler, G. and Milstein, C.; Nature 256:495, 1975.
2. Kennett, R.H., and Gilbert, F.; Science 203:1120, 1979.
3. Koprowski, H., Steplewski, Z., Herlyn, D.; Proc. Natl. Acad. Sci. USA 75:3405, 1978.
4. Yeh, M-Y., Hellstrom, I., Brown, J.P., et al., Proc. Natl. Acad. Sci. 76:2927, 1979.
5. Herlyn, M., Steplewski, Z., Herlyn, D., et al.; Proc. Natl. Acad. Sci. USA 76:1438, 1979.
6. Woodbury, R.G., Brown, J.P., Yeh, M.-Y., et al.; Proc. Natl. Acad. Sci. USA 77:2183, 1980.
7. Nadler, L.M., Stashenki, P., Hardy, R., et al.; J. Immunol. 125:570, 1980.
8. Brodsky, F.M., Parham, P., Barnstable, C.J., Crumpton, M.J. and Bodmer, W.F.; Immunological Reviews 47:3, 1979.
9. Quaranta, V., Ferrone, S., and Molinaro, G.A.; Transplant Proc. 11:1748, 1979.
10. Trucco, M.M., Stocker, J.W., Ceppellini, R.; Nature 273:666, 1978.
11. Reinherz, E.L., Kung, P.C., Pesando, J.M., et al.; J. Exp. Med. 150:1472, 1979.
12. Hansen, J.A., Martin, P.J., and Nowinski, R.C.; Immunogenetics 10:247, 1980.
13. Boumsell, L., Coppin, H., Pham, D., et al.; J. Exp. Med. 152:229, 1980.
14. Engleman, E.G. and Levy, R.; Clinical Research 28, 511A, 1980.
15. Hansen, J.A., Martin, P.J., Kamoun, M., et al.; Transplant Proc., in press.
16. Haynes, B.F., Mann, D.L., Hemler, M.E., et al.; Proc. Natl. Acad. Sci. USA 77:2914, 1980.
17. Howard, F.D., Ledbetter, J.A., Wong, J., et al.; Manuscript submitted.
18. Kamoun, M., Martin, P.J., Hansen, J.A., Brown, M.A., and Nowinski, R.C.; Manuscript submitted.
19. Martin, P.J., Hansen, J.A., Nowinski, R.C., and Brown, M.A.; Immunogenetics, in press.
20. Kung, P.C., Goldstein, G., Reinherz, E.L.; Science 201:347, 1979.
21. Reinherz, E., Kung, P., Goldstein, G., and Schlossman, S.F.; J. Immunol. 123:1312, 1979.

22. Wang, C.Y., Good, R.A., Ammirati, R., et al.; J. Exp. Med. 151:1539, 1980.
23. Royston, I., Majda, J.A., Baird, S.M., et al.; Manuscript submitted
24. Levy, R., Dilley, J., Fox, R.I., et al.; Proc. Natl. Acad. Sci. USA 76:5662, 1979.
25. McMichael, A.J., Pilch, J.R., Galfre, G., et al.; Eur. J. Immunol. 9:205, 1979.
26. Reinherz, E.L., Kung, P.C., Goldstein, G. et al.; Proc Nat Acad Sci 77:1588, 1980.
27. Breard, J., Reinherz, E.L., Kung, P.C., et al.; J. Immunol. 124:1943, 1980.
28. Ritz, J., Pesando, J.M., Notis-McConarty, et al.; Nature 283:538, 1980.
29. Thomas, E.D.; Presented at: 1980 International Symposium on Cancer
30. Storb, R.; Presented at: 1980 International Symposium on Cancer.
31. Santos, G.; Presented at: 1980 International Symposium on Cancer.
32. O'Reilly, R.; Presented at: 1980 International Symposium on Cancer.
33. Cerottini, J.C., Nordin, A.A., and Brunner, K.T.; J. Exp. Med. 134:553, 1971.
34. Elkins, W.L.; Prog. Allergy 15:78, 1971.
35. Bortin, M.M., Rimm, A.A., Rose, W.C., et al.; Transplantation 21:331, 1976.
36. Tulunay, O., Good, R.A., Yunis, E.J.; Proc. Natl. Acad. Sci. 72:4100, 1975.
37. Yunis, E.J., Fernandes, G., Smith, J., et al.; Transplant Proc. 8:521, 1976.
38. Korngold, R., and Sprent, J.; J. Exp. Med. 148:1687, 1978
39. Muller-Ruchholtz, W., Wottge, H.U., and Muller-Hermelink, H.K.; Transplant Proc. 8 (4):537, 1976.
40. Onoe, K., Fernandes, G., and Good, R.A.; J. Exp. Med. 151:115, 1980.
41. Rodt, H., Thierfelder, S., and Eultz, M.; Eur. J. Immunol 4:25, 1974.
42. vonBoehmer, H., and Sprent, J.; Transplant. Rev. 29:3, 1976.
43. Zinkernagel, R.M.; J. Exp. Med. 144(4):933, 1976.
44. Nathan, D.G., Chess, L., Hillman, D.G., et al.; J. Exp. Med. 147:324, 1978.
45. Torok-Storb, B., et al.; Blood 55:211, 1980.
46. Lipton, J.M., Reinherz, E.L., Kudisch, M.; J. Exp. Med. 152:350, 1980.
47. Deeg, H.J., Storb, R., Weiden, P.L.; Blood 53:552, 1979.
48. Storb, R.; Transplant Proc 11:1916, 1979.

49. Weiden, P.L., Doney, K., Storb, R., et al.; Transplantation 27:227, 1979.
50. Levey, R.H., Parkman, R., Rappeport, J.; Transplant Proc. 11:199, 1979.
51. Thomas, E.D., Buckner, C.D., Clift, R.A., et al., N. Eng. J. Med. 301(11)597, 1979.
52. Thomas, E.D., Sanders, J.E., Flournoy, N., et al.; Blood Vo. 54(2):468, 1979.
53. Bernstein, I.D., Tam, M.R., and Nowinski, R.C.; Science 207:68, 1980.
54. Bernstein, I.D., Nowinski, R.C., Tam, M.R., et al.; Monoclonal Antibodies, Plenum Press, pp 275-291.
55. Nadler, L.M., Stashenki, P., Hardy,R., et at.; Cancer Res. 40:3147, 1980.
56. Ritz, J., Pesando, J.M., Notis-McConarty, J., et al.; In: Cancer Treatment Reports, in press .
57. Boyse, E.A., Stockert, E., and Old, L.J.; Proc. Natl. Acad. Sci. 58:954, 1967.
58. Netzel, B., Haas, R.J., Rodt, H., et al.; Lancet I:1330, 1980.
59. Nowinski, R., Berglund, C., Lane, J., et al.; Science, in press.
60. Olsson, L., and Kaplan, H.; Proc. Natl. Acad. Sci., USA, in press.

CURRENT STATUS OF AUTOLOGOUS MARROW TRANSPLANTATION

*George W. Santos, M.D., Herbert Kaizer, M.D. and
the Johns Hopkins University Bone Marrow Transplantation Team
Johns Hopkins University Oncology Center
Baltimore, Maryland 21205*

INTRODUCTION

The major limiting toxicity of intensive cytoreductive therapy in malignancy has been hematopoietic and attempts to lessen this complication have made the assumption that given enough time marrow regeneration would occur. The use of protective environments, platelet support, prophylactic and therapeutic granulocyte transfusions, and pharmacological rescue of hematologic function have met with some success in decreasing the morbidity and mortality associated with such treatment (1).

The preparative cytoreductive regimens applied in allogeneic marrow transplantation have been even more intensive, and irreversible hematopoietic stem cell toxicity has been accepted in this procedure. The initial results of this form of therapy for patients with "refractory" leukemia in relapse was encouraging (2). More recently, however, the therapeutic results in acute myelocytic leukemia (3) and to a lesser degree in acute lymphocytic leukemia transplanted in remission have been impressive (4). Although many problems remain that are peculiar to allogeneic marrow transplantation such as graft-versus-host disease and a significant incidence of fatal interstitial pneumonitis (5), these results have demonstrated that therapy which is lethal for neoplastic hematopoietic cells can be administered without irreversible toxicity to susceptible normal tissues and is followed by prompt hematopoietic recovery if marrow cell infusions are utilized.

Supported by Public Health Service Research Grants CA06973 and CA15396 from the National Cancer Institute, National Institutes of Health, Bethesda, Maryland

The use of monozygotic twin marrow donors for patients
with leukemia avoids several of the hazards associated with
allogeneic donors but is also devoid of the anti-leukemic
effects of graft-versus-host disease (6). In balance, however, the long term therapeutic results in acute leukemia in
relapse are better with syngeneic donors than that seen with
allogeneic transplantation (7). The therapeutic results in
chronic myelogenous leukemia, however, are truly remarkable
(8). Although patients with identical twin donors are rare,
transplants in this setting are of signal importance since
the therapeutic results of such transplants constitute an
important benchmark by which the results of autologous
transplants may be judged.

There was sporadic interest in autologous marrow transplantation in the fifties but it is only until recently that
this area of clinical research has attracted a much wider
interest among medical centers in the United States and
abroad and already a number of reviews of these early efforts have appeared (1,9,10). The purpose of this communication is to review the rationale, concepts, early clinical
results and future directions of autologous hematopoietic
stem cell transplantation.

The successful application of autologous marrow transplantation to the treatment of neoplastic disease has three
requirements. First, it must be possible to obtain and
viably store sufficient numbers of hematopoietic stem cells
to ensure recovery of hematologic and immunologic function.
Second, clonogenic tumor cells must be absent from the hematopoietic stem cell inoculum. Third, the tumor remaining in
the patient must be sensitive to an intensive pulse of
pretransplant therapy at doses which have acceptable extra
medullary toxicity.

Collection and Storage of Viable Hematopoietic Cells

Prior animal studies as well as more recent studies in
man indicate that marrow may be collected, processed and
cryopreserved in a viable state such that when thawed it
will safely reconstitute the hematopoietic and lymphoid
system in animals and man that have received otherwise
marrow lethal preparative regimens. In addition, animal
studies have shown that hematopoietic stem cells in the
peripheral blood are capable of reconstituting the lymphohematopoietic system. These matters have been reviewed in
more detail elsewhere (1).

Despite the many technical problems that need to be
solved, the use of stem cells from the peripheral blood
might offer several potential advantages not offered by

marrow collection. For instance, eventually this might
allow repeated collections without the hazards of anesthesia.
In addition, it is possible that such collections might be
less contaminated with tumor or that such cell suspensions
might be more easily fractionate.

Clonogenic Tumor Cells

There are certain "responsive" tumors where the marrow
is not involved such as ovarian carcinoma. However, in
other malignancies such as lymphomas and small cell carcinoma
of the lung this may be a significant problem. Clearly it
is reasonable to consider that marrow collected from patients
with acute leukemia in remission will have a high probability of containing tumor cells. Before discussing possible methodologies for cleansing cell suspensions of tumor
cells it is useful to consider the time of harvesting hematopoietic stem cells.

The risks to be balanced in making a decision about the
time of harvest are the possible effects of cytoreductive
therapy in reducing stem cell pool size versus the risk of
tumor cell contamination. In patients with marrow involvement at the time of diagnosis, one must, of course, delay
the collection of stem cells at least until no tumor cells
can be detected in the marrow. There is, on the other hand,
some evidence that prolonged chemotherapy may reduce the
chance of obtaining sufficient stem cells. One small group
of patients with acute leukemia whose marrows were obtained
after multiple relapses and prolonged chemotherapy showed no
evidence of hematologic recovery after autologous transplantation (11). On the other hand, there is evidence that stem
cells, as measured by CFU-c, remain in the normal range in
the early stages of cytoreductive therapy (12). In leukemia,
for instance, we have adopted the approach of harvesting
marrow for storage as soon after conventional remission
induction therapy as possible. In the future, one might be
able to exploit potential differences in hematopoietic stem
cell to clonogenic tumor cell ratios that may exist in the
blood versus marrow at various time points during a given
clinical course. For example, is it possible that blood may
have a more favorable ratio in this regard than the marrow
in a patient with acute myelogenous leukemia in remission?

With presently available methodology one might be able
to cleanse or "purge" marrow suspensions of residual tumor
cells by physical, pharmacologic and immunological techniques.
Dicke et al. (13) devised discontinuous albumin gradients
for the separation of human marrow cells in patients with
acute leukemia. On the basis of cytogenetic and electron

microscopy examinations they were able to show a one log
reduction in leukemia marker-positive cells in density
fractions containing the bulk of stem cells as measured by
CFUc (14). Ten of twenty-one evaluable patients received
autologous transplants with remission marrows fractionated
prior to storage (15). No difference in post-transplanted
remission duration was seen between patients receiving
fractionated versus unfractionated marrow. This indicates
that the fractionation was incomplete or that the pretransplant therapy was ineffective in eliminating all leukemic
cells prior to marrow infusion. In view of these findings
and the lack of testing of this principle in animal models
the validity of this approach at present must remain in
question.

     Pharmacologic methods for eliminating tumor cells in
vitro from stem cell-tumor cell mixtures have not been
extensively investigated despite the classical work of Bruce
in a mouse lymphoma model showing significant differential
sensitivity of lymphoma cells versus hematopoietic stem
cells (16).

     We recently have reported that a congener of cyclophos-
phamide 4-hydroperoxycyclophosphamide (4HC) is able to
eliminate rat AML tumor cells from normal marrow-tumor cell
suspensions with a short incubation. Dose response studies
were performed and at the higher dose levels the treated
marrow was able to protect lethally irradiated syngeneic
animals. Furthermore, these animals did not develop leukemia after adequate followup (17). These results suggest
that further studies using other chemotherapeutic agents are
desirable.

     Attempts to clear marrow-tumor cell mixtures of tumor
cells without destroying hematopoietic stem cells by immunologic means has been confined to the use of xenogeneic
(rabbit) antibody and complement. This approach has been
used successfully both in murine (18,19) and rat model
leukemia systems (20). Analogous clinical studies have been
reported. One patient was treated by our group. Although
he exhibited rapid hematologic recovery after the reinfusion
of antibody treated marrow, a relapse occurred soon after
engraftment (20). Although the antibody treatment did not
destroy significant amounts of stem cell function, leukemic
cells may also have not been destroyed and be responsible
for the relapse. In three cases investigated by the UCLA
marrow transplant group (21), all patients died of complications related to therapy. While two of these patients died
too early for complete evaluation, one patient survived for

four months with good recovery of hematologic function and
no evidence of recurrent tumor.   Netzel et al. (22) have
transplanted two children with advanced stages of acute
lymphocytic leukemia following intensive combination chemotherapy and total body irradiation (TBI) with remission
marrow previously treated with antiserum and cryopreserved.
There was evidence of take in the first patient who died on
day 7 of cardiac failure.   The second patient rapidly recovered hematologic competence and was in complete remission of
greater than 50 days at the time of writing.

The above studies at least indicate the clinical feasibility of incubating marrow with anti-sera designed to kill
tumor cells.   It should be pointed out, however, that the
successful application of this technique does not require
antibody highly specific for tumor cells.   The requirements
are that all tumor cells have surface markers capable of
reacting with the antibody and complement for completion of
lysis and that the hematopoietic stem cells be operationally
devoid of these surface markers and, therefore, not susceptible to lysis.

Pretransplant Therapy

Ideally tumors selected for autologous marrow transplantation should occur in a younger age population, have a low
likelihood for bone marrow metastases and not have prior
pelvic or other extensive irradiation.   In addition, these
tumors should be potentially responsive to high intensity
pulse therapy.   Ovarian, testicular, soft tissue sarcomas,
breast, lymphomas, and Hodgkin's disease would appear to fit
these criteria.   Acute and chronic leukemia, some lymphomas
and small cell carcinoma of the lung would fit these criteria
except for the marrow involvement with tumor.

Although attempts have been made to provide a more rational basis for the development of combination cytoreductive
protocols, this exercise still remains an empiric art.   TBI
used in combination with chemotherapy remains a mainstay of
many current transplantation protocols.   Critical questions
regarding dose fractionation and timing of the radiation
modality have been explored in a preliminary way (23), but
much more needs to be done before optimum dose fractionation
and scheduling can be demonstrated.

An alternative approach to pretransplant therapy without the use of TBI is represented by the work of Graw and
his colleagues with refractory Burkitt's lymphoma given
pretransplant therapy with combination chemotherapy alone.
These studies documented that autologous marrow transplantation resulted in a more rapid hematologic reconstitution

since the marrow-sublethal properties of the treatment
regimen permitted them to examine a non-transplanted group
(24). Four of 22 patients so treated exhibited prolonged
disease-free survival and probable cure as a consequence of
the intensive pulse therapy (25). These studies have established that it is possible to carry out autologous transplants in patients with lymphoma who do not have detectable
marrow involvement and not reinfuse tumor cells. Some of
the treatment failures may have been due to the reinfusion
of tumor cells but it is equally possible that the pretransplant cytoreductive therapy was inadequate in eliminating
most or all tumor cells in the majority of these patients.

The development of new treatment protocols with chemotherapeutic agents requires a careful study of their properties in the high doses made possible in autologous transplant protocols. This information should include data on
the pharmacokinetics, anti-tumor response, extra medullary
toxicities and possible drug interactions when the dose
range is significantly extended. Studies such as those
reported by Phillips et al. (26) investigating the effects
of escalating doses of BCNU, those reported by McElwain (27)
using high dose melphalan and those reported by the UCLA
group (28) employing high dose mitomycin C represent a first
step in this process and are critical to the development of
new and more effective pulses of cytoreductive therapy prior
to transplantation with cryopreserved autologous marrow.

Current Clinical Trials

Although most studies have published preliminary results
(12,29,30) some have only been described in abstracts of
recent meetings (31-33), and a few have been described more
extensively (15,25). The limited number of patients thus
far studied and the short duration of follow-up makes any
conclusions quite tentative. Summary of the salient features
of these reports does, however, provide a basis for establishing future research priorities.

As noted above, many of the current clinical trials
have employed marrow-lethal doses of TBI especially in the
treatment of leukemias and lymphomas. The total doses have
been between 800-1200 rads given as a single or fractionated
dose at a dose rate of 5-20 rads/min. Although most of the
transplanted patients showed hematological recovery, there
was considerable patient variability in the rate and pattern
of recovery. In general, evidence of hematologic recovery
by marrow biopsy was noted 1-2 weeks following transplantation. The time to reach 500-1000 granulocytes/mm^3 has
averaged 3-4 weeks. Platelet recovery to 50,000 plate-

lets/mm^3 took 4-6 weeks. Although these recovery rates are somewhat slower than has been observed with fresh marrow, the consistency of recovery suggests at least that the methods used for cryopreservation were adequate.

Estimates of extra medullary toxicities must await further experience with the individual treatment protocols employed. In general, some tentative generalizations can be made. Most patients showed significant gastrointestinal (GI) toxicity (particularly nausea, vomiting and diarrhea), life-threatening or irreversible GI toxicity has been rare (20) except perhaps with mitomycin C (28). Life-threatening or irreversible renal, hepatic and CNS toxicities have also been rare except for hepatic and CNS toxicity with BCNU (26). Rarely cardiotoxic deaths have been seen, particularly in patients with a history of having received large cumulative doses of anthracycline antibiotics (15,30). The major life-threatening complications have been related to infections and pulmonary toxicity. Pulmonary failure related to lung irradiation (possibly related in part to prior chemotherapy) has been observed (15,30). Fractionation of the radiation dose has resulted in a considerable decrease in the incidence of this complication (34), although interstitial pneumonitis related to herpes-type virus infection continues to be a problem (12,21) as in allogeneic transplantation, the incidence of such extra medullary complications is related in part to the intensity and duration of the prior treatment history (15,30).

As has already been emphasized, clinical studies to date have been phase I trials and evaluation of therapeutic efficacy has been complex. In lymphomas and leukemias, for example, the relapses can either be due to failure of the pretransplant therapy or failure to infuse marrow free of tumor. Certain preliminary observations, however, are pertinent to this question. Although some patients with acute leukemia receiving an autologous transplant are still in complete remission at the time of this writing, none has exhibited prolonged disease-free survival equivalent to those reported for several patients with non-Hodgkin's lymphoma (12,25,32). In these latter cases, tumor was not detected in the marrow prior to storage. It would seem, therefore, that the problem of tumor cell contamination of cryopreserved autologous marrow appears to be supported at least in the hematological malignancies. If most relapses in leukemia were the result of reinfused tumor cells, one would expect at least a rough correlation of time of relapse and duration of their initial remission (i.e., subsequent to

marrow storage). This is not necessarily so. This suggests
that the pretransplant therapy itself plays a significant
role in determining the time of relapse following transplantation. This is not surprising in view of the fact that the
relapse rate in refractory acute leukemia patients receiving
identical twin transplants is 60-70%. Indeed, the relapse
rate in identical twin transplants provides the best measure
as to therapeutic efficacy. For example, an effective in
vitro method for eliminating tumor from stem cell suspensions must show relapse rates that do not exceed those
achieved in the identical twin studies.

Conclusions and Future Goals

In the case of non-hematologic malignancies, particularly those without marrow involvement, entirely new treatment protocols will, of necessity, have to be developed
along lines somewhat different from the more responsive
hematologic malignancies. Phase 1 trials of agents known to
be "active" will have to be carefully examined as to possible increased anti-tumor effects when given at marrow
lethal doses. These studies will, of course, have to carefully explore new limiting toxicities. Furthermore, possible interactions of various single agents on extra medullary toxicities will have to be examined and in many situations with bulky tumor masses the role of localized radiotherapy and surgical debulking will of necessity have to be
examined.

Factors likely to require further investigation and
definition include: marrow reserve after intensive therapy
and autologous marrow infusion, the role of peripheral blood
stem cells in autologous reconstitution, the possibility of
repeated courses of marrow ablative therapy and autologous
reconstitution and the role of post-transplant therapy in
the control of tumor.

It is clearly established that marrow even after chemotherapy is able to be collected, cryopreserved in a viable
manner such that the infusion of these collections are able
to ensure in the majority of patients lymphohematopoietic
reconstitution following marrow-lethal cytoreductive therapy.

In the case of hematologic malignancies and in particular acute leukemia there is at present no sure way to eliminate clonogenic tumor cells from the marrow suspensions.
Animal data indicate that tumor may be purged of residual
tumor cells with the use of immunologic or pharmacologic
agents and clearly physical separation methods have been
able to reduce the percentage of tumor cells. It is possible that a combination of methods may eventually be best.

At present, there is no way in man to detect a minute population of tumor cells in a normal bone marrow population as is afforded in animals with sensitive bioassays. Clearly efforts to develop more sensitive techniques for the in vitro detection of residual tumor cells in human marrow suspensions should have a high priority. At present, however, the effectiveness of "purging" marrow will have to be gauged indirectly by the design of creative clinical trials.

The potential cures of non-Hodgkin's lymphoma who may never have had tumor invasion of the marrow or who may have had microscopic foci of tumor cleared by prestorage cytoreductive therapy have been reported. Thus, even without further development of methods for "purging" tumor-marrow mixtures, some patients with hematologic malignancy may achieve lasting benefit from autologous transplantation.

REFERENCES

1. Deisseroth, A., and Abrams, R.A. Cancer Treat. Rep. 63 (3): 461, 1979.
2. Thomas, E.D., Buckner, C.D., Banaji, M. et al. Blood 49: 511, 1977.
3. Thomas, E.D., Buckner, C.D., Clift, R.A. et al. N. Engl. J. Med. 301: 597, 1979.
4. Thomas, E.D., Sanders, J.E., Flournoy, N. et al. Blood 54: 468, 1979.
5. Santos, G.W. In Advances in Internal Medicine (G.H. Stollerman,Ed.) Year Book Medical Publishers, Inc. Chicago, Illinois, Vol. 24, pp 157-182, 1979.
6. Weiden, P.L., Flournoy, N., Thomas, E.D. et al. N. Engl. J. Med. 300: 1068, 1979.
7. Fefer, A., Buckner, C.D., Thomas, E.D. et al. N. Engl. J. Med. 297: 146, 1977.
8. Fefer, A., Cheever, M.A., Thomas, E.D. et al. N. Engl. J. Med. 300: 333, 1979.
9. Graze, P.R., and Gale, R.P. Transplant. Proc. 10: 177, 1978.
10. Tobias, J.S., and Tattersall, M.N.H. Europ. J. Cancer 12: 1, 1976.
11. Graw, R.G., Jr. Personal Communication.
12. Kaizer, H., Wharam, M.D., Munoz, L.L. et al. Exp. Hematol. 7: 309, 1979.
13. Dicke, K.A., McCredie, K.B., Stevens, E.E. et al. Transplant. Proc. 9: 193, 1977.

14. Dicke, K.A., Zander, A., Spitzer, G. et al. Exp. Hematol. 7: 170, 1979.

15. Dicke, K.A., Zander, A., Spitzer, G. et al. Lancet 1: 514, 1978.

16. Bruce, W.R., Mecker, B.E. and Valeriote, F.A. J. Nat. Cancer Inst. 37: 233, 1966.

17. Sharkis, S.J., Santos, G.W. and Colvin, M. Blood 55: 521, 1980.

18. Thierfelder, S., Rodt, H., Netzel, B. Transplantation 23: 459, 1977.

19. Economou, J.S., Shin, H.S., Kaizer, H. et al. Proc. Soc. Exp. Biol. Med. 158: 449, 1978.

20. Kaizer, H., Wharam, M.D., Johnson, R.J. et al. Blut Supple. Immunobiology of Bone Marrow Transplantation, Thierfelder, S., Rodt, H. and Kolb, H.J. (Eds.), Springer-Verlag Berlin Heidelberg, 1980, pp 285-296.

21. Wells, J.R., Billing, R., Herzog, P. et al. Exp. Hematol. 7: 164, 1979.

22. Netzel, B., Hass, R.J., Rodt, H. et al. (abst) F12.5. VII Inter. Congress of the Trans. Soc. June 29-July 5, 1980, Boston, Mass.

23. Peters, L.J., Withers, H.R., Jackson, H.C. et al. Radiol. 131: 243, 1979.

24. Appelbaum, F.R., Herzig, G., Ziegler, J.L. et al. Blood 52: 85, 1978.

25. Appelbaum, F.R., Herzig, G., Graw, R.E. et al. Exp. Hematol. 7: 297, 1979.

26. Phillips, G.L., Fay, J.W., Wolff, S.N. et al. Proc. Am. Assoc. Ca. Res. 21: 721, 1980.

27. McElwain, T.J., Hedley, D.W., Gordon, M.Y. et al. Exp. Hematol. 7: 360, 1979.

28. Champlin, R., Sarna, G., Stitzel, K. et al. ASCO Proc. (abst) 21: C-135, May 26-27, 1980, San Diego, Cal.

29. Fay, J.W., Silberman, H.R., Moore, J.O. et al. Exp. Hematol. 7: 302, 1979.

30. Gale, R.P., Graze, P.R., Wells, J. et al. Exp. Hematol. 7: 351, 1979.

31. Fay, J.W. and Huang, A.T. Blood 52 (Suppl. 1): 288, 1979.

32. Herzig, G.P., Phillips, G.L., Mill, W. et al. Blood 52 (Suppl. 1): 257, 1979.

33. Spitzer, G., Verma, D.S., Zander, A. et al. Blood 52 (Suppl. 1): 232, 1979.

34. Lichter, A.S., Tutschka, P.J., Wharam, et al. Transpl. Proc. 11: 1492, 1979.

HLA FACTORS AND BONE MARROW GRAFTING

BO DUPONT

Member and Professor
Human Immunogenetics Section
Memorial Sloan-Kettering Cancer Center
New York, New York   10021

Introduction:

Knowledge of transplantation antigens was first developed from experimental work on allotransplantation of normal tissues and tumors. A major breakthrough in transplantation immunology came in 1938 when the British scientist Peter Gorer discovered the serology of alloantigens belonging to the Major Histocompatibility Complex (MHC) of the mouse. These alloantigens were found to be strongly implicated in tissue rejection and the genetic system that they identified in the mouse was named H-2 (Snell, 1948). The antigens of the major histocompatibility complex are more immunogenic than other transplantation antigens and matching for the MHC gene products result in a delay of rejection of allografts.

The major histocompatibility complex in man and in a large number of other species has been found to consist of a number of closely linked genes that constitute a genetic system. Since the products of the MHC genes interact together in many functions and normally are inherited as a bloc of genes, they can be considered a genetic unit. Alleles of the different genetic loci of MHC occur together in non-random associations which is called genetic linkage disequilibrium. Therefore, the MHC can be considered to be a super-gene.

The importance for marrow transplantation of compatibility between donor and recipient for the genetic determinants of the MHC has been evident since the early studies in mice by Uphoff & Law, 1958. The innoculation of immunocompetent cells into allogeneic immunoincompetent recipients leads to the development of Graft-versus-Host Reaction (GVHR). The classical GVHR model has been the injection of parental cells into the immunosuppressed F_1 mouse (Simonsen

1962).   The involvement of the H-2 complex in GVHR is well
established.
        The different components of H-2 are not equally important
in GvH development.   It has now been demonstrated that incompatibilities at the K-end of the H-2 complex and especially I-region incompatibilities are of particular importance
for GVHR.   Several other H-2 regions are, however, also
involved.   Some studies have suggested that the in vitro
tests for allogeneic lymphocyte responses (i.e. the Mixed
Lymphocyte Culture (MLC) and the Cell-Mediated Lympholysis
(CML)) were models for predicting GVHR (reviewed by J.
Klein, 1975).   Studied in the mouse have, however, also
demonstrated the influence of non-H-2 differences on GvHR.
Almost any minor H locus difference can induce GvHR under
special conditions and the main factors involved are the dose
of donor cells, preimmunization of the recipient and the route
of injection (Cantrell and Hildemann, 1972).
        The dog was the first random bred animal where histocom-
patibility testing was used to predict the outcome of bone
marrow transplantation (Epstein et al, 1968).   Littermates
identical for the DLA determinants (i.e. the MHC of dogs)
survived better than incompatible transplants (Storb et al,
1971).   Further studies in unrelated dogs demonstrated
that successful long-term survival could be achieved in some
recipients of histocompatible marrow (Storb et al, 1977).
        The purpose of this paper is to review the present
status of histocompatibility testing in man in relation to
clinical bone marrow transplantation.   It is now evident that
long-term survival can be achieved following allogeneic
bone marrow transplantation even in situations where the
donor and recipient are not HLA genotypically identical
siblings.   Most frequently, such histocompatible donors
are identified within the patient's family, but a few successful cases of unrelated allogeneic bone marrow grafting have
now been performed.

The MHC in Man: HLA

        The identification of the major histocompatibility
complex in man, HLA, and the gene products of the different
HLA loci have evolved as a result of large scale international collaborations during the last 20-25 years.   A brief
history of major discoveries is summarized in Table I.   The
development of allogeneic bone marrow transplantation (BMT)
as a viable therapy is intimately related to the possibility
for proper HLA genotyping.   The early clinical attempts
resulting in marrow repopulation by allogeneic grafts were
practically invariably followed by a lethal GvHR (reviewed

in Thomas et al, 1975). The first successful allogeneic bone marrow transplant with complete hemopoietic reconstitution was achieved in a patient with Severe Combined Immunodeficiency (SCID) (Gatti et al, 1968). This transplant coincided with the discovery of the first two HLA-loci (HLA-A and B) which allowed for HLA genotyping in families. The patients with SCID do not require immunosuppression to accept the graft and the myeloid marrow function is present. Therefore, rapid marrow engraftment is not mandatory, and such patients can be treated repeatedly with small numbers of marrow cells.

TABLE I

HISTORY OF HLA

1953 - 1958	Leukocyte-agglutinating antibodies are found in sera of alloimmunized individuals.
1958	The first human lymphocyte antigen MAC is described.
1962 - 1963	The first allelic lymphocyte antigen systems LA and FOUR are identified.
1963 - 1964	The in vitro mixed lymphocyte culture (MLC) assay is developed.
1964	Development of the microlymphocytotoxity test.
1964 - 1966	Evidence of relevance of leukocyte-antigen matching within families for kidney transplantation and skin grafting.
1967	HLA seroidentical siblings have nonreactive MLC. First evidence for HLA and disease association. (Hodgkin's Disease and acute lymphocytic leukemia).
1968	Identification of two, closely linked HLA loci: HLA-A and HLA-B.
1970	Identification of a third HLA-locus: HLA-C.
1971	Identification of a separate genetic locus (HLA-D) controlling stimulation in MLC. Development of the in vitro cell-mediated lympholysis test.
1973	Identification of B-lymphocyte specific antigens (HLA-DR).
1974 - 1975	Linkage of HLA with serum-complement components Bf, C2 and C4.
1972 - 1980	Large number of HLA associated and/or HLA linked diseases.
1979	Identification of HLA-associated T-lymphocyte antigens.

In order successfully to transplant patients with aplastic anemia (AA) or Acute Leukemia (AL) additional progress
in the prevention and management of GvHR and in supportive
measures for patients with no marrow function was required.
It is now well established that the preferred bone
marrow transplant donor is the HLA genotypically identical
sibling. Many patients receiving such transplants succumb,
however, from GvHR, graft rejection and their complications
(see Thomas et al and Storb et al, this issue). While many
factors obviously contribute to these complications, it should
be kept in mind, that the donor and recipient are identified
as HLA genotypically identical only for the presently known
HLA determinants. It is, however, established in studies of
H-2, that the I-region is composed of several subregions,
while HLA typing presently can only identify the HLA-D and DR
determinants in the homologous genetic region. Also, a series
of H-2 linked histocompatibility determinants are found coding
for cell surface antigens expressed on subsets of T-lymphocytes (the Qa-antigens and the TLa antigens). Typing for
the homologous human antigens are not yet developed, even
though such antigens probably do exist (Gazit et al, 1979; Kim
et al, 1980) (Figure 1).

Selection of Related Donor for Patients Without HLA
Genotypically Identical Siblings

The discovery by Yunis and Amos, 1971 of a separate
genetic locus within HLA which was responsible for stimulation
in the in vitro mixed lymphocyte culture reaction resulted
in that studies were undertaken to test, if compatibility in
MLC between donor and recipient reflected sufficient degree
of histocompatibility to allow successful clinical bone
marrow transplantation. A study of a large pedigree of a
patient with SCID (III.2 in Figure 2) demonstrated that the
patient was MLC compatible with the mother (II.4) and her two
brothers (II.5 and II.6). (Dupont et al, 1972). This patient
was subsequently transplanted with bone marrow from one of
the maternal uncles (Fig 2) and long-term T-cell reconstitution was obtained (Koch et al, 1973). The same immunogenetic
principle (i.e. MLC compatibility) was later applied for the
transplantation of the patient's sister, who also suffers from
SCID. This patient was also successfully immunologically
reconstituted (Ramsoe et al, 1978).

COMPARATIVE GENE MAP OF
H-2 (MOUSE) AND HLA (MAN)

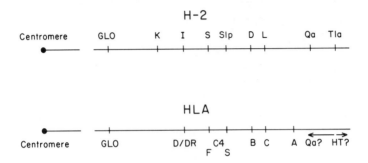

H-2

| Centromere | GLO | K | I | S Slp | D L | Qa Tla |

HLA

| Centromere | GLO | D/DR | C4 | B C | A Qa? HT? |
| | | | F S | | |

Figure 1

HLA Haplotypes in Copenhagen Family KJ (SCID)

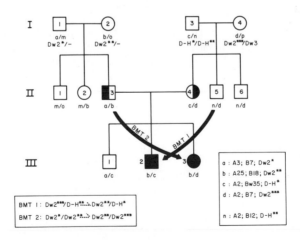

BMT 1: Dw2***/D-H**...→ Dw2**/D-H*
BMT 2: Dw2*/Dw2**...→ Dw2**/Dw2***

a : A3; B7; Dw2*
b : A25; B18; Dw2**
c : A2; Bw35; D-H*
d : A2; B7; Dw2***

n : A2; B12; D-H**

Figure 2

TABLE II

SEVERE COMBINED IMMUNODEFICIENCY: RELATED DONOR
AND RECIPIENT (NOT HLA GENOTYPICAL IDENTITY)

HISTOCOMPATIBILILTY TESTING			DONOR	OUTCOME
HLA				
A	B	D		
≠	=	=	SIBLING	WELL
≠	≠	=	UNCLE	WELL
=	=	=	FATHER	WELL
=	=	=	FATHER	DECEASED
=	=	=	MOTHER	DECEASED
≠	=	=	FATHER	WELL
≠	≠	=	FATHER	WELL

A summary of the seven reported bone marrow transplants, which have been performed in patients with SCID, using MLC compatibility between the related donor and the recipient as the criterion for selection is presented in Table II. Five of the 7 patients are well and long-term chimeras (reviewed in Dupont et al, 1980).   This material is very small and represents results from several different transplant groups. It can be concluded that compatibility for HLA-D as judged by weak or non-reactive MLR between donor and recipient (when the underlying disease is SCID) can result in long-term chimerism in spite of several incompatibilities for HLA-A and -B determinants.   No systematic study of the reverse situation i.e. compatibility for HLA-A,B but incompatibility for HLA-D has been performed.   The early reports on BMT in SCID by Buckley, 1971 and Park et al, 1973 indicate, however, that such transplants in most cases will result in fatal GvHR.

In order to offer bone marrow transplantation to patients with AA and AL, when an HLA identical sibling is not available, a number of transplant centers have begun to search for other related potential donors.   The most common approach has been to limit the number of genetically determined HLA incompatibilities between donor and recipient to a minimum by selecting a donor, who share at least one complete HLA haplotype with the patients.   Because of the considerable genetic linkage disequilibrium which exists for the alleles of the different HLA loci, some HLA-A,B,D/DR haplotypes occur with frequencies up to 0.005 - 0.008 in the Caucasian population in spite of the fact that more than 30 million different and identifiable HLA phenotypes should exist. Many individuals therefore will carry one rare HLA haplotype and in addition carry a second more common HLA haplotype or a part of a more common haplotype (i.e. common for the HLA-A,B segment or common for the HLA-B,D segment). It is therefore sometimes possible within a family to a patient to identify an individual who genetically share the infrequent HLA haplotype with the patient and in addition fortuitously is phenotypically identical with the patient for the second haplotype. In some cases, the relative may only share the HLA-A,B segment or the HLA-B,D segment on this second haplotype with the patient. Most frequently, such donors will be identified within the immediate family (i.e. parents or siblings). This will frequently be the case in families where both parents by coincidence both carry the same, common HLA haplotype (e.g. HLA-A3;B7;DR2 or A1;B8;DR3).

The most common donor and recipient combinations which have been used successfully for BMT when an HLA identical sibling was not available, are shown in Table III. (For review of the individual cases see Dupont et al 1980 and Clift et al, 1979.)

TABLE III

RELATED DONOR - RECIPIENT COMBINATIONS
FOR PATIENTS WITHOUT HLA IDENTICAL SIBLINGS

HLA IDENTITY FOR ONE HAPLOTYPE AND:

I. Phenotypic identity for HLA-A,B,C,D/DR on second haplotype

II. Phenotypic identify for HLA-D/DR on second haplotype

III.Phenotypic identity for HLA-A,B,C on second haplotype

IV. HLA homozygous recipient but HLA-heterozygous donor

V. Sibling transplants where donor or recipient carry one intra-HLA recombinant haplotype

This table also emphasizes two unique donor-recipient combinations: (1) the HLA homozygous recipient who may accept a bone marrow graft from a related donor, who is heterozygous for the same haplotype (O'Reilly et al, 1978) and (2) the sibling donor, who only differs from the recipient for a small segment of the HLA complex on one haplotype because of an intra HLA-recombination.

The case reported by O'Reilly et al 1978, is a patient with aplastic anemia, who was HLA-D homozygous. She received a bone marrow graft from her HLA-D heterozygous sister. The patient is now chimeric and hematologically normal. This transplant has been interpreted to correspond to the classical F_1 - parental transplant situation, where the graft should be accepted.

A particularly interesting case involving a transplant between siblings, where the donor differed from the patient for the HLA-D/DR region because of genetic recombination has been reported by Clift et al 1979. This patient (case report UPN 762) with acute myelogenous leukemia is well and in remission more than 500 days and had only mild GvHR in spite of strong pre-transplantation MLR between donor and recipient. This case demonstrates that long-term survival can be obtained in spite of HLA-D and MLC incompatibility.

TABLE IV

MARROW GRAFTING FROM RELATED DONORS
OTHER THAN HLA IDENTICAL SIBLINGS
Aplastic Anemia and Acute Leukemia

Aplastic Anemia	Total Transplants	Long-Term Survivors
Single Case Reports[1]	8	2
Seattle-Transplant Team[2]	10	1

Acute Leukemia	Total Transplants	Long-Term Survivors
Single Case Reports[1]	6	1
Seattle-Transplant Team[2]	27	11

1)   Original references to individual case reports are provided in Dupont et al, 1979 and 1980.
2)   Data from Hansen, Clift, Storb and Thomas, Amer. J. Clin. Pathol. (in press)

The overall worldwide experience in marrow grafting from related donors other than HLA identical siblings in AA and AL are shown in Table IV. The data demonstrates surprisingly, that the acute leukemia group seems to accept this kind of transplant better than the aplastic anemia group. The table demonstrates in addition that donor selection according to the principles, which have been outlined are feasible.

Marrow Grafting Between Unrelated Individuals
    Two patients with AA have been transplanted unsuccess-
fully with allogeneic bone marrow from unrelated donors (Speck
et al, 1973 & Lohrmann et al, 1975). The first long-term
survival following allogeneic bone marrow grafting was reported for a patient with SCID (L'Esperance et al, 1975 and
O'Reilly et al, 1977). Another patient with SCID was transplanted with unrelated marrow graft but died from post-trans-
plantation infection (Horowitz et al, 1975). Recently, Hansen
et al, 1980 have reported a case with acute leukemia, that was
sucessfully transplanted with unrelated, HLA-phenotypically
identical marrow. The histocompatibility testing data on
these two long-term survivors are given in Table V. It is
evident, that both cases involve patients with quite common
HLA haplotypes.

TABLE V

BONE MARROW TRANSPLANTATION WITH UNRELATED DONOR
(Long-term Survivors)

DISEASE	HLA STATUS DONOR - RECIPIENT		REFERENCE
SCID[1]	DONOR	A1;B8;Dw3 A2;B15;Dw4	O'Reilly et al (1977)
	RECIPIENT	A1;B8;Dw3 A1;B15;Dw4	
Acute Leukemia[2]	DONOR	A1;B8;Dw3 A3;B7;Dw2	Hansen et al (1980)
	RECIPIENT	A1;B8;Dw3 A3;B7;Dw2	

1) Chronic GvH particularly involving skin.
2) No significant GvH.
   >300 days in remission as chimera

    Table VI lists some of the most common HLA-A,B,D/DR
haplotypes in the Caucasian population. It must now be
considered feasible to attempt to identify an unrelated bone
marrow transplant donor for a patient, who requires bone
marrow transplantation if (1) no related donor can be identi-

fied, who fulfills any of the donor options listed in Table
III and (2) if the patient can be shown to carry two of the
common HLA-A,B,D/DR haplotypes listed in Table VI.

TABLE VI

STRONG HLA-A,B HAPLOTYPE ASSOCIATIONS TO
HLA-D/DR DETERMINANTS

HLA - DR	HLA - A ; B Haplotype
DR 1	A3 ; Bw35
	A11 ; Bw35
	- ; B14
DR 2	A2 ; B7
	A3 ; B7
	A25 ; B18
DR 3	A1 ; B8
	Aw30 ; B18
DR 4	A2 ; Bw62(15.1)
	A2 ; Bw44
DR 5	?
DRw 6	?
DR 7	Aw23 ; Bw44
	A29 ; Bw44
	Aw19 ; B13
	A1 ; B17

Conclusions

The progressive development of histocompatibility testing
during the last 10 years, the development of measures for
prevention and management of GvH disease, and the development
of supportive care for patients without marrow function have
allowed the possibility for bone marrow transplantation for
many patients who do not have HLA genotypically identical
sibling donors. The relative strength of the different
components of HLA for development of GvHR is not yet known.
The studies in patients with SCID indicate, however, that the
HLA-B;D region plays a major role and that matching for this
region may be of particular importance.

Acknowledgement: Original work supported in part by U.S.
Public Health Services, N.I.H.-N.C.I. CA 19267; CA 08748;
CA 17404, CA 23766 and CA 22507.

Buckley RH: In Amos DB (ed) Progress in Immunology.
  New York, London, Academic Press, 1971, p. 1061.
Cantrell JL, Hildemann WH: Transplantation 14:761, 1972.
Clift RA, Hansen JA, Thomas ED, et al: Transplantation
  28:235, 1979.
Dupont B, Andersen V, Hansen GS, Svejgaard A: Trans-
  plantation 14:557, 1972.
Dupont B, O'Reilly RJ, Pollack MS, Good RA: Transplant
  Proc 11:219, 1979.
Dupont B, O'Reilly RJ, Pollack MS, Good RA: In Thierfelder
  S, Rodt H, Kolb HJ (eds) Immunobiology of Bone Marrow
  Transplantation. Berlin, Springer, 1980, p 121.
Epstein RB, Storb R, Ragde H, Thomas ED: Transplantation,
  6:45, 1968.
Gatti RA, Meuwissen HJ, Allen HD et al: Lancet 2: 1366, 1968.
Gazit E, Terhorst C, Yunis EJ: Nature 284: 275, 1980.
Hansen JA, Clift RA, Thomas ED, et al: N Engl J Med
  303:565, 1980.
Horowitz SD, Groshong T, Bach FH et al: Lancet 2: 431, 1975.
Kim SJ, Christiansen FT, Gosar I, et al: Hum Immunol
  1980 (in press).
Klein J: Biology of the Mouse Histocompatibility-2 Complex.
  New York, Springer, 1975.
Koch C, Henriksen K, Juhl F, et al: Lancet 1:1146, 1973.
L'Esperance P, Hansen JA, Jersild C, et al: Transplant Proc
  7, suppl 1:823, 1975.
Lohrmann HP, Dietrich M, Goldmann SF, et al:Blut 31:347,
  1975.
O'Reilly RJ, Dupont B, Pahwa S, et al: N Engl J Med
  297:1311, 1977.
O'Reilly RJ, Pahwa R, Kirkpatrick D, et al: Transplant Proc
  10:957, 1978.
O'Reilly RJ, Kapoor N, Pollack MS, et al: Transplant Proc
  11:1934, 1979.
Park BH, Biggar WD, Yunis EJ, Good RA: Transplant Proc
  5:899, 1973.
Ramsøe K, Skinhøj P, Andersen V, et al: Transplantation
  26:369, 1978.
Snell GD: J Genet 49:87, 1948.
Speck B, Zwaan FE, Rood JJ van, Eernisse JG: Transplanta-
  tion 16:24, 1973.
Storb R, Rudolph RH, Thomas ED: J Clin Invest 50:1272, 1971.
Storb R, Weiden PL, Graham TC, et al: Transplantation
  24:165, 1977.
Thomas ED, Storb R, Clift RA, et al: N Engl J Med 292:832
  & 895, 1975.
Uphoff DE, Law LW: J Natl Cancer Inst 20: 617, 1958.
Yunis EJ, Amos DB: Proc Natl Acad Sci USA 68:3031, 1971.

Advances in Supportive Measures

ADVANCES IN SUPPORTIVE MEASURES

Paul Sherlock, M.D.

Memorial Sloan-Kettering Cancer Center

The past decade has been characterized by major advances in the treatment of the patient with cancer. More extensive surgery, combination chemotherapy and sophisticated radiotherapy in addition to multimodality treatment have resulted in regression of disease and increased remission and cure rates in a variety of cancers. However, many of these advances would have been impossible were it not for concomitant advances in the medical support systems which have enabled the patient to withstand the major complications associated with cancer and its treatment.

Supportive measures are vital to the total care of the patient with cancer. Advances in the control of pain, nutritional management, psychological support, infection control with new antibiotics and protected environment, and the development of the critical care unit with its respiratory, cardiac, hepatic and renal support technologies have been vital for the development and implementation of more intensive therapies that have resulted in more cures.

Since cancer and cancer treatment can interfere with the optimal functioning of the immune system, patients are much more susceptible to a variety of infections that the normal host can handle very well. In addition, opportunistic infections frequently occur. A sterile environment and combination antibiotic therapy have enabled higher doses of chemotherapy. This increased chemotherapy has resulted in more remissions, particularly in some of the leukemias and lymphomas.

Malnutrition is a serious problem in patients with cancer, with loss of appetite, changes in taste and alteration in gastrointestinal structure and function as a result of their disease and its treatment. Various surgical procedures may result in loss of the esophagus with diarrhea resulting from vagal transection; loss of the reservoir function of the stomach; loss of pancreatic enzymes; malabsorption from resection of the small bowel or the development of a blind loop and gastrointestinal bypass relating to fistula formation.

Radiotherapy may cause decreased appetite, nausea and vomiting as well as effects on the small and large intestine which
result in diarrhea and malabsorption. The various chemotherapeutic agents may have profound effects on nutrition by
producing anorexia, nausea, vomiting, diarrhea, ileus, gastrointestinal ulceration and malabsorption. The patient with
cancer may have multiple mineral and vitamin deficiencies
which may be accentuated by the effects of treatment.

Newer concepts regarding hyperalimentation have resulted in the technique of total parenteral nutrition which
allows the patient to receive all essential calories, protein
and fat in the presence of gastrointestinal malfunction or
bypass. Improved tube formulae as well as better and thinner
tubes have also made it possible to provide better enteral
nutrition.

Patients with cancer may require extensive psychological support to cope with their disease. Their psychological
needs vary with the underlying stability of the patient; the
presence of previous psychiatric disease; the severity of the
illness; and the availability of social and emotional support
that can be drawn from friends and relatives. The role of a
psychiatric service in assessing the needs of patients with
cancer, analyzing and dealing with the psychologic effects
and the quantitation of psychologic parameters in a research
setting has resulted in the emerging field of psychosocial
oncology. Advances in this field will help patients to cope
with their disease.

Pain is one of the most feared effects of cancer and is
a debilitating force in about one-half of patients. The control of pain is a vital part of any treatment approach.
Careful attention to the causes of the pain and attempts at
elimination of the cause such as by the use of palliative
radiotherapy and relief of obstruction can result in a functioning patient with minimal hospitalization time. Synergistic effects can be accomplished by the use of combination
analgesic narcotics and can be effective in the vast majority
of patients. Newer knowledge of endorphins, natural substances endogenously produced which control pain, will result in
the ability to alter the perception of pain.

The critical care unit with its advanced support technology has enabled the use of more intensive surgery and
chemotherapy. The development of sepsis, shock, renal failure, respiratory failure and cardiac dysfunction from the use
of these modalities would have severely affected their use.

However, patients who manifest these problems can be segrega-
ted in a special area and can be managed effectively with
complete cardiac and respiratory monitoring, new ventilatory
devices to support respiration in patients whose lungs have
become impaired from the effects of chemotherapy, hemo- and
peritoneal dialysis equipment for renal failure and intensive
management of massive gastrointestinal hemorrhage.

The next series of five papers will outline in some
detail advances in supportive management of patients with
cancer, which have been as important as advances in the primary treatment of the disease.

PROTECTED ENVIRONMENTS

Gerald P. Bodey, M. D., Victorio Rodriguez, M. D.,
Emil J. Freireich, M. D.,
Kenneth B. McCredie, M. D.,
Manuel Valdivieso, M. D.,
Fernando Cabanillas, M. D. and
Linda S. Martin, R. N.

The University of Texas System Cancer Center
M. D. Anderson Hospital and Tumor Institute
Houston, Texas   77030

The cancer patient often experiences prolonged
periods of neutropenia as a consequence of his
disease or its therapy, which increases his risk of
becoming infected. The presence of infection often
delays the administration of anti-tumor agents.
Furthermore, since most anti-tumor agents cause
myelosuppression, the risk of infection is the
factor which limits the amount of drug which can be
administered. Hence, methods for protecting
against infectious complications have been of considerable interest to oncologists. The introduction of the plastic tent isolator, and subsequently, the laminar air flow (LAF) room, provided
a method for reducing exposure to environmental
contamination (1). The air supply in these units
passes through high efficiency particulate air
filters which remove 99.97% of microbial contamination. Plastic curtains create a barrier between
the patient and hospital personnel and allow most
nursing care to be given to the patient without
entering the room. The rooms are cleaned routinely
with germicidal solutions to further reduce the
amount of microbial contamination.

Prophylactic regimens have been developed to
reduce the patients' endogenous microbial flora.
These regimens include the ingestion of oral non-
absorbable antibiotics, application of antibiotic
ointments and sprays to body orifices and bathing
with bacteriostatic soap solutions. Since food may

serve as a source of colonization by potential
pathogens, it is specially prepared to reduce
microbial contamination to a minimum. Sterile
linens, clothing, equipment and furnishings are
provided. Cultures of the patients and the protected environment (PE) units have been collected
routinely to monitor the prophylactic program.
Details of the operation of the units and the prophylactic regimens have been reported elsewhere (7).
      The majority of patients entered on the pro-
tected environment-prophylactic antibiotic (PEPA)
program receive several courses of remission induction chemotherapy, requiring 6 to 10 weeks of
isolation. Initially, considerable concern was
manifested over patients ability to tolerate the
sensory deprivation required by this type of isolation, but only a few patients have developed
psychological abnormalities. Also concern was
expressed that the use of intensive prophylactic
antibiotics would facilitate overgrowth by resistant organisms and cause nutritional deficiencies
but these potential difficulties have seldom
occurred in patients on the PEPA program.
      Microbial monitoring of the PE units has demon-
strated that they substantially reduced the amount
of environmental contamination (3). Settling
plates have proven useful when placed in the LAF
rooms for 8 hours daily (TABLE 1). Whereas no samples from regular hospital rooms were sterile, 57%
from LAF rooms were sterile. Potentially, pathogenic organisms were isolated much less frequently
from LAF rooms. However, the amount of contamination in a PE unit depends upon the type of unit
utilized and whether or not the patient is receiving oral non-absorbable antibiotics (8). When LAF
rooms were occupied by patients taking oral non-
absorbable antibiotics, 5% of samples from permanent LAF rooms contained pathogens whereas 12% of
samples from portable LAF rooms contained pathogens.
Only 12% of settling plates contained pathogens
when the portable LAF rooms were occupied by patients taking oral non-absorbable antibiotics whereas 32% of samples contained pathogens when the
rooms were occupied by patients who were not taking
these antibiotics.
      The original objective of the prophylactic regi-

TABLE 1
MICROBIOLOGICAL MONITORING OF LAF ROOMS
Settling Plate Cultures

Type of Room	Perm[1]	Perm	Port[2]	Port	Hosp[3]
Prophylactic Antibiotics	Yes	No	Yes	No	No
Patients	51	13	74	10	-
Samples	3634	687	5648	798	54
Sterile Samples(%)	57	46	46	25	0
Samples with Pathogens(%)	5	9	12	32	26
Organism Deposited/Hr	0.3	0.4	1.3	1.8	13

[1]Perm=Permanent   [2]Port=Portable   [3]Hosp=Hospital

mens was to eliminate as much as possible of the
patients' endogenous microbial flora. The most
frequently used regimens have been gentamicin
(tobramycin) plus vancomycin and nystatin. These
regimens have been very effective in suppressing
the stool flora, although they have had a lesser
impact on the throat flora. For example, in one
study, 24% of patients had persistently sterile
stool cultures and only 16% had potentially pathogenic bacteria persisting in the stools during prophylaxis (7). Antifungal prophylaxis was much less
effective and 66% of patients had fungi persisting
in the stools during prophylaxis.

Most studies designed to evaluate the PEPA program have been conducted in patients undergoing remission induction chemotherapy for acute leukemia.
The first reported study compared 33 patients on
the PEPA program to 2 sets of controls selected by
biostatisticians who were treated concomitantly
with the same antileukemic regimens and had a similar prognosis (2). Subsequently, several prospective randomized trials of the PEPA program were
conducted (11,13,15). Table 2 summarizes the results of 4 of these studies. In all of these
studies, the frequency of major infectious complications was substantially higher among the control
patients than among the PEPA patients. Likewise, a
higher proportion of the control patients died of

infectious complications in each of these studies.
In 3 of these studies, the frequency of infection
was related to neutrophil count and the PEPA patients spent significantly less time with major infection when they were severely neutropenic (<100
neutrophils/mm^3).

TABLE 2
SEVERE INFECTIONS DURING REMISSION INDUCTION
THERAPY FOR ACUTE LEUKEMIA ON THE PEPA PROGRAM

	PEPA Patients	Control Patients
Patients Studied	107	154
% with Major Infection	21	56
% with Fatal Infection	7	27

    The use of the PEPA program might be expected to
improve the complete remission rate by 2 effects.
First, since the fatality rate from infection
during remission induction therapy was lower, more
patients would be expected to survive long enough
to achieve remission. Secondly, since the risk of
infection was lower, it should be possible to administer higher doses of chemotherapy which might
improve the complete remission rate. The complete
remission rate was significantly higher for the
PEPA patients only in the study of Schimpff et al
(TABLE 3). In the study of Bodey et al, the PEPA
patients received higher doses of chemotherapy than
the control patients but this was not studied on a
systematic basis. The PEPA patients had only a
slightly higher complete remission rate in this
study, but the duration of remission curve was significantly longer (median, 55 wks vs 26 wks, p<.05).
In this study, the median duration of survival was
34 wks for the PEPA patients compared to 23 wks for
the control patients (p≈.02). The improvement in
duration of survival existed throughout the period
of observation, reflecting the lower fatality rate
from infection during remission induction, the
higher remission rate and the longer duration of
remission for the PEPA patients.
    Subsequently, in a prospective randomized study,
we evaluated not only the PEPA program but also 2
different prophylactic antibiotic regimens, an oral

TABLE 3
REMISSION INDUCTION THERAPY OF ACUTE LEUKEMIA ON
THE PEPA PROGRAM

| | PE Group | | Control Group | |
	Patients	%CR	Patients	%CR
Bodey et al(2)	33	61	66	48
Levine et al(11)	22	45	28	43
Yates and				
Holland(15)	28	33	39	31
Schimpff et al(13)	24	54	21	24

(PA) regimen and a parenteral (SA) regimen (12).
The oral regimen included both oral non-absorbable
antibiotics and a rotating sequence of absorbable
antibiotics. The parenteral regimen consisted of a
rotating schedule of gentamicin, colistin, amphotericin B, chloramphenicol, ampicillin, clindamycin
and cephalothin. The patients initially received
antileukemic therapy with vincristine, prednisone
and cytosar, but later adriamycin and BCG immunotherapy were added. The study was designed so that
when a PE unit was available, patients were randomized to enter the PE unit and receive PA or SA, or
to receive SA in a regular hospital room. If a PE
unit was not available, the patient was randomized
to receive either SA or PA in a regular hospital
room. A control group with no prophylactic antibiotics was not included because most patients have
required frequent and prolonged therapeutic antibiotic regimens.

Table 4 shows the results for the patients who
were randomized when a PE unit was available. The
complete remission rate was highest for the PESA
patients and the difference between this group and
the SA group was statistically significant (p<0.01).
The SA group had the highest frequency of major infectious complications whereas the PESA group had
the lowest frequency (p=.004). Although the duration of remissions was similar for all 3 groups,
the duration of survival was significantly longer
for the PESA patients due to the lower fatality
rate from infection and the higher complete remission rate.

Groups of patients could be combined because
antibiotic prophylaxis was randomly assigned and

TABLE 4
RANDOMIZED STUDY OF THE PEPA PROGRAM IN ACUTE
LEUKEMIA
Patients Entered on Study When PE Unit
was Available

	PEPA	PESA	SA
Patients Entered	29	34	29
Complete Remissions(%)	59	82	48
Patients with Major Infection(%)	48	35	55
Episodes of Infection/ Patient	0.66	0.41	0.79
Median Duration of Remission(wks)	52	72	64
Median Duration of Survival(wks)	64	94	47

the availability of a PE unit was a random event
(TABLE 5). The complete remission rate was significantly higher for those patients treated in the
PE units than for those patients treated out of the
PE units (p<.01). A logistic regression equation
was used to predict the prognosis for all patients.
Both those patients with the poorest and best prognosis who were treated in a PE unit had significantly higher complete remission rates than their
counterparts treated out of a PE unit. Fewer patients treated in the PE units developed major infections (p=.08) and the fatality rate from infection was significantly lower among these patients (p=.04). There was no difference between
the 2 groups in their durations of remission,
however, the patients treated in the PE units had
significantly longer durations of survival (median,
72 wks vs 42 wks, p<.01).
    This was the first study to evaluate different
approaches to antibiotic prophylaxis in a large
group of patients. Although the results tended to
favor the group of patients receiving parenteral
antibiotics, there were no statistically significant differences. It is interesting that the
parenteral regimen was as effective as the oral
regimens. The former patients' endogenous microbial flora was not as greatly affected by their
prophylactic regimen. Furthermore, because their

TABLE 5
RANDOMIZED STUDY OF THE PEPA PROGRAM IN ACUTE
LEUKEMIA
Effect of Treatment in a PE Unit

	In	Out	PA	SA
Patients Entered	63	82	55	90
Complete Remissions(%)	71	43	45	61
Poor Prognosis Only(%)	60	29	35	46
Good Prognosis Only(%)	90	53	67	74
Patients with Major Infection(%)	41	57	53	49
Patients with Fatal Infection(%)	13	28	24	20
% Days Spent with Major Infection When Neutrophils <100/mm^3	18	28	23	23

gastrointestinal flora was not greatly reduced,
they shed more organisms into the environment
causing increased environmental contamination.

Subsequently, in order to confirm the excellent
results observed among the patients with the best
prognosis, we admitted all patients 14 to 50 years
old who had received no prior therapy on the PEPA
program if a PE unit was available (4). Remission
induction therapy consisted of 3 courses of the Ad-
OAP regimen. Twenty-seven of the 30 (90%) evaluable patients achieved a complete remission, including all 9 patients with acute lymphocytic
leukemia and 18 (86%) of the 21 patients with acute
myelogenous leukemia. However, only 3 (11%) of the
patients who achieved complete remission remain in
remission at 39 to 53 months. Only 7 patients
(23%) developed major infectious complications and
none died of infection despite spending 36% of
their time in the PE units with a neutrophil count
<100/mm^3. During the periods when their neutrophil
count was this low, they spent only 7% of their
time with major infection.

The encouraging results in patients with acute
leukemia led to the evaluation of the PEPA program
in patients with malignant lymphoma, sarcomas and
small cell carcinoma of the lung. The objectives
of our lymphoma and sarcoma studies were to determine whether the PEPA program reduced the risk of

major infection, and permitted the administration
of higher doses of chemotherapy and whether higher
doses of chemotherapy resulted in higher response
rates and longer durations of response and survival.
Patients were randomly assigned to receive 3
courses of remission induction therapy on the PEPA
program or as controls. The lymphoma patients received the CHOP-Bleo regimen and the sarcoma patients received the CYVADIC regimen (5,6). All patients were required to receive dosage escalation
during the second and third courses if they did not
develop a major infectious complication, regardless
of the degree or duration of myelosuppression
during the preceding course.
     The complete remission rate for all 58 evaluable
patients with lymphoma was 74%, and there was no
difference between the PEPA patients and the control patients (TABLE 6).

TABLE 6

PEPA PROGRAM IN MALIGNANT LYMPHOMA[1] AND SARCOMA[2]

	PEPA[1]	Control[1]	PEPA[2]	Control[2]
Patients Evaluable	30	28	24	27
Complete Remissions(%)	77	71	33	15
Patients with Major Infection(%)	7	29	12	26
% Days Spent with Major Infection when Neutrophils <100/mm^3	3	27	3	16

The control patients experienced a higher frequency
of infectious complications (p=.06) and one of
these patients died of infection. Also the control
patients spent a greater proportion of their time
with infection when severely neutropenic (p<.001).
Since infection occurred less often among the PEPA
patients, they were able to receive more intensive
chemotherapy. Only 4% of the PEPA patients were
prevented from receiving full dosage escalation due
to infectious complications compared to 23% of the
control patients (p=.09). The ability to receive
the highest doses of the CHOP-Bleo regimen did not
appear to convey any advantages when compared to
the intermediate doses. However, patients who received the lowest dose had the lowest complete re-

mission rate, highest relapse rate and highest
fatality rate (p=.004).

Among the evaluable patients with sarcoma, who
received the CYVADIC regimen, the response rate was
71% for the 24 PEPA patients whereas it was 67% for
the 27 control patients. However, 33% of the PEPA
patients achieved a complete remission compared to
15% of the control patients (TABLE 6). Although
this difference is not statistically significant,
the 33% complete remission rate for the PEPA patients is the highest ever reported for the CYVADIC
regimen. Major infection occurred more often among
the control patients and they spent a significantly
greater proportion of their time with infection
when they were severely neutropenic (p=.00001).
Eight percent of the PEPA patients could not receive full dosage escalation because they developed
major infections compared to 26% of the control patients (p=0.20). The median duration of complete
remissions was 52 wks for the PEPA patients and 35
wks for the controls. The projected median duration of survival was 78 wks for the PEPA patients
and 52 wks for the control patients. Neither of
these differences are statistically significant.
The patients who received the highest dosage of
CYVADIC had the highest complete remission rate,
lowest relapse rate and lowest death rate. The
median survival for patients receiving the lowest
dosage was 46 wks, whereas it was 70 wks for patients receiving the intermediate dosage (p=.05).
Patients receiving the highest dosage had a median
survival of 56 wks.

Cohen et al evaluated the role of the PEPA program and high dose chemotherapy (CCNU, cyclophosphamide and methotrexate) in small cell carcinoma
of the lung (10). Patients were randomized to high
dose chemotherapy on the PEPA program (12 patients),
high dose chemotherapy without prophylaxis (11
patients) or conventional dose chemotherapy without
prophylaxis (9 patients). Antibiotic prophylaxis
consisted of a non-absorbable regimen. Only one
patient who received high dose chemotherapy developed major infection and he was on the PEPA program. Of the 23 patients receiving high dose
chemotherapy, 7 achieved a complete remission and
15 achieved a partial remission. Of the 9 patients

receiving conventional doses, none achieved a complete remission and 4 achieved a partial remission
(p<.05). We have been evaluating the PEPA program
in small cell carcinoma, using an induction regimen consisting of adriamycin, ifosfamide, VP-16 and
vincristine (14). Preliminary results suggest that
prophylactic non-absorbable antibiotic regimens are
ineffective in reducing infectious complications.
Systemic antibiotics administered prophylactically
to patients in or out of a PE unit do reduce infectious complications. Patients treated on the
PEPA program have received more intensive chemotherapy, but this does not appear to improve the
complete remission rate or duration of disease-
free survival.

It has been clearly demonstrated that the PEPA
program has been evaluated in
a prospective randomized trial in patients undergoing bone marrow transplantation for acute leukemia or aplastic anemia (9). Major local infection
occurred in 22 of the 44 control patients but in
only 3 of the 46 PEPA patients. Septicemia
occurred in 23 of the former patients but in only
10 of the latter patients. The need for granulocyte transfusions was substantially reduced by the
PEPA program (5 vs 22 patients, p<.0001). Nineteen of the 46 PEPA patients remained alive at the
time of analysis compared to 6 of the 44 control
patients. Among the 17 patients in each group
with aplastic anemia, 13 PEPA patients and 4 control patients remained alive.

It has been clearly demonstrated that the PEPA
program effectively reduces the frequency of infection among patients at high risk during periods
of myelosuppression. Although several studies
have shown that prophylactic antibiotic regimens
alone can accomplish the same objective, they
probably are not as effective. Furthermore, the
profligate use of prophylactic antibiotics in patients who are not isolated from the hospital environment is likely to encourage the emergence of
resistant organisms. These resistant organisms
will pose a threat not only to the patients receiving the regimens but also to other hospitalized
patients. The PEPA program permits the safe administration of high doses of myelosuppressive
anti-tumor agents. The impact of high dose chemo-

therapy on complete remission rates and duration of disease-free survival has been somewhat disappointing thus far. However, it would be premature to draw final conclusions from the few studies currently completed. Additional studies in other malignant diseases and with other regimens need to be initiated to resolve this important issue.

REFERENCES

1. Bodey, G. P., Freireich, E. J and Frei, E. III: Studies of patients in a laminar air flow unit. Cancer 24:972-980, 1969.
2. Bodey, G. P., Gehan, E. A., Freireich, E. J et al: Protected environment-prophylactic antibiotic program in the chemotherapy of acute leukemia. Am. J. Med. Sci. 262:138-151, 1971.
3. Bodey, G. P. and Johnston, D.: Microbiological evaluation of protected environments during patient occupancy. Appl. Microbiol. 22:828-836, 1971.
4. Bodey, G. P., McCredie, K. B., Keating, M. J. et al: Treatment of acute leukemia in protected environment units. Cancer 44:431-436, 1979.
5. Bodey, G. P., Rodriguez, V., Cabanillas, F. et al: Protected environment-prophylactic antibiotic program for malignant lymphoma. Randomized trial during chemotherapy to induce remission. Am. J. Med. 66:74-81, 1979.
6. Bodey, G. P., Rodriguez, V., Murphy, W. K. et al: Protected environment-prophylactic antibiotic program for malignant sarcomas. Randomized trial during remission induction chemotherapy. Cancer. In Press.
7. Bodey, G. P. and Rosenbaum, B.: Effect of prophylactic measures on the microbial flora of patients in protected environment units. Medicine 53:209-228, 1974.
8. Bodey, G. P. and Rosenbaum, B.: Microbiological monitoring of protected environment units. Effects of antibiotic prophylaxis and type of unit. Europ. J. Cancer 16:67-75, 1979.
9. Buckner, C. D., Clift, R. A., Sanders, J. E. et al: Protective environment for marrow trans-

plant recipients. A prospective study. Ann.
Intern. Med. 89:893-901, 1978.

10. Cohen, M. H., Creaven, P. J., Fossieck, B. E.
    et al: Intensive chemotherapy of small cell
    bronchogenic carcinoma. Cancer Treat. Rep. 61:
    349-354, 1977.

11. Levine, A. S., Siegel, S. E., Schreiber, A. D.
    et al: Protected environments and prophylactic
    antibiotics. A prospective controlled study
    of their utility in the therapy of acute
    leukemia. New Eng. J. Med. 288:477-483, 1973.

12. Rodriguez, V., Bodey, G. P., Freireich, E. J
    et al: Randomized trial of protected environ-
    ment-prophylactic antibiotics in 145 adults
    with acute leukemia. Medicine 57:253-266,
    1978.

13. Schimpff, S. C., Greene, W. H., Young, V. M.
    et al: Infection prevention in acute non-
    lymphocytic leukemia. Laminar air flow room
    reverse isolation with oral, non-absorbable
    antibiotic prophylaxis. Ann. Intern. Med. 82:
    351-358, 1975.

14. Valdivieso, M., Cabanillas, F., Barkley, H. T.
    et al: Intensive induction chemotherapy of
    extensive small cell bronchogenic carcinoma in
    protected environment-prophylactic antibiotic
    units. A preliminary report. Int. J. Radiat.
    Oncol. Biol. Phys. 6:1087-1092, 1980.

15. Yates, J. W. and Holland, J. F.: A controlled
    study of isolation and endogenous microbial
    suppression in acute myelocytic leukemia pa-
    tients. Cancer 32:1490-1498, 1973.

Nutritional Support of the Cancer
Patient

Maurice E. Shils, M.D., Sc.D.

Director of Clinical Nutrition and Attending Physician
Department of Medicine
Memorial Sloan-Kettering Cancer Center
New York, New York

Professor of Medicine
Cornell University Medical College
New York, New York

Before discussing methods of nutrition support of the cancer
patient, it is desirable to consider briefly some of the
reasons why it is desirable to provide such support. Three
major influences may be operative. The first is the generalized or systemic effects of cancer under which I would include the psychological impact of the disease on the patient.
The second influence is the local effects of the tumor and
the third is the effect of various treatments of neoplastic
diseases.
    In considering systemic effects, perhaps the most strik-
ing and presently unexplained manifestation of active and
especially disseminated neoplastic disease in a significant
number of patients is the marked anorexia, that is loss of
appetite, with consequent depressed food intake. If persistent, this will lead to the severe wasting of body mass which
we call cancer cachexia. Although the anorexia is not unique
to cancer, its high incidence and prolonged and deleterious
effect make it of special concern. In my opinion, this is
the primary cause of weight loss experienced by many patients. It is common for the anorectic hospitalized patient
to ingest breakfast fairly well and then eat progressively
less with each succeeding meal. Often the anorexia is associated with alterations in taste leading patients to ascribe
diminished appetite to the unpleasant taste of one or more
foods or to an unpleasant taste which lingers in the mouth
between meals. The latter is more common in patients on

711

certain chemotherapy regimens. In my opinion, there is no
consistent pattern of taste changes in cancer patients. Consequently each individual must be considered on the basis of
his own likes and dislikes in providing specific foods in an
effort to improve intake. In my opinion, alterations in taste
are probably not primary factors but are associated with more
basic changes initiated by the malignancy in association with
psychosomatic factors and with chemotherapy when given.
There is reasonable evidence that some cancer patients do
have a moderate increase in resting metabolic expenditure;
others have expenditures similar to that of controls.[1] For
those who do have increased metabolic expenditure, the simultaneous presence of anorexia depressing caloric intake
creates a double problem since there is both an increased
need and a decreased intake; the combination obviously will
speed up the rate of weight loss. The possible basis for increased caloric expenditure in terms of altered substrate
metabolism has been discussed;[2] however, the nature and significance of the modifications, if any, are presently unclear.

A common cause of serious malnutrition is the localized
effects of tumor interfering with food intake as a result of
partial or complete obstruction of some portion of the alimentary tract. Relief of obstruction by one or another antitumor modality is necessary before the patient can again ingest adequate amounts of food. Prior to and during radiation
therapy and chemotherapy and for a period after intervention,
nutrition support may be critical in sustaining the patient.
There is often impaired digestion in patients with tumor of
the pancreas as a result of blockage of the pancreatic duct.
Lymphoma and carcinoma may involve the small bowel wall leading to malabsorption. Infiltration of the lamina propria of
the small intestine lymph nodes with obstruction of lymphatic
channels is associated with protein losing enteropathy with
hypoalbuminemia, hypoglobulinemia and lymphocytopenia. Secretion by tumors of ectopic hormones (including steroids, PTH,
ADH, gastrin, calcitonin, glucagon, serotonin, kinins, prostaglandins and others) may lead to a variety of problems of
fluid and electrolyte imbalance. The resulting syndromes are
often associated with anorexia and malnutrition adding to the
complexity of the physiologic situation. A major cause of
fluid and electrolyte imbalance in cancer patients is the
vomiting and diarrhea secondary to partial or complete obstruction or to intestinal fluid losses through a fistula. In
addition to the loss of sodium, potassium, chloride and bi-
carbonate, that of magnesium and zinc must be considered.

Significant nutritional problems may arise as a result of
a specific treatment of the neoplastic disease. (Table 1)

TABLE 1
Consequences of Cancer Treatment Predisposing to Nutrition
Problems 8/*

1. Radiation treatment.
    A. Radiation of oropharyngeal area.
        (1) Destruction of sense of taste; xerostomia and
            odynophagia; loss of teeth.
    B. Radiation to lower neck and mediastinum.
        (1) Esophagitis with dysphagia.
        (2) Fibrosis with esophageal stricture.
    C. Radiation of abdomen and pelvis.
        (1) Bowel damage, acute and chronic, with diarrhea,
            malabsorption, stenosis and obstruction, fistul-
            ization.
2. Surgical treatment.
    A. Radical resection of oropharyngeal area.
        (1) Chewing and swallowing difficulties.
        (2) Tube feeding possibly required.
    B. Esophagectomy and esophageal reconstruction.
        (1) Gastric stasis and hypochlorhydria secondary to
            vagotomy.
        (2) Steatorrhea.   (3) Diarrhea.
    C. Gastrectomy (high subtotal or total).
        (1) Dumping syndrome.   (2) Malabsorption.
        (3) Achlorhydria and lack of intrinsic factor.
        (4) Hypoglycemia.
    D. Intestinal resection.
        (1) Jejunum.
            (a) Decreased efficiency of absorption of many
                nutrients.
        (2) Ileum.
            (a) Vitamin B_{12} deficiency.   (b) Bile salt losses
                with diarrhea.   (c) Hyperoxaluria.
        (3) Massive bowel resection.
            (a) Life-threatening malabsorption.
            (b) Malnutrition.   (c) Metabolic acidosis.
        (4) Ileostomy and colostomy.
            (a) Complications of salt and water balance.
    E. Blind-loop syndrome.
    F. Pancreatectomy.
        (1) Malabsorption.   (2) Diabetes Mellitus.
3. Chemotherapy treatment.
    A. Corticosteroids.
        (1) Fluid and electrolyte problems.   (2) Nitrogen and
            calcium losses.   (3) Hyperglycemia.
    B. Antimetabolites, alkylating agents and other drugs.

*Reprinted with the permission of Lea and Febiger.

Since treatments are combined there may be multiple adverse effects. A combination of surgery and radiation to the head and neck often causes loss of taste, dry mouth and problems in chewing and swallowing as well as psychological reactions secondary to disfiguring surgery. Tube feedings may be necessary for those patients with chewing or swallowing problems or a tendency for aspiration of food.

The epithelium of the small bowel is second only to bone marrow in its sensitivity to radiation. A small but significant portion of individuals given external and/or internal radiation will develop chronic changes which may manifest themselves months to years after the radiation is completed. Flattening an ulceration of the mucosa, telangiectasia with bleeding, hyalinization of arterioles, fibrosis, strictures, obstruction and fistulization of the intestine may occur. Resection or by-pass of the involved intestine may be necessary; not uncommonly, if radiation damage is severe, obstruction and/or fistula may recur with progressive resection or by-pass of bowel to the point of the severe malabsorption (short bowel syndrome).

Resection of segments of the alimentary tract or modification of its normal continuity has adverse nutritional consequences depending on the specific segments involved and the extent of resection or by-pass (Table 1). This is a complex subject and has been reviewed elsewhere.[3,4] Adequate nutritional management of the affected patient depends upon an understanding of the nature of the changes imposed by a specific surgical procedure upon normal digestive and absorptive processes.

Many of the chemotherapeutic agents in use have deleterious effects on the mucosa of the alimentary tract. A number of these agents and their effects are listed in Table 2. The increasing use of combinations of chemotherapeutic agents in cyclical fashion - while increasingly effective against various malignancies - often results in anorexia, nausea, altered taste, mucositis and diarrhea and other changes with resultant impairment of food intake. Since such treatments may be given over months or years, weight loss may be severe. These undesirable reactions are intensified when radiation therapy to the abdomen or surgical resection of a portion of the intestinal tract impair intestinal function. Adequate nutritional support may make a major contribution in permitting patients on these regimens to maintain weight and strength.

NUTRITION THERAPY IN THE CANCER PATIENT

Malignant diseases must be viewed as potential or actual

chronic diseases and as a matter of concern for long periods
by the patient and physician either in terms of persistent
treatment or prolonged side effects of one type or another.
The short bowel syndrome following surgery or severe persistent radiation enteritis often induces nutritional problems
lasting a life-time. The requirement for repeated chemotherapy schedules similarly imposes long-term problems.
These factors often combine to affect adversely the quality
of life of the patient.

TABLE 2
Alimentary Tract Effects of Cancer
Chemotherapeutic Agents 8/**

Drug	Effect*	Drug	Effect*
Adriamycin	A,N,V,N	Daunorubicin	A,N,V,M
Asparaginase	A,N,V	CDDP ("Cis-Pt")	A,N,V
BCNU	A,N,V	Hydroxyurea	N,V,M,D
Bleomycin	M	Methotrexate	A,N,U,P,M
Busulfan	N.V	Mithramycin	A,N,V,D
Cyclophosphamide	A,N,V,P	Procarbazine	A,N,V
Cytarbine	N,V,M,U	Vinblastine	N,V
Dactinomycin	A,N,V,D,M,P	Vincristine	P,O

*A = anorexia, N = nausea, D = diarrhea, M = mucositis,
 P = abdominal pain, O = obstipation, U = intestinal ulcer-
 ation
**Reprinted with the permission of Lea and Febiger.

Table 3 lists some of the undesirable effects of malnutrition. It is obvious that many of these effects are deleterious and contribute to increased morbidity and mortality.
Progressive weight loss and debility are often frightening to
the patient and family members.

ROUTES AND MODALITIES OF NUTRITIONAL THERAPY

It is desirable to utilize the alimentary tract if it is
functioning adequately. The first approach, of course, is
the voluntary ingestion of an adequate oral diet. Care in
the provision of the types of food, frequency of feeding and
use of supplements can improve intake and meet special absorptive and metabolic problems. Often the cancer patient will
not take sufficient food voluntarily no matter how one tries.
Tube feeding: When oral intake is unsatisfactory and
when the alimentary tract is functioning, tube feeding is an
attractive alternative to intravenous feeding. Tube feeding
is relatively inexpensive, easy to perform and relatively

free of hazard.[5] However, it is contraindicated in the
patient with intestinal obstruction or persistent nausea and
vomiting or when entry of food into the alimentary tract
intensifies negative fluid and electrolyte balance in those
with severe malabsorption or small bowel fistula. Tube
feeding may be contraindicated when there is the liklihood of
aspiration unless the tube tip is placed into the small bowel.
The composition of the formula to be administered will depend
upon the functional state of the gastrointestinal tract and
the metabolic needs of the patient. There are now available
a large variety of complete defined formula liquid diets for
tube feeding which flow easily through the finest caliber
tube.[6] Such small caliber tubes are available and very well
tolerated for long periods. Patients and family members can
be trained to insert the tubes themselves at home so that a
constant indwelling tube is not necessary. For the individual with a serious risk of aspiration, these tubes can be
placed into the upper small bowel and fed slow drip to minimize the risk of regurgitation.

TABLE 3
CLINICAL EFFECTS OF MALNUTRITION 9/*

Weight loss	Protein depletion
Fat utilization	Progressive weakness
Skin breakdown	Apathy/irritability
Prolonged bedrest	Impaired wound healing
Endocrine changes	Electrolyte-fluid imbalance
Secondary nutrient	Decreased hypoxic response
depletion	

Depressed immune mechanisms:
   Impaired phagocytosis
   Decreased macrophage mobilization
   Depressed lymphocyte function

Delay in diagnostic and therapeutic program

Increased morbidity and mortality
*Reprinted with permission of the American Cancer Soc.

Tubes may be placed surgically through an esophagostome,
gastrostome or an enterostome for special indications, particularly when the alimentary tract is obstructed at a higher
level. Esophagostomy or gastrostomy feeding tubes are useful
for the patient unable or unwilling to utilize a naso-

pharyngeal tube for any reason.

Debilitated patients or those with gastrostomy, short bowel syndrome or radiation enteritis often do not tolerate lactose well. Hence, lactose-low or lactose-free diets should be given initially. Milk or milk products may then be tested and given if tolerated.

There is a tendency to underestimate the caloric needs of patients on tube feeding; the same criteria should be applied as in oral or intravenous feeding. Too rapid feeding will result in vomiting or diarrhea. Special formulations and slow rate of feeding are often beneficial in meeting the needs of patients with serious digestive or absorptive problems secondary to pancreatic insufficiency or malabsorption, partial obstruction or colon fistulas. Special formulations are useful in the presence of various types of organ failure that modify nutritional requirements e.g. pancreatic, renal or hepatic dysfunction.[5]

Oral and tube feeding serve as a stimulus to maintenance of intestinal structure and function and help induce hyperplasia of the villi when resection of bowel has occurred.[7]

Despite the proven value of enteral feedings in suitable patients, our experience indicates that it has limited value for patients on high dose cyclical chemotherapy and abdominal radiation because of the high prevalence of nausea and mucositis. Aversion to tube feeding by these patients is marked. There is serious reservation by physicians to the passage of feeding tubes into the alimentary tract of patients with marked thrombocytopenia with the argument that tubes - no matter how flexible and narrow - will induce bleeding. In my opinion, this is an unproven position and should be studied.

Parenteral feeding: Nutrition may be supplied intravenously either through a peripheral or a central vein. Use of a peripheral vein requires an isotonic or only slightly hypertonic solution to minimize phlebitis and thrombosis. To obtain a significant number of calories it is necessary to use isotonic 10% or 20% sterile stable fat emulsions providing 1100 to 2200 kcal per liter together with amino acids, some glucose and minerals and vitamins. Drawbacks to this technique include the high cost of intravenous fat relative to glucose, the inability of some patients to tolerate continuous high fat infusions and the scarcity of suitable peripheral veins in many hospitalized patients who have been on routine intravenous fluids for some time. Peripheral parenteral nutrition is very useful when smaller amounts of fat together with adequate amino acids and other nutrients which provide about 1000 kcal per day are given as a rela-

tively short term supplement to partially anorectic patients
capable of taking 800 to 1000 kcal by mouth and who are
opposed to tube feeding.

For the malnourished or hypermetabolic patients unable to
ingest any appreciable amount of food orally or enterally,
support is provided by total parenteral nutrition (TPN)
through a central vein.

The procedures, equipment and precautions for minimizing
complications are now well established.[10,11] Previously
used primarily for patients with surgical problems, TPN is
now widely used in our institution in maintaining patients
during intensive chemotherapy, radiation therapy or in the
prolonged treatment of severe malabsorption.

TPN is applicable not only in hospitals but also at home.
Two groups of patients may benefit from TPN at home. One
group is exemplified by the individual whose alimentary tract
has been so damaged or so obstructed by cancer and its
treatments that adequate nutrition cannot be maintained by
the oral or tube routes and the patient would otherwise have
to remain in the hospital for very long periods or for the
duration of life or else die of malnutrition. The other
type is exemplified by the individual with serious but reversible dysfunction secondary to high dose chemotherapy or
radiation therapy or combination or one who is awaiting
surgical treatment for an underlying problem but who is so
debilitated that further surgery must await nutritional rehabilitation. Such a patient may be maintained at home on
TPN during treatment or during the rehabilitation period at
much reduced expense as far as hospital costs are concerned.
This type of support is presently used infrequently because
of its expense to the patient and the need for increased
personnel and facilities in-hospital.

Since the first patient was sent home from Memorial Hospital in December, 1969, this technique has spread throughout
the United States and other countries so that many hundreds
of patients have been sent home in the interval.

While it is expensive - with the cost ranging between
$40-$100 a day - this is appreciably cheaper than the cost
of an average day in North American big-city hospitals.

A number of decisions must be made and problems solved
before home TPN can or should be undertaken. These include
a decision on a) whether there is a "reasonable" probability
of a significant period of survival at home with a satisfactory quality of life, b) the ability of the patient and/or
family to execute the program at home, c) the nutritional
needs related to long term intravenous feeding. Once an
affirmative decision is made there must be an educational
program to teach the patient and family the necessary tech-

niques and provision for adequate hospital support in the event of catheter problems and infection. Experience indicates that this is a worthwhile and useful technique which enables the patient meeting the criteria to join his family and be maintained in good nutritional status and, in a number of instances, to carry on a significant proportion, if not all, of his/her previous activities for a period commensurate with the nature of the underlying disease process. Basic to success of this program is the availability of an experienced nutrition team available to do the training and follow the patients with emergency support available when necessary 24 hours per day everyday.

The principles of nutritional therapy in the cancer patient have been presented.[9] These may be summarized as follows:

1. Malnutrition is not an obligatory response of the host to cancer. It is relatively uncommon to find a cancer patient who cannot be either maintained in good nutritional status or improved when previously malnourished by means of appropriate therapeutic nutritional modalities (i.e. oral, tube or intravenous feeding).

2. A rational nutritional therapeutic program for a patient requires analysis of the factors inducing depletion in that patient. Every patient should have an early and then periodic assessment of nutritional status so that the already malnourished patients or those at risk of developing malnutrition are detected early.

3. Nutritional therapy should be instituted early when the patient is deemed to be at risk for malnutrition since it is much easier to maintain a reasonably good state of nutrition than it is to try to rehabilitate the already malnourished individual.

4. It is essential that the patient who has had improvement in nutritional status in the hospital be followed as an out-patient for assurance that the nutrition therapy is not neglected after discharge.

5. Who is to be given aggressive nutritional therapy? If antitumor therapy of one type or another is to be undertaken, the patient deserves nutritional therapy so long as the treatment is applied and is being evaluated. If, on the other hand, the patient is not considered a suitable candidate for any further type of treatment, aggressive nutritional therapy is not to be instituted or continued except in rare instances.

6. Nutritional therapy can be divided into: a) supportive b) adjunctive and c) definitive. Supportive therapy is exemplified by the patient with bowel obstruction who is deemed a poor surgical risk because of malnutrition and who will be

clinically improved by nutritional means to the point where surgery can be undertaken at appreciably lower risk. Adjunctive nutrition therapy is the type where nutrition becomes a part of the therapeutic program. Examples of this are: a) improving resistance to infection by improving immune status; b) permitting more rapid application and better adherence to a proposed antitumor therapeutic regimen by improved nutrition; or c) inducing spontaneous closure of an intestinal fistula as a result of nutritional therapy. Definitive nutrition therapy is defined as that where the therapy becomes the modality upon which the longer-term existence of the patient depends, i.e., when the nutritional program permits survival of a patient in good condition who has had a massive bowel resection or severe radiation enteritis or both and where debility or death will result without such therapy. This may be a short-time or long-term endeavor. The therapeutic modalities necessary to achieve these objectives should be available for in-patients and out-patients.

7. Nutritional status, tumor growth, and antitumor treatment are intimately related. Many of the most potent cytoxic agents used in antitumor therapy have optimum activity against cells that are in the process of division. Hence, malignancies are most susceptible to chemotherapeutic measures where a high percentage of the cells are in that state. Nutrition plays a role in the rate of cell growth and mitosis. Increased growth of residual tumor would be expected in patients as a result of improved nutrition since tumor cells have a dependency on good nutrition as do host cells although clinical experience indicates it is a rare patient who has marked acceleration of growth of tumor during a period of improved nutrition. Improved nutrition may be a therapeutically useful occurence since actively dividing tumor cells are more likely to be more sensitive to radiation therapy and chemotherapy than are slowly dividing cells. It is the opinion of the author that it is not in the interest of the tumor-bearing patient who is a candidate for treatment to be maintained on nutritional therapy without at the same time institutioning appropriate antitumor therapy.

REFERENCES

1. Warmold I, Lundhold, K, Schursten, T.: Energy balance and body composition in cancer patients. Cancer Res. 38: 1081, 1978.
2. Young, VR: Energy metabolism and requirements in the

cancer patient. Cancer Res. 37: 2336, 1977.

3. Lawrence W Jr: Nutritional consequences of surgical resection of the gastrointestinal tract for cancer Cancer Res. 37: 2379, 1977.

4. Shils ME: Effect on nutrition of surgery of the liver, pancreas and genitourinary tract. Cancer Res. 37: 2387, 1977.

5. Shils ME: Enteral nutrition by tube. Cancer Res. 37: 2432, 1977.

6. Shils ME, Bloch AS, Chernoff R: Liquid formulas for oral and tube feeding. 2nd ed. 1980. Available from the authors.

7. Williamson RCN: Intestinal adaptation. New Engl. J. Med. 298: 1393 and 1444, 1979.

8. Shils ME: Nutrition and Neoplasia, in Goodhart RS, Shils ME (eds): Modern Nutrition in Health and Disease 6th ed. Phila. Lea and Febiger 1980 pp 1153-1192.

9. Shils ME: Principles of nutritional therapy. Cancer 43: 2093, 1979.

10. Shils ME: Parenteral Nutrition, in Goodhart RS, Shils ME (eds): Modern Nutrition in Health and Disease. 6th ed. Phila. Lea and Febiger 1980 pp 1125-1152.

11. Dudrick SJ, Long JM III: Applications and hazards of intravenous hyperalimentation. Ann. Rev. Med. 28: 517, 1977.

12. Shils ME: A program for total parenteral nutrition at home. Am. J. Clin. Nutr. 28: 1429, 1975.

Advances in Psychologic Support

JIMMIE C. HOLLAND, M.D.

Chief, Psychiatry Service
Department of Neurology
Memorial Sloan-Kettering Cancer Center
New York, New York

Supportive care of cancer patients now includes increasing
attention to their psychologic wellbeing. This emphasis was
encouraged by the National Cancer Plan of 1970 which placed a
priority upon new research studies in rehabilitation and cancer control. In part as a consequence, information has accumulated over the past 10 years about the nature of the psychiatric and psychosocial problems which cancer patients experience. A range of supportive measures have also developed.
The composite of this information constitutes a developing new
subspecialty of psychiatric and psychosocial oncology. Typical
of a new field in which research methods are developing and
the problems are being defined, many studies have of necessity
been descriptive. A primary focus was required to delineate
and define the clinical problems. This review of recent advances in the psychologic area of supportive care outlines
three major areas: 1) the nature and prevalence of psychiatric syndromes in cancer patients; 2) current research in
specific psychologic problems of informed consent, coping
strategies, measurement of psychosocial variables; and 3) the
range and availability of psychologic supportive measures.

PSYCHIATRIC SYNDROMES IN CANCER

The increasing use of psychosocial and multidisciplinary
rounds and conferences, usually including the liaison psychiatric consultant to oncology units, is providing both clinical
experience and documentation of the day to day psychologic
problems and psychiatric syndromes seen in cancer patients.
The identification of the patient with psychologic difficulties is more readily apparent to staff when rounds include

discussion of psychologically difficult patients; appreciation
of the nature of a patient's psychologic problem promotes development of a therapeutic plan which can be more readily carried out by a clinic or ward staff.

It is clear that cancer diagnosis produces stress upon the
individual which relates both to the actual symptoms of the
disease and to the psychologic meaning that cancer carries.
The patient manages the stresses depending on prior level of
emotional adjustment, the presence of emotionally supportive
persons in his or her environment and the variables of symptoms, site and outcome which depend upon the disease and its
treatment (Holland, Mastrovito 1980). Any single significantly negative factor, or combination of these factors, places
the individual at higher risk of psychologic distress and possible decompensation. When the emotional distress exceeds
that which we identify as an expected "normal" level of distress associated with having cancer (a difficult problem to
assess in a physically ill person), the psychiatric symptoms
must be evaluated, and the type, severity, and need for treatment assessed. The clusters of symptoms make up the psychiatric syndromes in cancer.

These syndromes have been studied by the Memorial Hospital
Psychiatry Service by a review of the psychiatric consultations requested over the first year of a full time service.
(Massie et al, 1979). Five percent of new admissions were referred. Depression was the commonest diagnosis, present in
about half of the patients referred. Significantly, however,
the depression was usually regarded as a part of a stress response to the illness, that is, reactive depression. Infrequently was it severe enough to fall within the level of depression encountered in a psychiatric population. A review of
100 consecutive psychiatric consultations for cancer patients
at Dartmouth yielded similar data (Levine et al, 1979).

Anxiety was a frequent accompaniment of the depression in
many of the cancer patients. In the Memorial Hospital study,
anxiety was the primary diagnosis in 15% of patients referred.
It was predominantly, again, reactive to stress and was considered part of a stress response.

The second most common diagnosis in both studies mentioned
above was cerebral dysfunction, usually secondary to encepha-
lopathy associated with organ failure, metabolic derangement,
idiosyncratic response to a drug, or metastatic tumor spread.
These patients were the most frequently misdiagnosed by medical staff who did not recognize the changes in mental state
consistent with delirium.

The question of prevalence of significant depression in
hospitalized cancer patients who had not been referred for
psychiatric consultation was addressed last year by Bukberg at

Memorial Hospital (Bukberg et al, 1980). By interviewing
every fourth admission to two medical wards for a two month
period, and using depression scales and DSM-III clinical diagnostic criteria, 24% met criteria for significant depression;
another 18% had a dysphoric syndrome, but did not have clinical depression. Importantly, despite having cancer, 44% showed no depression at all. The more severely medically ill
tended to be those with more severe depression. These data
are consistent with the findings of Plumb and Holland in two
studies at Roswell Park which identified 20-25% of a randomly
selected cancer group as having significant depression (Plumb
and Holland, 1977). In summary, it would appear that up to a
quarter of cancer patients may be experiencing significant
emotional distress, largely depressive. However, in the two
studies of psychiatric consultations cited, the percent of
patients with depression who had been referred for consultation
was less than 3% of hospitalized patients. A study of psychotropic drug prescriptions in cancer patients found only 1% of
prescriptions were for antidepressants (Derogatis et al, 1979).

These studies of psychiatric consultations, prevalence of
depression, and treatment practices, in relation to antide-
pressant drug use have enabled us to recognize that a significant percent of cancer patients are depressed, yet many may go
unrecognized and their depressions are untreated. The need
for a prospective controlled study of antidepressants has been
recognized and is being pursued by the Psychosocial Collaborative Oncology Group (see Psychopharmacologic Management below).

The most commonly observed psychiatric syndromes in cancer
patients can be classified as follows:

1. Acute stress responses (reactive to illness)
   a. Reactive Depression
   b. Reactive Anxiety
2. Organic Mental Disorders
   a. Delirium
   b. Dementia
3. Major Psychiatric Disorders (antedating onset of cancer)
   a. Schizophrenia
   b. Affective Disorders
4. Psychiatric Emergencies
   a. Disruptive behavior (often related to delirium)
   b. Suicidal
   c. Homicidal
5. Anxiety Disorders
   a. Phobias related to illness (needles, hospitals)
   b. Panic Reactions

6. Somatoform Disorders
   a. Conversions, dissociative states
   b. Factitious
7. Psychosexual Disorders
   a. Adjustment reactions to illness resulting in sexual
      dysfunction (impotence, frigidity, fears)
   b. Adjustment reactions to sexual impairment resulting
      from cancer or treatment
8. Personality Disorders that Complicate Medical Management:
   Paranoid   Narcissistic
   Histrionic   Dependent
   Antisocial   Compulsive
   Schizoid   Introverted
   Borderline   Passive-aggressive

RESEARCH STUDIES IN SPECIFIC PSYCHOSOCIAL ISSUES

Doctor-patient Relationship and Acceptance of Treatment

The giving of informed consent to accept treatment by
chemotherapeutic agents that are investigational has been increasingly regulated to protect patients' rights. The requirements of current consent forms place great emphasis on
risks and side effects; considerably less emphasis is placed
on possible benefits. A study of 87 patients being treated
at 3 institutions represented in the Psychosocial Collaborative Oncology Group were questioned 1 to 3 weeks after accepting a new chemotherapy treatment, as to their recall and perception of the interview with the doctor in which they agreed
to treatment by a chemotherapy protocol and indicated acceptance by signing a form indicating their consent (Penman et al,
1980). The doctor's perception of the interview was also requested. The patients' answers reflected that greater than
80% of them recognized the seriousness of their illness and
uncertain outcome without treatment, and that they believed
that the proposed treatment offered hope of benefit to their
disease. Trust in the doctor was the most important reason
given for accepting treatment by 54% of the patients. Despite
the fact that protocols listed between 6 to 18 side effects
(mean of 11), at up to 3 weeks, patients remembered none at
all, or at most 6 (mean 3).

The study suggests that trust, fear and hope are the primary emotions of patients which weigh in the decision to
accept a new treatment; heavy reliance on the physician's
advice was evident. Much information was lost to memory at
3 weeks and the consent form was regarded by most as playing
little or no role in their decision to accept treatment.

These data indicate that current procedures which have evolved
in relation to largely legalistic protection of patient's
rights have failed to reflect adequate concern for the psychological parameters which influence acceptance of treatment.
The procedures should be reviewed to take into account this
parameter, as it becomes clearer that acceptance of more
treatments can result in cure.

Coping Strategies

The manner in which patients cope with cancer has an effect
upon their ability to maintain psychic equilibrium, and to
avoid emotional distress. Weiman and Sobel have studied which
coping strategies were effective and which proved to be ineffective, thus increasing the patient's vulnerability to psychologic distress (Weisman and Sobel, 1979). They are studying
the possibility that adaptive coping strategies may be taught
to patients. Penman found that women who demonstrated active
coping strategies which were apparent immediately after mastectomy had a better psychologic state at 4 months than those
women who had initially used passive, avoiding or capitulating
techniques (Penman, 1979). Clearly, irrespective of other contributing factors, the attitudes and behaviors which are used
to master the emotional crisis which cancer presents are important in psychologic outcome; they may be utilized in the
near future as helpful predictors to allow early intervention.

Measurement of Psychosocial Variables
in Multidisciplinary Research

A major drawback to more rigorous study of psychosocial and
psychiatric problems in cancer patients has been the dearth of
psychologic assessment techniques which could be used with
medically ill patients. The extensive assessment instruments
developed for evaluation of physically healthy but psychiatrically disturbed patients ordinarily are geared for evaluation of greater levels of psychopathological symptoms than
cancer patients exhibit, and they do not allow for consideration of the effects of medical illness which may produce spuri-
ous results with standard tests. Entirely new instruments
have had to be devised, tested and validated, along with
adapting instruments developed for use with psychiatric patients to this population. The Psychosocial Collaborative
Oncology Group, funded by the Division of Cancer Control and
Rehabilitation of the National Cancer Institute, has over the
past 3 years, identified this as a key psychosocial issue and
has directed studies toward development of psychologic instruments for assessment of cancer patients. Two studies have been

carried out using videotaped interviews of oncology staff with
cancer patients to identify the most useful brief global assessment instruments which could be used easily by busy oncology staff. Attention is also being given to development of a
brief and acceptable technique from which patients can provide
a ready self-assessment of their psychologic state.

The Cancer and Leukemia Group B, though its Psychiatry
Committee, has addressed the quantification of psychologic
data from which psychiatric and psychosocial variables can be
correlated with other clinical variables, particularly outcome
and treatment. (Holland, Bahna et al, 1980). The clinical
trial groups have traditionally monitored all aspects of tumor
response and toxicity, including neurotoxicity. However, the
"psychologic toxicity", the limiting effect which treatment
may have on psychosocial function, and how patients emotionally tolerate the therapy, have not been part of the assessment. Since psychiatry was added in the multimodality approach of Cancer and Leukemia Group B in 1976, data have been
collected in 10 protocols which now include evaluation of
psychosocial function. Two types of psychosocial data are
collected: observer (by the research nurse) report and self-
report (by the patient). The observer rates level of psychosocial function in three major areas: global, social and job.
The patients report their own psychologic function by means of
the Profile of Moods Scale, a brief adjective check list.
These simple "quality of life" measures are now numerically
entered into the data bank with other medical and treatment
variables which can be analyzed over time. Patients have
rarely refused to participate and overall, compliance is between 60-70% in the ongoing protocols. Preliminary data on
305 patients in 3 protocols demonstrated that psychosocial
function could be differentiated by treatment regimen, site,
disease stage and by treatment over time. Our current preliminary data suggest that psychologic and social function
during cancer treatment is quantifiable independently by
patient and staff, and that data can discriminate between
treatment regimens. The potential for correlation of psychologic and medical treatment variables will permit study of
patients who, stratified for disease and treatment, can be
assessed for level and type of psychologic adjustment and
coping techniques. It will then be possible to correlate
psychologic variables with response to cancer therapy. The
question frequently raised of whether psychologic state contributes to response to treatment can be answered in the near
future with the availability of multidisciplinary studies
which include psychiatric assessment. New supportive measures
can also be tested for effectiveness in patients who are stratified and receiving identical therapeutic regimens.

The potential value from adding psychosocial variables to multidisciplinary clinical trials research is just beginning to be recognized. The need exists for a system to test supportive methods in the psychologic area since currently, much is being made of relaxation, visual imagery and personality factors as influences upon survival, yet most of these studies have not taken into account the uncontrolled treatment and tumor variables which could account for any observed differences in outcome, which may be ascribed incorrectly to psychologic differences or interventions.

STATUS OF PSYCHOLOGIC SUPPORTIVE MEASURES

Stage and Site-Related Psychosocial Interventions

Terminal Care
Many psychosocial supportive measures have developed to aid patients at a specific stage of cancer, or with problems resulting from a specific tumor and its treatment. The most notable of the stage-specific interventions is the hospice movement, which, following the European model, has attempted to provide more humane care for terminally ill patients. The approach combines development of special care units and support for families in caring for their dying relative at home. Inadequate financial support has been available to explore these alternatives to hospital care. A current evaluation of hospice units, with a view to establishing reimbursement rates, may begin to address this issue. Better insurance plans for home-related care would also encourage families to accept the burden of home care. A change in emphasis is needed in oncology centers to develop active home care programs; oncology nurses are particularly adept at management of pain through home visits, with telephone consultation from the responsible physician who has managed the patient through his or her illness and can offer most appropriate medical and emotional support.

Self-Help Care
Self-help groups have been an important recent development. They are focused in two ways: those which related to help for patients with the same stage of cancer, as represented by the Make Today Count and, the Cured Cancer Club, (perhaps the earliest of these groups in the 1950s). Other groups relate to support of patients with specific tumors and treatment, represented by Reach to Recovery for mastectomy patients, groups for laryngectomees and their families, and Ostomy clubs. Some groups have been developed which relate by age -- teenage can-

cer groups. Surviving spouses have also formed groups for mutual help. The permutations seem as endless and as varied as
the range of problems which bring persons toward a shared
identity when they have like problems, and mutually can seek
solutions to the difficulties encountered. The consensus is
that, far from being detrimental, as often feared in the past,
groups provide important support which can only be appreciated
by those who have shared the same experience.

A modification of this model has been evolving at Memorial
Hospital where "veteran patients" with tumors of various
sites have given their time as volunteers to work with a core
of professionals from psychiatry and social work. The opportunity to support one another in assuming a counseling role
with other patients has appeared valuable, as well as beginning to evaluate novel and useful counseling approaches (Mastrovito, Moynihan, Lee, Fisher, 1980).

Psychotherapeutic interventions are based on a crisis-in-
tervention model aimed at helping the patient to retain his or
her sense of self esteem and worth, and to offer emotional
support with insight into adaptation to perceived losses associated with cancer and its treatment.

Interventions increasingly include the significant other
relative, the person who is key to social support. The evidence for positive value in both medical outcome and in retained sense of well-being can be found in literature from other
medical areas; the conclusions may be applicable with equal
assurance to cancer patients.

Psychopharmacologic Management

The psychiatric syndromes outlined above are often best
managed by a combined psychotherapeutic and psychopharmacologic approach. Gorzynski, Massie and Holland have outlined the
use of the major psychotropic drugs in the psychiatric syndromes often seen in cancer patients (Gorzynski, Massie, Holland, 1980). The acute stress responses, characterized by depression and/or anxiety, are managed by directing attention to
treatment of the predominant symptoms. It has been the experience of the Psychiatry Service that reactively depressed patients respond well to low doses of antidepressants in the
same pattern that would be expected in psychiatrically depressed patients, and often more rapidly and at lower doses.
When sedating effects are desired, amitriptyline is the drug
of choice; when stimulating effects for a retarded depression
are desired, then imipramine or desipramine are indicated.
The anxiolytic drugs, diazepam and Chlordiazepoxide, are giv-
en in dose levels sufficient to control distressing anxiety.
Some newer agents, such as doxepin, are useful in control of

combined anxiety and depressive symptoms.

Disruptive behavior related to delirium is managed by small doses of haloperidol or trifluoperazine, given by mouth, if possible. For acutely disturbed behavior, haloperidol can be given intramuscularly or intravenously at a rate not exceeding 1 mg per minute up to 5 mg. Haloperidol is preferable to phenothiazines in part because of the low frequency of hypotension and cardio-vascular effects.

When a patient with cancer has a history of schizophrenia or manic-depressive disorder, the medication on which they have been maintained should be continued, since they are at risk of exacerbation of their psychiatric illness resulting from attempts to adapt to the stress imposed by cancer therapy. Lithium can be successfully continued, monitoring in the same way for side effects and blood level. Phenothiazines should be used in effective doses to control schizophrenic symptoms with medical management by the oncologist and the psychiatrist serving as consultant.

Behavioral Approach

Hypnosis appears, especially in children, to have a role in pain control, and possibly in stimulation of appetite and promotion of a sense of well-being.

Relaxation techniques to reduce tension and anxiety have a role in patients who find these approaches helpful. These techniques combined with behavior modification, may be helpful in diminishing the conditioned nausea and vomiting of chemotherapy when it occurs prior to therapy.

SUMMARY

Patients with cancer today experience more attention to their psychologic state and optimal well-being despite illness. Psychiatric syndromes common in cancer have been delineated and management principles developed. A range of specific psychosocial issues have been studied: doctor-patient interaction around informed consent, identification of adaptive coping strategies and development of psychologic assessment techniques for patients with cancer to enhance the potential for collaborative research. Psychologic supportive measures have developed for stage and site-related self-help, veteran patient counseling, and psychotherapeutic, psychopharmacologic and behavioral interventions. In the 1980's psychosocial research area should increase in quality with development of more effective psychosocial interventions which can be tested in clinical trials.

REFERENCES

1. Bukberg, J.B., and Holland, J.C. A prevalence study of
    depression in a cancer hospital. (Abstract) Proceedings
    of AACR and ASCO, (ASCO), 1980, 21, 382.
2. Derogatis, L.R., Feldstein, M., Morrow, G., Schmale, A.,
    Schmitt, M., Gates, C., Murawski, B., Holland, J.,
    Penman, D., Malisaratos, Enelow, A.J., and Adler, L.M.
    A survey of psychotropic drug prescriptions in an oncol-
    ogy population. Cancer, 1979, 44, 1919-1929.
3. Gorzynski, G., Massie, M.J., Holland, J. Diagnosis and
    management of psychiatric syndromes in cancer patients.
    In L. Derogatis (Ed.), Psychopharmacology in clinical
    practice. Addison-Wesley Press, 1980, in press.
4. Holland, J., Bahna, G., McKegney, P., Silberfarb, P.,
    Tross, S. and Glidewell, O. Psychiatric research in
    mutli-modal cancer clinical trials in CALGB. (Abstract)
    Proceedings of AACR and ASCO (ASCO), 1980, 21, 354.
5. Holland, J. and Mastrovito, R. Psychologic adaptation to
    breast cancer. Cancer, 1980, 46, 187-194.
6. Levine, P.M., Silberfarb, P.M. and Lipowski, Z.J. Mental
    disorders in cancer patients, a study of 100 psychiatric
    referrals. Cancer, 1978, 42, 1385-1391.
7. Massie, M.J., Gorzynski, G., Mastrovito, R., Theis, D.,
    and Holland, J. The diagnosis of depression in hospital-
    ized patients with cancer. Proceedings of AACR and ASCO,
    (Abstract), 1979, 20, 432.
8. Mastrovito, R., Moynihan, R., Lee, J., Fisher, R. The
    veteran patient counseling program. National Conference
    on Rehabilitation, 1980, Williamsburg, Va.
9. Penman, D. Coping strategies in adaptation to mastectomy.
    Unpublished doctoral dissertation, 1979, Yeshiva Univer-
    sity, New York.
10. Penman, D., Bahna, G., Holland, J.C., Morrow, G., Morse,
    I., Schmale, A., and Derogatis, L. Patients' perception
    of giving informed consent for investigational chemo-
    therapy. (Abstract) Proceedings of AACR and ASCO (AACR)
    1980, 21, 188.
11. Weisman, A.D. and Sobel, H.J. Coping with cancer through
    self-instruction: a hypothesis. Journal of Human Stress
    1979, 5(1), 3-8.

Critical Care of the Cancer Patient

GRAZIANO C. CARLON, M.D.

Clinical Chief
Department of Critical Care
Memorial Sloan-Kettering Cancer Center
New York, New York   10021

Before considering clinical aspects of intensive care in a cancer institution, some philosophical considerations are necessary. In a world of limited resources, equitable distribution of a commodity as precious as life support represents a staggering ethical problem. In the belief that a strictly pragmatic approach represents the best solution, all patients admitted to our Institution are classified into four categories, according to their disease status;[1] unlimited life support is provided to those in the first two groups, while those in the fourth group only receive pain medications and supportive measures to provide maximum comfort. The third category is that of patients with unfavorable short term prognosis who have received experimental chemotherapy. This group reflects the human and clinical need for flexibility, when the chances of a patient's survival are small, but the efficacy of a new therapy which could benefit many, must be fully tested. We do not mean that a patient should needlessly suffer, so that information useful to others be obtained; rather, when experimental therapy has been administered, we feel morally obliged to support the patient through its complications. On occasion patients have survived dire side effects of new drugs, and recovered completely cured of their underlying neoplasm. It is apparent that in such cases refusal of exceptional therapy on the ground that it would have prolonged misery rather than life would have been unjustified.

A basic distinction should be drawn between a critically ill patient, who also has a neoplastic disease, and the individual who has developed a life-threatening complication because of cancer or its therapy.

For instance, the care of a patient with an early stage of a
colon carcinoma who is admitted to an Intensive Care Unit with
severe head injury need not take into account the presence of a
neoplastic disease. On the other hand, respiratory support for
a patient who has received bleomycin, alkylating agents or
radiation therapy may differ substantially from that applied to
other forms of respiratory failure.[2,3] Time limitation prevents discussion of all aspects of management of critically ill
cancer patient. I will therefore address some of the more
serious problems that set cancer patients apart from other
critically ill individuals.

Respiratory Failure

The most common causes of respiratory failure in a general
ICU are sepsis, trauma and massive hemorrhage. Through a final
common pathway of injury, pulmonary capillary permeability
increases, fluids accumulate in the loose perialveolar interstitial space, proteinaceous material accumulates within the
alveoli, surfactant production ceases and Type II alveolar
pneumocytes are replaced by immature forms of Type I pneumocytes. The result is increased lung weight and decreased lung
compliance and lung volume. In most cases, application of
positive end-expiratory pressure restores lung volume at higher
transpulmonary pressure, providing proper matching of ventilation and perfusion.[4]
In cancer patients, the major sources of acute respiratory
failure are sepsis during episodes of neutropenia, lung-
specific drug toxicity, intrapulmonary hemorrhage and hypersensitivity pneumonitis. Although some recent evidence suggests that complement mediated leukoagglutination plays an
important role in the development of pulmonary infiltrates,[5] it
is apparent that alternative mechanisms must exist, since
diffuse bilateral infiltrates develop in patients with absolute
polymorphonuclear counts of less than 100 cells/mm^3. Regardless of the mechanism, the limitations of therapy of
respiratory failure associated with sepsis in neutropenic patients are severe. In as many as 50% of the patients, we are
unable to determine an etiologic diagnosis. Usually, broad
spectrum antibiotic coverage is initiated when temperature
increases above 38° in patients with less than 1,000 polymorphonuclear cells. Accordingly, subsequent blood cultures
and sputum cultures are usually negative, even though some
parts of the lungs or of other organs may harbor infectious
agents not exposed to adequate concentration of antibiotics.
In some patients the etiology of pulmonary infiltrates may be
viral; rapid diagnosis is then usually impossible and causal
therapy non-existent.

Supportive measures are limited to mechanical ventilation and empiric antibiotic treatment. When fever does not subside or respiratory failure is not improved within a few days despite broad spectrum antibiotic therapy, intravenous antifungal agents (Amphotericin B) are added. Intravenous sulfamethoxazole is also given if the clinical history is suggestive of Pneumocystis Carini pneumonia (Hodgkin's disease, long-term steroid therapy). Transfusion of white cells is only administered when an etiologic microbial agent is positively identified. We have observed transient deterioration of respiratory function, with increase of pulmonary artery mean pressure and peak inspiratory pressure immediately after white cell transfusion. This event represents agglutination of white cells activated by the plastic container in the pulmonary capillaries. This reaction is uncommon and rarely severe or prolonged; in susceptible patients, increasing PEEP by 3-5 cmH_2O for 2-3 hours after white cell transfusion eliminates the detrimental effects of leukoagglutination on capillary permeability and lung volume. Regardless of the etiologic agents of the respiratory failure, survival of the patients is strictly a function of recovery of hematopoeitic function.

Bleomycin, alkylating agents, methotrexate and radiation therapy represent the forms of cancer therapy more commonly associated with lung damage.[6]

Bilateral infiltrates, usually localized at the basis of the lung can develop after therapy with the antineoplastic antibiotic bleomycin.[7] Although the pulmonary disease is usually benign, there is no specific therapy, if severe respiratory failure develops. The development of pulmonary toxicity after bleomycin therapy is more common with doses exceeding 350 mg/m^2. However, much larger doses have been administered with impunity, while severe infiltrates have been reported after less than 100 mg/m^8. Prevention appears the best approach to bleomycin lung injury. Determination of forced vital capacity and carbon monoxide diffusion are sensitive early tests of developing lung injury. Development of combined restrictive and obstructive lung disease, with decreased diffusion capacity mandates discontinuation of the drug. Although spirometric and diffusion studies normalize within 4-12 months after termination of bleomycin therapy, many reports exist of continued sensitivity to non-specific noxious agents. Exposure to high oxygen concentration, massive transfusions, prolonged surgical procedures have resulted in respiratory failure in patients who had received bleomycin many months before.[2,9] Bilateral confluent pulmonary infiltrates rapidly progress in the absence of positive sputum cultures or febrile episodes. Death usually occurs within 5-10 days, regardless of the degree of respiratory support. In a series of patients we studied, 5 of 17 patients with dysgerminonas, who had received large doses of bleomycin ($>$ 500 mg/m^2) 8-12 months before a surgical procedure for removal of retroperitoneal lymphnodes, died of respiratory failure in the postoperative period. In each case, the higher intraoperative F_{IO_2} administered to the patients who had died seemed a major contributing factor.[2] Since then, the policy at our Institution has been to manage all patients who have received $>$ 300 mg/m^2 of bleomycin with $F_{IO_2} <$ .35 intra- and postoperatively, and to carefully monitor their fluid balance. Methotrexate has been associated with development of lung infiltrates and a pathologic picture of non-desquamating interstitial pneumonia and non-caseating granulomas.[10] Usually self-limited, this form of lung injury rarely requires intensive care.

A more severe lung damage may follow therapy with alkylating agents and irradiation. Ionizing radiation may cause acute pneumonia during the course of therapy, especially when single doses $>$ 500 rads are applied to pulmonary fields. More frequently, infiltrates accompanied by fever and marked respiratory distress develop 3-9 months after a course of radiation therapy.[11] Sometimes, bilateral infiltrates may follow unilateral irradiation, "mantle" therapy to the supraclavicular region or radiation of the mediastinum.[12] An hypothesis explaining the diffuse pulmonary injury resulting from a limited area of direct insult suggests that bradykinins and/or prostagladins are released from the areas of the lung primarily affected, ultimately altering capillary permeability in both lungs. Accumulation of proteinaceous material in the interstitium of the lung and enhanced proliferation of fibroblasts follow. Hyaluronic acid, secreted by the fibroblasts, increases the oncotic activity of interstitial lung fluids, further aggravating fluid extravasation from the capillaries. Fibroblastic proliferation results in pulmonary fibrosis. An additional observation is that after exposure to radiation therapy alveolar cells may become unable to synthetize reducing enzymes, such as peroxidase or superoxide dismutase. High energy radicals cannot be eliminated, and their accumulation results in damage to phospholipidic membranes (lipid peroxidation), compromising cellular integrity.[13]

Similar damages are observed after therapy with alkylating agents, especially busulfan, which is associated with irreversible lung fibrosis that sometimes develops insidiously over many years.[14]

The critical care physician must provide respiratory support to patients who develop acute respiratory failure, requiring mechanical ventilation, after exposure to radiation or alkylating agents. Pulmonary fibrosis, a consequence of chemotherapy and radiation, primarily affects the loose interstitial collagen, which provides the greatest lung distensibility and elastic recoil. The tight collagen surrounding the alveoli has an elastic module of 1.5-2 only, so that it cannot be stretched to more than twice its original length without severe loss in compliance and elastic recoil as in an overstretched spring, so that expiration requires active effort.[15] In such patients PEEP, the single most important therapy for many forms of acute respiratory failure may not be effective, since lung volume cannot be increased; indeed, overdistension of the lung will actually increase the expiratory work of breathing. Since the degree of fibrosis of different areas of the lungs often varies, the stress applied to the lung structures during positive pressure ventilation readily results in barotrauma (pneumothorax, pneumomediastinum, intrapulmonary air dissection). To further complicate the problem, when acute infection precipitates the respiratory failure, ventilation without PEEP cannot maintain the function of those parts of the lung, which are affected by the infectious process more severely than by fibrosis.

A special case of this problem is represented by patients who have received homologous bone marrow transplantation. They usually receive total body irradiation and high doses of cyclophosphamide. Three-to-six months after the transplant, when the hematopoietic function has resumed but B-lymphocyte activity is still depressed, some patients develop acute respiratory failure. We have observed six such cases in the last three years. In each instance, a definite etiology for the pulmonary infiltrates could not be identified, despite open lung biopsy in four patients. Acute viral titers were elevated in one patient suggesting adenovirus infection, and herpetic pneumonia seemed a strong possibility in a second. In yet another patient, respiratory failure followed therapy for pneumococcal meningitis. In all cases, respiratory failure was a consequence of the lung damage caused by radiation therapy and alkylating agents, complicated by precipitation in the lung capillaries of insoluble immunocomplexes in a situation of overwhelming antigenic predominance.

The pathological picture demonstrated by the lung biopsy was that of an acute inflammatory reaction of the interstitial space, alveolar flooding with monocytes and marked lung fibrosis. The predicament of patients with this clinical picture is exemplified in Figure 1. Normally in acute respiratory failure pulmonary venous admixture decreases with application of PEEP. In many cases a critical value must be reached before large groups of alveoli are recruited to ventilation, so that oxygenation may improve. Occasionally, arterial blood gases only improve when PEEP levels of 30-40 cmH$_2$0 are reached.[16] In patients with lung fibrosis combined with acute infection, however, PEEP therapy can be unsuccessful. Although pulmonary shunt fraction initially decreases when PEEP is applied, a point is rapidly reached when further increases of PEEP result in higher peak inspiratory pressure without improvement in venous admixture. In most patients, barotrauma develops and death rapidly follows.

Pneumocystis carinii pneumonia is another cause of severe respiratory failure in adult cancer patients, that poses considerable therapeutic problems. A recently completed survey at our Institution suggests that the reduction in mortality for Pneumocystis pneumonia observed in recent years is a function of greater awareness and earlier recognition, rather than im- proved therapy.[17] When respiratory failure develops, mortality is extremely high; indeed in the last 15 years none of the pa-

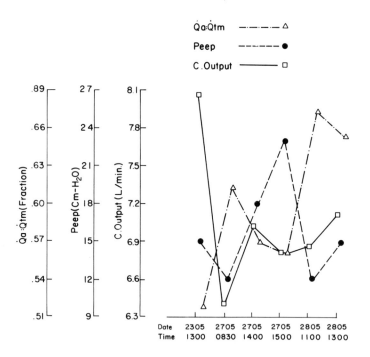

Figure 1. Changes of pulmonary venous admixture (Q̇a:Q̇t), positive end-expiratory pressure (PEEP) and cardiac output in a patient with severe lung fibrosis and acute respiratory fail- ure. Increasing PEEP initially resulted in decreased venous admixture, at constant cardiac output. Further increase in PEEP, however, did not improve shunt fraction.

tients who required > 5 days of mechanical ventilation, or PEEP
>10 cmH$_2$0 survived, regardless of the type of respiratory
support. The course of the disease was characterized by early
improvement with PEEP therapy, followed by development of
elevated peak inspiratory pressures with barotrauma as the most
common terminal complication.

In an attempt to solve some of the problems described, we
have been experimenting with a new type of mechanical support,
high frequency jet ventilation (HFJV), which maintains alveolar
ventilation without increasing airway pressure.[18] Initial clinical experience has been limited to preterminal patients, a
sort of Phase I trial for the device; within the limit
associated with such a poor risk population, initial results
appeared encouraging.[19] We are now beginning a more extensive
trial, randomizing patients who require high peak inspiratory
pressure on mechanical ventilation either to conventional
mechanical support or HFJV. We hope to demonstrate a reduced
incidence of pulmonary disruption on HFJV, thanks to lower
inspiratory pressures and a decrease of the fibroblastic
proliferation which is associated with high distending airway
pressure.

Intrapulmonary hemorrhage is a potentially lethal complication of thrombocytopenia and other coagulation abnormalities that follow chemotherapy. The diagnosis is sometimes
difficult, since rusty sputum or frank hemoptisis may be absent
and the radiographic picture is undistinguishable from that of
diffuse patchy bilateral infiltrates.[20] Fever may be absent or
follow, rather than precede, the development of infiltrates.
These patients often respond favorably to PEEP and mechanical
support, as long as hemorrhages can be controlled. Aggressive
transfusion therapy with platelets and coagulation factors is
necessary. By increasing intra-alveolar pressures, mechanical
ventilation with PEEP may be helpful in decreasing the rate of
bleeding. However, some caution is necessary, since PEEP may
have unpredictable effects on interstitial lung pressure. When
lungs are hyperinflated, PEEP may actually cause negative
interstitial pressure at the end of inspiration.[21] Furthermore, in order to significantly increase intrapleural pressure,
a higher PEEP than that necessary to restore lung volume must be
applied. Accordingly, impairment of cardiac function may
occur. In general, however, patients who respond positively to
mechanical support, and do not have repeated bleeding episodes,
have a benign course.

In addition to those with specific lung toxicity, an extraordinary variety of chemotherapeutic agents have been associated with hypersensitivity reaction. Bleomycin, methotrexate, nitrogen mustard, cyclophosphamide, more recently 2,3

deoxycuphramycin; the list of drugs that may cause allergic reactions in the lungs is continuously expanding.[14]   The clinical picture is characterized by rapidly evolving pulmonary infiltrates, hardly distinguishable from those of other forms of acute respiratory failure. A history of recent exposure to a chemotherapeutic agent is of course the most relevant element for diagnosis. Usually, the epidose follows the administration of a new substance by 1-7 days. Pathognomic features, such as high concentration of eosinophils or increased IgG immuno-globins in the sputum may be absent in pancytopenic patients or in those with depressed humoral immunity.   Frequently, the diagnosis is only tentative and confirmation can be obtained by response to empirical therapy (discontinuation of the offending agents, high dose corticosteroids).

In this review, I have only addressed some of the respiratory problems that are unique to cancer patients. I have concentrated on the lungs, as the organ whose failure more commonly requires extreme supportive measures. All intensive care physicians should be aware of the severe complications that cancer therapy can cause.

REFERENCES

1. Turnbull AD, Carlon GC, Baron R et al: The inverse relationship between cost and survival. Crit Care Med 7:30, 1979.
2. Goldiner PL, Carlon GC, Cvitkovic E et al: Factors influencing postoperative morbidity and mortality in patients treated with bleomycin. Brit Med J 1:1664, 1978.
3. Carlon GC: Respiratory failure in cancer patients. Curr Prob in Cancer 4:3:47, 1979.
4. Gallagher TJ, Civetta JM, Kirby RR: Terminology update: optimal PEEP. Crit Care Med 6:323, 1978.
5. Hammerschmnidt DE, Weaver LJ, Hudson LD et al: Association of complement activation and elevated Plasma C50 with adult respiratory distress syndrome. The Lancet 1:947, 1980.
6. Friedman MA, Carter JB: Serious toxicities associated with chemotherapy. Semin Oncol 5:193, 1978.
7. Luna MA, Bedrosian CWM, Lichtiger B et al: Interstitial pneumonitis associated with bleomycin therapy. Am J Clin Path 58:501, 1972.
8. Iacovino JR, Leitner J, Abhas AK et al: Fatal pulmonary reaction from low doses of bleomycin. JAMA 235:1253, 1976.
9. Nygaard K, Smith-Ericksen N, Hatleran R et al: Pulmonary complications after bleomycin, irradiation and surgery for esophageal cancer. Cancer 41:17, 1978.
10. Claysse RM, Cathey WI, Cartwright GF et al: Pulmonary disease complicating intermittent therapy with methotrexate. JAMA 209:1861, 1969.
11. Braun SR, Dopico A, Olsen OE et al: Low dose radiation pneumonitis. Cancer 35:1322, 1978.
12. Cohen Y, Gelle B, Robinson E: Bilateral radiation pneumonitis after unilateral lung and mediastinal irradiation. Radiol Clin Biol 43:465, 1974.
13. McCord JM, Fridovich I: The biology and pathology of oxygen radicals. Ann Int Med 89:122, 1975.
14. Rosenow EC III: The spectrum of drug-induced lung disease. Ann Int Med 77:971, 1972.
15. Peters RM: Pulmonary physiology studies in the perioperative period. Chest 76:5, 1979.
16. Kirby RE, Downs JB, Civetta JM et al: High level positive end-expiratory pressure (PEEP) in acute respiratory insufficiency. Chest 67:156, 1975.
17. Carlon GC, Turnbull AD, Parker S et al: Respiratory failure in Pneumocystis Carinii Pneumonia. Crit Care Med 8:238, 1980.
18. Sjostrand U: High frequency positive pressure ventilation (HFPPV): A review. Crit Care Med 8:345, 1980.

19. Carlon GC, Ray C, Klain M et al: High frequency positive
    pressure ventilation in a patient with bronchopleural
    fistula. Anesthesiology 52:160, 1980.
20. Thomas HM, Irwin RS: Classification of diffuse in-
    trapulmonary hemorrhage. Chest 68:483, 1975.
21. Caldini P, Leith JD, Brennan MJ: Effect of continuous
    positive pressure ventilation (CPPV) on edema formation in
    dog lung. J Appl Physiol 39:672, 1975.

Cancer Control

The Role
Of The Hospital Cancer Program
In Cancer Control

ROBERT J. McKENNA, M.D.

Clinical Professor of Surgery, USC
Director of Regional Activities
LAC-USC Comprehensive Cancer Center
Los Angeles, California

The goal of every cancer control program should be to decrease the morbidity and mortality of all patients with cancer. Almost all cancer is initially either diagnosed in, or treated in a hospital, often in the facility nearest the patient's home. The hospital is the logical setting where the majority of cancer control activities should be centered since cancer management is best accomplished by an interaction of a multidisciplinary physician group of surgical, radiation, and medical oncologists, with the assistance of the primary physician, oncologic nurses, social workers, physiatrists, rehabilitationists, etc.

A Hospital Cancer Program is intended to encourage the proper atmosphere and organization within each institution to deliver optimal care for the cancer patient. In special situations this will include the referral of some cancer patients to more specialized cancer-treating centers. Each hospital should be responsible for its own attending staff educational programs, quality-care evaluation, and the monitoring of its own experiences in the treatment of cancer patients. Included in a complete Hospital Cancer Program is a

cancer data base or registry which may be used for medical
resource planning, physician education and research, as well
as encouraging the systematic life-time re-examination of
cancer patients.

At this time in the United States, there are 864 hospitals
with approved cancer programs; this represents 14.6% of all
hospitals in the United States, but more importantly, 32.1% of
all hospital beds in the United States. The most important
figure is that currently 54.3% of all new cancer cases in the
United States are seen in hospitals with approved cancer programs. These approved hospitals are located in 49 states
(none in Nevada) and in the District of Columbia and Puerto
Rico (1). The Western and Eastern areas of the United States
have the largest percent of approved hospital cancer programs
(Table 1-1).

TABLE 1-1
Percent Approved Hospital Cancer Programs
By Hospital Bed Size and Region of the United States

Area	500+	400-499	300-399	200-299
Western	63	62	58	32
Eastern	54	50	45	27
Southern	46	42	24	13
Mid-Western	53	31	29	19

The approval of a Hospital Cancer Program assures that the
necessary program elements are established and are functioning
at a satisfactory level, thereby meeting certain minimal requirements. However, each institution should strive to exceed

these requirements in order to benefit from an optimal program.
The approval process is carried on by the Commission on Cancer
of the American College of Surgeons, and is co-sponsored with
the two co-sponsors of this meeting, namely, the American
Cancer Society, Inc. and the National Cancer Institute.

HISTORY OF THE
HOSPITAL CANCER PROGRAM

The Cancer Program of the American College of Surgeons was
instituted in 1932 to improve the care of the patient with
cancer at the hospital level. From 1932 to 1952, cancer
programs were primarily concerned with the establishment of
cancer clinics directed toward the diagnosis and treatment of
indigent patients. In 1956, cancer registries were incor-

porated in the Hospital Cancer Program enabling hospitals to
document their results in the diagnosis and management of all
cancer patients. In 1966, multidisciplinary cancer conferences and/or tumor boards were added to the hospital cancer program, and in 1976, patient-care evaluation studies were
also made a part of the approval requirement.

The Commission on Cancer

In 1963 appropriate cancer management was recognized to be
a multidisciplinary activity and membership in the Cancer
Commission was expanded. Presently, there are 23 representatives of organizations other than the American College of
Surgeons serving on the Commission on Cancer. At the present
time, two-thirds of the members of the Approvals Committee
of the Commission on Cancer are non-surgeons, emphasizing that
this program is no longer the exclusive program of its founder,
the American College of Surgeons, but of the Commission on
Cancer with representation from all organizations involved in
cancer management.

Since 1932, the American Cancer Society has provided financial support for the Hospital Cancer Program. Since 1957
the National Institute of Health has done likewise. Funding
at the present time for the administration of this program is
approximately one-third from the American Cancer Society, one-
third from the National Cancer Institute, and one-third from
the American College of Surgeons.

It is important to emphasize that participation in the Hospital Cancer Program is strictly voluntary and is designed
primarily to improve the care of the patient with cancer at
the hospital level. It should be emphasized that the
Commission on Cancer does not tell physicians how to treat
their patients, and does not measure or rate the quality of
cancer care in each hospital. The Commission does insist
that each Cancer Committee oversees cancer management in the
hospital, and measures the quality of its cancer care.

The Cancer Committee

The Cancer Program leadership rests with the Cancer Committee Chairman and the multidisciplinary Cancer Committee.
The membership of the Committee should include credentialed
representatives from all medical specialities involved in
the care of the cancer patient, within the limits of those
disciplines available to the institution. The Committee
should also include members from hospital administration,
nursing service, rehabilitation, and the cancer registry.
Ideally, the tumor registrar should serve as a cancer program

coordinator.

The Cancer Committee's duties are to plan, initiate, supervise, and evaluate all cancer activities in the hospital. The Committee must insure that patients have access to consultative services in all disciplines. The Cancer Committee is responsible for assuring that educational programs, conferences, and other clinical activities cover the entire spectrum of cancer. The Cancer Committee must actively supervise the cancer data base for quality control of abstracting, staging, and reporting of all cancer cases in the hospital. The Cancer Committee should provide cancer care audits, either directly or by reviewing audit data supplied by other committees regarding cancer patient care.

Cancer Conferences. Patient oriented, multidisciplinary cancer conferences or tumor boards can improve the care of patients with cancer within an institution through education. These conferences should be multidisciplinary and should involve all hospital departments in one common setting. Physicians in training, students, health professionals, and other cancer-related personnel are encouraged to attend these meetings. Over the course of a year, conferences should cover all the major cancer sites. These conferences should be held at least monthly in the smallest hospital and with greater frequency in the larger hospitals. In the large teaching hospitals, at least weekly conferences should be held, and in the largest centers, including the Comprehensive Cancer Centers, meetings will often be daily. These larger institutions may hold site-oriented conferences such as head and neck, bone and soft part, GU, GYN, etc., tumor conferences which must be multidisciplinary. Although differing opinions may be expressed by the many disciplines attending the conferences, the ultimate therapeutic decision should rest with the referring physician.

Patient Care Evaluation. A basic requirement of the approved cancer program is a system of patient-care evaluation with documentation of its operation. This evaluation should be a meaningful review of the hospital's process (short-term) and outcome (long-term) patient-care studies covering a variety of cancer sites. Should these audits be done by others than the Cancer Committee, it is the duty of the Cancer Committee to review the findings and to analyze their results and implement appropriate educational and other measures to correct any deficiencies.

Cancer Patient End Results Reporting. The objective of a cancer data system (registry) is to improve cancer management by acquiring, organizing, analyzing, and interpreting information on all cancer patients in the hospital. In order to be effective, the registry must have the support and supervision of a well organized, enthusiastic Cancer Committee and the endorsement of the medical staff, and the governing body of the hospital. The Cancer Committee is responsible for the

technical supervision of the cancer registry, including development, organization, utilization, continuity, quality control, and data analysis. The hospital administrator or his representative on the Cancer Committee should provide administrative supervision for the registry. Approximately 75% of cancer registries are manually operated with the remainder computerized. Computerization does not make a registry better, but can be cost-effective and make utilization of registry data more accessible and feasible.

All cancer cases diagnosed, either clinically or histologically, and/or treated in the hospital (both inpatient and outpatient) must be recorded in the registry. It is not required that basal cell or squamous cell carcinomas of the skin be included. A brief registry abstract of the hospital medical record should include specific core information, including the extent of the disease, treatment, and type of rehabilitation.

A follow-up system is essential to assure that the patient continues to see his or/her physician for examinations at intervals after treatment and to record any evidence of recurrent or continuing disease, further treatments given, and the quality of patient survival.

The annual report of the Cancer Committee to the hospital staff and administration should contain a narrative by the

Committee describing the activity and goals of the cancer program, a summary of the registry activity, and an in-depth report of at least one major cancer site complete with survival data and critique. The registry should be used for reports at staff conferences and for the preparation of

manuscripts for publication where appropriate.

Benefit of Hospital Cancer Program. The Cancer Program is an integral function of all hospitals electing to treat cancer patients and the cost of its operation is considered to be a reimbursable item in the administrative budget.

The benefits of a Hospital Cancer Program may be summarized as follows: *For the patient* the program promotes continuous care through follow-up with the potential for cure if recurrent or metastatic tumors are detected. It assures that a summary abstract can be easily forwarded to another treatment facility, if necessary, should the patient elect

to transfer to another institution. It encourages screening
for a second cancer and it helps to identify complications of
primary cancer treatment. *For the physician* the Hospital
Cancer Program encourages multidisciplinary consultations,
assistance with the management of the problem case, as well
as a continuing update through continuing education
of newer modalities of cancer therapy. *The housestaff* may
be assured that educational activities are optimized, and
that a data base is available for research and preparation
of scientific papers. *For the hospital administrator* the
Hospital Cancer Program provides the data base for resource
planning, facility renovation and expansion, and the
assurance that optimal cancer care is possible in their hospital. *The nursing service* benefits by a Hospital Cancer
Program by better facilities, quality patient care, the
establishment of oncology units, and continuing educational
opportunities. *The community* benefits by a Hospital Cancer
Program by the provision of optimal diagnostic and
treatment facilities as well as health education in prevention
and screening. *Everyone* benefits by evaluating treatment
results of cancer care in the hospital with the outcome that
areas which need improvement are identified. *The American
Cancer Society* often provides considerable assistance to the
Hospital Cancer Programs by program funding, assistance with
service and rehabilitation, and often with professional
education and research.

CHALLENGE FOR THE 80's

The minimum requirements of the Hospital Cancer Program are
constantly updated by the Commission on Cancer. A new manual
for operation is presently being printed and will outline
the direction that this program is expected to take in the
coming years (2). It is expected in the 80's that each
clinical program will be expanded to include appropriate
activities in cancer prevention, screening, diagnosis, treatment, follow-up, rehabilitation, and continuing care.
In the areas of prevention it is hoped that active involvement in smoking cessation clinics and patient health
education, especially as it relates to cancer, will be undertaken. In the areas of screening it is hoped that high-
risk groups will be offered special detection programs.
High-risk groups include those who are not in the mainstream
of health care, those who are at high risk to develop cancer
of the cervix, breast, colon, and thyroid because of a family
history of cancer, etc., as well as those individuals at high

risk to develop cancer because of their occupation. Health
fairs based at a community hospital can serve both an
educational and a screening function.
     Improved diagnostic activities should include more careful
treatment evaluation with appropriate staging, using the AJC

(American Joint Committee) classification where practical.
Professional education through conferences and tumor boards
is a mechanism by which updated cancer knowledge may be made
available to the medical staff. Improved hospital resources
for both diagnosis and treatment must be planned for by the
Cancer Committee working in consortium with the hospital
administration. Best cancer treatment results from cancer
management guidelines established by the Cancer Committee. The
in-hospital patient management may be best coordinated through
the development of oncology units. Comprehensive review or
auditing of the cancer patient care will demonstrate
deficiencies which may be present, and the Cancer Committee
can correct such deficiencies by a planned educational process. Coordinated discharge planning will assist in a better
quality of life for the cancer patient.
     Rehabilitation activities should involve team work between
the physician, oncology nurse, social worker, occupational
and vocational therapist, enterostomal therapist,
psychiatrists, nutritionists, etc., coordinating their
activities with the patient and the family through education,
referral, and coordinated assistance. The follow-up of the
patient after cancer treatment is essential for the detection
of recurrences which may still be curable as well as for the
detection of a second cancer in these high-risk patients.
     Continuing care activities include the coordination of the
visiting nurse and home health-care providers, hospices,
support group counseling referral to the appropriate
specialized centers for the management of complicated difficult problems such as pain, prosthetics, reconstruction, etc.,
An expanded clinical program for the 80's should include more
case presentations of hospitalized patients and outpatients
with diagnostic and therapeutic management problems.
Didactic conferences fail to provide the intellectual
challenge that the patient-oriented conferences offer.
Continuing staff education in oncology should be an on-going
activity of interest to all physicians, regardless of
specialty, and is often the best attended medical-staff
conference. A well-organized hospital registry should be
able to record the size, type, and stage of all cancers which
are diagnosed and treated in the hospital. The registrar
should be able to compare the incidence and cancer stage of
the hospital cases with national experience. The data base

should be used to evaluate treatment, both singly or in
combination, for at least the major cancer sites in comparison to national norms. A study of patient survival by
stage and treatment will determine if comparable end results
are being achieved in the community hospital setting. A
well-organized cancer registry should document the patterns
of recurrence of cancer, and determine the success rate
of further treatment. The documentation of multiple primary
malignancies in an individual patient is important because
of a common carcinogenic effect as well as the possibility
that primary surgical, radiotherapeutic or chemotherapeutic
therapy may induce second cancers. The continual evaluation
of the quality of life of cancer patients after treatment is
essential to update and upgrade newer treatment modalities
which may avoid complications of therapy.

COOPERATIVE STUDIES USING DATA
FROM
HOSPITAL CANCER PROGRAMS

In 1976 the National Cancer Advising Board asked the Commission on Cancer to assist in collecting data on a national
scale on liver tumors in order to study a possible relationship to the use of oral contraceptives. Through a network of
Liaison Fellows and Associates, a voluntary effort collected
543 cases, both male and female, in the age group 15-45 years
diagnosed during 1970-75 from 477 hospitals. Three hundred
seventy-eight cases were in women, and 56% of these tumors
were benign. This study comprised the largest series of liver
tumors to date, and appeared to support an association between
hepatic cell adenomas and focal nodular hyperplasia, and the
usage of oral contraceptives (3).
In 1977 a patterns of care study in colon cancer was done in
two parts. The short-term evaluation included patients with
histologically confirmed carcinoma of the colon and rectosigmoid with no prior definitive treatment. Twenty-five
consecutive cases were submitted from 491 hospitals for a total
of 11, 659 cases. There was great similarity of patient
symptoms, stage of disease, treatment (67% for cure), complications and mortality in hospitals of all sizes, whether community, teaching or university designation.
A long-term evaluation of colon cancer was done on 38,884
cases (treated in 1971) which were submitted from 327 hospitals. Thirty-six percent of all patients were alive five
years, a figure which was 58% for the Duke's A cases. The
reader is referred to the complete report for analysis according to stage, hospital size and category of hospital cancer

program. Never before has such complete data been available
from so many representative hospitals to study present-day
patterns of care of colon cancer (4)(Table 1-2).

TABLE 1-2
Number of Hospitals Voluntarily Participating in the
Surveys of the Commission on Cancer

Survey	Year	# of Hospitals	# of Cases
Liver Tumors	1976	477	543
Colon Long-Term	1977	327	38,884
Short-Term		491	11,659
Breast Long-Term	1978	498	24,125
Short-Term		629	15,468
Rectum Long-Term	1979	441	20,371
Short-Term		716	7,023
Prostate	1980	---In Progress-----	
Melanoma	1981	---Prospective in Process	

In 1978 a national study on breast cancer was done on
24,125 cases from 498 hospitals (5). The age at diagnosis
seemed to be somewhat younger than was demonstrated in the
Third National Cancer Survey. One-half of one percent had
bilateral breast cancer. Fifty-one percent of tumors were localized to the breast. Seventy percent of tumors were detected by the patient and only five percent by mammography.
About 60% were treated by modified radical mastectomy, a dramatic change from 24% so treated five years earlier. Forty-
four percent of the tumors had estrogen receptors studies, 55%
of which were positive. There was no evidence that the stage
of disease differed in the five-year span of this study. Five-
year survival decreased with an increasing number of axillary
node metastases, decreasing significantly with three or more
nodes.
A fourth national site study was done voluntarily in 1979 on
rectal cancer involving 716 hospitals, the most ever. Sixty
percent of white females with localized rectal cancer were
alive at five years, which is better survival than a similar
stage of rectal cancer in white males and blacks, both male
and female. Much more extensive data is available from this
patterns of care study (6).
A fifth national study is now in progress on prostate cancer.
The sixth study in 1981 will be on melanoma. Other studies
on two million cases of all sites have been completed. This
data may be analyzed according to cancer site, state of
residence, etc. The potential for more complex studies is even

greater if all cancer registries were computerized and compatible, and if data collected was more extensive.

The Hospital Cancer Programs of the Commission on Cancer
could be expanded to mount a nation-wide CHOP (Combined Hospital Oncology Program) program. If such were accomplished,
cooperative clinical trials could be undertaken with cost
savings and a wider selection of clinical material. Eventually cost effectiveness of staging and treatment must be
analyzed in relation to patient survival as well as in relation to patient quality of life.

SUMMARY

Some of the achievements of the approved Hospital Cancer
Programs in the United States have been documented. Eight
hundred sixty-four such programs exist at present and are in
the institutions which treat more than 54% of all patients
with cancer. There has been a continued improvement in the
quality of cancer care through tumor boards, cancer conferences, lectures, patient-care audits, etc., all of which
are components of an approved Hospital Cancer Program.
Nation-wide patterns of care studies of breast, colon, and
rectal cancers have been accomplished, and studies of prostate
cancer and melanoma are in progress.

The challenges for the 80's include expanded community-
health education in prevention and screening through an expanded Hospital Cancer Program. Pre-treatment staging and
multidisciplinary treatment planning for all cases of cancer
is a goal for the 80's. The institution of cooperative
clinical treatment protocols is possible in hospitals with
Hospital Cancer Programs. Improved rehabilitation efforts in
each community hospital is also a goal. Nation-wide evaluation of current cancer management in at least 15 sites
should be possible in this decade.

Prospect For The Future. A common or uniform cancer-data
system from all hospitals in the USA with approved cancer programs maintaining confidentiality of patient and hospital is
the ideal to allow nation-wide sharing of treatment practices
and end results reporting. An analysis of the patterns of care
of all cancer patients should be used as a basis for continuing medical education in the community hospital setting, as
well as in regional conferences. The rapid transfer of new
technologies through the community hospital program is practical. A cost-effective analysis of various staging and
diagnostic procedures as well as treatment methods must be
undertaken in order to assist with cost-containment while
maintaining quality cancer care with improved survival with

decreased morbidity.

REFERENCES

1. Bulletin of the American College of Surgeons (ACOS),
    September 1980, Vol. 65 No. 9.

2. Cancer Program Manual, American College of Surgeons
    (ACOS), Commission on Cancer, 1980.

3. Study of Association Between Liver Tumors and Oral
    Contraceptive Use. American College of Surgeons (ACOS),
    Commission on Cancer, 1976.

4. Carcinoma of Colon-Pattern of Care. American College
    of Surgeon (ACOS), Commission on Cancer, 1977.

5. Patterns of Care-Carcinoma of the Female Breast.
    American College of Surgeons (ACOS), Commission on Cancer,
    1978.

6. Patterns of Care-Carcinoma of the Rectum. American
    College of Surgeons (ACOS), Commission on Cancer, 1979.

WHAT IS CANCER CONTROL?

JOSEPH T. PAINTER, M.D.

Vice President and Professor of Medicine
The University of Texas System Cancer Center
M.D. Anderson Hospital and Tumor Institute
Houston, Texas

The emergence of cancer as a major public health problem has lent emphasis to the efforts to develop programs for control of the disease. Unlike communicable diseases, prolonged latency, diversity of presentation, and multiple site tendencies in cancer have made development of public health approaches difficult. Responsibility for the detection, diagnosis and treatment of cancer has rested primarily with practicing physicians. As improvements have occurred in each of these areas, the need to transmit this information to the health care community for general application has been recognized. In the communities of the nation, special skills and knowledge have often been lacking, making the incorporation of advances into patient care slow. Many citizens have remained out of the mainstream of medical care, however, and, as social programs evolved for the medically disadvantaged, the focus of programs to control cancer broadened. Further recognition of the importance of individual health habits as major contributing causes to cancer added the dimensions of motivation and compliance to this mix of activities.

Each of these facets of cancer control - the physician, the community, the health care system, societal forces and the individual person - has presented different priorities in different geographic areas. However, the available interventions for control of cancer, i.e., prevention, detection, diagnosis, treatment, continuing care and rehabilitation, remain unchanged.

Given agreement on target groups and intervention areas, the mechanism used to effect better control of cancer at the community level has been public and professional education.

The broad scope and the array of options available to develop cancer control programs have led to confusion as to exactly what cancer control is.

Significant Federal Developments

The passage of the National Cancer Institute Act in 1937 established cancer control as an important element in the national program. Section Two of the Act directed the Federal Cancer Control Program to procure, use and lend radium, to provide NCI fellowships and oncology training to physicians and nurses and to coordinate the programs with state health departments.[1] A decade later, the National Advisory Cancer Council outlined the components of a complete cancer control program. Included in the outline were statistical research, public and professional education, provision of prevention, detection, diagnostic and treatment clinics, consultation, tissue diagnostic services and an unprecedented directive for "special facilities and services for patients in terminal condition at hospitals or in their homes."[2] In 1960, the Advisory Committee to the Cancer Control Program recommended restriction of research to that applied directly to the program. The National Cancer Act of 1971 emphasized federal cooperation with state and other health agencies in control activities and urged a reduction in cancer morbidity and mortality through prevention, diagnosis, treatment and rehabilitation.

Working Group 8 of the National Cancer Program Planning Conference proposed in 1975 that cancer control be a distinct entity in the comprehensive National Cancer Program. The aims of the program were to identify potential cancer control methods and techniques, conduct necessary testing, evaluate applicability for community use and promote those methods found useful. Methods cited included as approaches developmental research and community demonstration.[3]

In 1977, the National Cancer Institute sponsored a comprehensive documentation of the history of cancer control in the United States. The document describes cancer control as beginning with the identification of potentially

effective technology, progressing from the formulation of a
strategy for its use through testing for safety and efficacy
and to promotion of applicable technology via public and
professional education. The renewal of the National Cancer
Act in 1978 incorporated specific directions from Congress
to emphasize detection, stress locally initiated community
programs, add local educational networks for physicians
and initiate programs to inform the public of unproven
cancer remedies.

Significant Program Development

The National Cancer Advisory Board reviewed the cancer
control program in 1978. The resulting material provides a
sense of cancer control as it had evolved under the direction
of the Division of Cancer Control and Rehabilitation. In
general, the programs were catagorized as contributing
directly to improved patient care (technology transfer, treatment networks, pain control, patient rehabilitation and
family counselling and care of the terminal patient), education (public and professional) and related issues (cost,
quality control, followup, etc.).

Some Impediments

Cancer control programs are new. The scope of interventions is broad, and the mechanisms for implementing
successful projects are not well delineated. At the operational level, program development has been impeded by the
absence of professional personnel with the management
experience necessary for leadership roles. Problems have
also been caused by an instability of core staff funding.
Furthermore, program initiation at the community level has
raised expectations and challenged the "turf" of existing
influential groups. In general, cancer control programs
have suffered a lack of personnel trained in the special
skills required for cancer control, exclusion of applied
research and demonstrations from the national program, and
an absence of effective evaluation mechanisms.

Fundamental to all of these operational problems,
however, is a lack of understanding of the definition of
cancer control.

What Is Cancer Control?

      Cancer control program directors have been wrestling
with this question for the past several years and agree
that the lack of a consensus definition is a serious deficiency which impairs both communication and development. Meeting as members of the Association of American
Cancer Institutes, program directors developed the following working definition:

      Cancer Control constitutes those activities which
      (1) facilitate the diffusion of existing and new
      biomedical technology, skills and knowledge from
      the cancer centers to the communities, (2) identi-
      fy cancer control methods and techniques, field
      test in the community, evaluate the applicability
      of use in the community, demonstrate the effective-
      ness of methods and techniques found applicable,
      and promote appropriate and widespread use of use-
      ful methods and techniques.

These elements follow in large part those recommended by
Working Group 8 of the National Cancer Program Planning
Conference.

      The scope of interventions under cancer control was
modified to emphasize the increasing importance of prevention, detection and diagnosis, and is as follows:

      prevention, screening, detection, diagnosis, and
      management (treatment, continuing care and rehabili-
      tation).

      Approaches for accomplishing cancer control were de-
fined as including:

      developmental research (identification, field test-
      ing, and evaluation of cancer control methods and
      techniques), demonstrations (determination of appli-
      cability, acceptability, cost/effectiveness, and
      risks) and education.

Working within this definition, a framework of broad program
guidelines can be developed and brought to bear upon the
priorities required. That cancer control will change is inevitable; that priorities will shift is desirable. However,

common understanding of a working definition can facilitate both progress and change. Do we need a definition? Only in order to think clearly.

Some Conclusions

Cancer control is not an exact science but is an amalgam of professional, institutional, social, educational, and communication sciences operating in a setting of extraordinary variability, the community. While much of the impetus for cancer control has been a perceived need to transfer technology from academic centers to the community, what has not been emphasized is the role which individual motivation and group dynamics play in the end results achieved.

Some Outstanding Opportunities

While a clear definition will be useful in communicating what cancer control is, some program decisions - and opportunities - remain:

o   Shift from modelling and limited funding to an integrated system of coordinated programs which will impact favorably upon cancer control

o   Change to high priority for prevention and detection with less emphasis upon other interventions

o   Increase emphasis upon developing mechanisms which alter the behavioral patterns of individuals and groups

o   Focus on the individual's responsibility for health through health education and through individual risk identification and surveillance

o   Collaborate with other categorical disease programs to integrate control efforts

Is cancer controllable? It is, if we get about it.

FOOTNOTES

1   Senate Bill 2067. 75th Congress. Public Law
     244. Approved August 5, 1937

2   J Nat Cancer Inst 6:243, April, 1946

3   Working Group Report: National Cancer Program
     Planning Conference, Summary Report for Cancer
     Control. USDHEW, PHS, NIH, NCI, June, 1975

Value Of A Communications Office
At A Comprehensive Cancer Center

MIRIAM ADAMS

*Director of Office of Cancer
Communications
Memorial Sloan-Kettering
Cancer Center
1275 York Avenue
New York, New York*

The National Cancer Act of 1971 underscored the efforts to
place all usuable information and skills in the hands of
health professionals by providing for additional ways of
expanding and expediting the translation of research results
into effective clinical practice. Specifically, the act
authorized the development of comprehensive cancer centers
and specialized cancer centers. The 21 comprehensive cancer
centers have the additional responsibility of providing
coordination and leadership within their geographic region.

THE NATIONAL CANCER PROGRAM

In communication, education and outreach, the most visible
participants in the National Cancer Program are the National
Cancer Institute, the American Cancer Society, and the
comprehensive cancer centers. Other participants in the
National Cancer Program include academic and non-profit
institutions, hospitals, and clinics, industry, state and

local governments, federal agencies other than the National
Cancer Institute, other volunteer groups and health
professionals.

With the comprehensive cancer centers serving as focal
points, a communications network was established with the
coordination and support of the other National Cancer
Program members. Its goal is to help make cancer knowledge
quickly and easily available to the public and health
professionals. The comprehensive cancer centers communications network is now in its sixth year of funding by the
National Cancer Institute, with communications offices
existing in 20 of the 21 comprehensive cancer centers.

COMPREHENSIVE CANCER CENTERS
COMMUNICATIONS NETWORK

The goal of the network is to engage in the dissemination
and interpretation of new and existing knowledge produced by
all constituents of the National Cancer Program to the
concerned communities. These communities include researchers,
practicing physicians, other health professionals and the
general public.

The specific objectives of the network are:

1. Provide the public with timely, useful and accurate cancer
    control knowledge.
2. Provide health professionals with information useful in
    the detection, diagnosis, pretreatment, evaluation and
    treatment of cancer as well as rehabilitation and
    continuing care of patients with cancer.
3. Increase and improve methods of referring the public to
    physicians and other consultants and resources, and to
    convenient institutions capable of diagnosis and
    treatment of specific cancers.
4. Increase in quantity and quality the interchange among
    health professionals of up-to-date cancer knowledge and
    techniques for application at the community level.
5. Assist the public to perceive cancer as not necessarily
    fatal, leading to attitudes and practices toward cancer
    and the patient with cancer which reflect a better under-
    standing of the nature of the disease and what is being
    done about it.

MEMORIAL SLOAN-KETTERING CANCER CENTER
COMMUNICATIONS OFFICE

At Memorial Sloan-Kettering Cancer Center the Communications
office was extablished in 1975 under the auspices of the
center's cancer control program. In addition to its goal
of making knowledge about cancer more available to the
general public and to health professionals, the communications office is vitally concerned with the development of
techniques to motivate these audiences to make greater use
of this knowledge.

The communications office has played a leadership role in
the establishment of numerous cancer center and city-wide
programs in the fields of health communications, school
health, health education, public information and nursing
education. Through television and radio features, public
service radio and television announcements, the press, as
well as other media channels, the residents of New York City
have become aware of the center's communications office and
its many programs, including the New York City Cancer
Information Service.

The following will highlight the major programs designed,
implemented, and evaluated by the communications office.

CANCER INFORMATION SERVICE

The most visible program of the communications office is
the Cancer Information Service telephone inquiry system,
known as the CIS. This program component is common to all
the network communications offices funded by the National
Cancer Institute. The Memorial Sloan-Kettering Cancer
Information Service opened in July, 1976, with 30 telephone
calls the first month. The service now handles from 1,000
to 1,500 calls per month with five incoming lines, three
of which are for the metropolitan New York City area and
two toll-free WATS lines for northern New Jersey. The
phones are answered "live" Monday through Friday from 9 a.m.
to 5 p.m. An answering machine responds to telephone calls
at all other times. Callers can either leave a brief
message or call the National Cancer Institute's toll free
number which is given by the taped message. The CIS is
supervised by a registered nurse with a master's degree in
community health education.

Fear of cancer and confusion about the disease were
reasons leading to the formation of the CIS. The service
was created to provide rapid access to the latest

information about cancer, to address the particular needs of
the population served by each CIS office and to bridge the
gap between cancer knowledge and personal action.

A Gallup Poll conducted for the American Cancer Society
found that cancer is the number one disease concern of the
public. Approximately 60 percent of Americans polled
ranked cancer number one, compared with 32 percent for heart
disease, the second greatest. Thus, an important objective
of the CIS is to reduce the public's fear of cancer by
providing information to assist in coping with the disease.

The CIS telephone system provides specific information on
particular cancer sites, detection programs, local
resources for cancer patients -- treatment and rehabilitation
facilities, home care assistance, availability of trans-
portation -- and facts about the process of patient referral
to physicians and consultation among health professionals.
Information about possible causes of cancer, how to help
prevent cancer, and how different forms of the disease are
detected and treated is also provided.

Questions received in CIS offices range from "Is cancer
contagious?" and "How can I get interferon?" to requests for
information about local self-help groups for cancer patients
and their families.

Approximately 60 percent of calls to CIS offices are
inquiries about cancer of five major body sites: breast
(24%), lung (16%), colon/rectum (10%), female reproductive
system (6%) and skin (4%). No single body site outside of
these five accounts for more than 2 percent of total
questions. The remaining 38 percent of the calls are
questions about other body sites and a wide range of other
subjects, from the known causes of cancer, the side effects
of radiation therapy, to the herditary factors associated
with cancer, or available resources for patients. And of
course, many requests for specific information result from
stories in the news media.

CANCER INFORMATION SERVICE
EVALUATION

The guaranteed anonymity of each caller makes it difficult
to make generalizations about users of the service or to
categorize them demographically. But information gathered
from an ongoing CIS evaluation indicates that callers are a
mix of cancer patients, families and friends of cancer
patients, the general public and health professionals. Of
particular significance this year is the increased number of

health professionals -- that is physicians, researchers,
nurses, social workers, physical therapists, etc., using
the CIS. Approximately 9 percent of our callers are now
health professionals, compared to less than one percent in
1977 and approximately 2 percent in 1978. The Memorial
Sloan-Kettering CIS is now reaching 92 per 1,000,000
individuals per year or an average of 38 calls for each day
the CIS is open. Calls have increased 30 percent in the
first half of 1980 versus the same time period in 1979.

Two months have been selected -- May and November -- as
periods during which all callers are asked for their names
and addresses to participate in a "user satisfaction"
survey. In November, 1979, 257 questionnaires were mailed
to those callers who provided us with their names and
addresses out of a total of 614 calls that were received that
month. Of the 257 questionnaires mailed, 127 individuals,
or 49.4 percent returned the survey. Highlights of this
evaluation are:

1. 42 percent of individuals who responded said that they
    were calling for themselves; 53 percent were calling
    for someone else; and 5 percent were students who wanted
    information for school reports.
2. 90 percent of individuals responding said that they were
    either "very satisfied" or "satisfied" with the service.
3. Of the 10 percent who indicated that they were not
    satisfied, most gave reasons not related to functions
    of the CIS.
4. 63 percent of individuals responding reported a specific
    action taken as a result of contact with the CIS.
    Specifically, 20 percent reported that they saw a
    physician as a result of calling the service.
5. 96 percent of those who responded said they would refer
    a friend or relative to the service.
6. 95 percent of those who responded reported that the
    materials mailed to them were useful.
7. 25 percent of callers had called the service at least
    once before.

Additional evaluative studies have been undertaken to
ascertain impact changes over time as well as to compare
the New York City population and CIS callers by ethnic
groups. Our most current data indicates that approximately
3.5 percent of callers are Hispanic in orgin while during a
previous period some 8.7 percent of callers were Black.

Under the supervision of the CIS coordinator mentioned
previously, the CIS is staffed by cancer communications

interns; students from public health and health education
programs in the New York City area. During this past year,
15 students completed the program, providing 1,651 unpaid
hours of service to the communications office. The program,
which was initiated in 1977, has graduated 31 cancer
communications interns to date through affiliations with
nine schools and universities.

CANCER INFORMATION SERVICE
PROMOTION

   Promotion of the CIS is achieved through utilization of a
wide variety of communications channels. Radio and
television public service spots are produced, pre-tested, and
placed by the Office of Cancer Communications on a regular
basis to both promote the CIS as well as to educate the
public about issues relating to occupational health, smoke
cessation, cancer prevention, nutrition, etc. New York City
stations -- both radio and television -- are currently using
these spots. During the past year it is estimated that more
than $100,000 was donated to us by the electronic media in
this region.
   Special promotional programs to reach both Black and
Spanish-speaking New Yorkers have included subway car card
campaigns as well as the development and placement of public
service radio announcements. Measurement of the impact of
these programs on the target population through appropriate
evaluation surveys is ongoing. Close to 5,000 colorful cards
promoting the CIS were placed on all lines of the New York
City subway system. Surveys conducted indicate that
the awareness level of the CIS more than doubled in the two
months following the posting of the car cards. Statistics
compiled by the New York City Subway Advertising Company
indicate that subway advertising is an effective way to
reach large proportions of Blacks, Hispanics, senior citizens
and lower income groups presently underutilizing the CIS.
   Flyers and other materials promoting the CIS or providing
an educational message are prominently displayed at health
fairs and other health-related public events.
   Print public service advertisements are also utilized to
promote the CIS and are distributed to weekly newspapers in
the region.

PUBLIC AWARENESS CAMPAIGNS

The Office of Cancer Communications has participated in several special public awareness campaigns in cooperation with the National Cancer Institute. New York City was designated as one of 16 priority markets for participation in the public awareness campaign on asbestos exposure. The communications objective of this campaign was to increase public awareness and understanding of the health risks of asbestos exposure; the importance of getting regular medical check ups; the need to stop smoking; the need for prompt medical treatment for respiratory illness and the need for additional information. The audience was defined as former workers (approximately 75 percent of those exposed are former workers and over half of these individuals were exposed by working in shipyards during World War II) as well as present workers (about 25 percent of those exposed are currently employed in an asbestos-related industry).

The communication strategies included informing the high risk target audience and the general public about the nature, extent and seriousness of asbestos exposure, instructing the target audience what to do and encouraging current workers to utilize available safety measures to reduce asbestos exposure.

Campaign elements included radio and television spots, print public service advertisements, materials for the media such as fact sheets and news releases, and brochures both for the general public as well as for the professional including the health communications specialist.

In addition, two Gallup Polls were conducted in an attempt to measure the impact of HEW's campaign to inform the public about the hazards of asbestos exposure. Results of a national survey conducted during the campaign's mid-point indicated that 62 percent of adult Americans had heard or seen something recently on the hazards of asbestos exposure, compared to 50 percent in an identical survey taken before the campaign was initiated.

Another public awareness campaign was executed in January 1979 to coincide with the release of the Surgeon General's report on smoking and health. Television slides were designed and distributed to all New York City stations encouraging viewers to call the CIS for information on local stop smoking programs as well as to receive appropriate printed materials on this subject.

HEALTH EDUCATION PROGRAMS

Numerous other health promotion and health education projects are currently coordinated by the Memorial Sloan-Kettering communications office including the establishment of a city-wide Task Force on Smoking to design and implement a plan to introduce a new tobacco education curriculum into the New York City school system. Two seminars geared to assist principals, district coordinators of health and directors of school-based drug prevention programs have been held. A one-day conference on Smoking and Health, targeted toward New York City school teachers is planned for this November.

Mass distribution of selected cancer-related reading materials to large groups of individuals via mailings to senior citizen centers, community health agencies, and libraries, is routinely carried out. The communications office also provides bulk materials to community health education centers throughout the city. A record of the number of publications distributed as well as anticipated usage of this material is maintained by us as part of our mandate to evaluate individual program components.

National Cancer Institute-produced materials such as annotated bibliographies as well as information for physicians on irradiation-related thyroid cancer and DES exposure, are also distributed to health professionals by the communications office.

The Office of Cancer Communications participates in the National Cancer Institute's supermarket campaign which distributes cancer-related brochures and pamphlets -- all listing the telephone numbers of the CIS offices -- in some 125 supermarkets in New York City and some 250 supermarkets in the New Jersey area. Accompanying supermarket television public service announcements have been provided to the Office of Cancer Communications by the National Cancer Institute and are now being distributed to encourage public usage of the racks. Overall, the supermarket distribution system appears to be reaching a broad range of individuals in terms of age and sex.

A newsletter written for hospital employees is produced by the Office of Cancer Communications and distributed to employees at Memorial Sloan-Kettering Cancer Center and at the 12 institutions within our Affiliated Hospital Network. This employee newsletter has a distribution of 3,000 copies monthly. Each issue contains information about recent developments in cancer control and lists new educational materials available free through the communications office.

A newsletter for health professionals is also produced by the communications staff and is distributed in a similar manner to the same institutions.

The communications office assists with the publication of ONCOLOGY TIMES, a monthly newspaper for specialists in cancer. The publication has a circulation of approximately 23,000 physicians and researchers. A mailing list was developed which encompases all members of the major cancer-related specialty societies. An editorial board and a group of associate editors have been brought together, representing numerous scientific and medical disciplines. In addition, the directors of communications offices at five other comprehensive cancer centers serve as regional associates. Readership surveys to evaluate the usefulness and effectiveness of this new publication are now being designed.

SPECIAL AUDIENCE PROGRAMS

Special audience programs are also coordinated by the communications office. The objectives of these programs are to:

1. Increase realistic awareness of cancer's impact among these special, and often high-risk, groups.
2. Reduce myths and sense of fears or fatalism toward cancer.
3. Provide specific information on actions individuals can take to guard against cancer.
4. Increase prevention, self-detection and medical consultation practices.

The development of communications strategies to reach Black women with information about breast cancer, breast self-examination and breast screening are included in this broad category of special audience projects. Program components include focus group studies to determine knowledge and attitudes among Black women of central Harlem toward breast cancer and breast cancer screening, and telephone and central location interviews to further define the underutilization of cancer-related services in the Harlem area.

These studies were conducted on behalf of the Harlem Breast Examination Center, a New York State Department of Health-funded screening and education program. The project was implemented with the assistance of the National Cancer Institute's Office of Cancer Communications.

Three main reasons for the underutilization of this center were cited most frequently in the study: lack of awareness

of the center and its location; confusion regarding Black
women's susceptibility to breast cancer; and lack of
awareness and misinformation regarding breast examinations
and BSE.

These studies, conducted to determine attitudes and
knowledge among women in the Harlem community related to
breast cancer, will be utilized by the communications office
in the development of communications strategies to reach
this target audience. Promotional materials are now being
produced to motivate women to utilize the facilities of the
center; to promote early breast cancer detection to Black
women in central Harlem; to increase awareness of the
potential threat of breast disease among women, particularly
among the less educated; and to initiate and promote
utilization of BSE programs in the central Harlem community.

SUMMARY

Over the past 5 years the programs of the Office of Cancer
Communications have made a definite impact in the fields of
public education, school health education, hospital employee
education, professional education and minority health
communication. The total program is perceived as an integral
part of the cancer-related services available to the
residents of the metropolitan New York area and the
communications office serves as the focal point to which the
general public and health professionals can turn for
information, help and advice -- both from within the cancer
center as well as from the community-at-large.

A National Planning Program for
Cancer Rehabilitation

Lawrence D. Burke

"I have always believed, during my many years in
Rehabilitation that hope is the priceless ingredient if
we are to achieve success in any type of Rehabilitation
for individuals. The individuals own hope is vitally
important and the hopeful outlook of therapists,
physicians and counselors is equally so. It is hope
that keeps the spark of life alive and moves people
forward to achieve their optimum progress."[1]

Mary E. Switzer, 1968

It is indeed a pleasure and a privelege to review with you
the early development, the progress and the future
challenges in planning the National Cancer Institute's
Rehabilitation program for cancer patients. The concept of
rehabilitation specifically for cancer patients is perhaps
a very late arrival on the medical scene. Diagnosis and
treatment have historically been the primary focus and
major emphasis in the war against cancer. Rehabilitation
being designated as the third phase in cancer management.
Time and results have certainly justified this emphasis.
It is precisely because of the advances in cancer treatment
that clinicians now call for supporting advances in cancer
rehabilitation. For while treatment advances enable an
increasing number of cancer patients to live longer, with
or without evidence of disease, residual impairments in
physical, behavioral and social functioning frequently
occur and must be treated if the real benefits from cure
and/or longer survival are to be realized by the patient
and society.

Having spent literally thousands of dollars to eradicate
the patient's cancer, we have a further responsibility.
We must prevent having that patient sit alone and lonely, a
social isolate, economically unproductive--growing ever
more pale, thin and debilitated. When rehabilitation
skills and resources are not available this is all too
frequently the lot of cancer patients.

Mary E. Switzer, who in 1965 was commissioner of the
Vocational Rehabilitation Administration, set this
phenomenon in historical perspective:

> "I was around when the National Cancer Council was
> created and when the first program of grants for
> research was set up in the Public Health Service
> back in 1937. Almost from the beginning there has
> been ..A failure to take full advantage of what is
> going on in rehabilitation for the benefit of the
> cancer patient and the baffling psychological
> atmosphere that surrounds the whole area of cancer
> as a condition of man."[2]

These quotes are from the Keynote Address given at the
first major conference on research from cancer. It was
hosted by Dr. Howard Rusk at the Institute of Physical
Medicine and Rehabilitation in New York City.

During the following 15-year period, there has been some
recognition of the specialized rehabilitative needs of
cancer patients. But negative attitudes of hopelessness
still persist and interfere with real programmatic
progress. As recently as 1971, of 260,000 people
rehabilitated in State Vocational Rehabilitation programs,
only 1,000 had a diagnosis of cancer.[3]

The Evolvement of the National Cancer Rehabilitation Program

The need for and role of rehabilitation in a total national
cancer plan was recognized in 1971 while legislation was
being developed in the White House and Congress for an
unprecedented national effort against cancer.
Dr. Carl Baker, then Director of NCI and the Committee of
Consultants on cancer to Senator Ralph Yarborough, while

considering elements that should go into a National Cancer
Program Plan, included rehabilitation of the cancer patient
as an area ready for development, research and
demonstration. The National Cancer Act of 1971 was signed
by the President on December 23, 1971. The National Cancer
Program Plan was formulated in a series of strategic
planning meetings. Two hundred and fifty laboratory and
clinical scientists met in a series of 40 planning sessions
and two major review sessions between October 1971 and
March 1972 to develop recommendations for a National Cancer
Plan. Objective 7 of this plan focused on cancer patient
rehabilitation and stressed the need:

 "to develop the means to improve the rehabilitation
 of cancer patients."

The next step was a National Cancer Rehabilitation Planning
Conference sponsored by the National Cancer Institute,
December 4-8, 1972. Eighty-six participants including
biomedical and rehabilitation experts, cancer patients,
union representatives, insurance carriers, ACS staff
members and social scientists attended this 4-day
conference. It was chaired by Dr. Guy Robbins, then Chief
of the Breast Service at Memorial Sloan-Kettering and
Dr. Jack Healy, then Head of the Department of Physical
Medicine and Rehabilitation at M.D. Anderson Hospital and
Tumor Institute.

This was indeed a landmark conference because it
acknowledged that rehabilitation does not automatically
accompany or follow successful cancer treatment, but cancer
treatment to be successful must be accompanied by
rehabilitation. Thus, Conference delegates were charged
with identifying general areas of concern, specific
rehabilitative problems and needs that historically and
currently beset the cancer patient during the course of
treatment. The group struggled for consensus on:

(1) A working definition of cancer rehabilitation; (2)
basic concepts of cancer rehabilitation; and (3) current
areas ready for demonstration and/or research. Following
the plenary session the conference delegates were divided
into six panels for detailed consideration and

recommendations on specific subject areas. The six areas
designated as basic for a comprehensive program in cancer
rehabilitaton were:

    o palliative and supportive care;
    o physical restoration - head and neck;
    o physical restoration - breast, extremities;
      gastrointestinal and genitourinary;
    o psychosocial needs;
    o vocational needs; and
    o educational needs.

The panels proceeded to define and establish priorities for
a total of 120 projects, 90 in the area of cancer control
(i.e., techniques, concepts ready for field testing,
demonstration or clinical evaluation) and 30 in the area of
research.

The individual panel reports and the chairman's summary
served as guidelines to NCI staff and remain a part of the
current rehabilitation program direction.

To the initial Objective 7 the rehabilitation conference
delegates added three additional objectives for a National
Cancer Rehabilitation Program;

    o develop the national capability to provide
      rehabilitation to all cancer patients;

    o develop improved means to restore maximum
      physical and educational capabilities to
      cancer patients; and

    o develop improved means to restore cancer
      patients' lifestyle and reinforce re-entry
      into the community.

As the conference delegates explored the state of cancer
rehabilitation and sought to formulate a proper program
content, these major concerns emerged.

o   The first emphasized that treated cancer
     patients, especially successfully treated
     patients, do have residual effects from
     the disease and the consequences of
     treatment. The residual impairments must
     be met through aggressive, structured
     rehabilitation if optimal restoration is
     to be achieved.

o   The next considered that the multifacet
     rehabilitative needs of the cancer patient
     be recognized openly and that uniform
     protocols be developed to apply both
     existing and emerging techniques to meet
     these needs.

o   The third concern was that the multifacet
     needs of the treated cancer patient must
     be met through programs that are
     integrated with the total medical plan.

The planning conference, the working groups, and the panels
produced a wealth of reports, documents and summaries.
These were made available to the NCI Rehabilitation Program
staff. In addition, the participants of the conference
subsequently became a valuable resource as advisors and
consultants in particular areas of expertise.

These recommendations were now to be implemented into a
nationwide program of funded projects, demonstrating, field
testing and evaluating rehabilitation concepts, techniques
and practices that would ultimately insure adequate and
available rehabilitation to every treated cancer patient.

Thus in 1972, with limited staff, uncertain funding,
dissimilar interests within the biomedical community, how
did the program actually get started?

The National Cancer Program Plan, which was regularly
reviewed and modified by representatives of the National
Cancer Advisory Board, was organized into a hierarchical
format:

Goal, Objectives, Approaches, Approach Elements, Project
Areas.

The National Cancer Program Plan set out seven major
research objectives (See Appendix A), spelling out an
Approach, Approach Elements and Project Areas for each
objective.

Using Objective 7 as an illustration.

GOAL

Reduce the Morbidity From Cancer

OBJECTIVE 7

Develop the means to improve the rehabilitation of
cancer patients.

APPROACH 7.1

Increase the national capacity to provide cancer
rehabilitation services.

Approach Element 7.1.1

Expand Rehabilitation Facilities

PROJECT AREAS WITHIN APPROACH ELEMENT 7.1.1

7.1.1.1   Assess morbidity -- determine and quantify disease
          effects amenable to rehabilitation.

7.1.1.2   Assess the current availability and utilization of
          cancer patient rehabilitation services.

7.1.1.3   Expand existing rehabilitation and associated
          educational facilities.

7.1.1.4   Develop additional rehabilitation facilities for
          the cancer patient.

7.1.1.5   Develop criteria for evaluation of rehabilitation
          efforts.

Each approach element could be achieved via a number of projects. These were step units in a logical progression toward the overall objective. This hierarchical format provided for continuity and a basis for the subsequent evaluation, recommendation and revision by future planning or advisory committee. It also served as a guide for staff to measure its progress within a given time period. The NCI staff then had the task of selecting project areas within the Approach, coordinating them with NCI program policy and determining the funding levels and method.

The contract method of funding was initially chosen because we wanted those early projects carried out according to the guidelines recommended by the planning committee and certain NCI specifications. It was a program decision that major cancer centers would be encouraged to respond to the initial procurement offerings. In the first full year of the Cancer Control and Rehabilitation program 24, 3-year contracts were awarded within a funding level of $5 million.

Without providing reason or rationale, it might be interesting just to note the titles of the first five project areas funded. (See Appendix B for brief description)

> o Demonstration of Cancer Rehabilitation
>   Facility and/or Departments
>
> o Training of Professional Teams in Cancer
>   Rehabilitation
>
> o Implementation of a Training Program for
>   Physical and/or Occupational Therapists
>
> o Training of Maxillofacial Prothodontists and
>   Maxillofacial Dental Technicians
>
> o Demonstration of Integrated Cancer
>   Rehabilitation Services

These were basic bread and butter projects oriented toward developing and organizing resources for increasing the

number and variety of professionals competent and committed
to working with cancer patients. Fortunately, major cancer
centers responded enthusiastically to our procurement
offers so that rehabilitation programs were immediately
mainlined into the prescribed services of cancer care
centers. Pragmatic problems involving logistics, discharge
patterns and treatment assumptions as they related to
clinical rehabilitation surfaced and were fed back to NCI
program staff. New RFPs were generated to study, more
clearly identify the problems surfaced and to test
solutions effective for enabling the rehabilitation program
to function as a discreet, regularized component of routine
oncology care.

One later project grew directly out of the experience with
the demonstration projects. Patients, following definitive
treatments, were frequently discharged from the cancer ward
to outpatient status and could no longer participate in the
hospital based rehabilitation program. Neither public nor
private insurers would pay the cost of follow-up visits for
rehabilitation alone. Thus, the patient was separated from
the rehabilitation resource when the need was greatest and
the time optimal.

An RFP entitled <u>Cancer Rehabilitation on an At Home Basis</u>
was issued to explore this need and to develop
rehabilitation protocols effective for patients living in
their own homes. An at-home training manual and special
training curriculum was developed to expedite the training
of "at-home rehabilitation teams." This is but one example
of program expansion based on experience and data from
ongoing projects.

Each funded project produced a Final Report with
observations and/or tentative conclusions. Some of these
follow.

        o Once a rehabilitation program is instituted and
           identified as such, the number of patients
           referred to the rehabilitation unit increases
           from month to month.

This finding was consistent for the ten
<u>Demonstration of Cancer Rehabilitation</u>
<u>Facilities and/or Departments</u> projects whether
or not the medical team initially believed a
formalized rehabilitation unit was needed.

o Patients in general did not find the increased
   time required by hospital rehabilitation
   programs to be a burden or inconvenience as
   indicated by their continued participation in
   the program.

o In one project 467 patients were studied and
   reported that those patients who received
   integrated rehabilitative service benefitted
   over and above those who did not. Shortened
   hospital stays by an average of 6.7 days:
   decreased hospital costs, increased survival
   rates (28%) and patients better able to follow
   prescriptions for self-care, self-examination
   and keeping appointments were used as benefit
   criteria.

o Several studies emphasized the need for more of
   a balance between attention to physical and
   emotional health in cancer rehabilitation.
   Institutions tended to emphasize one or the
   other.

o There was no evidence of conflict or lack of
   cooperation/coordination between the oncology
   treatment team and the rehabilitation treament
   team.

It is not possible to discuss all the findings, the
information and the data provided by the many funded
projects. The task of reviewing Final Reports, and the
analysis and consolidation of study data into
generalizations with widespread applicability is an ongoing
staff function. Currently, the NCI rehabilitation program
has funded 56 contracts.

To ensure that significant areas of research or unique
study approaches were not lost to the rehabilitation
endeavor, the grant funding mechanism has been utilized
along with contract funding. Investigator-initiated
research grant applications are encouraged and have made a
substantive contribution to the total program.
Approximately 70 grants related to rehabilitation research
have been funded to date.

The use of grant funding has expanded the cancer
rehabilitation program into a variety of new areas not
traditionally associated with rehabilitation. Some
examples are:

- o Nutritional support as a rehabilitation
  modality;
- o Improved management in terminal cancer;
- o Coping characteristics of pediatric cancer;
  patients;
- o Free flap trachea and esophageal
  reconstruction - microsurgical techniques;
- o Assessing and reducing the morbidity of the
  cancer patient's survivors; and
- o Counselling strategies for cancer patients

Five years is not a long time to implement a national
program, yet we feel the effort to date has been markedly
successful.

Over 100 professional papers, in addition to pamphlets and
monographs have been written as a result of the
rehabilitation program.

Other federal agencies have evinced interest in cancer
rehabilitation initiating studies and sponsoring workshops
and conferences.

The private sector has organized numerous workshops and
continuing education courses dealing specifically with
aspects of cancer rehabilitation.

As an example, one notes that the American Congress of
Rehabilitation Medicine (ACRM) has formally approved and

appointed an ad hoc committee on cancer rehabilitation.
The Annual Conference Program (October 1980) of the ACRM
list two courses on cancer rehabilitation. One based on
the summary of data from NCI funded research and
demonstration projects. The present action of this most
relevant professional group is directly related to the
stimulation and support of the National Cancer
Rehabilitation Program.

Evidence of increased public awareness is reflected in the
many inquiries to NCI (Average 6 per day), and the
proliferation of articles on cancer rehabilitation in the
lay press and professional journals.

An increased number of health disciplines have initiated
courses in cancer rehabilitation in their professional
schools or in programs of continuing education. Nursing,
social work, psychology, physical therapy come readily to
mind.

There were early growing pains and problems which if
detailed might make for a sizable book but, the initial
recommendations from the planning conferences, the
continued input from the many expert consultants and the
collaboration with cancer centers' staff combined to ensure
that a national program of cancer rehabilitation would be
implemented successfully.

I believe it is only proper to acknowledge the support and
continued guidance from two major cancer centers that had
rehabilitation programs long before the implementation of
the National Cancer Act of 1971. These are M.D. Anderson
Hospital and Tumor Institute and Memorial Sloan-Kettering
Cancer Center. Because cancer is not one but many
diseases, cancer rehabilitation by definition must have
access to a variety of experts knowledgeable on services
and resources related to impairments and disabilities. We
found it necessary to call upon the scientists and
clinicians at these institutions time and time again. They
gave freely of their time and expertise. By freely I mean
they were not always on a professional service contract.

The task of implementing a national cancer rehabilitation
program was further complicated by the fact that
rehabilitation is such a poorly defined specialty area in
medicine. It is like many other clinical activities that
seek to benefit the patient but yet it is "different
somehow." Because any rehabilitation treatment requires a
combination of services, skills and resources the primary
responsibility can never be assigned solely to one
discipline. It is axiomatic that nobody can do
rehabilitation alone, and nobody can be the single expert
in all its departments. Such an axiom does not promote a
strong constituency.

Enthusiasm for a national program was not completely devoid
of cautions seemingly because the word rehabilitation is
tainted with negative implications. Except for the clearly
congenital handicapped and accident-impaired person, the
public view of rehabilitation is that it is sought for and
applied to an "unsavory lot." Further complicating, is the
linguistic ubiquity of the term. Rehabilitation has been
used to denote any activity that sought change from an
undesirable to a desirable state.

> "Sommerville suggested that its first use in common
> British parlance was to denote re-adoption of
> denominational dress by transgressors who had been
> deprived of the privilege of wearing it."[4]

Currently, the term is applied to clean-up projects of
slums and country swamps. Undesirable social states
require rehabilitation. Both criminals and their victims
require rehabilitation. Alcoholics, drug addicts,
delinquents, unemployed, etc., all require rehabilitation.
A disturbing fact is that rehabilitation endeavors for
people or projects all too often profit too little from the
rehabilitationists expenditure of energy, time and funds.

There is a philosophy of pessimism common to rehabilitation
and a historical hopelessness common to cancer--Cancer
Rehabilitation as a program entity provoked a four-fold
intensification of these feeling in many. A major
responsibility of the NCI staff was to recognize this
negative philosophy and develop positive and constructive
ways to deal with it. We defined rehabilitaton as simply
"making able to do again - to some degree." The "different
somehow" of rehabilitation from other helpful clinical
activities is that in rehabilitation the patient is also
the therapist. The patient is the only one who can
rehabilitate him/her self.

Granville states it beautifully:

> "Effective rehabilitation depends more than anything upon
> the intelligent cooperation by patients themselves, and
> that depends ultimately upon the attitudes of mind that
> they can be encouraged to generate and maintain support
> for themselves often through weeks or months
> interspersed with small triumphs, disappointments,
> painful times, the fear and uncertainties that will
> haunt them on the way to recovery or building a new
> life." (5)

I submit that the historical lack of effectiveness in many
rehabilitation endeavors might be directly related to the
attempt to rehabilitate persons, for society's sake, who
did not want to be rehabilitated for their own sake.

Future challenges and goals: We must refine the focus of
the cancer rehabilitation research, and increase the
knowledge based on methods for achieving intelligent
cooperation and maintaining high motivation in cancer
patients. This must be done as opposed to sponsoring
demonstrations of known techniques with known effectiveness.

o We must help the health professional, including the
   oncologists, to understand the biosocial model of
   disease as well as the current biological model.
   The complex intertwining of psychosocial elements of
   illness are especially pertinent to the
   rehabilitation area.

o   We must continue the conceptualization and testing
    of a vastly newer role for the cancer
    rehabilitationists - which might include greater
    involvement of relatives in the interactional team
    that provides patient support.

o   There is the need to develop newer, more
    sophisticated techniques for measuring cancer
    disability and evaluating the effectiveness of
    rehabilitation.

o   We have to ensure that every comprehensive cancer
    center has a functional rehabilitation program -
    each providing the same types of service, employing
    uniform protocols. Such centers should be funded
    for ongoing research and clinical studies in
    rehabilitation.

o   We need to develop and implement a system for the
    regular dissemination of rehabilitation information
    among cancer centers, cancer hospitals and federal
    agencies. To share on wider bases what we have
    already learned is an obvious need.

o   Regional state of the art conferences are necessary
    to capitalize on the current research and interest
    in cancer rehabilitation. Regional conferences in
    cancer rehabilitaion could be co-sponsored with the
    American Cancer Society (ACS), private medical
    facilities, volunteer associations, etc.

o   There is a requirement for the development of
    program cooperatives involving community wide
    participation and employer involvement designed to
    mainstream cancer patients back into the economic
    life of America.

o   There must be greater involvement and utilization of
    the community hospital as a focus for
    rehabilitation, educational seminars of a
    multispecialty, interdisciplinary nature. This is
    especially indicated since the vast majority (80%)
    continue to receive care there.

Legislative Needs Include:

   ...legislation for the provision of third-party
   payments for services of health professionals which are
   necessary for the achievement of the goals of cancer
   rehabilitation.

   ...the establishment of rehabilitation research and
   training centers for cancer rehabilitation or to more
   clearly authorize the cancer rehabilitation emphasis in
   existing research and training centers.

   ...to establish and maintain minimum standards of
   cancer rehabilitation in institutions where cancer
   treatment is federally funded.

   There is a need for the investigation of how many
   dollars are lost to the commercial sector because of
   emotional disorders secondary to the diagnosis and
   treatment of cancer.

This list is not meant to be exhaustive, but merely
suggestive of broad general areas for future consideration.

The impact of cancer is felt in lives cut short, in income
lost by prematurely ended working lives, in the cost of
treatment and care and and in the physical and emotional
pain the disease brings. Rehabilitation addresses all of
these problems and is thus urgently needed.

The NCI Director's Report of 1979 sums it up:

   "The other issue is the quality of life of persons who
   have or have had cancer and are now living normal life
   spans free of disease. Many persons suffer needlessly
   because of attitudes of friends, employers, and even
   family that sometimes place the cancer patient in a
   class of "non-persons" who are shunned or avoided.
   Cancer patients may be disabled as a consequence of the

disease and may need assistance to restore their psychological well-being. For those who have been incapacitated, appropriate rehabiliation can often restore self-confidence, self-care, and a sufficient degree of independence to enable the individual to resume satisfactory social and business involvements. With greater numbers of cancer survivors each year, improving rehabilitation is now one of the major objectives of the National Cancer Program."

APPENDIX A

NATIONAL CANCER PROGRAM RESEARCH OBJECTIVES

OBJECTIVE 1

Develop the means to reduce the effectiveness of external agents
for producing cancer.

OBJECTIVE 2

Develop the means to modify individuals in order to minimize the
risk of cancer development.

OBJECTIVE 3

Develop the means to prevent transformation of normal cells to
cells capable of forming cancers.

OBJECTIVE 4

Develop the means to prevent progression of precancerous cells to
cancers, the development of cancers from precancerous conditions,
and spread of cancers from primary sites.

OBJECTIVE 5

Develop the means to achieve an accurate assessment of (a) the
risk of developing cancer in individuals and in population groups,
and (b) the presence, extent and probable course of existing
cancers.

OBJECTIVE 6

Develop the means to cure cancer patients and to maintain control of
cancer in patients who are not cured.

OBJECTIVE 7

Develop the means to improve the rehabilitation of cancer patients.

APPENDIX B

Demonstration of Cancer Rehabilitation Facilities and/or Departments

This project is to develop a model system of total rehabilitation services for cancer patients. The system shall provide for education in the rehabilitation team concept and the implementation of new approaches to the rehabilitation of cancer patients. Prospective offerors must have at least a basic operational rehabilitation department and a wide range of para-medical specialties related to rehabilitation. The program is primarily directed toward major medical centers or comprehensive cancer care centers.

Training of Professional Teams in Cancer Rehabilitation

This project provides for the establishment of a cancer rehabilitation personnel training program coordinated by one center for the training of 12 professional teams from selected geographically distributed health institutions. It is anticipated that 12 teams composed of 5 members per team will be trained under this contract, and that these teams, upon returning to their respective institutions, will be capable of providing, on site, rehabilitative care and treatment as well as conducting secondary training programs.

The one ongoing project funded by DCCR is M.D. Anderson.

Cancer Training Programs for Physical Therapists and/or Occupational Therapists

These programs provide for the development, demonstration and evaluation of basic and/or advanced training curricula

for physical/occupational therapists to enable these
disciplines to work more effectively with cancer patients.
An average of 25 therapists per institution are to be
trained under these contracts.

Training Programs for Maxillofacial Prosthodontists and Laboratory Technicians

This project solicits proplsals for the development of
training programs to increase the number of maxiloofacial
prosthodontists to increase the number of maxillofacial
prosthodontists to provide the necessary facial restoration
secondary to the surgery for the head and neck.
Comprehensive rehabilitation of patients with cancer of the
head and neck requires the highly specialized techniques
and skills of maxilloracial prosthodontists and
maxillofacial technicians. Training must be provided
within an accredited program. Offerors must have or have
access to the necessary physical facilities and teaching
staff, as well as accessibility to prospective trainees.

Integrated Cancer Rehabilitation Services

This project is to develop and demonstrate the
effectiveness of coordinated cancer rehabilitation services
among community hospitals or medical facilities within a
given catchment area. While this effort includes selection
and training of rehabilitation coordinators, prospective
offerors must have access to trained rehabilitation
professionals, staff, and facilities for training of
supporting personnel, and the ability to develop a patient
referral system responding to the requirement of this
project. This contract program is primarily directed
toward the community and nonspecialty hospitals with a
patient flow of 350 new cancer patients per year.

References

1. Leonard G. Perlman, Ed., The Role of Vocational
    Rehabilitation in the 1980's, A Report of the Third
    Mary E. Switzer Memorial Seminar, Dec 1978, National
    Rehabilitation Association, Washington, D.C., Dec 1978

2. Conference on Research Needs in the Rehabilitation of
    Persons with Disabilities Resulting From Cancer. U.S.
    DHEW, URA and N.Y.U. Medical Center, Nov. 1965.

3. Switzer, Mary E. The Health Memorial Lecture:
    Rehabilitation-An Act of Faith.   In M.D. Anderson
    Hospital Staff (Eds.) _Rehabilitation of the Cancer
    Patient. Chicago: Yearbook 1972

4. Sommerville, J.G., Workshop on Disablement and
    Rehabilitation in Developing Countries, Medical
    Rehabilitation, Gelly Oak Colleges, Birmingham 29, V.K
    April 1975.

5. Ganville, H.J., What is Rehabilitation? An Inaugurial
    Lecture. Rehabilitation: Journal of the British
    Council for Rehabilitation of the Disabled, Number One
    Hundred, Jan-March 1977.

Readings

McGann, Leona M. The Cancer Patient's Needs: How Can We
Meet Them? Journal of Rehabilitation, Nov.-Dec. 1964.

McAlerr, Charles A. and Kluge, Charles, Why Cancer
Rehabilitation? Rehabilitation Counseling Bulletin 21,3,
1978

Cromes, G., Fred Jr., Implementation of Interdisciplinary
Cancer Rehabilitation. Rehabilitation Counselling Bulletin
21,3, 1978.

Perlman, Leonard G. And Burke, Lawrence D., Cancer Rehab:
New Directions and New Attitudes, American Rehabilitation,
Volume 4, Number 5. May-June 1979

Dietz, J.H. Jr., "Rehabilitation of the Cancer Patient"
Med. Clinics of North America. Vol. 3, No. 3, May 1969:
607-624

Diller, Leonard, Gordon, Wayne, A., Final
Report-Demonstration of the Benefit of Early Identification
of Psvchosocial Problems and Earlv Intervention Toward
Rehabilitation of Cancer Patients.

Isler. L. "Emerging in Cancer Care-The Regional Ambulatory
Center" RN, Feburary 1977 33-46.

Kluge, Charles A. and McAleer, Charles. Factors that
Predict Successful Outcome in a Cancer Rehabilitation
Program--A Pilot Study, "Rehabilitation Counseling
Bulletin, March 1978 246-252

Sever, R. "Cancer: More than a Disease, For Many a Silent
Stigma," New York Time, May 4, 1977

Current Progress and Future Trends

SURGERY AND CANCER   1970 to 1980

Edward J. Beattie, Jr., M.D.
General Director
Memorial Hospital
New York, New York

INTRODUCTION

Surgery has been the prime treatment modality for the cure of cancer. The operations developed for cure of cancer assumed that the primary tumor should be widely excised along with its lymph node drainage area. This principle underlay the Halstead operation (the classic radical mastectomy) and the Miles operation for cancer of the rectum. If the tumor had spread to the regional lymph nodes, it was expected that some patients would be cured, but this would be more serious. If the tumor might spread past the lymph nodes a block excision usually could not be carried out for cure. Surgery for cancer spread beyond these limits was used for palliative benefit only.

The pattern of spread is different dependent upon whether one is treating a carcinoma or a sarcoma. Usually the carcinoma spreads to its regional lymph nodes and from there becomes blood borne and systemic. The location of the tumor in the body determines where the metastases will develop. If it is in the abdomen, liver metastases may develop since the liver is the filter for the portal venous circulcation. If the carcinoma drains into a systemic vein, lung metastases may occur. Liver metastases may further metastasize into the lungs before developing widespread systemic metastases.

Sarcomas tend not to spread to the regional lymph nodes, but spread via the venous drainage. Sarcomas in the abdomen can spread to the liver but the sarcomas otherwise metastasize to the lungs.

Surgeons were loathe to attack metastases to the lungs until the first successful operation on a pulmonary metastasis by Churchill[1] in 1939. He performed a right middle lobe lobectomy for a lung mass which was found to be a solitary metastasis from the kidney. Subsequently a nephrectomy was done for the primary kidney cancer. The patient survived for many years thereafter. Thoracic surgeons came to realize that provided the primary tumor was controllable, a solitary pulmonary metastasis could be resected with a 30% "cure". Since most metastases to the lungs tend to be multiple and/or bilateral, surgeons did not take an aggressive approach to

bilateral multiple pulmonary metastases of whatever source.
Solitary metastases in the liver can likewise be resected
with a chance for cure. This fact was realized later since
it is easier to evaluate the lungs by chest x-ray than it is
to evaluate the liver. The development of liver isotope
scans and more recently CTT scans, as well as angiograms provide an improved way of assessing the liver. At thoracotomy,
a surgeon can determine fairly accurately by palpation and
inspection metastases in the lung. This is more difficult in
palpating and inspecting the liver.

MATERIALS

The tumor registry at Memorial Hospital has collected
over the past 25 years 14,372 cancers to be surveyed in this
paper. These are cancers from white patients only since the
number of black patients was much smaller. Five-year survival
curves have been used throughout except in breast cancer where
a 10 year period has been used. The five periods under study
are A-1950-1954, B-1955-1959, C-1960-1964, D-1965-1969, and
E-1970-1974. "Localized" and "regional" tumors have been the
subject of study although this classification has serious
staging drawbacks as will be discussed.

COLON AND RECTAL CANCER

There are approximately 170,000 cases of gastrointestinal
cancer in the United States annually, of which 110,000 are new
cases of cancer of the colon and rectum. Attempts to diagnose
colon cancer early by screening and to eliminate polyps by
polypectomy increased the number of stage A (local) and/or B
(regional) colon cancers from 30% to 80%. The Strang[2] Clinic
in their cancer detection program found that 80% of colon
cancers detected by sigmoidoscopy was "localized". Recently
early detection is stressed more using studies with stool
guaiac. Significant progress is being made since a survival
rate of 80% is anticipated with Duke's A lesions confined to
the bowel and 70% survival with Duke's B lesions spread
regionally. The U.S. national survival[3] figures for colon and
rectal surgery at community hospitals still approximate 30%.
At specialized centers, patients with colon cancer and positive lymph nodes have increasing numbers of reports reflecting
a 60% to 70% five-year survival rate. Sphincter preserving
surgery has been done for all but the lowest of rectal cancers. Now only 15% to 20% of patients with rectal cancer
require a permanent colostomy. Better antimicrobial drugs

have been valuable in decreasing the risk of sepsis in colon surgery.

In males with localized colon cancer treated at Memorial Hospital during the past 25 years, there is a five-year survival rate varying from 59% to 73% (Graph 1). There is no obvious improvement in later periods (0.5853). In the female with localized colon cancer, the survival varied from 67% to 83% (Graph 2). There was some slight improvement in the last two periods. The significance was only 0.257.

Colon cancer regionally spread in the male showed a five-year survival from 27% to 69%. The last five-year period was the highest and was better than the previous years (Graph 3). The significance is 0.0297. Colon cancers regionally spread in the female were closer together in their end results and varied from 46% to 55%. The significance is 0.7927 (Graph 4).

Survival of cancer of the rectum localized in the male for the five periods varied from 60% to 65%. The curves are very similar and there is no statistically significant difference (Graph 5). In the female with localized rectum cancer, survival rates varied from 62% to 73%. The results were similar over the five-year period although the last five-year period has the highest survival (Graph 6). Its significance was 0.4783. Carcinoma of the rectum regionally spread in the male showed that the five-year survival rates varied from 26% to 41%. There was no significant difference in the periods (0.2417) (Graph 7). Carcinoma of the rectum regionally spread in the female showed five-year survival rates of 31% to 42%. There was no significant difference in the groups at 0.4793 (Graph 8).

UTERUS

Carcinoma of the uterine cervix localized in the female shows similar survival rates for all the five-year periods. The survival rate has varied from 61% to 66% (Graph 9). These differences are not significant at 0.9095. Carcinoma of the uterine cervix regionally spread in the female shows differences. The period 1950-54 showed a five-year survival of 20%, whereas the period 1965-69 indicates a 38% survival, and 1970-74 shows a 58% survival (Graph 10). The early curves were the period of Dr. Alexander Brunschwig, Chief of the Gynecology Service. At that time, all cervix cancers were operated upon and were surgically pathologically staged. During the last two periods under Dr. John Lewis, Chief of the Gynecology Service, the cervix cancer presumed to be

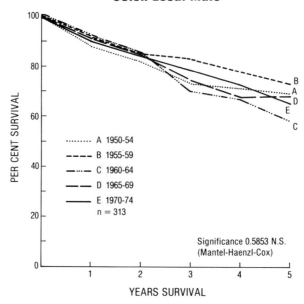

GRAPH 1

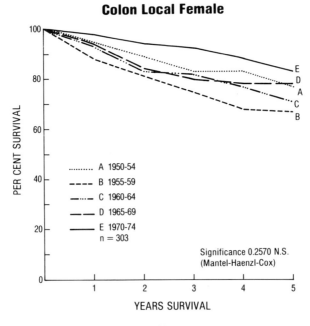

GRAPH 2

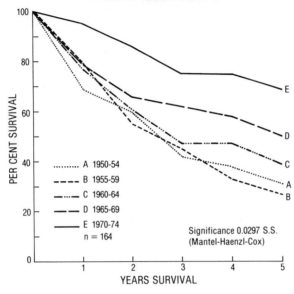

GRAPH 3

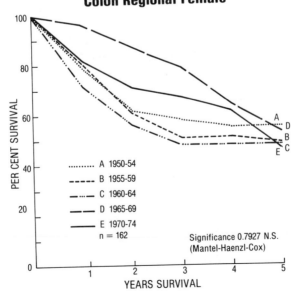

GRAPH 4

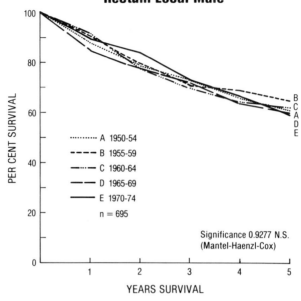

GRAPH 5

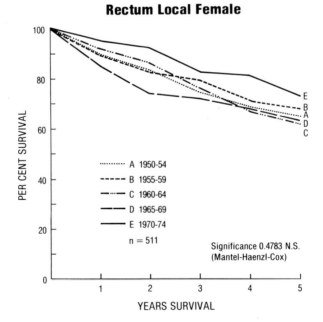

GRAPH 6

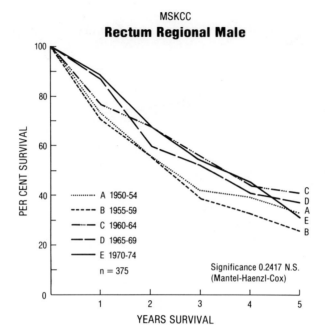

MSKCC
Rectum Regional Male

GRAPH 7

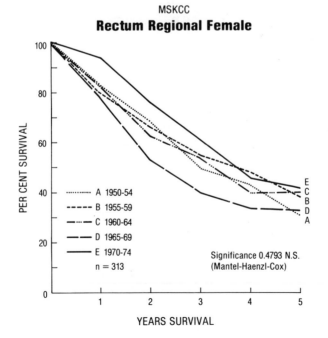

MSKCC
Rectum Regional Female

GRAPH 8

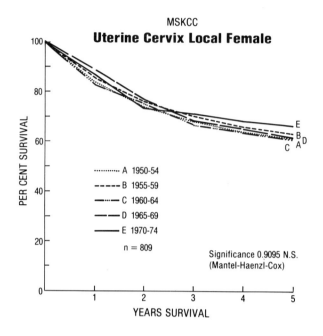

MSKCC
Uterine Cervix Local Female

A 1950-54
B 1955-59
C 1960-64
D 1965-69
E 1970-74
n = 809

Significance 0.9095 N.S.
(Mantel-Haenzl-Cox)

PER CENT SURVIVAL

YEARS SURVIVAL

GRAPH 9

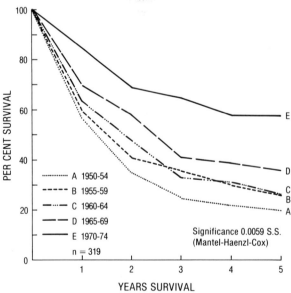

MSKCC
Uterine Cervix Regional Female

A 1950-54
B 1955-59
C 1960-64
D 1965-69
E 1970-74
n = 319

Significance 0.0059 S.S.
(Mantel-Haenzl-Cox)

PER CENT SURVIVAL

YEARS SURVIVAL

GRAPH 10

regionally spread was treated with preoperative radiotherapy and then treated surgically. In some of these patients, there was clinical staging. However, the differences in the survival rates are considered significant at the 0.0059 level.

The most recent data for carcinoma of the body of the uterus confined to the uterus (stage I) where the policy of the Gynecology Service is to carry out hysterectomy after preoperative radiation therapy, has exhibited a five-year survival rate in excess of 90%.[4]

The importance of regular pelvic examination and Pap smears of vaginal secretions cannot be stressed too highly. In this way tumors of the cervix can be detected in a pre-malignant or non-invasive stage. If carcinoma does develop, the stage I variants of cervix and body of uterus carcinoma are highly curable.[5]

LUNG

The data shows that localized carcinoma of the lung in the male had a five-year survival rate from 13% to 26% (Graph 11). The last 2 periods were higher than the other three periods with a significance of approximately 0.018. The data for localized lung cancer in the female showed an improvement over the males with a five-year survival rate from 21% to 48% (Graph 12). The last period of 1970-74 was 33% and the statistical difference for the whole group was 0.145.

Results of lung cancer regionally spread in the male were poor. Survival rates ranged from 3% to 10% and the statistical significance of change was 0.0118 (Graph 13). In the female with lung cancer regionally spread survival rates ranged from 5% to 18% (Graph 14) The last two periods were slightly better for a significance of 0.1160.

These relatively poor statistics with the staging commonly in vogue for lung cancer were about similar to the U.S. national average. Lung cancer is the most common cancer responsible for deaths in the U.S. and more than 100,000 lung cancer deaths are expected in 1980. Lung cancer is the leading cancer responsible for deaths in males, and it is rapidly increasing in females. By 1983 lung cancer will pass breast cancer and be the most common cancer responsible for death in females.

The staging method listing lung cancer as localized or regionalized is an obsolete staging system and interferes with the proper study of lung cancer. The TNM system advocated by the American Joint Committee is a superior

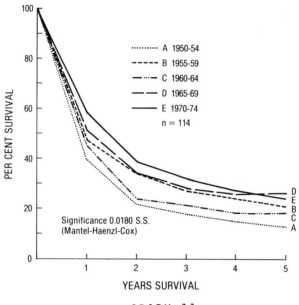

MSKCC
Lung Local Male

A 1950-54
B 1955-59
C 1960-64
D 1965-69
E 1970-74
n = 114

PER CENT SURVIVAL

Significance 0.0180 S.S.
(Mantel-Haenzl-Cox)

YEARS SURVIVAL

GRAPH 11

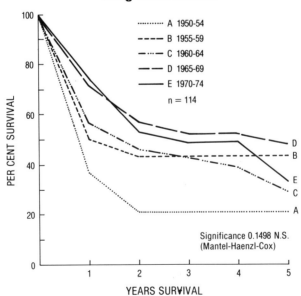

MSKCC
Lung Local Female

A 1950-54
B 1955-59
C 1960-64
D 1965-69
E 1970-74
n = 114

PER CENT SURVIVAL

Significance 0.1498 N.S.
(Mantel-Haenzl-Cox)

YEARS SURVIVAL

GRAPH 12

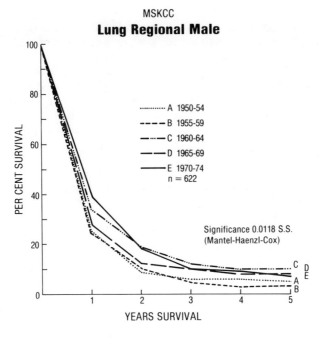

MSKCC
Lung Regional Male

GRAPH 13

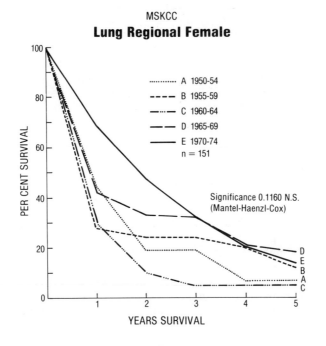

MSKCC
Lung Regional Female

GRAPH 14

803

system and has been in use at Memorial Hospital since 1972.
Also, in that year we developed a staging map for the mediastinum. It is required that during thoracotomies the
operating surgeon fill out a chart. The lymph nodes removed
from the mediastinum and lung are numbered and classified for
the pathologist. Single digit numbers represent mediastinal
lymph nodes. The upper mediastinum is numbered 2, 3 and 4;
the bifurcation of the trachea (subcarinal node) is 7; and
lymph nodes 8 and 9 extend inferiorly along the esophagus and
the inferior pulmonary ligaments. Lymph nodes outside the
mediastinal pleura, in the hilum of the lung, of the lobes,
or of the segments are given double digit numbers.

A present important observation relates to monitoring
males at high risk for lung cancer. Memorial Hospital
started a National Lung Program sponsored by the National
Cancer Institute in 1974. 10,000 male volunteers over the
age of 45 who smoked more than 1 pack of cigarettes a day for
20 years were enrolled. The enrolment was completed by 1977.
The compliance and followup has been good. All receive an
annual PA and lateral chest x-ray, and half in matched pairs
give a sputum for cytology examination each four months. As
of early 1980, 159 lung cancers were detected. Fifty-five of
the patients entered with undetected lung cancer found in
their first examination. The others developed incidental
lung cancers at the rate of over 30 patients per 100,000 per
year. Sixty-five patients were staged as stage I lung cancer
and were promptly treated with surgical excision of their
cancers. The survival curve for these males showed a survival rate in excess of 90% from one to five years. The stage
II and stage III lung cancer patients totaled 94. They
showed a survival curve which had dropped to less than 10%
survival at 2 1/2 years post treatment. Thus 38% of the lung
cancers discovered were stage I with over 90% survival rates.
This is statistically highly significant. Epidermoid carcinoma and adenocarcinoma gave similar survival curves. In the
incidental cases found in the series, 25% were oat cell carcinoma; 75% were non-oat cell carcinoma. Of the non-oat cell
carcinomas, 60% were stage I.[6]

In 1977, Martini and Beattie[7] reported 691 non-oat cell
lung cancers seen at Memorial Hospital during 1972-1976 in-
clusively. 216 patients were clinically staged as stage I.
After surgical pathologic staging, there were 125 stage I
patients. Of these, 10 were so-called occult lung cancers
with positive sputum and negative chest x-rays. This relatively rare group of lung cancers has a cure rate in excess
of 90% and were not used in the analysis. The survival curve
of the 115 stage I cancers showed 90% survival at 36 months,

with 83% free of disease at 36 months. When the stage I
patients were subdivided into T1 (less than 3 cm in diameter)
versus T2 (over 3 cm in diameter), the survival curves were
markedly different at 4 years. T1 tumors had a 92% survival
rate at 4 years whereas T2 tumors showed a 68% survival rate.
We anticipate that this group of stage I lung cancers will
have a five-year survival rate of 60% to 70%. We must have
accurate TNM surgical pathologic staging to understand the
true nature of the various stages of lung cancer. Further,
it has been our experience that the TNM staging is far more
important than cell types after the division into oat cell
and non-oat cell. Our adenocarcinomas and epidermoid carcinomas have fared similarly when one compares similar TNM
stages.

There are a considerable number of lung cancer patients
where one cannot surgically remove all the cancer either because of the physiological status of the patient, or because
of involvement of major mediastinal structures. An advance
that we feel has been very significant has been the use of
internal radiotherapy in these non-resectable lung cancers.

Internal radiotherapy has the following advantages.[8] It
is of greater curative potential. It gives good palliation by
quick and prolonged tumor shrinkage. There is no further
therapy or hospital stay after the patient has recovered from
the operation. The technique converts an otherwise useless
operation into an effective therapeutic procedure.

The technique consists of exposing the tumor, placing
hollow needles 1 cm equidistant throughout the tumor, and as
the needles are withdrawn, a radioactive seed is left every
1 cm in the tumor. The radiation therapy persists over the
course of 1 year with 80% of the dose being given the first
60 days. A more recent technique of leaving hollow catheters
across the mediastinum permits the introduction or radioactive iridium postoperatively. This isotope supplements the
implanted internal radiotherapy. Subsequently, additional
external radiotherapy can be given. This technique affords
control in 80% of the cancers in the chest. The major cause
of failure is disease outside the chest.

There has been common usage of the mediastinoscope to
stage lung cancer. If mediastinal lymph nodes were found
involved with cancer, especially with adenocarcinoma, surgery
was considered contraindicated and the treatment has been
external radiation therapy alone.

In 1980, Martini and Beattie[9] reported their experience
with surgical treatment of N2 mediastinal lymph nodes. From
1974 to 1978, 998 lung cancers were staged. 2% were the
so-called TX occult. 32% were stage I. 3% were stage II.

63% were stage III. Of the 998 patients, 445 had positive
(N2) mediastinal lymph nodes. No surgery was done on 204 of
the 445 because of extensive disease outside of the chest
with M1 metastases. 241 patients were surgically explored.
In 80 of these patients it was possible to remove all the
mediastinal lymph nodes for cure. All received postoperative
radiation therapy. The survival curve at 36 months was 49%
overall. The adenocarcinoma had a 56% survival rate at 3
years compared to epidermoid carcinoma which had a 44% rate.
This result confirms our impression that the TNM stage of
lung cancer is more important than the cell type in non-oat
cell tumors. The 21 patients staged as T1N0M0 but who had N2
positive nodes, had a 74% survival rate at 3 years. The 26
patients clinically staged T2N0M0 but who had N2 positive
nodes had a 52% 3 year survival rate. It is our conclusion
that any patient clinically staged as having no tumor in the
mediastinum should not have a mediastinoscopy since one could
expect up to a 75% 3 year survival rate following surgical
resection and postoperative radiation therapy.

The major challenge consists of patients with N2 positive nodes where all the N2 nodes can not be totally resected
but where there are no known metastases outside the chest.
We are presently treating these patients with surgery, internal radiotherapy and external radiotherapy, and it is planned
to use adjuvant chemotherapy. Our best chemotherapy protocol
has been high dose cis-Platinum plus Vindesine in the
disseminated advanced non-oat cell lung cancer. Drs. Gralla[10]
and Golbey have found a 43% complete and partial remission
rate. The responders have a median survival rate of 22
months compared to similar patients without chemotherapy
where the median survival rate is 6 months. We feel that we
can begin to use prophylactic, adjuvant chemotherapy with
success. Oat cell carcinoma has been chemotherapy sensitive
with about a 40% survival rate after 24 months[11] and with an
occasional cure. An even more aggressive combined treatment
plan is needed if we are to cure the oat cell carcinomas.

METASTATIC LUNG TUMORS

McCormack[12] has presented data from Memorial Hospital on
the surgical treatment of pulmonary metastases. From 1970 to
1976, 409 patients were operated upon with a total of 622
thoracotomies. There were 220 patients with metastatic carcinoma from colon, melanoma, breast, testes, head and neck,
kidney, bladder, and ovary. There were 189 sarcomas from
bone, chondrosarcoma, leiomyosarcoma, rhabdomyosarcoma,

synovial sarcoma, schwannoma, liposarcoma, fibrosarcoma, and alveolar soft part sarcoma. The surgical procedures were wedge or segmental resection 69%, lobectomies 19%, pneumonectomies 3%, implants 3%, and exploration only 6%. The maximum number of thoracotomies per patient was 10 on one patient. Overall these patients had a five-year survival rate of 25%. It was further confirmed that in a large variety of carcinomas and sarcomas, bilateral and multiple pulmonary metastases have a survival rate above 15% with surgery alone. In the next decade, better combination chemotherapy should improve these results.

METASTATIC BRAIN TUMORS

The brain is a frequent site of metastases from tumors elsewhere in the body, especially from the lung. At times the primary tumor can be controlled, and the cause of death is the brain metastasis. Posner[13,14] and Galicich[15,16] at Memorial Hospital have studied this problem. Metastases to the brain treated with whole brain radiation therapy plus corticosteroids have a median survival rate of 12 weeks. 24% of patients treated in this fashion survived over 6 months, but only 7% survived for over one year. Galicich reported that from July 1977 through December 1978, 33 patients with solitary brain metastases underwent surgical resection and postoperative radiation therapy. The median survival rate of the entire group is 8 months with a 1 year survival rate of 44%. Of those patients with no evidence of systemic cancer at the time of craniotomy, 80% lived for 1 year. This data shows that recurrence in the central nervous system following craniotomy and radiation therapy for a single brain metastasis is low. The serial CT scanner provides a better way to follow these patients. 13 of the original 33 patients were alive 18 months after treatment. A surgical approach plus radiotherapy seems much better than radiation therapy alone in this condition.

BREAST

The results with localized carcinoma of the breast show considerable improvement. In 1950-54 the 5 and 10 year survival rates were respectively 77% and 63%. By 1965-69, the 5 and 10 year survival rates were 87% and 74%. The most recent period of 1970-74 shows a 5 year survival rate of 90% and an 8 year survival rate of 80%. These differences are significant at 0.0000 (Graph 15).

MSKCC

Breast Female Local

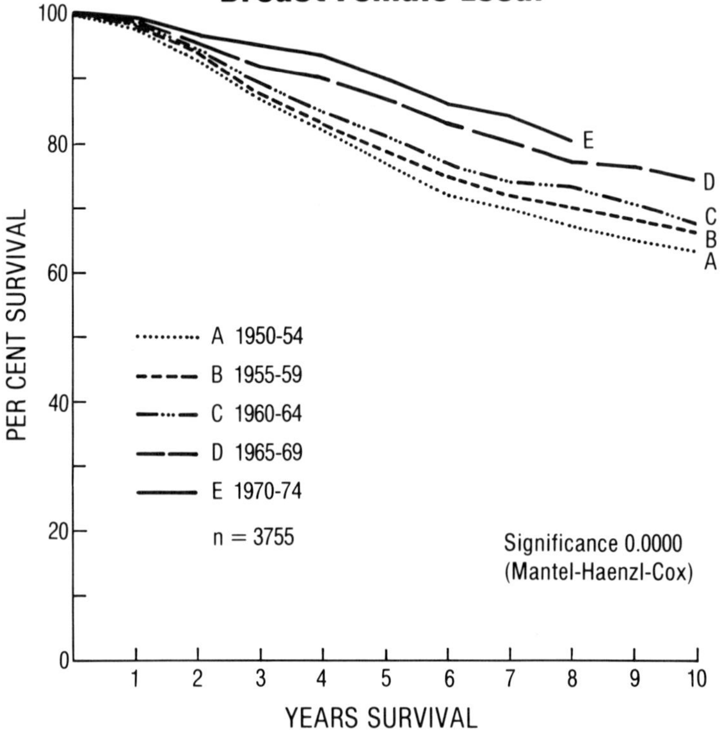

100
80
60
40
20
0
PER CENT SURVIVAL
1
2
3
4
5
6
7
8
9
10
YEARS SURVIVAL
E
D
C
B
A
A 1950-54
B 1955-59
C 1960-64
D 1965-69
E 1970-74
n = 3755
Significance 0.0000
(Mantel-Haenzl-Cox)

GRAPH 15

Breast cancer regionally spread has also been analyzed.
The five-year survival rates in the periods under evaluation
have risen from 45%, to 48%, to 52%, to 57%, and to 65% in
the most recent period. Likewise, there has been steady rise
in the 10 year survival rates from 28% to 30%, to 34%, to 39%
in the last period of 1965-69. The 10 year survival statistics are not yet available in the 1970-74 period. This is
statistically significant at the level of 0.0000 (Graph 16)
There is clearly an improvement in the survival rate of the
woman coming to Memorial Hospital with regional spread of
breast cancer treated by surgery alone. This is probably
related to less advanced stage of regional disease.

In analyzing the survival rates for breast cancer, the
status of the tumor and of the lymph nodes in the TNM system
are paramount. It is important that breast cancer survival
statistics be at least of 10 years duration. Thus any survival data quoted in 1980 must be from patients treated prior to
1970. Analysis by Robbins[17] of the breast cancers treated
at Memorial Hospital in 1964 and analyzed in 1975 show that
tumors measuring less than 3 cm in diameter with no metastases to the regional lymph nodes had an 80% 10 year survival
rate. Additional data at Memorial Hospital indicates that
tumors under 1 cm in diameter have a 10 year survival rate of
95%.[18] Therefore early diagnosis of breast cancer treated surgically has an excellent survival rate. The big advance of
the decade 1970-1980 was the use of adjuvant chemotherapy for
women at increased risk from breast cancer, namely, those who
had metastases to axillary lymph nodes. The contributions of
Fisher, et al[19] that patients with 4 or more lymph nodes invaded with metastatic breast cancer in the axilla were at
quite high risk were valuable. The introduction of the CMF
protocol by Bonadonna[20] where he gave one year of CMF chemotherapy prophylactically to women following radical mastectomy improved the survival rate by 30% in the premenopausal
women. Present studies at Memorial Hospital indicate that
women with breast cancer at high risk who are on two years of
CMF chemotherapy have improved survival in both premenopausal
and postmenopausal women.

Adair, et al,[21] from Memorial Hospital analyzed the survival rate 30 years later in 1,458 women with breast cancer
treated by radical mastectomy from 1940 to 1943. The
patients were analyzed by the size of the tumor in centi-
meters and the status of the axillary lymph nodes. The
axillary lymph nodes were designated as negative or positive
at level I (with nodes at the bottom of the axilla), positive
at level II (nodes at the middle of the axilla), or positive
at level III (nodes at the apex of the axilla). The survival

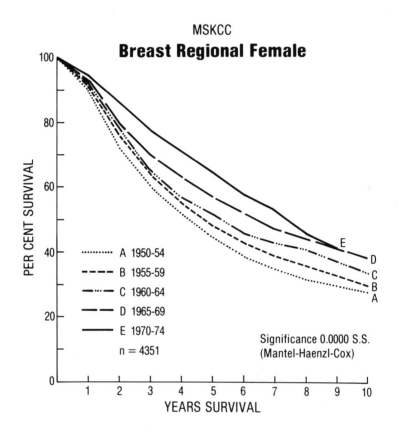

MSKCC
Breast Regional Female

PER CENT SURVIVAL

.... A 1950-54
----- B 1955-59
--·--·-- C 1960-64
-- -- D 1965-69
——— E 1970-74

n = 4351

Significance 0.0000 S.S.
(Mantel-Haenzl-Cox)

YEARS SURVIVAL

GRAPH 16

810

curves in all these classifications fell for 10 years, but
after 10 years all survival curves regardless of stage of
disease leveled off. In general there was less than 10%
difference between the survival rates at 10 years and 30
years. In no combination of factors was there zero survival
rate at 30 years, except in one classification with a limited
number of patients. This paper was important in the concept
that patients should be followed for life in tumor registries. These results are not consistent with the thought
that breast cancer is always systemic at the time of diagnosis, and that all women with breast cancer will die of breast
cancer.

Another interesting observation was that in 1960, 55% of
women coming to Memorial Hospital with breast cancer had
negative lymph nodes at the time of operation. In 1979, 63%
of the women presenting themselves at Memorial Hospital with
breast cancer had negative lymph nodes. This demonstrates
slow but steady improvement in earlier diagnosis.

A major surgical advance in the last decade has been the
increase in the number of patients with breast cancer who
received plastic reconstruction postoperatively. The
utilization of myocutaneous flaps has been a distinct advance
when skin and muscle are deficient, as after the classic
radical mastectomy. These flaps transfer skin using the
underlying muscle as the vascular supply. The myocutaneous
flap from the latissimum dorsi permits an incision in the
brassiere line which can then take this flap from posterior
to anterior to fill in the missing breast skin and muscle
contour. The addition of a silicone implant and the
reconstruction of the nipple creates a more normal appearing
breast.

In the past decade, clinical trials have been developed
to see if lesser forms of treatment for breast cancer with
primary operable breast cancer will achieve the same results
as with more radical surgery alone. One such study is
Veronisi's[22] project where in clinical stage I breast cancer
the patients are randomized to either radical mastectomy or
to partial mastectomy with axillary dissection plus radiation
therapy to the remaining breast. In both arms of this study,
those patients with positive axillary nodes also receive
adjuvant CMF chemotherapy. With a median followup that
approximates 5 years, there is presently no difference in
recurrence or survival in either group. The Fisher NSABP[23]
group is presently studying a protocol with three arms,
comparing modified radical mastectomy with a partial mastectomy plus axillary dissection without radiation therapy and
compared to a partial mastectomy, axillary dissection and

radiation therapy to the breast. In all three arms those
patients with positive axillary lymph nodes are being treated
with adjuvant chemotherapy. This study is being done in an
attempt to answer the biological importance of the multicentricity of breast cancer in the breast. Studies at Memorial
Hospital have shown that even small breast cancers (2 cm or
less in diameter) have multi-focal cancer in 60% of the
instances. This is why the so-called lumpectomy or segmental
resection of an early carcinoma of the breast appears to have
a 40% 10-year survival rate.

The development of estrogen and progesterone receptor
determinations has improved the response rate in selecting
patients for ablative endocrine surgery from 30% success to
60%. This has been an important development.

The progress in the decade is that breast cancer can be
found earlier. Early breast cancer has a relatively high
cure rate, and it may be that lesser surgical procedures with
proper use of adjuvant therapy will give equally satisfactory
high cure rates.

HEAD AND NECK

In localized supraglottic laryngeal cancer in the male,
the five year survival curves in this 25 year period ranged
from 57% to 74% and overall are just under 70%. There is no
statistical significant difference between these five periods
(Graph 17). In the female with localized supraglottic laryngeal cancer, there is a wider variation in survival ranging
from 33% to 83% in the last period (Graph 18). The numbers
are too small for statistical significance.

Supraglottic laryngeal cancer regionally spread in the
male has less curability. The 5-year survival rate in the
five periods varied from 12% to 28%. The 1970-74 period and
the 1960-64 period were better than the other periods, and
there was a slight significance of 0.1204 (Graph 19). The
supraglottic laryngeal cancers regionally spread in the female have a 5-year survival range from 12% to 51%. The last
five years 1970-74 were better, but the significance was not
great (Graph 20)

Local glottic laryngeal cancer in the male had a better
survival rate in the recent five year periods. This survival
rate improved from 62% to 82% in the last five year period.
This is significant at 0.05 (Graph 21). Local glottic laryngeal cancer in the female shows a good survival rate. The
range of five year survivals runs from 75% to 92% (Graph 22).
There is not a clear trend of improvement over the 25 years.

Larynx Supraglottic Local Male

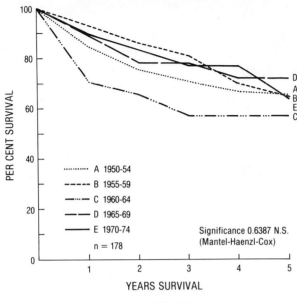

GRAPH 17

Larynx Supraglottic Local Female

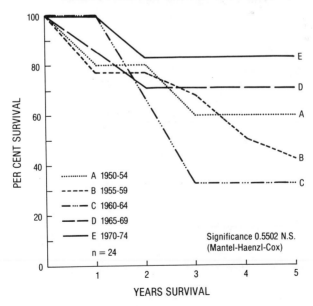

GRAPH 18

Larynx Supraglottic Regional Male

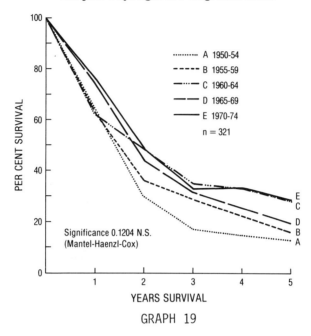

GRAPH 19

Larynx Supraglottic Regional Female

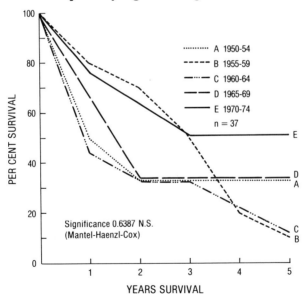

GRAPH 20

814

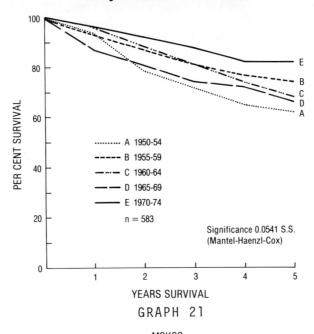

MSKCC
Larynx Glottic Local Male

PER CENT SURVIVAL

.... A 1950-54
----- B 1955-59
—··— C 1960-64
— — D 1965-69
——— E 1970-74
n = 583

Significance 0.0541 S.S.
(Mantel-Haenzl-Cox)

YEARS SURVIVAL

GRAPH 21

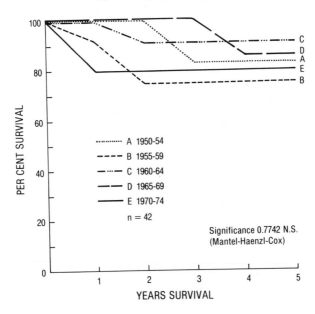

MSKCC
Larynx Glottic Local Female

PER CENT SURVIVAL

.... A 1950-54
----- B 1955-59
—··— C 1960-64
— — D 1965-69
——— E 1970-74
n = 42

Significance 0.7742 N.S.
(Mantel-Haenzl-Cox)

YEARS SURVIVAL

GRAPH 22

815

Glottic laryngeal cancer spread regionally in the male
has a lesser 5-year survival rate varying from 30% to 57%
(Graph 23). The last 5-year period, 1970-74, was at the 57%
level. The numbers are small and the significance not great.
The numbers in the female were too low to make a definite
statement (Graph 24).

The main advances in head and neck cancer in the last
decade have been more conservation in treating cancers of the
larynx and pharynx. In the reconstructive field, the advent
of myocutaneous flaps has revolutionized the reconstruction
of may patients with advanced head and neck cancer. These
flaps have greatly assisted in expeditious, prompt reconstruction of major defects. One of the most valuable techniques is preservation of speech following laryngectomy utilizing the puncture technique devised by Blom and Singer.[24]
This procedure consists of the creation of a surgical fistula
between the trachea and hypopharynx which is kept open by a
plastic one-way prosthesis. This device enables these
patients to gain the ability to speak in the immediate postoperative period.

LIVER AND PANCREAS

Progress in surgery of cancer of the liver in the decade
1970 to 1980 has been outstanding. The works of Fortner[25] and
Starzl have lead the field. Analysis of the data from
Fortner at Memorial Hospital shows that in the period 1970 to
1980, 436 patients with liver disease were operated upon.
124 patients had resection for malignant tumor in the liver.
In the period 1975 to 1980, there was a 30-day hospital
operative mortality rate of 6%. In the resection of metastatic colo-rectal cancer to the liver, there was a 73% 3-year
survival rate in 27 patients with colo-rectal metastases which
were localized to liver parenchyma. A relatively low
operative mortality rate with resection of metastatic liver
disease combined with a high percentage of 3-year survivals
in carcinoma confined to the liver bodes well for the future.
Liver survery for metastatic disease is at the stage where
metastatic pulmonary sarcoma was a decade ago. It seems logical to predict that as chemotherapy improves for colon cancer,
there will be an increasing long-term survival rate of colon
cancer metastatic to the liver treated by surgery and
chemotherapy.

The other serious problem in the abdomen is cancer of the
pancreas which has had a poor curability and survival rate.
The Memorial Hospital figures for cancer of the pancreas in

Larynx Glottic Regional Male

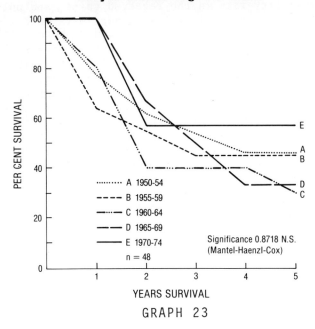

A 1950-54
B 1955-59
C 1960-64
D 1965-69
E 1970-74
n = 48

Significance 0.8718 N.S.
(Mantel-Haenzl-Cox)

GRAPH 23

MSKCC
Larynx Glottic Regional Female

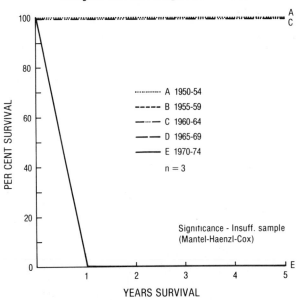

A 1950-54
B 1955-59
C 1960-64
D 1965-69
E 1970-74
n = 3

Significance - Insuff. sample
(Mantel-Haenzl-Cox)

GRAPH 24

the past have shown that 15% were resectable, there was a 15% operative mortality rate in the resected cases, and only 15% of the resected cases survived for 3 years with no 5-year survivors. Fortner[26] has devised a procedure he has called regional pancreatectomy. This is the en bloc resection of the pancreas along with the portal vein and the regional lymph nodes. In some instances, he has also resected the superior mesenteric artery. In 1972-1977, Fortner performed 40 of these regional pancreatectomies with a 30-day surgical mortality rate of 15% overall. Thirty-six of the patients had periampullary or pancreatic cancer, and 4 had benign disease. Of the 30 patients with cancer who survived the operation, 10 are currently alive and well (33%). 27% died of other causes without evidence of recurrent cancer. Two of the 15 patients with adenocarcinoma are presently alive, and 8 patients of 15 with other types of malignant tumors are currently alive. The mortality rate for total pancreatectomy alone is 7%. It seems that with this approach, the survival rate will be increased over previous procedures and some 5-year cures will result. Here it is possible that effective adjuvant chemotherapy used in combination with this more aggressive surgical approach might turn the tide. It is a major problem for the 1980s.

UROLOGY

Localized bladder cancer in the male over the past 25 years has survival rates ranging from 29% to 62%. The most recent period, 1970-1974, exhibits the 62% survival rate. This is a considerable improvement and has a significance of 0.0009 (Graph 25). In the female with localized bladder cancer, the survival rates have ranged from 25% to 66% with the best results in the period 1970-74. The significance in this series is 0.2030. (Graph 26)

Bladder cancer spread regionally in the male is a serious problem. The survival rates vary from 0% to 30% and there was no apparent improvement in the recent years (Graph 27). Bladder cancer spread regionally in the female varies from 0% to 36% survival (Graph 28). There was some significance in the fact that the only survivors in the females with regional disease were in the past two periods, and were 17% and 36% respectively for the periods 1965-69 and 1970-74. This is significant at the 0.0058 value.

A major advance however in urologic surgery has been in the management of deeply invasive bladder cancer.[27] Here the use of moderate doses of radiation preoperatively has doubled

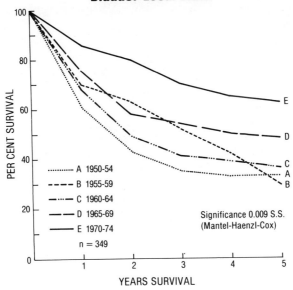

MSKCC
Bladder Local Male

A 1950-54
B 1955-59
C 1960-64
D 1965-69
E 1970-74
n = 349

Significance 0.009 S.S.
(Mantel-Haenzl-Cox)

GRAPH 25

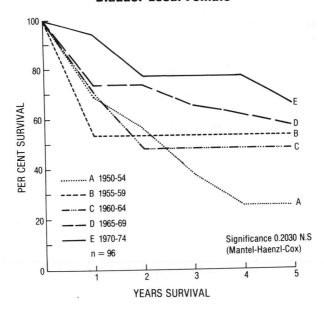

MSKCC
Bladder Local Female

A 1950-54
B 1955-59
C 1960-64
D 1965-69
E 1970-74
n = 96

Significance 0.2030 N.S
(Mantel-Haenzl-Cox)

GRAPH 26

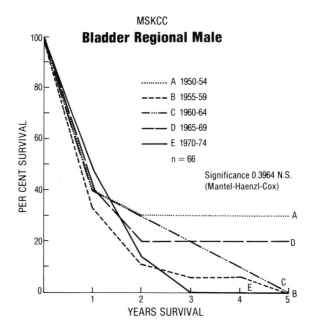

GRAPH 27

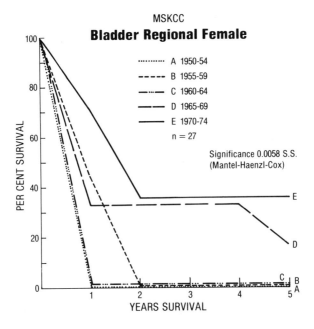

GRAPH 28

the five-year survival rate from 20% to 40%.

Localized prostate cancer has shown a very significant improvement in recent years. The most recent period of 1970-74 shows that the survival rate has risen to 87% (Graph 29). This is statistically significant at 0.0005. This is due to the improved treatment with the internal radiotherapy technique.

In prostate cancer regionally spread, the numbers treated are small and the survival rate has varied from 0% to 55%. The last three time periods have shown the most improvement. They were respectively 50%, 33% and 48%. This is significant at 0.0501, and appears to be due to a more aggressive therapeutic approach. (Graph 30)

Whitmore and Hilaris[28] over the past 10 years have been treating non-metastatic prostate cancer with laparotomy pelvic lymph node dissection, and I-125 implantation of the prostate. Over 600 patients were treated. The advantages are that it gives accurate staging and has a low morbidity and mortality rate compared to radical prostatectomy. There is no incontinence with the internal radiotherapy technique and sexual potency is unchanged. There is more rapid treatment during a hospital stay averaging 9 days, and there is less undesirable radiation therapy given to normal tissue compared to external radiotherapy alone.

The survival results are comparable to the best of the other treatment modalities of external beam therapy or radical prostatectomy. The procedure has a 5-year survival of better than 90% in disease confined to the prostate alone. Overall results in clinical stage B and C cancer of the prostate were 83% survival at 5 years, and 58% survival free of disease at 5 years.

Ten years ago, embryonal cell carcinoma of the testis metastatic to the abdomen and chest had a survival rate near zero. The outstanding development in the last decade has been the VAB chemotherapy program by Golbey and his colleagues. With surgical resection of the testis followed by intensive chemotherapy (now VAB VI) and utilizing repeat surgical operations for any persistent disease in the abdomen or chest along with radiation therapy as indicated, a 5-year survival of 80% is anticipated. This is the sensational story of Brian Piccolo where the National Football League, the Chicago Bears Football Club, Joy Piccolo and Jeannie Morris (who wrote "Brian Piccolo: A Short Season"), all contributed so much in supporting the development of the VAB program.[29,30,31,32]

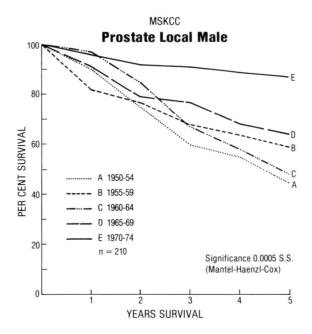

GRAPH 29

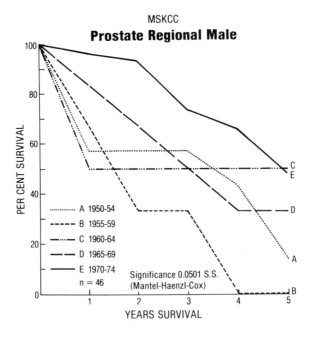

GRAPH 30

PEDIATRIC SURGERY

The improvement in the treatment of pediatric tumors over the last decade has been remarkable. Hodgkin's Disease, Wilm's Tumor, Ewing's Sarcoma, rhabdomyosarcoma, osteosarcoma and non-Hodgkin's lymphoma have risen from cure rates of 0% to 30% in 1960 to cure rates of 60% to 80% in 1975. This advance was achieved by the combination of surgery, radiotherapy and chemotherapy. Two tumors which have not advanced as well as the previous group are brain tumors and nerve tumors in children which are still below the 30% survival rate.[33]

Cure rates in Wilm's tumor are around 90% and rhabdomyosarcoma about 80%. Surgery has concentrated on resecting the tumor for cure, and at the same time preserving the anatomy of the child and the physiologic function as much as possible. This has meant doing more complicated procedures, often during periods of severe myelosuppression from chemotherapy. The timing of surgery, the selection of corrective procedures and the use of supportive measures have permitted operations on children who would have been abandoned 10 years ago. Now the challenge is to achieve the same results with less mutilating surgery. The best example of the benefit of a combined approach to a tumor system relates to the osteosarcomas of childhood. The osteosarcomas of the extremities of persons under the age of 21 have been serious tumors. A review by Marcove of the Memorial Hospital experience showed that 145 consecutive osteosarcomas treated by amputation had a 5-year survival rate of 15%.[34]   Beginning in 1966 we adopted an aggressive approach to the osteosarcoma pulmonary metastases. In 1971, Martini, et al,[35] reported 28 children operated upon with pulmonary metastases mostly multiple and/ or bilateral. In 22 of the 28 children it was possible to clear the lesions from the lungs although multiple thoracotomies were frequently needed. Of these 22 children, 45% were alive and well 3 years after amputation. In the control series of 118 patients where the pulmonary metastases were not resected, there was a 5% survival rate 3 years after amputation. Now in 1980, 6 of the original 22 children (30%) are alive and well more than 10 years later. A typical example is J.S., a 10 year old girl who had a hemipelvectomy in May 1968. She had 6 thoracotomies from May 1969 until July 1972 with removal of 12 metastatic tumors from the lungs. She received 9 months of chemotherapy which was completed in February 1974. She is now alive and well.

After Rosen developed the Memorial Hospital chemotherapy protocol for osteosarcoma, results began to improve further.

Our present treatment is: patients are biopsied for diagnosis. They then receive a 2 month chemotherapy protocol while
a steel prosthesis is custom made for the individual. Since
most of the tumors occur in the distal femur, most of the
replacements have consisted of a total femur, knee and upper
tibia. Limb conservation surgery is performed as developed
by Marcove provided the neurovascular bundle is not involved.
Huvos grades the chemotherapy effect on the tumor. Grading
is 1 through 4, with 1 and 2 showing insignificant tumor
necrosis and 3 and 4 showing significant tumor necrosis.
Rosen reports that children who have chemotherapy sensitive
tumors have a 5-year survival rate of almost 100%. With
resistant osteosarcoma, the 5-year survival rate was 30%.
With a new chemotherapy protocol adding high-dose cis-Platinum to the high-dose Methotrexate, Adriamycin, Vincristine
and Cytoxan regimen, Rosen found a 24 month survival rate of
90% in tumors that were resistant to the four-drug protocol.

A worse group of patients with osteosarcoma present with
pulmonary metastases already present. Here the treatment
plan is the same except that persistent lung lesions must be
removed surgically. Chest x-rays cannot tell whether the
pulmonary metastases are necrotic. Thoracotomy is indicated
to clear the lungs of tumor so that the chemotherapy is not
unduly prolonged. This approach can save 50% to 80% of
children with pulmonary metastases.[36]

Another malignant bone tumor in children which has responded well to the multidisciplinary treatment has been the
Ewing's sarcomas. Rosen, Marcove and Lane reported 20 cases
of pelvic Ewing's sarcoma treated with combined therapy.
There were 13 males and 7 females from 10 to 27 years old.
The local treatment was en bloc resection plus radiation
therapy in 12 patients, and intensive radiation therapy alone
in 8 patients. In the 20 cases there is a survival rate of
60%. Those cases treated surgically with radiotherapy show a
40% survival rate. Rosen has also reported 86 patients with
diverse Ewing's sarcoma treated in a multidisciplinary fashion
with an 80% survival rate at 5 years.[37]

This program in two very difficult tumor systems in
children points the way for what we hope to do with adult
solid tumors.

REFERENCES:
1. Barney, J.D., Churchill, E.D., Adenocarcinoma of the
Kidney with Metastases to the Lung, Cured by Nephrectomy and
Lobectomy. J.Urol. 42: 269, 1939.
2. Hertz, R.E., Deddish, M.R., Day E.: Value of Periodic
Examination in Detecting Cancer of the Rectum & Colon.
Postgraduate Medicine, Vol 27, 290-294, 1960

3. Enker, W.B., Laffer, U.T., Block G.: Enhanced survival of patients with colon and rectal cancer based upon wide anatomic resections. Annals of Surgery, 190: 350-360, September 1979.

4. Lewis J.L.: Stage I cancer of the body of the uterus; preoperative radiotherapy plus surgery with 93% survival. (Personal Communication)

5. Lewis J.L.: Stage 1b Cancer of the cervix with 90% survival. (Personal Communication)

6. Melamed, M.R., Flehinger, B.J., Zaman, M.B., Heelan, R.T., Hallerman, B.S., and Martini, N.: Detection of true pathologic Stage I lung cancer in a screening program and the effect on survival. Cancer (In Press)

7. Martini, N., and Beattie, E.J.: Results of surgical treatment in Stage I lung cancer. J.Thorac & Cardiovasc. Surg. 74: 499-505, October 1977.

8. Hilaris, B.S., Martini, N., Batata, M., and Beattie, E.J.: Interstitial irradiation for unresectable carcinoma of the lung. Ann. of Thoracic Surg., 20: 491-500, November 1975.

9. Martini,N., Flehinger, B.J., Zaman, B., Beattie, E.J.: Prospective study of 445 lung carcinomas with mediastinal lymph node metastases. J.THorac & Cardiovasc.Surg., 80: 390-399, 1980.

10. Casper, E., Gralla, R., Golbey, R.: Vindesine (DVA) and cis-dichlorodiammineplatinum II (DDP) combination chemotherapy in non-small cell lung cancer (NSCLC). Proc. AACR and ASCO, 20: Abstract No. C-190, 1979.

11. Natale,R., Hilaris, B., Wittes, R.: Prolonged remission of small cell lung carcinoma (SCLC) with intensive chemotherapy induction and high-dose radiation therapy without maintanence. Proc. AACR and ASCO, 21: C-525, 1980.

12. McCormack, P., Martini, N.: The changing role of surgery for pulmonary metastases. Ann.of Thoracic Surg., 28: 139-145, August 1979.

13. Posner, J.R., Chernik, N.L.: Intracranial metastases from systemic cancer, in Schoenberg, B.S. (ed): Neurological Epidemiology: Principles and Clinical Applications. Advances in Neurology, Vol. 19, Raven Press, 1978, pp 579-592.

14. Posner, J.B., Shapiro, W.R.: The management of intracranial metastases,in Morley, T.P. (Ed): Current Controversies in Neurosurgery. W.B. Saunders, pp 356-366, 1976.

15. Galicich,J.H., Sundaresan,N., and Thaler, H.T.: Surgical treatment of single brain metastasis: evaluation of results by computerized tomography scanning. J.Neurosurg., 53: 63-67, July 1980.

826 Edward J. Beattie, Jr.

16. Galicich, J.H., Sundaresan, N., Arbit,E., and Passe, S.: Surgical treatment of single brain metastasis: factors associated with survival. Cancer, 45,2: 381-386, January 1980.
17. Schottenfeld,D., Nash, A.G., Robbins, G.F., and Beattie, E.J.: Ten year results of the treatment of primary operable breast carcinoma. A summary of 304 patients evaluated by the TNM system. Cancer, 38: 1001-107, August 1976.
18. Kinne D.: Minimal breast cancer with 95% survival rate. (Personal communication).
19. Fisher, B., etal: L-phenylalanine mustard (L-PAM) in the management of primary breast cancer: an update of earlier findings and a comparison with those utilizing L-PAM plus 5-fluoruracil (5-FU). Cancer (Supp) 39: 2883-2903, June 1977.
20. Bonadonna, G., Rossi, A., Pinucchia, V., Banfi, A., Veronisi, U.: The CMF program for operable breast cancer with positive axillary nodes: updated analysis on disease-free interval, site of relapse, and drug tolrance. Cancer (Supp), 39: 2904-2915, June 1977.
21. Adair, F., Berg, J., Joubert, L., Robbins, G.F.: Long-term followup of breast cancer patients: 30-year report. Cancer: 33,4: 1145-1150, April 1974.
22. Veronisi, U., Banfi, A., Saccozzi,R., Salvadori, B., Zucali, R., Uslenghi, C, Greco, M., Luini, A., Rilke, F., Sultan, L.: Conservative treatment of breast cancer: a trial in progress at the Cancer Institute of Milan. Cancer (Supp) 39: 2822-2826, 1977.
23. Fisher, B., etal: Comparison of radical mastectomy with alternative treatments of primary breast cancer. Cancer (Supp) 39: 2827-2839, June 1977.
24. Singer, M.I., Blom, E.D.: An endoscopic technique for restoration of voice after laryngectomy. Presented at the Annual Meeting of the American Laryngologic Association, April 1980. (to be published).
25. Fortner, J.G., Kim, D.K., MacLean, B., Barrett, M.K., Iwatsuki, S., Turnbull, A.D., Howland, W.S., and Beattie, E.J: Major hepatic resection for neoplasia: personal experience in 108 patients. Ann. of Surg., 188: 363-371, September 1978.
26. Fortner, J.G.: Surgical principles for pancreatic cancer: regional, total and subtotal pancreatectomy. Cancer (In Press)
27. Whitmore, W.F. : Integrated irradiation & cystectomy for bladder cancer. Brit.J. of Urology, 52: 1-9, 1980.

28. Sogani, P.C., Whitmore, W.F., Hilaris, B.S., Batata, M.A.: Experience with interstitial implanation of Iodine-125 in the treatment of prostatic carcinoma. Scandinavian J. of Urology and Nephrology (In Press).

29. Silvay, O., Yagoda, A., Wittes, R., Whitmore, W., and Golbey, R.: Treatment of germ cell carcinomas with a combination of actinomycin-D, vinblastine, and bleomycin. Proceed. of the Amer.Association for Cancer Res. 14:68, March 1973, (Abstract)

30. Cvitkovic,E., Wittes, R., Golbey, R., and Krakoff, I.H.: Primary combination chemotherapy (VAB II) for metastatic or unresectable germ cell tumors. Proceed. of the Amer.Assoc. for Cancer Res. 16:174, March 1975.

31. Cvitkovic, E., Hayes, D., and Golbey, R.: Primary combination chemotherapy (VAB III) for metastatic or unresectable germ cell tumors. Proceed. of the Amer.Asso. for Cancer Res. 17:296, March 1976 (Abstract).

32. Hayes, D.M., Cvitkovic, E., Golbey, R., Scheiner, E., Helson, L., and Krakoff, I.H.: High dose cis-platinum diammine dichloride: amelioration of renal toxicity by mannitol diuresis. Cancer, 39: 1372-1381, April 1977.

33. Hammond, D., Bleyer, A., Hartmann, J., Hayes, D., Jenkins, R.: The team approach to the management of pediatric cancer. Cancer, 41: 29-35, 1978.

34. Marcove, R., Mike, V., Hajek, J.V., Levin, A.G., and Hutter, R.V.P.: Osteogenic sarcoma under the age of twenty-one: a review of 145 operative cases. J.Bone Joint Surg. (Amer.) 52: 411, 1970.

35. Martini, N., Huvos, G., Mike, V., Marcove, R. and Beattie, E.J.: Multiple pulmonary resections in the treatment of osteogenic sarcoma. Ann. of Thora. Surg., 12,3: 271-280, September 1971.

36. Rosen, G., Bone tumors. Presented at International Symposium on Cancer, New York City, September 1980.(In press, Grune & Stratton)

37. Rosen, G., Caparros, B., Niernberg, A., Marcove, R., and Huvos, A., Kosloff, C., Lane, J., Murphy, L.: Ewing's sarcoma: 10 years experience with adjuvant chemotherapy. Cancer (In Press).

Progress in Radiation Therapy
of Cancer

HENRY S. KAPLAN

Maureen Lyles D'Ambrogio Professor of Radiology
Director
Cancer Biology Research Laboratory
Stanford University Medical Center
Stanford, California

Radiation therapy was introduced as a new treatment modality at about the turn of the century, almost immediately after the discovery of x-rays by Röntgen,[119] of radioactivity by Becquerel,[9] and of radium by the Curies.[25] The initial responses of skin cancers treated with the primitive early x-ray tubes were so dramatic that it was at first thought that a miraculous cure for cancer had finally been discovered.[17] This unrealistic view was soon succeeded by a wave of disillusionment and pessimism when tumor recurrences and injuries to normal tissues began to appear. Yet, it would have been remarkable indeed if such failures and difficulties had not occurred during that early era; the first 25 years of this new discipline were indeed its "dark ages". The early radiation therapists had no understanding of the physical nature of the new and mysterious agents with which they worked, nor did they have any comprehension of their biological effects. There were no reliable methods with which to measure dose, and no generally agreed unit of dose existed. Equipment was primitive, temperamental, and too limited in energy to permit any but the most superficial neoplasms to be

treated. The initial crude treatment techniques involved
massive exposures, aimed at the eradication of tumors in a
single treatment, comparable to the extirpation of tumors by
surgery.[125] The primary morbidity, and even the acute mortality, of such massive-dose treatment was often comparable
to those of major surgery of that day. Patients who survived
the immediate post-irradiation period sometimes experienced
complete regression of their tumors, but these initial responses were all too often followed by major complications,
as well as by high rates of tumor recurrence. Indeed, much
of the clinical research of that era was directed toward the
description and analysis of hitherto unknown forms of tissue
injury.[15]

Radiation therapy was born again in the 1920's as a result
of the pioneering laboratory and clinical research of the
group at the Fondation Curie in Paris, headed by Claude
Regaud. Regaud and his co-workers performed a classical
series of experiments demonstrating that spermatogenesis in
the testis of experimental animals could be permanently
eradicated by the administration of successive daily doses of
fractionated radiotherapy, whereas single massive doses
failed to elicit the same biological response without concomitant permanent and often intolerable injury to the overlying skin.[114,116] Regaud suggested by analogy that radiotherapy should be similarly fractionated in the treatment of
cancers. He and his colleague, Henri Coutard, introduced
these techniques in the treatment of patients with cancers
arising in the head and neck region, and others used this
new approach in the treatment of cancer of the cervix uteri.
Within a few years, the Fondation Curie group began to report
5-year survival data for a variety of primary cancers of the

oral cavity, pharynx, and larynx which were indeed revolutionary.[24,115]   Equally impressive results soon followed
from programs using fractionated radiotherapy in the treatment of patients with cancer of the cervix. Long-term
relapse - free survival data indicated that many of these
patients had been permanently cured, some for the first time
in history. Thus, fractionation of radiation treatments
became a universally accepted technique which remains in use
to the present day.

The third decade of this century also witnessed important
technological and physical advances.[136] Reliable x-ray
therapy apparatus finally became available after the invention by Coolidge[21] of a vacuum x-ray tube capable of operation at hitherto unattainable energies as high as 200 kilo-
volts (200 kVp). Meanwhile, radiological physicists were
developing quantitative methods for the measurement of
radiation dose and defining the first physical unit of dose,
the roentgen.[127] During the next two decades, dosimetric
techniques were extensively developed and refined,[112] and in
1956, the present unit of absorbed dose, the rad, was adopted.[73]

The kilovoltage era was one of great achievement.[14] Centers in many parts of the world reported substantial cure
rates for cancers of the skin, the lip, the tonsil, the
anterior tongue, the larynx, and the cervix uteri. However,
the physical dose distribution of 200 kVp x-rays severely
limited the efforts of the radiotherapists of that era to
apply the new modality to more deeply seated tumors. By
about 1940, it was clear that beams of higher energy had to
be developed.

Soon after World War II, several groups of physicists
responded to this need by the introduction of imaginative new
devices of much higher energy. The unfolding of the "supervoltage" or, more properly, the megavoltage era of radiotherapy has been chronicled by Schulz.[124] Radioactive cobalt
(^{60}Co) provided by nuclear fission reactions made available
unlimited quantities of a cheap manmade substitute for radium.
This artificial isotope was first introduced for interstitial and intracavitary therapy, but as larger quantities
became available, ^{60}Co teletherapy apparatus with beam
energies equivalent to those of 3 MV x-rays was designed.
Electronic devices such as the betatron[90] and the linear
electron accelerator[48] were capable of yielding beams of very
high energy while operating at quite nominal voltages.
Linear electron accelerators were soon adapted to medical
radiotherapeutic use in England[102] and at Stanford University.[49] The linear accelerator proved to be a remarkably
versatile, reliable, and efficient clinical instrument[87] and
has today become the standard of excellence of megavoltage
equipment. Such accelerators, as well as cobalt teletherapy
units, are now found in radiation therapy departments throughout the world.

The high-energy beams generated by these new megavoltage
sources liberated radiation therapists from the physical
constraints of the kilovoltage era. Beams of megavoltage
energies produce their maximal ionization at significant
depths beneath the skin surface, thus effectively eliminating
the radiation tolerance of the skin as a dose-limiting factor.
The beams have sharply defined, knifelike edges, thus greatly
diminishing lateral scatter, and enabling these beams to be
used in the treatment of very small lesions in the eye, the

larynx, and other sites in close proximity to vital structures.[87] The much greater penetration of these high-energy
beams made it relatively easy to deliver tumoricidal doses
to neoplasms deep within the body, even in very obese patients. Finally, the very high beam intensities provided by
linear electron accelerators enabled their operation at much
longer target-patient distances, thus permitting quite large
fields which could encompass multiple areas of tumor involvement in contiguity. Taken together, these physical advantages have greatly increased the versatility and precision of
modern radiation therapy. For example, they made it possible
to develop entirely new and highly effective radiotherapy
techniques for Hodgkin's disease and other malignant lymphomas.[50,76,86,123] They have also enlarged the scope of
modern radiotherapy by permitting the definitive treatment
of neoplasms such as carcinoma of the prostate,[3,4,87] a
widely prevalent cancer which could not be effectively
treated earlier because of the severe skin reactions induced
in the perineal and inguinal regions by kilovoltage x-ray
beams. Significantly improved cure rates have now been
reported with megavoltage radiotherapy for several types of
cancers, especially those arising in the pelvis, the head
and neck region, and the lymphomas.[4,42,43,45,83]

Radiation therapists during this period also created the
foundations of modern clinical oncology through meticulous
and detailed studies of the patterns of spread of carcinomas,
sarcomas, and lymphomas arising in a variety of sites.[42,43,81]
In some instances, such studies led to the development of new
therapeutic strategies linked to the natural history of the
corresponding neoplasms. A key example is the evolution of
total lymphoid radiotherapy for Hodgkin's disease and other

malignant lymphomas.[76,85,86] Radiation therapists have also
carefully recorded the acute and chronic complications of
treatment, gradually compiling a body of data on which
current guidelines concerning the radiation tolerance of
various tissues and organs are based.[38,129] In many instances, recognition of the hazard of a complication, such as
radiation hepatitis,[72] radiation nephritis,[98] radiation
pneumonitis,[74] or radiation pericarditis,[128] was promptly
followed by refinements and modifications of technique which
mitigated or eliminated the problem.[16,105]

The radiotherapeutic armamentarium today includes a wide
variety of radiation sources: linear electron accelerators
and ^{60}Co teletherapy apparatus capable of providing external
x-ray and gamma ray beams of megavoltage energies are supplemented by interstitial and intracavitary capsules, needles,
tubes, and hollow sutures containing natural or artificial
radioactive isotopes permitting intense, highly localized
deposition of ionizing radiation in various tissues deep
within the body. Afterloading techniques now permit such
containers to be placed within the tumor initially, their
physical distribution checked and adjusted as necessary, and
then filled with the radioactive sources after homogeneous
dose distributions have been assured.[64,108] Such interstitial techniques have been particularly useful in the
treatment of cancers of the oral cavity, pharynx, and other
sites in the head and neck region. Intracavitary techniques
have been an extremely effective part of the management of
carcinoma of the cervix and other gynecological neoplasms.
Interstitial implantation is now being used also to supplement external beam therapy in the primary management of
cancers of the breast, localized carcinomas of the bronchus,

and other selected situations involving neoplasms of limited
volume. Radioactive isotopes have also been administered
intravenously, taking advantage of the phagocytic activity of
the reticulo-endothelial system to achieve selective localization in the liver, spleen, and/or bone marrow.[95] Intra-
lymphatic infusion of radioactive materials has been of
limited value because of the variability of lymph node
filling. Finally, beams of particulate radiations are now in
use or are being developed for ultra high energy radiation
therapy. These ionizing particles include electrons, pro-
tons, deuterons, neutrons, heavy ions, and π^- mesons. It is
anticipated that the high linear energy transfer (LET) of
some of these particles will confer substantial physical and/
or radiobiological advantages.[5,6,47,113,135]

It has required many years for radiation therapy to live
down the unfortunate reputation which it acquired during the
first decades of the century. During that dismal era, many
physicians concluded that radiotherapy was useful as a form
of palliative treatment but had no curative potential. This
erroneous notion became deeply entrenched, and could not be
effectively dispelled by the substantial achievements which
radiation therapists were able to report later in the kilovoltage era. In the modern megavoltage era, cure rates have
substantially increased and the scope of curative radiotherapy has been extended to types of malignant neoplasms
which, for technical reasons, could not be effectively
treated with lower energy equipment. Today, the radiation
oncologist can cite an extensive and convincing mass of
evidence to justify his use of the term "cure" with the same
degree of assurance as the surgeon.[83] Many patients treated
25 or more years ago with kilovoltage x-rays and/or radium

for carcinoma of the cervix uteri, or for cancers in the
head and neck region, survived into old age with no subsequent manifestations of their tumors, or died of natural
causes with no evidence of persistent neoplasm at autopsy.
Although such individual cases suffer from the limitation of
being anecdotal, there can be no question that they represent
true cures. Meaningful assessment of the curative potential
of modern radiation therapy requires, however, the systematic
long-term study of large numbers of consecutive, unselected
patients with biopsy proved malignant neoplasms of various
types. Analyses of actuarial survival curves based on such
large series,[42,52,86] as well as studies of the temporal
distribution of relapses following radiotherapy,[79,147] have
today provided unambiguous evidence that radiotherapy can
indeed yield permanent cure in substantial proportions of
patients with malignant neoplasms of various primary sites.

   The improvement in prognosis which occurred with the
transition from kilovoltage to megavoltage beam energies
may be illustrated with a few representative examples. Five-
year survival in patients with cancer of the cervix, considered tantamount to permanent cure, has increased from around
35-45% in the kilovoltage era to approximately 65% with megavoltage radiotherapy.[42,43] Survival has more than doubled,
from about 25% to more than 50%, in cancer of the nasopharynx.[65] Similar gains have been noted with respect to
other head and neck primary sites.[43] Cervical lymph node
metastasis from primary tumors in the oral cavity and
pharynx can now be eradicated by techniques made possible by
megavoltage beam energies.[59] Long-term survival in invasive
cancer of the urinary bladder has increased from near zero to
about 30%.[52] Carcinoma of the prostate can now be treated

with curative intent with external megavoltage beam radiation therapy, with long-term survival rates which compare very favorably with those of radical extirpative surgery.[4] Perhaps the most dramatic example of improvement is that seen in Hodgkin's disease, in which 5-year survival in the kilo-voltage era was only about 25-30% for patients with all stages of disease. With the aid of diagnostic techniques such as lymphangiography and staging laparotomy, the development of total lymphoid megavoltage radiotherapy, and the introduction of combination chemotherapy, 5-year survival for patients with Hodgkin's disease of all stages now exceeds 80%.[86] Moreover, a very high proportion of these patients are relapse-free for more than 5 years after initial treatment and may thus be considered permanently cured.[79,86] Long-term relapse-free survival of patients with highly radio-sensitive testicular seminomas has improved to 90% or more with the advent of external beam megavoltage radiotherapy.[36] Impressive gains have also been recorded in the treatment of the more resistant embryonal carcinomas of the testis, even in instances involving spread to the retroperitoneal lymph nodes.[36,103] Most patients successfully treated with megavoltage radiotherapy are not only cured of their neoplasms but are restored to essentially normal functional capacity for work and for the enjoyment of a full normal span of life, with few or no symptomatically significant sequelae of treatment. Collectively, these accomplishments attest convincingly to the fact that modern radiotherapy has taken its place firmly alongside of surgery as a major curative modality for cancer.

The radiobiological foundations of radiotherapy remained largely unexplored until about 25 years ago, when the

development of new techniques for the clonal cultivation of
mammalian cells in vitro opened the way to quantitative
analysis of radiation dose-cell survival relationships,
revealing exponential survival curves with an initial
"shoulder" region.[111] Subsequent research revealed that this
initial shoulder was due to recovery from sublethal damage in
the low-dose range.[37] The existence of other reparable types
of injury, such as potentially lethal damage, was also documented.[107] Studies at the molecular level demonstrated
convincingly that the lethal effects of ionizing radiation in
bacterial and mammalian cells are in large part the consequence of strand breakage and other damage produced in chromosomal DNA.[78] Enzymatic repair of single strand breaks in
DNA is an efficient process,[77,100] whereas breaks induced in
both strands of DNA are largely nonreparable,[77] and are
probably the single lesion most directly associated with
lethality.[33] Enzymatic misrepair may also contribute
significantly to radiation-induced cell death.

Fundamental laboratory investigations in molecular and
cellular radiobiology have now suggested several promising
approaches to the differential modification of radiation
responses in tumors vs. normal tissues (Table I). The
studies of Gray and his colleagues[53,54,134] first called
attention to the possible relevance of the existence within
many tumors of hypoxic foci at sites where tumors had out-
grown their blood supply. The radiosensitivity of mammalian
cells decreases about 3-fold when they are irradiated in an
atmosphere of nitrogen rather than air or oxygen. Oxygen
appears to be involved in instantaneous reactions which
convert the initially reversible forms of chemical alteration
induced by ionization to irreversible secondary forms, thus

TABLE I
Differential Modification of Radiosensitivity

A. Increased Yield of Irreversible Radiochemical Lesions

  1. Oxygen: atmospheric; hyperbaric
  2. Nitric oxide, organic nitroxides
  3. Metronidazole, misonidazole, and derivatives
  4. High LET particulate radiations

B. Increased Intrinsic Sensitivity of Target DNA

  1. Halogenated pyrimidine analogs (BUdR, BCdR, IUdR)
  2. Possible potentiation of BCdR by tetrahydrouridine
  3. Inhibition of dehalogenation by 5-diazouracil

C. Inhibition of Repair

  1. Chemical inhibitors (actinomycin D, quinacrine, lucanthone, acriflavine)
  2. High LET particulate radiations
  3. Hyperthermia

D. Optimization of Dose Fractionation Schedules

  1. Large increment paucifractionation for tumors of high D_Q
  2. Radiation-induced partial synchronization of mitosis
  3. Drug-induced partial synchronization of mitosis (colchicine, vinca alkaloid mitotic spindle poisons)

E. Differential Radioprotection of Normal Tissues

  1. Thiophosphate compounds (WR-2721)
  2. Tourniquet hypoxia

F. Selective Delivery of Radionuclides to Tumor Cells

  1. Radiolabeled human monoclonal anti-tumor antibodies

fixing the radiation damage within the cell.

Radiotherapy of patients breathing pure oxygen at hyperbaric pressures[20] and the converse procedure, treatment of
tumors on the extremities under tourniquet hypoxia,[130,141]
were the first approaches adopted in efforts to circumvent
the problem apparently posed by the existence of hypoxic foci
within tumors. Randomized clinical trials have recently
indicated that hyperbaric oxygen can indeed significantly improve the results of radiotherapy for cancers of
the head and neck regions.[62,63] However, the method is so
unwieldy and time consuming as to be quite impractical.
Accordingly, investigators have turned their attention to
other approaches. Large cyclotrons and proton accelerators
are being used to generate beams of neutrons, π^- mesons,
and heavy ions which, due to their high LET, are substantially less oxygen-dependent than x-rays or electrons.[5,6,47,
58,113,135] Encouraging reports have recently emerged from
clinical studies with fast neutrons.[18,55,70]

A much less expensive alternative approach is that
provided by the electron affinic chemical radiosensitizers.[1]
Many of these compounds are stable radicals, thus mimicking
the action of oxygen. However, the fact that they are not
metabolized should permit them to diffuse longer distances
within tissue than is the case for oxygen. It is therefore
believed that they will reach hypoxic zones within tumors in
sufficient concentration to restore radio-responsiveness.
The organic nitroxides first tried were highly toxic for
mammalian cells,[39] but more encouraging results were obtained
with nitrofurans and nitroimidazoles.[13,19,28] Compounds such
as metronidazole and misonidazole have now been introduced
into clinical trials,[30,138] and new chemical derivatives of

these compounds, designed to have less toxicity, have been
developed and are undergoing preliminary testing. Meanwhile,
it has been demonstrated[61,69,131,133,142,143] that the cells
of many tumors can undergo reoxygenation during the interval
between successive doses of fractionated radiotherapy.
Indeed, it has been suggested[75] that this phenomenon may well
account for the greatly increased efficacy of fractionated
radiotherapy observed so many years ago by Regaud and his
colleagues. Nonetheless, the electron affinic radiosensitizers may well have a significant role to play in those
tumors in which reoxygenation is sluggish or deficient.

Other classes of radiosensitizers have been identified.
The halogenated pyrimidines 5-bromo- and 5-iodo-deoxyuridine
are analogs of the DNA precursor, thymidine. Under appropriate conditions, they may be incorporated into cellular
DNA in place of thymidine, and then induce an approximately
three-fold increase in sensitivity to the lethal effects of
ionizing radiations.[31,88,89] These compounds were initially
administered intra-arterially during radiotherapy of advanced
cancers of the oral cavity.[2,80] Tumor radiosensitization
was observed, but there was also significant radiosensitization of the normal mucous membranes, resulting in reactions
of undesirable severity. More recently, these agents have
been intra-arterially infused during fractionated radiotherapy of gliomas of the brain[68] and sarcomas of bone or
soft tissue origin,[51] with encouraging results. Technical
difficulties and increased complication rates associated with
the intra-arterial infusions have limited this approach.
However, the analogs 6-aminothymine[96] and 5-diazouracil[22]
can block the dehalogenation of these compounds, thus reopen-
ing the possibility that they could be administered

effectively by the intravenous route. Another possibility
is the use of 5-bromodeoxycytidine, a precursor of 5-bromo-
deoxyuridine, in conjunction with another analog, tetrahydrouridine, which prevents its deamination in the blood
stream.[23] The halogenated pyrimidine analogs are not presently
available in quantities sufficient for clinical investigation.

Other chemical agents are known to bind to DNA, and may
thus interfere with the enzymatic repair of radiation-induced
DNA damage. The best studied examples are Actinomycin D,[7,27]
lucanthone,[8] chloroquine,[140] and quinacrine.[144] Actinomycin
D has been reported to potentiate the radiation response of
pediatric solid tumors, especially Wilms' tumor.[26,97]
Lucanthone, used in conjunction with radiation therapy in
the treatment of advanced head and neck tumors, has been
reported to increase the rate and extent of tumor regression.[137] These chemical inhibitors of repair have demonstrated sufficient promise to warrant additional clinical
investigation.

The pattern of fractionation in clinical radiotherapy has
long been relatively standardized, with most radiotherapy
centers delivering consecutive daily treatments on five days
per week for four to six weeks. Serious questions have been
raised as to whether this pattern of daily fractionation is
indeed optimal for all tumors.[46] Split-course and other
modifications of fractionation schedule have been investigated clinically in patients with cancers of the head and
neck region.[35,122] Preliminary studies have also been
carried out in which patients have been treated with more
than one fraction per day.[126,132] Laboratory investigations
indicate that osteogenic and soft tissue sarcomas may exhibit

an extremely wide shoulder region in their dose-response
curves, due to an increased capacity for recovery from
sublethal damage.[40,41,117,146] If this phenomenon also
occurs in the clinical setting, it could well account for the
extreme radioresistance of many such tumors. Accordingly,
some groups have begun to experiment with paucifractionated
radiotherapy, delivering larger individual doses of up to
600-700 rad per fraction at intervals of 4 to 5 days. Preliminary results in the treatment of patients with osteogenic
and soft tissue sarcomas have been quite encouraging.[51]
Similar observations have been reported in the treatment
of malignant melanomas,[56] suggesting that this neoplasm may
not be as radioresistant as is generally believed.

Hyperthermia was first reported to enhance cellular
responses to ionizing radiation some 15 years ago.[10] Subsequent studies by other investigators[106] indicated that
hyperthermia alone also has substantial tumoricidal effects.
However, serious interest in hyperthermia as a new therapeutic modality and as a possible radiosensitizer has developed
only during the past several years.[11,29,60,93,118] Hyperthermia has also been shown to enhance responses of mammalian
cells to certain cancer chemotherapeutic agents.[12,57]
Autochthonous tumors arising in accessible sites in dogs and
cats have been successfully treated with hyperthermia alone
or with combinations of hyperthermia and radiotherapy.[101]
These encouraging experimental studies have now led to systematic clinical investigations in which the potential of
hyperthermia, used either alone or in conjunction with radiotherapy and/or chemotherapy, is being explored in a variety
of human malignant neoplasms.[34,67,91,92,99] The dramatic
responses observed in some instances have suggested the

possible desirability of reviving the technique of intraoperative radiotherapy in conjunction with hyperthermia for
the treatment of abdominal and thoracic neoplasms discovered
at exploratory surgery to be inoperable.[84]

Differential radioprotection is also a valid approach to
the improvement of therapeutic gain. Recent interest has
centered on thiophosphate compounds such as WR-2721, which
have been shown to yield differential radioprotection of normal tissues as contrasted with tumor tissues, most probably
due to differential rates of diffusion of the protective
compound.[139,145,148] It is also noteworthy that such radioprotective compounds have been used together with some of
the electron affinic radiosensitizers with an improvement in
therapeutic gain.[199]

Recent advances in experimental immunology also have
important implications for radiotherapy. The "hybridoma"
technique, first developed for mouse antibody-producing cells
a few years ago by Köhler and Milstein,[94] has now been
successfully extended to human antibody-producing cells by
Olsson and Kaplan.[104] In a hybridoma, B-lymphocytes immunized against a specific antigen are fused with myeloma cells
pre-adapted to permanent growth in culture, and the selected
hybrids are then cloned, thus yielding immortal cell factories producing limitless quantities of monospecific antibodies. The availability of human hybridomas opens the way
to the use of their antibody products in clinical diagnosis
and treatment. Efforts are now under way to generate human
hybridoma antibodies against the cell membrane antigens
which comprise the distinctive "signature" of each type of
cancer. Such antibodies could readily be radiolabeled with
various radionuclides for use in diagnostic imaging, in the

detection of micrometastases, and perhaps in the eradication of such micrometastases ("immunoradiotherapy"). Alternatively, chemotherapeutic agents or toxins could be conjugated to the antibody molecules and thus selectively delivered to cancer cells.

Combined modalities of treatment are also being explored in those clinical situations in which the results of any one form of treatment alone appear to have reached their limits.[84] The rationale for the use of combined radiotherapy and surgery in the management of squamous cell carcinomas arising in the oral cavity and pharynx, and of their cervical lymph node metastases, has been well stated.[44] Preliminary radiotherapy is aimed at reducing tumor bulk to levels at which subsequent surgical extirpation can be accomplished with greater ease and reliability. Preoperative radiotherapy followed by surgery is also being used extensively in the management of primary colorectal carcinomas. "Sandwich" techniques involving both preoperative and postoperative radiotherapy with intervening surgical extirpation of retroperitoneal lymph node chains are being tried in the management of embryonal carcinoma and teratocarcinoma of the testis.[103] In primary bronchogenic carcinoma, however, combined external beam radiotherapy and radical surgery have yielded disappointing results[110] and have been largely abandoned.

Radiotherapy is being used in combination with chemotherapy in a widening spectrum of neoplasms. The rationale for this combined modality approach has been presented in detail elsewhere.[84] Significant improvement in survival has been reported in patients with a variety of pediatric neoplasms (Wilms' tumor, Ewing's tumor, and rhabdomyosarcoma)

treated with combined modality therapy.[26,32,109,120]
Craniospinal irradiation, or cranial irradiation plus intrathecal chemotherapy, used in conjuction with intensive
systemic chemotherapy, has contributed to the dramatic
improvement in prognosis of children with acute leukemia.[71]
Sequential or alternating regimens of radiotherapy and
combination chemotherapy have clearly yielded substantial
reductions in relapse rates of patients with advanced
Hodgkin's disease.[66,121] As new chemotherapeutic agents
with demonstrable efficacy against a variety of epithelial
neoplasms become available, combined modality therapy is
likely to come into increasingly widespread use.

References

1. Adams GE, Asquith JC, Watts ME: Electron-affinic sensitizers for hypoxic cells irradiated in vitro and in vivo: current status. In: Advances in chemical Radiosensitization. Vienna, Intl Atomic Energy Agency, 1974, pp 1-12.

2. Bagshaw MA, Doggett RLS, Smith KC, et al: Intra-arterial 5-bromodeoxyuridine and x-ray therapy. Am J Roentgenol 99:886-894, 1967.

3. Bagshaw MA, Kaplan HS, Sagerman RH: Linear accelerator supervoltage radiotherapy. VII. Carcinoma of the prostate. Radiology 85:121-129, 1965.

4. Bagshaw MA, Ray GR, Pistenma DA, et al: External beam radiation therapy of primary carcinoma of the prostate. Cancer 36:723-728, 1975.

5. Barendsen GW: Responses of cultured cells, tumours and normal tissues to radiations of different linear energy transfer. In: Current Topics in Radiation Research. Ebert M, Howard A (eds.). Amsterdam: North-Holland. 1968, pp 295-356.

6. Barendsen GW, Broerse JJ: Experimental radiotherapy of a rat rhabdomyosarcoma with 15 MeV neutrons and 300 kV x-rays. I. Effects of single exposures. Eur J Cancer 5:373-391, 1969.

7. Bases RE: Modification of the radiation response determined by single-cell technics: Actinomycin D. Cancer Res 19:1223-1229, 1959.

8. Bases R: Enhancement of x-ray damage in Hela cells by exposure to lucanthone (Miracil D) following radiation. Cancer Res 30:2007-2011,1970.

9. Becquerel H: Emission of the new radiations by metallic uranium. Compt Rend Acad Sci 122:1086-1088, 1896.

10. Belli JA, Bonte FJ: Influence of temperature on the radiation response of mammalian cells in tissue culture. Radiat Res 18:272-276, 1963.

11. Ben-Hur E, Bronk BV, Elkind MM: Thermally enhanced radiosensitivity of cultured Chinese hamster cells. Nature New Biol 238:209-211, 1972.

12. Braun J, Hahn GM: Enhanced cell killing by bleomycin and 43° hyperthermia and the inhibition of recovery from potentially lethal damage. Cancer Res 35:2921-2927, 1975.

13. Brown JM: Selective radiosensitization of the hypoxic
    cells of mouse tumors with the nitroimidazoles metro-
    nidazole and RO 7-0582. Radiat Res 64:633-647, 1975.
14. Buschke F: Radiation therapy: the past, the present,
    the future; Janeway lecture, 1969. Am J Roentgenol
    108:236-246, 1970.
15. Cantril ST: The contributions of biology to radiation
    therapy; Janeway lecture, 1957. Am J Roentgenol 78:
    751-768, 1957.
16. Carmel RJ, Kaplan HS: Mantle irradiation in Hodgkin's
    disease. An analysis of technique, tumor eradication,
    and complications. Cancer 37:2813-2825, 1976.
17. Case JT: History of radiation therapy. Buschke F (ed):
    Progress in Radiation Therapy. New York: Grune and
    Stratton, 1958, pp 13-41.
18. Catterall M: First randomized clinical trial of fast
    neutrons compared with photons in advanced carcinoma
    of the head and neck. Clin Otolaryngol 2:359-372, 1977.
19. Chapman JD, Reuvers AP, Borsa J, et al: Nitrofurans
    as radiosensitizers of hypoxic mammalian cells. Cancer
    Res 32:2616-2624, 1972.
20. Churchill-Davidson I, Sanger C, Thomlinson RH: High-
    pressure oxygen and radiotherapy. Lancet 1:1091-1095,
    1955.
21. Coolidge WD: A powerful roentgen-ray tube with a pure
    electron discharge. Physical Rev 2:409-413, 1913.
22. Cooper GM, Greer S: Irreversible inhibition of dehalo-
    genation of 5-iodouracil by 5-diazouracil and rever-
    sible inhibition by 5-cyanouracil. Cancer Res 30:
    2937-2941, 1970.
23. Cooper GM, Greer S: The effect of inhibition of cyti-
    dine deaminase by tetrahydrouridine on the utilization
    of deoxycytidine and 5-bromodeoxcytidine for DNA
    synthesis. Molec Pharmacol 9:698-703, 1973.
24. Coutard H: Roentgenotherapy of epitheliomas of the
    tonsillar region, hypopharynx and larynx from 1920 to
    1926. Am J Roentgeno 28:313-331, 1932.
25. Curie P, Curie MS: Sur une substance nouvelle radio-
    active, contenue dans la pechblende. Compt Rend Acad
    Sci 127:175-178, 1898.
26. D'Angio GJ, Evans AE, Breslow N, et al: The treatment
    of Wilms' tumor. Results of the National Wilms' Tumor
    Study. Cancer 38:633-646, 1976.
27. D'Angio GJ, Farber S, Maddock CL: Potentiation of
    x-ray effects by actinomycin D. Radiology 73:175-177,
    1959.

28. Denekamp J, Fowler JF: Radiosensitization of solid tumors by nitroimidazoles. Int J Radiat Oncol Biol Phys 4:143-151, 1978.

29. Dewey WC, Hopwood LE, Sapareto SA, et al: Cellular responses to combinations of hyperthermia and radiation. Radiology 123:463-474, 1977.

30. Dische S, Saunders MI, Flockhart IR: The optimum regime for the administration of misonidazole and the establishment of multi-centre clinical trials. Br J Cancer 37:318-321, 1978.

31. Djordjevic B, Szybalski W: Genetics of human cell lines. III. Incorporation of 5-bromo- and 5-iodo-deoxyuridine into the deoxyribonucliec acid of human cells and its effect on radiation sensitivity. J Exp Med 112:519-531, 1960.

32. Donaldson SS, Castro JR, Wilbur JR, et al: Rhabdomyo-sarcoma of head and neck in children. Combination treatment by surgery, irradiation, and chemotherapy. Cancer 31:26-35, 1973.

33. Dugle DL, Gillespie CJ, Chapman JD: DNA strand breaks, repair and survival in x-irradiated mammalian cells. Proc Nat Acad Sci US 73:809-812, 1976.

34. Dutreix J, LeBourgeois JP, Salama M: Hyperthermia in the treatment of cancer. J Radiol Electrol Med Nucl 59:323-334, 1978.

35. Dutreix J, Wambersie A: Radiobiologic data obtained from clinical observation of the regression of epithelioma of the tonsil under different fractionation regimes. Am J Roentgenol 108:37-43, 1970.

36. Earle JD, Bagshaw MA, Kaplan HS: Supervoltage radiation therapy of testicular tumors. Am J Roentgenol 117:653-661, 1973.

37. Elkind MM, Sutton H: Radiation response of mammalian cells grown in culture. I. Repair of x-ray damage in surviving Chinese hamster cells. Radiat Res 13:556-593, 1960.

38. Ellis F: Relationship of biological effect of dose time fractionation factors in radiotherapy. In: Ebert M, Howard A (eds.) Current Topics in Radiation Research. Amsterdam: North-Holland, 1968, pp 382-397.

39. Emmerson PT, Howard-Flanders P: Sensitization of anoxic bacteria to x-rays by di-t-butylnitroxide and analogues. Nature 204:1005-1006, 1964.

40. Fischer JJ, Moulder JE: The steepness of the dose-response curve in radiation therapy. Theoretical considerations and experimental results. Radiology 117:179-184, 1975.

41. Fischer JJ, Reinhold HS: The cure of rhabdomyosarcoma BA 1112 with fractionated radiotherapy. Radiology 105: 429-433, 1972.

42. Fletcher GH: Cancer of the uterine cervix; Janeway lecture, 1970. Am J Roentgenol 111:225-242, 1971.

43. Fletcher GH: The evolution of the basic concepts underlying the practice of radiotherapy from 1949 to 1979; Erskine Memorial Lecture, 1977. Radiology 127: 3-19, 1978.

44. Fletcher GH, Jesse RH: The contribution of supervoltage roentgenotherapy to the integration of radiation and surgery in head and neck squamous cell carcinomas. Cancer 15:566-577, 1962.

45. Fletcher GH, MacComb WS, Chau PM, et al: Comparison of medium voltage and supervoltage roentgen therapy in the treatment of oropharynx cancers. Am J Roentgenol 81:375-401, 1959.

46. Fowler JF, Thomlinson RH, Howes AE: Time-dose relationships in radiotherapy. Eur J Cancer 6:207-221, 1970.

47. Fowler PH, Perkins DH: The possibility of therapeutic applications of beams of negative π mesons. Nature 189:528, 1961.

48. Ginzton EL, Hansen WW, Kennedy WR: A linear electron accelerator. Rev Sci Inst 19:89-108, 1948.

49. Ginzton EL, Mallory KB, Kaplan HS: The Stanford medical linear accelerator. I. Design and development. Stanford Med Bull 15:123-140, 1957.

50. Goffinet DR, Glatstein E, Fuks Z, et al: Abdominal irradiation in non-Hodgkin's lymphomas. Cancer 37: 2797-2805, 1976.

51. Goffinet DR, Kaplan HS, Donaldson SS, et al: Combined radiosensitizer infusions and irradiation of osteogenic sarcomas. Radiology 117:211-214, 1975.

52. Goffinet DR, Schneider MJ, Glatstein EJ, et al: Bladder cancer: results of radiation therapy in 384 patients. Radiology 117:149-153, 1957.

53. Gray LH: Oxygenation in radiotherapy. I. Radiobiological considerations. Br J Radiol 30:403-406, 1957.

54. Gray LH, Conger AD, Ebert M, et al: The concentration of oxygen dissolved in tissues at the time of irradiation as a factor in radiotherapy. Br J Radiol 26:638-648, 1953.

55. Griffin TW, Laramore GE, Parker RG, et al: An evaluation of fast neutron beam teletherapy of metastatic cervical adenopathy from squamous cell carcinomas of the head and neck region. Cancer 42:2517-2520, 1978.

56. Habermalz HJ, Fischer JJ: Radiation therapy of malignant melanoma. Experience with high individual treatment doses. Cancer 38:2258-2262, 1976.

57. Hahn GM, Braun J, Har-Kedar I: Thermochemotherapy: synergism between hyperthermia (42-43°) and adriamycin (or bleomycin) in mammalian cell inactivation. Proc Nat Acad Sci USA 72:937-940, 1975.

58. Hall EJ, Roizin-Towle L, Theus RB, et al: Radiobiological properties of high-energy cyclotron-produced neutrons used for radiotherapy. Radiology 117:173-178, 1975.

59. Hanks GE, Bagshaw MA, Kaplan HS: Management of cervical lymph node metastasis by megavoltage radiotherapy. Am J Roentgenol 105:74-82, 1969.

60. Harisiadis L, Hall EJ, Kraljevic U, et al: Hyperthermia: biological studies at the cellular level. Radiology 117:447-452, 1975.

61. Hawkes MJ, Hill RP, Lindop PJ, et al: The response of C_3H mammary tumours to irradiation in single and fractionated doses. Br J Radiol 41:134-141, 1968.

62. Henk JM, Kunkler PB, Smith CW: Radiotherapy and hyperbaric oxygen in head and neck cancer. (Final report of first controlled clinical trial.) Lancet 2:101-103, 1977.

63. Henk JM, Smith CW: Radiotherapy and hyperbaric oxygen in head and neck cancer. Interim report of second clinical trial. Lancet 2:104-105, 1977.

64. Henschke UK, Hilaris BS, Mahan GD: Afterloading in interstitial and intracavitary radiation therapy. Am J Roentgenol 90:386-395, 1963.

65. Hoppe RT, Goffinet DR, Bagshaw MA: Carcinoma of the nasopharynx: Eighteen years experience with megavoltage radiation therapy. Cancer 37:2605-2612, 1976.

66. Hoppe RT, Portlock CS, Glatstein E, et al: Alternating chemotherapy and irradiation in the treatment of advanced Hodgkin's disease. Cancer 43:472-481, 1979.

67. Hornback NB, Shupe RE, Shidnia H. et al: Preliminary clinical results of combined 433 megahertz microwave therapy and radiation therapy on patients with advanced cancer. Cancer 40:2854-2863, 1977.

68. Hoshino T, Sano K: Radiosensitization of malignant
     brain tumors with bromouridine (thymidine analogue).
     Acta Radiol (Ther) 8:15-26, 1969.
69. Howes AE: An estimation of changes in the proportions
     and absolute numbers of hypoxic cells after irradiation
     of transplanted C_3H mouse mammary tumours. Br J Radiol
     42:441-447, 1969.
70. Hussey DH, Fletcher GH, Caderao JB: Experience with
     fast neutron therapy using the Texas A & M variable
     energy cyclotron. Cancer 34:65-77, 1974.
71. Hustu HO, Aur RJA, Versoza MS, et al: Prevention of
     central nervous system leukemia by irradiation. Cancer
     32:585-597, 1973.
72. Ingold JA, Reed GB, Kaplan HS, et al: Radiation hepa-
     titis. Am J Roentgenol 93:200-208, 1965.
73. International Commission on Radiological Units and
     Measurements, Handbook 62. Washington, D.C.: U.S.
     Natl. Bureau of Standards, 1956.
74. Jennings FL, Arden A: Development of radiation pneu-
     monitis. Time and dose factors. Arch Path 74:351-360,
     1962.
75. Kallman RF: The phenomenon of reoxygenation and its
     implications for fractionated radiotherapy. Radiology
     105:135-142, 1972.
76. Kaplan HS: Role of intensive radiotherapy in the
     management of Hodgkin's disease. Cancer 19:356-367,
     1966.
77. Kaplan HS: DNA strand scission and loss of viability
     after X-irradiation of normal and sensitized bacterial
     cells. Proc Nat Acad Sci US 55:1442-1446, 1966.
78. Kaplan HS: Macromolecular basis of radiation-induced
     loss of viability in cells and viruses. In: Haissinsky
     M (ed). Actions Chimiques et Biologiques des Radia-
     tions. Paris: Masson, 1968, pp 69-94.
79. Kaplan HS: Prognostic significance of the relapse-free
     interval after radiotherapy in Hodgkin's disease.
     Cancer 22:1131-1136, 1968.
80. Kaplan HS: Radiosensitization by the halogenated
     pyrimidine analogues: laboratory and clinical investi-
     gations. In: Moroson HL, Quintiliani M (eds.).
     Radiation Protection and Sensitization. London, Taylor
     and Francis, 1970, pp 35-42.
81. Kaplan HS: On the natural history, treatment, and
     prognosis of Hodgkin's disease. In: Harvey Lectures,
     Series 64, 1968-1969. New York: Academic Press, 1970,
     pp. 215-259.

82. Kaplan HS: Hodgkin's disease and other human malignant lymphomas: advances and prospects. GHA Clowes Memorial Lecture. Cancer Res 36:3863-3878, 1976.

83. Kaplan HS: Present status of radiotherapy of cancer: an overview. In: Becker FF (ed) Cancer--A Comprehensive Treatise. New York: Plenum Press, Vol. 6, 1977, pp 3-38.

84. Kaplan HS: Fundamental mechanisms in combined modality therapy of cancer; Janeway Lecture, 1977. Am J Roentgenol 129:383-393, 1977.

85. Kaplan HS: Hodgkin's disease: unfolding concepts concerning its nature, management and prognosis. Cancer 45:2439-2474, 1980.

86. Kaplan HS: Hodgkin's disease. (Ed. 2). Cambridge, Mass.: Harvard University Press, 1980.

87. Kaplan HS, Bagshaw MA: The Stanford medical linear accelerator. III. Application to clinical problems of radiation therapy. Stanford Med Bull 15:141-151, 1957.

88. Kaplan HS, Smith KC, Tomlin PA: Effect of halogenated pyrimidines on radiosensitivity of E. coli. Radiat Res 16:98-113, 1962.

89. Kaplan HS, Tomlin PA, Smith KC: Radiosensitization of E. coli by purine and pyrimidine analogs incorporated in deoxyribonucleic acid. Nature 190:794-796, 1961.

90. Kerst DW: The acceleration of electrons by magnetic induction. Physical Rev 60:47-52, 1941.

91. Kim JH, Hahn EW, Tokita N: Combination hyperthermia and radiation therapy for cutaneous malignant melanoma. Cancer 41:2143-2148, 1978.

92. Kim JH, Hahn EW, Tokita N, et al: Local tumor hyperthermia in combination with radiation therapy. I. Malignant cutaneous lesions. Cancer 40:161-169, 1977.

93. Kim SH, Kim JH, Hahn EW: The radiosensitization of hypoxic tumor cells by hyperthermia. Radiology 114: 727-728, 1975.

94. Köhler G, Milstein C: Continuous cultures of fused cells secreting antibody of predefined specificity. Nature 256:495-497, 1975.

95. Kraut JW, Kaplan HS, Bagshaw MA: Combined fractionated isotopic and external irradiation of the liver in Hodgkin's disease. A study of 21 patients. Cancer 30:39-46, 1972.

96. Langen P, Etzold G, Bärwolff, et al: Inhibition of thymidine phosphorylase by 6-aminothymine and derivatives of 6-aminouracil. Biochem Pharmacol 16:1833-1837, 1967.

97. Lemerle J, Donaldson SS: Wilms' tumor: current concepts in diagnosis, prognosis, and treatment. Paediatrician 1:220-230, 1972.

98. Luxton R: Radiation nephritis. Quart J Med 22:215-242, 1953.

99. Marmor JB, Pounds D, Postic TB, et al: Treatment of superficial human neoplasms by local hyperthermia induced by ultrasound. Cancer 43:188-197, 1979.

100. McGrath RA, Williams RW: Reconstruction in vivo of irradiated Escherichia coli deoxyribonucleic acid; the rejoining of broken pieces. Nature 212:534-535, 1966.

101. Miller RC, Connor WG, Heusinkveld RS, et al: Prospects for hyperthermia in human cancer therapy. I. Hyperthermic effects in man and spontaneous animal tumors. Radiology 123:489-495, 1977.

102. Newbery GR, Bewley DK: The performance of the Medical Research Council 8 MeV linear accelerator. Br J Radiol 28:241, 1955.

103. Nicholson TC, Walsh PC, Rotner MB: Lymphadenectomy combined with preoperative and postoperative cobalt 60 teletherapy in the management of embryonal carcinoma and teratocarcinoma of the testis. J Urol 112:109-110, 1974.

104. Olsson L, Kaplan HS: Human-human hybridomas producing monoclonal antibodies of predefined antigenic specificity. Proc Nat Acad Sci US, in press.

105. Palos B, Kaplan HS, Karzmark CJ: The use of thin lung shields to deliver limited whole-lung irradiation during mantle field treatment of Hodgkin's disease. Radiology 101:441-442, 1971.

106. Palzer RJ, Heidelberger C: Studies on the quantitative biology of hyperthermic killings of HeLa cells. Cancer Res 33:415-421, 1973.

107. Phillips RA, Tolmach LJ: Repair of potentially lethal damage in x-irradiated HeLa cells. Radiat Res 29:413-432, 1966.

108. Pierquin B, Chassagne D, Cox J: Toward consistent local control of certain malignant tumors: Endoradiotherapy with Iridium 192. Radiology 99:661-667, 1971.

109. Pratt CB, Hustu HO, Fleming ID, et al: Coordinated treatment of childhood rhabdomyosarcoma with surgery, radiotherapy, and combination chemotherapy. Cancer Res 32:606-610, 1972.

110. Preoperative irradiation of cancer of the lung. Preliminary report of a therapeutic trial. Collaborative

study. Cancer 23:419-430, 1969.

111. Puck TT, Marcus PI: Action of x-rays on mammalian cells. J Exp Med 103:653-666, 1956.

112. Quimby EH: The specification of dosage in radiation therapy. Janeway lecture, 1940. Am J Roentgenol 45:1-16, 1941.

113. Raju MR: Heavy particle radiotherapy. New York: Academic Press, 1980.

114. Regaud C: Sur les principes radiophysiologiques de la radiotherapie des cancers. Acta Radiol 11:456-486, 1930.

115. Regaud C, Coutard H, Hautant A: Contribution au traitement des cancers endolaryngés par les rayons-X. Proc 10th Int'l Congr of Otolaryngology, 1922, pp 19-22.

116. Regaud C, Ferroux R: Discordance des effets des rayons X, d'une part dans la peau, d'autre part dans le testicule, par le fractionnement de la dose; diminution de l'efficacité dans le peau, maintien de l'efficacité dans le testicule. Compt Rend Soc de Biol 97:431-434, 1927.

117. Reinhold HS: Quantitative evaluation of the radio-sensitivity of cells of a transplantable rhabdomyosarcoma in the rat. Eur J Cancer 2:33-42, 1966.

118. Robinson JE, Wizenberg MJ: Thermal sensitivity and the effect of elevated temperatures on the radiation sensitivity of Chinese hamster cells. Acta Radiol (Ther) 13:241-248, 1974.

119. Röntgen WC: Über eine neue Art von Strahlen. Erste mitteilung. Sitzgsber. physikal-med. Gesellschaft (Würzburg), Dec. 28, 1895, pp 132-141.

120. Rosen G, Wollner N, Tan C, etal: Disease-free survival in children with Ewing's sarcoma treated with radiation therapy and adjuvant four-drug sequential chemotherapy. Cancer 33:384-393, 1974.

121. Rosenberg SA, Kaplan HS, Glatstein EJ, et al: Combined modality therapy of Hodgkin's disease - a report on the Stanford trails. Cancer 42:991-1000, 1978.

122. Sambrook DK: Split-course radiation therapy in malignant tumors, Am J Roentgenol 91:37-45, 1964.

123. Schultz HP, Glatstein E, Kaplan HS: Management of presumptive or proven Hodgkin's disease of the liver: a new radiotherapy technique. Int J Rad Oncol Biol Phys 1:1-8, 1975.

124. Schulz MD: The supervoltage story; Janeway lecture, 1974. Am J Roentgenol 124:541-559, 1975.

125. Seitz S, Wintz H: Uber die Beseitigung von Myom - und
     Wechselblutungen in einmaligere Sitzung durch Zink-
     filter intensivbestrahlung. Munchen Med Wchnschr
     63:1785-1787, 1916.
126. Shukovsky LJ, Fletcher GH, Montague ED, et al:
     Experience with twice-a-day fractionation in clinical
     radiotherapy. Am J Roentgenol 126:155-161, 1976.
127. Siegbahn M, Ownen EA, Holthusen H: Report from Inter-
     national X-ray Unit Committee. Am J Roentgenol 20:470-
     471, 1928.
128. Stewart JR, Cohn KE, Fajardo LF, et al: Radiation
     induced heart disease. A study of twenty-five patients.
     Radiology 89:302-310, 1967.
129. Strandqvist M: Studien über die Kumulative Wirkung der
     Rontgenstrahlen bei Fraktionierung. Acta Radiol (Suppl)
     73:1-300, 1944.
130. Suit HD, Lindberg R: Radiation therapy administered
     under conditions of tourniquet-induced local tissue
     anoxia. Am J Roentgenol 102:27-37, 1968.
131. Suit HD, Schiavone J: Effect of a first dose of radia-
     tion on the proportion of cells in a mouse mammary
     carcinoma which are hypoxic. Radiology 90:325-328,
     1968.
132. Svoboda VHJ: Radiotherapy by several sessions a day.
     Br J Radiol 48:131-133, 1975.
133. Thomlinson RH: Changes of oxygenation in tumours in
     relation to irradiation. Front Radiat Ther Oncol
     3:109-121, 1968.
134. Thomlinson RH, Gray LH: The histological structure of
     some human lung cancers and the possible implications
     for radiotherapy. Br J Cancer 9:539-549, 1955.
135. Tobias C, Lyman J, Lawrence T: Some consideration of
     physical and biological factors in radiotherapy with
     high-LET radiations including heavy particles, pi
     mesons, and fast neutrons. Adv Nucl Med 3:167-218,
     1971.
136. Trout ED: History of radiation sources for cancer
     therapy. Buschke F (ed) In: Progress in Radiation
     Therapy. New York: Grune and Stratton, 1958, pp 42-61.
137. Turner S, Bases RE, Pealman A, et al: The adjuvant
     effect of lucanthone (Miracil D) in clinical radiation
     therapy. Radiology 114:729-731, 1975.
138. Urtasun RC, Band P, Chapman JD, et al: Clinical phase
     I study of the hypoxic cell radiosensitizer RO-07-0582,
     a 2-nitroimidazole derivative. Radiology 122:801-804,
     1977.

139. Utley JF, Phillips TL, Kane L: Differential radioprotection of euoxic and hypoxic mammary tumors by a
thiophosphate compound. Radiology 110:213-216, 1974.
140. Utley JF, Sachatello CR, Maruyana Y, et al: Radiosensitization of normal tissue by chloroquine.
Radiology 124:255-257, 1977.
141. Van den Brenk HAS: The oxygen effect in radiation
therapy. In: Ebert M, Howard A (eds.) Current
Topics in Radiation Research. Amsterdam: North-
Holland, 1969, pp 197-254.
142. Van Putten LM: Tumor reoxygenation during fractionated
radiotherapy: studies with transplantable mouse osteosarcoma. Europ J Cancer 4:173-182, 1968.
143. Van Putten LM, Kallman RF: Oxygenation status of a
transplantable tumor during fractionated radiation
therapy. J Natl Cancer Inst 40:441-451, 1968.
144. Voiculetz N, Smith KC, Kaplan HS: Effect of quinacrine
on survival and DNA repair in X-irradiated Chinese
hamster cells. Cancer Res 34:1038-1044, 1974.
145. Washburn LC, Carlton JE, Hayes RE, et al: Distribution
of WR-2721 in normal and tumor tissues of mice and
rats: dependence on tumor type, drug dose, and
species. Radiation Res 59:475-483, 1974.
146. Weichselbaum R, Little JB, Nove J: Response of human
osteosarcoma in vitro to irradiation: evidence for
unusual cellular repair activity. Int J Radiat Biol
31:295-299, 1977.
147. Weller SA, Glatstein E, Kaplan HS, et al: Initial
relapses in previously treated Hodgkin's disease. I.
Results of second treatment. Cancer 37:2840-2846, 1976.
148. Yuhas JM, Storer JB: Differential chemoprotection of
normal and malignant tissues. J Nat Cancer Inst 42:
331-335, 1969.
149. Yuhas JM, Youconic M, Kligerman MM, et al: Combined
use of radioprotective and radiosensitizing drugs in
experimental radiotherapy. Radiation Res 70:433-443,
1977.

ESTIMATION OF THE NUMERICAL AND
ECONOMIC IMPACT OF CHEMOTHERAPY
IN THE TREATMENT OF CANCER

VINCENT T. DEVITA,Jr.
JANE E. HENNEY
SUSAN M. HUBBARD

National Cancer Institute
National Institutes of Health
Bethesda, Maryland

In 1971, the National Cancer Act was passed by the
Ninety Second Congress. Funding appropriated for an
increased level of effort and research into the cause, prevention, and treatment of cancer did not begin to reach
investigators until 1972. In eight years the activities
of the National Cancer Program have generated significant
information in all aspects of cancer. This paper will focus
only on those accomplishments that have been achieved in
cancer treatment, particularly with chemotherapy.

After examining the data, our primary conclusion is that
the impact of chemotherapy on patients with cancer while
numerically modest, is of extraordinary biologic importance.
Secondly, we have concluded that these modest gains coupled
with widespread application of chemotherapy has created a
backlash in the mind of the public, since the majority of
patients receive chemotherapy are unlikely to acheive significant clinical benefit.

The Development of Methods to Treat Cancer

The roots of effective cancer treatment have their ori-
gins in four major discoveries that occurred since the turn
of the century (1).

1. The development of the principles of cancer surgery,
which led to en-bloc resection, the radical mastectomy
procedure in 1894.

2. The discovery of roentgen rays by Wihelm Conrad Roentgen.

3. The demonstration that experimental animals could be inbred and that tumors could be consistently transplanted
   into these animals. This system thus provided a useful
   model for identifying and developing new types of systemic
   therapy.

4. The development of the randomized clinical trial, first
   used successfully in the evaluation of antitubercular
   drugs.

Transplantable tumors in syngeneic animals led to three
major events which influenced the development and application of systemic therapy in humans with cancer.

1. The first event occurred when Dr. Howard Skipper and his
   colleagues performed seminal studies during 1960-1963.
   These studies established the quantitative relationship
   between drugs and the killing of tumor cells (2). This
   fractional kill hypothesis had its roots in the effect of
   antiseptics on skin bacteria. Subsequent experiments in
   rodents related the successful systemic treatment to drug
   dose and tumor cell number.

2. The second event occurred when numerous investigators
   initiated clinical studies to test Skipper's hypothesis,
   that drugs alone could cure patients with advanced cancer.
   By the early 1970's, this was adequately demonstrated as
   will be evident from the data presented below (3).

3. The third major event, the increased appreciation of the
   power of the study of the pharmacology of antitumor
   agents, is still in progress. In the early 1960's techniques available for studying the pharmacokinetics and
   intermediary metabolism of anticancer drugs were crude.
   Drugs and their active metabolites were not easily measured. With the advent of radioimmuno- and competitive
   binding assays, high pressure liquid chromatography, and
   the gas chromatographic mass spectrophotometric techniques, it has now become possible to measure the active
   principles of anticancer drugs and the range of their
   biologic activity (4).

When the success of chemotherapy in patients with advanced hematologic malignancies (5,6) was coupled with the
relationship between cytotoxicity and number of cancer
cells, investigators hypothesized that the application of
chemotherapy in patients who had a high risk of recurrence

after surgery would also be successful. This hypothesis has proven to be true in a number of cancers. It should be emphasized that by necessity, the widespread application of chemotherapy in the post-operative period awaited the proof that drugs alone could cure patients with advanced cancer, because "adjuvant" studies require the administration of toxic and potentially carcinogenic drugs to some patients who are cured by localized forms of treatment. This fact explains the lag of almost one decade from the identification of potentially curative chemotherapy to its use as an adjuvant.

Estimates of the Number of Patients Who Receive and Benefit from Chemotherapy

The purpose of this review is to provide a numerical estimate of the breadth of the use of chemotherapy and its impact on cancer treatment. Two points should be emphasized. With few exceptions, the numbers are best estimates that have been calculated using figures from texts and review articles (7-15). These figures are not meant to be absolute, but approximations. The second point is, in the data cited, we assume nationwide application of chemotherapy, which is suggested by the reduction in national mortality in patients under the age of 55 years (16,17).

We have used the 1977 American Cancer Society data (18) on the incidence of cancer for two reasons: it was the year that approximately one million new cases of cancer occurred in the United States; and it was the year closest to the Public Health Service Report on cancer patient survival Report #5 (19). This report was published in 1976 and is the source of the relative survival rate (41%) which is used in part for the calculations of cancer patient survival.

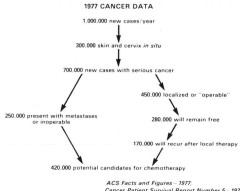

1977 CANCER DATA

1,000,000 new cases/year

300,000 skin and cervix *in situ*

700,000 new cases with serious cancer

450,000 localized or "operable"

250,000 present with metastases or inoperable

280,000 will remain free

170,000 will recur after local therapy

420,000 potential candidates for chemotherapy

ACS Facts and Figures – 1977;
Cancer Patient Survival Report Number 5 – 1976

It is necessary to divide patients with cancer into two major groups to understand the impact of chemotherapy: those with apparently localized disease; and those with disseminated disease. Of the one million new cases of cancer in 1977, approximately 300,000 patients had easily curable skin cancer or in situ carcinoma of the cervix (Fig. 1). Unfortunately, patients with easily curable cancers are often excluded from considerations of survival. The availability of the Pap test led to early diagnosis and successful treatment led to the cure of in situ cervical cancer. Surgery and topical chemotherapy, such as 5 fluorouracil, have yielded high cure rates in skin cancers (20).

When these 300,000 patients are excluded from the cases diagnosed in 1977, 700,000 patients with "serious" cancers remain. To estimate the fraction of the 700,000 patients who present to their physician with apparently localized cancer and those curable with local treatment, we referred to the relative survival rate in Report # 5 (19). This figure is 41% but was reduced by 1% because we reasoned that the 41% figure includes patients who survive as a result of treatment with chemotherapy. Forty percent of the 700,000 patients with serious cancers (280,000) represents the number successfully treated with surgery and/or radiation therapy or both plus chemotherapy.

The number of patients who have localized or "operable" cancers (450,000) was also derived from standard textbooks (7-15). We identified the annual incidence of the major cancers and the fraction that are treated with surgery or radiotherapy and exhibit no residual disease following this treatment. When the number curable, 280,000, is subtracted from the number of patients with operable or localized disease, it can be estimated that 170,000 patients will develop tumor recurrence and are therefore potential candidates for adjuvant chemotherapy. We will return to the discussion of this group shortly.

The difference between 700,000 (total serious cancers) and 450,000 (localized or operable cases) provides an estimate of patients (250,000) who present with inoperable tumors or with evidence of distant metastasis (Fig. 1). This estimate was then corroborated by checking the annual incidence of systemic cancers (leukemia, lymphoma, myeloma, etc.) and the number of patients with solid tumors who present with metastatic disease, such as breast cancer. The addition of the 250,000 patients who present with inoperable or metastastic disease to the 170,000 patients who recur after local therapy, provides a total of 420,000 patients who are potential candidates for chemotherapy.

Survival rates in patients with localized or operable cancers have improved over the past thirty years. This can be attributed, in part, to improvements in surgical techniques but is primarily due to widespread use of increasingly sophisticated radiotherapy equipment (21).

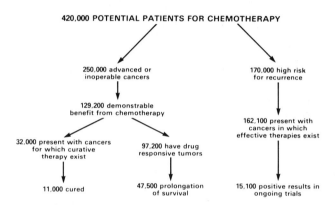

As previously stated, of the 420,000 potential patients for chemotherapy, 250,000 patients have metastatic disease. This group has always been the first to receive new forms of chemotherapy. When estimating the impact of chemotherapy on these 250,000 patients we divide them into two subsets: those who experience demonstrable benefit from chemotherapy and those who do not (Fig. 2).

Benefit is defined as evidence that prolongation of survival occurs in patients who respond to chemotherapy compared to those who do not respond. A response rate of 20 percent was used to define drug responsive tumors. While a partial response rate of 20% produces minimal clinical benefit, it is often the starting point for the identification of therapeutic programs that, when refined, may prove to be more useful. Using these criteria, we estimate that nearly 129,000 of the 250,000 patients can derive demonstrable benefit from chemotherapy.

Patients who experience benefit from chemotherapy using this definition, can also be divided into two distinct groups. The fraction of patients with advanced disease who

can potentially be cured using chemotherapy (32,000); and
those who have drug responsive tumors and may experience
prolonged survival, but cannot be considered curable with
chemotherapy (97,000). These two groups are shown in Tables
1 and 2.

**TWELVE CANCERS IN WHICH A FRACTION OF
PATIENTS WITH ADVANCED DISEASE CAN
BE CURED WITH CHEMOTHERAPY**

Choriocarcinoma	Ovarian carcinoma
Acute lymphocytic leukemia in children	Acute myelogenous leukemia
	Wilm's tumor
Hodgkin's disease	Burkitt's lymphoma
Diffuse histiocytic lymphoma	Embryonal rhabdomyosarcoma
Nodular mixed lymphoma	Ewing's sarcoma
Testicular carcinoma	

44,500   New cases
11,000   Cured with current therapy

< 10% of all cancers per year
< 10% of all cancer deaths per year

In Table 1, 12 cancers are listed in which a fraction of
patients with advanced disease can now be considered curable
with chemotherapy. Data documenting this curability are
familiar to most investigators (21-44) and have been
described in detail at this symposium. The addition of
diffuse histiocytic lymphoma, nodular mixed lymphoma, and
ovarian cancer to this list are relatively recent achievements. Approximately 44,500 new cases of these twelve
cancers were diagnosed in 1977. Of these, we estimate 32,000
patients had advanced cancer at the time of presentation.
By applying the results of the best available treatment
program, and extrapolating this to nationwide application,
the fraction of patients who remain free of disease beyond
five years can be estimated. Those calculations resulted in
the identification of approximately 11,000 of the 32,000
patients as potentially curable with current drug programs
(21-44). This group represents less than 10% of all cancers
in 1977 and represent less than 10% of all cancer deaths.
Thus, our greatest successes have occurred in the least
common cancers. However, it is important to recall that
12,500 had localized disease (44,500 new cases minus 32,000
with advanced disease) and are curable as a result of the
use of combined modality treatment. As a result, these
12,500 patients are considered as part of the 280,000
patients (40%) derived from the 5 year survival in Report
#5. (Fig. 1)

ADVANCED CANCERS IN WHICH A FRACTION OF
PATIENTS RESPOND TO CHEMOTHERAPY AND
IMPROVED SURVIVAL IS DEMONSTRABLE

Breast carcinoma	Gastric carcinoma
Chronic myelogenous leukemia	Malignant insulinoma
Chronic lymphocytic leukemia	Endometrial carcinoma
Nodular poorly differentiated	Adrenal cortical carcinoma
lymphocytic lymphoma	Medulloblastoma
Multiple myeloma	Neuroblastoma
Small cell carcinoma of the	Polycythemia vera
lung	Prostatic carcinoma
Soft tissue sarcomas	Glioblastoma

~40%   All new cancers per year
~30%   All cancer deaths

Of considerable interest are the 97,200 patients shown
in Table 2 who have drug responsive tumors. In this group,
responding patients demonstrate survival benefit, however
brief. Complete remissions occur in 20-68% of treated
patients in this group (breast cancer 20%, nodular poorly
differentiated lymphocytic lymphoma 68%, small-cell carcinoma
of the lung 50%) (45,29,46). Using the overall response
rate in the current literature for each of the tumors listed
in Table 2, we estimate that 47,500 of these 97,200 patients,
or 49%, respond sufficiently to have some prolongation of
survival. If, as in the case of breast cancer which makes
up a majority of the cases in Table 2, the average prolongation of life is approximately one year, the use of chemotherapy may result in the addition of 47,500 person years of
life annually. While the issue of the quality of this prolonged life is debatable for some patients, it depends
largely on the type of chemotherapy, the stage of disease,
the motivation and age of the patients, and often the
attitude of the physician. It is not our intention to debate
this issue, but rather to emphasize that chemotherapy that
is effective in advanced disease may have its greatest
potential for success in the post-operative period. This
has certainly been true in the case of breast cancer as will
be discussed in more detail below. It is worthy of emphasis,
that the drugs that prolong life can sometimes be intolerable, and are often responsible for the backlash of public
opinion against chemotherapy. It should also be noted that
the tumors listed in Table 2 are among the most common and
comprise approximately 40% of all new cancers and approximately 30% of all cancer deaths.

**SOME ADVANCED CANCERS IN WHICH
A FRACTION OF PATIENTS RESPOND
BUT NO IMPROVEMENT IN SURVIVAL
HAS YET BEEN DEMONSTRATED**

Adenocarcinoma of lung	Malignant carcinoid tumors
Bladder carcinoma	Malignant melanoma
Carcinoma of cervix	Thyroid carcinoma
Colon carcinoma	Rectal carcinoma
Head and neck carcinoma	Hepatocellular carcinoma
Hypernephroma	Carcinoma of the penis

~ 35%   All new cancers per year
~ 30%   All cancer deaths

We have considered the 129,200 patients who experience survival benefit from chemotherapy. We will now discuss the remaining 121,000 patients who represent those who may respond to drug treatment but experience no demonstrable survival benefit. Table 3 lists some of these tumors. Patients in this group represent one-third of all cancers diagnosed annually and nearly 30% of all cancer deaths. Again, it is important to note that partial responses in these patients have not led to survival benefit, but use of the same therapies in the adjuvant setting has produced demonstrable benefit as will be discussed below.

Estimates of the Number of Patients Who may Benefit from Adjuvant Treatment

It is estimated that 170,000 patients will develop tumor recurrences following primary treatment. (Fig. 2) This population includes tumors that are often resectable, such as breast and colon cancers. Again, we assume that a drug regimen that produces partial responses in 20% of patients with metastatic disease should be considered a candidate for clinical trials in the adjuvant setting. We have identified therapies that meet this criteria. We calculated the number of patients in this group who are at great risk of developing recurrent tumor and identified 162,100 patients who may currently be candidates for post-operative chemotherapy (Table 4). A few examples will be cited below.

PATIENTS POTENTIALLY BENEFITING
FROM ADJUVANT THERAPY

	Patients with Local Disease	Numbers Benefitted
Breast carcinoma	35,600	7,120
Rectal carcinoma	14,600	2,920
Colon carcinoma	29,400	2,940
Gastric carcinoma	4,400	880
Melanoma	6,800	680
Soft tissue sarcoma	1,400	560
Lung carcinoma	17,600	—
Testicular carcinoma	2,000	—
Ovarian carcinoma	4,800	—
Bladder carcinoma	24,200	—
Cervical carcinoma	9,800	—
Head and neck carcinoma	11,500	—
TOTALS	162,100	15,100

The first modern adjuvant trials were undertaken by two separate groups of investigators: the National Surgical Adjuvant Breast Project (NSABP) under the leadership of Dr. Bernard Fisher; and the National Cancer Institute of Milan under, the leadership of Dr. Gianni Bonadonna. Both groups initiated studies in women with Stage II breast cancer and have demonstrated a significant improvement in pre-menopausal patients and in certain post-menopausal patients as will be discussed. The Milan group has reported elsewhere in this volume the improvement in relapse-free survival in pre-menopausal patients with the drug program known as CMF compared to untreated controls. At five years, relapse-free survival in treated patients is 69% and 44% for controls. Analysis at two years indicated a significant benefit for all women who received post-operative treatment. Subsequent analysis reported that this effect was not observed in the post-menopausal women. However, recent re-analysis indicates that the drug dose was more influential than menopausal status on the relapse-free and overall survival of patients who recieved CMF. When the percentage of projected drug doses received were analyzed, 79.3% of the post-menopausal patients and 75.3% of the pre-menopausal women who received at least 85% of optimal doses are disease-free at five years. Approximately 55% of both pre and post-menopausal women who received 65-85% of the drug dose, are disease free at five years. Women who received less than 65 percent of the optimal drug dose faired little better than the control group. Nodal status influenced all groups in a similar fashion. Women with the least tumor burden (less than 3 positive nodes) did consistently better than

the women with more than 3 positive nodes within each drug
dose and menopausal group. The NSABP has observed similar
results in the post-menopausal group in their second study
which compared 5-FU + L-PAM to L-PAM. The patients who have
demonstrated the greatest improvement in overall survival,
however, has been the group of post-menopausal women with
the greatest tumor burden (4 or more positive nodes) 76 vs.
55 percent respectively (47).

These investigators have developed sequential studies
to extend the benefit of adjuvant therapy to a larger portion
of breast cancer patients in a step-wise manner. The NSABP
followed the two trials cited above, with a third trial
comparing 3-drug therapy (L-PAM, 5-FU, Mtx) to 2 drugs
(L-PAM, 5FU). To date, no significant difference has been
observed in either groups except for toxicity (47). The
fourth study in this series is comparing the 2-drug combination and the antiestrogen tamoxifen to L-PAM + 5FU. This
study was undertaken when information regarding the importance of estrogen receptors was just emerging. Although
not fully analyzed, this study suggests that the addition of
tamoxifen to the combination provides benefit to women with
positive estrogen receptors (48). The NSABP has also
initiated one of the first randomized trials of immunotherapy
as another adjuvant agent. A protocol has been designed for
patients with Stage I breast cancer, the next step in their
series of clinical trials that will hopefully lead us closer
to our goal of the complete therapeutic experiment. Those
patients with estrogen receptor negative tumors will be
randomized to observation or a non-alkylating drug combination (5-FU alternating with methotrexate). The choice of
this combination is based on laboratory data which suggests
optimization of both drugs in this sequence (49). Patients
with estrogen receptor positive tumors will be randomized to
tamoxifen or observation. Dr. Bondonna's trials have been
documented elsewhere in this volume.

Patients with breast cancer are not the only population who have benefitted from post-operative chemotherapy.
Recent results from the Gastrointestinal Study Group (GITSG)
reported by Dr. Schein in this volume also indicate a clear
benefit for patients with rectal cancer who received treatment following surgery. Four treatments were compared in a
prospective randomized trial: 5FU and Methyl CCNU; radiotherapy; 5FU, Methyl CCNU, and radiotherapy; and surgery
alone. All three treatment arms are statistically superior

to surgery with respect to disease-free survival and the combination of two drugs and radiation is the superior arm. As yet, there is no significant difference in overall survival but clear trends for the superiority of two drugs and radiation can be appreciated when a disease-free survival of 75% is projected. For two drugs and radiation, this is 60 months; for the other treatment arms it is less than 20 months and for surgery alone it is 13 months.

Positive results are also being observed in the adjuvant chemotherapy of other tumors such as soft-tissue sarcoma, malignant melanoma and colon cancer. These results have been reported in detail elsewhere (50-55).

All patients with tumors listed in Table 4 are prime candidates for adjuvant chemotherapy. The number of patients who develop recurrences after local treatment is estimated on the left. The column on the right is an estimation of the number of patients that could benefit if existing adjuvant therapy were applied on a nationwide basis.

Summary of the Numerical Impact of Chemotherapy

Assuming widespread use of chemotherapy, long-term useful benefit can be expected in the following patients: the 11,000 patients with advanced cancers that are now curable by chemotherapy alone; the 12,500 patients with localized presentations of these tumors that are effectively treated with combinations of surgery, radiotherapy and chemotherapy; and the 15,100 patients who could benefit from widespread application of current adjuvant chemotherapy programs (Table 4).

Patients in Whom Future Progress May Occur First

The remaining 22,000 patients of the 32,000 who are diagnosed with one of the twelve cancers shown in Table 1 who are not cured with current drug programs are worthy of further consideration. They often respond magnificently to chemotherapy and quite frequently have prolongation of survival that is satisfactory in terms of quality of life. Because these patients have demonstrated sensitivity to chemotherapy, they are therefore likely to respond to future drug programs. One only has to recall the dramatic change in prognosis of patients with metastatic testicular cancer. The complete response rate in 1960 was approximately

20%, and only half remained free of their disease (56). Now,
over 70% of all patients with metastatic testicular cancer
have complete remissions and a majority remain disease free
(57). Thus, this disease has been highly vulnerable to
improvements in treatment.

The 49,700 patients in Table 2 who have not experienced
survival benefit represent another population of patients
that can be expected to experience marked improvements when
better therapeutic regimens are developed. All of these
patients represent the prime candidates for future chemotherapeutic trials.

The 147,000 patients with tumors listed in Table 4 who
are at great risk of developing recurrent tumor will
directly benefit from the development of new drug programs
and techniques that are identified in patients with advanced
stages of disease. Any survival benefit in advanced disease
will be magnified many fold as it is applied to the earlier
stages of disease.

Annual Economic Impact of Chemotherapy

Since Congress created the Cancer Institute's Drug Development Program in 1955, approximately 500 million dollars
have been invested. While the full impact of this program
is not yet appreciated, it is worthwhile to separate the
economic gains of chemotherapy from the human aspects of
the treatment of cancer. These data are shown in Tables 5
and 6.

ANNUAL ECONOMIC IMPACT OF CURATIVE DRUG THERAPY FOR PATIENTS WITH METASTATIC DISEASE IN USA

Number of patients with potentially
curable cancers diagnosed..............44,500

Number of patients—advanced
disease...............................31,500

Total Cures 11,000

Income to economy.............. ~$1,600,000,000

Taxes collected.................. ~$ 240,000,000

The emphasis in Table 5 is on the 11,000 patients who are curable with chemotherapy alone; these cancers occur primarily in young patients (refer to Table 1). We assumed that all adult males and one half of the adult females patients who are cured will work until the age of 65. We then subtracted the average age of these patients at diagnosis from age 65 to estimate work-years gained. Because some of these cancers occur almost exclusively in pediatric patients, we considered them as entering the work force at age 21. For pediatric patients we subtracted 21 from 65 to estimate work-years gained in this group. We then multipled the number of work-years by $10,000 for males and $6,000 for females, a conservative estimate of their earning potential in the United States. We, therefore, estimated that approximately 1.6 billion dollars is generated by each cured cohort of 11,000 patients. If one then assumes that each individual who works will pay a 15% income tax, the U.S. economy accrues approximately 240 million dollars in taxes each year as a result of successful cancer chemotherapy. This estimate does not take into consideration the gains to society in reduced costs for the hospitalization and care of patients who would have had debilitating illnesses eventuating in death.

ANNUAL ECONOMIC IMPACT OF EFFECTIVE POST-OPERATIVE CHEMOTHERAPY FOR BREAST CANCER PATIENTS

Cost of therapy* for all pre-menopausal
  Stage II patients........................$ 57,240,000

Cost of therapy* for recurrent disease in
  20% of pre-menopausal patients..........$341,939,700

Includes direct costs of therapy and time lost from work force as a result of disease and/or treatment.

Table 6 focuses on pre-menopausal women with breast cancer who clearly benefit from adjuvant chemotherapy. These cost/benefit calculations differ from those in Table 5 in that the costs of administering adjuvant drug therapy to all premenopausal women is included. Nationwide costs of drugs, laboratory work, x-rays, and annual income lost from work due to doctor's appointments, and illness related to

drug toxicity for all pre-menopausal women was estimated to
be $57,240,000. This total is contrasted to the cost requir-
ed to care for the 20% of women who would have been treated
for recurrent breast cancer had they not received adjuvant
therapy. This cost is estimated at $341,939,700. Again,
the cost of successful therapy is far less than the cost and
loss that occurs if such therapy is not provided.

These conservative estimates support the conclusion
that the financial investment in the development of drugs
for use in cancer treatment has been worthwhile. Substan-
tiating the value of drug treatment also required a rapid
expansion of the clinical trials program of the Cancer Institute after the passage of the National Cancer Act. This
program is now paying handsome dividends.

There are many areas of research in need of exploration
to complete the chemotherapeutic experiment. We must continue to identify more effective and less toxic drugs, screen
fewer compounds, yet continue to identify the same number of
drugs for clinical trials (58).

We need to identify new drugs and combinations that are
not cross-resistant to older established programs which will
improve response rates and disease-free survival in tumors
already known to be sensitive to chemotherapy. This approach
has already shown promise in advanced Hodgkin's disease
where alternating sequential combinations have been employed.
Bonadonna has reported that when MOPP chemotherapy is alter-
nated with the drug combination of adriamycin, bleomycin,
vinblastine, dacarbazine (ABVD), a significantly higher
complete remission rate and better relapse-free survival
can be observed (59). A similar approach is under investigation at the Clinical Center of the National Cancer
Institute (60).

Reference has already been made to the need to develop
more sensitive techniques of measuring both the active forms
of anticancer drugs and their targets in the cell. With
these tools, we can enter an era where specific chemotherapy
may be individualized for patients.

The delivery of drugs directly to the tumor site is
another area of intense investigation. This approach has
been explored at the NCI in patients with ovarian cancer.
These patients die with disease almost exclusively localized
to the abdomen. Failure of surgery and radiotherapy to cure
patients is often related to the persistence of occult tumor

patients is often related to the persistence of occult tumor cells within the abdominal cavity. It was hypothesized that administration of drugs in large volume utilizing dialysis techniques could reach microscopic foci that were not eradicated by systemic therapy. A series of experiments in rodents indicated that the peritoneal clearance of chemo-therapeutic agents was significantly less than renal clearance offering a pharmacologic advantage (61). Since drugs administered into the peritoneal cavity are absorbed into the portal venous system, agents such as 5 fluorouracil which are metabolized to an inactive form by the liver may undergo significant metabolic clearance.

INTRAPERITONEAL DRUG THERAPY

	Ratio of Mean Concentration Peritoneal Fluid to Plasma	Maximum Plasma Concentration
Methotrexate	23	$2\text{-}3 \times 10^{-7}\text{M}$
5 Fluoruracil	298	$1.67 \times 10^{-5}\text{M}$
Adriamycin	343	$1.1 \times 10^{-7}\text{M}$

Table 7 summarizes the data on the difference in peritoneal versus plasma concentrations in three drugs, methotrexate, 5 fluorouracil, and adriamycin. It can be seen that intraperitoneal administration of these drugs provides a significantly higher mean concentrations of chemotherapy in the peritoneal fluid as compared to plasma concentration (62). Therapeutic trials at the NCI are now underway to exploit the pharmacologic advantages of these drugs administered intraperitoneally in patients with ovarian cancer with minimal residual disease.

Because the major route of drug eggress is the portal venous system, investigators at the NCI have asked whether the intraperitoneal administration of drugs might prevent tumor recurrence in cancers that are known to metastatize almost exclusively to the liver. Since 50% of patients with colorectal cancer recur inside the abdomen or in the liver, a protocol was developed at the NCI which randomly allocates patients with Duke's C colorectal cancer to intraperitoneal administration of 5 fluorouracil or intravenous 5 fluorouracil.

In addition, different modalities are now being combined in many unique ways. Hyperthermia, in conjunction with radiotherapy, has been reviewed by Dr. Kaplan in this volume. Weinstein has also reported data that suggests hyperthermia can selectively cause the release of antitumor agents from heat sensitive liposomes in the heated area (63). Both the intraperitoneal administration of chemotherapy and the selective release of drugs from liposomes under the influence of heat may help future investigators to target the delivery of chemotherapeutic agents.

The 1980's abound with opportunities for chemotherapy. The ever increasing number of interesting biological modifiers, the identification of DNA recombinant technology, the availability of antibodies produced by hybridomas, the development of in vitro assays that may permit a rationale selection of cancer agents based on the sensitivity of the patient's own tumor cells, the development of protein indexing techniques that may permit identification of responsive and unresponsive patients, all offer opportunities to amplify the impact of chemotherapy.

Finally, a few words about the backlash of progress. Multilation, burns, poison are words often used by lay persons when referring to surgery, radiation, and chemotherapy. Current technology, particularly the use of combination modalities, have led to less mutilating surgery exemplified by the clinical studies in the sarcomas (50). With the availability of new radiation equipment, superficial skin burns are, in general, a complication of the past. The development of radiosensitizers which sensitize tumor tissue to the lethal effects of radiation, and the use of high energy particulate therapy, should make it possible to further diminish the side effects of radiotherapy.

The Cancer Institute is deeply concerned about the side effects of chemotherapy. From our estimates, chemotherapy is currently administered to over 200,000 patients a year. Using 1977 data, we can demonstrate clinically useful effects in approximately 38,000. Thus, the majority of the patients exposed to chemotherapy will have most of the side effects and little of the benefit. Understandably, this has led to a negative opinion of chemotherapy by the public. The side

effects of chemotherapy and the slowness of progress will
only be tolerated as long as there is continued evidence of
progress. This means that we must rapidly test new drugs
and new drug programs to improve on old results. Our emphasis should not be on the widespread application of therapies that have already been identified, but on the improvement
of these treatments. The upsurge in the field of medical
oncology has produced a curious paradox. The therapies
described in this paper are being widely applied in non-
research settings and clinical trials that have been identified to improve these results lack untreated patients. The
Cancer Institute, its constituent centers, and the clinical
trials programs face a serious problem if this situation is
not corrected. We must develop a means that effectively
includes the participation of private physicians and their
patients in our clinical trials programs. Such an approach
will require a greater cooperation on the part of the private oncologists in this country and a greater understanding
by the research community who develops new approaches to
therapy. The public has been and will remain sympathetic to
the support of research to improve treatment, but it is
doubtful that they will remain sympathetic to a medical
community that fails to put their best interests as its
first priority.

REFERENCES

1. DeVita, V. T.: The evolution of therapeutic research in
   cancer. N. Eng. J. Med. 298: 907-910, 1978.
2. Skipper, H. E., Schabel, F. M., and Wilcox, W. S.:
   Experimental evaluation of potential anti-cancer agents,
   XIII. On the criteria and kinetics associated with
   "curability" of experimental leukemia. Cancer
   Chemother. Rep. 35: 1-111, 1964.
3. DeVita, V. T. and Schein, P. S.: The use of drugs in
   combination for the treatment of cancer. Rationale and
   results. N. Eng. J. Med. 288: 998-1007, 1973.
4. Capizzi, R.L. (Ed.): Seminars in Oncology, Vol.4 No.2,
   June 1977.
5. DeVita, V. T.,Serpick, A. A., and Carbone, P. P.:
   Combination chemotherapy in the treatment of advanced
   Hodgkin's disease. Ann. Int. Med. 73: 881-895, 1970.
6. Aur, R. J. A, Simone, J. V., Husta, H. O., Vercosa,
   M. S., and Pinkel, D.: Cessation of therapy during
   complete remission of childhood acute lymphocytic
   leukemia. N. Eng. J. Med. 291: 1230-1234, 1974.

7. Holland, J. and Frei, E. (Eds.): Cancer Medicine
    Philadelphia, Lea & Febiger, 1973.
8. Sinkovics, J. G.: Medical Oncology: An Advanced
    Course. New York, Grune & Stratton, Inc., 1979.
9. Jones, S. E. and Salmon, S. E. (Eds.): Adjuvant Therapy
    of Cancer II. New York, Grune & Stratton, Inc., 1979.
10. Rubin, P. (Ed.): Clinical Oncology for Medical Students
    and Physicians: A Multidisciplinary Approach.
    New York, American Cancer Society, 1978.
11. _____ Cancer: A Manual For Practitioners (Fifth
    Edition). Boston, American Cancer Society, 1978.
12. Ackerman, L. V. and del Regato, J. A.: Cancer,
    Diagnosis, Treatment and Prognosis, Fifth Edition.
    St. Louis, C. V. Mosby Co., 1977.
13. Pinedo, H. M.: Cancer Chemotherapy 1980. Amsterdam,
    Exerpta Medica, 1980.
14. Hoogstraten, B. (Ed.): Cancer Research: Impact of the
    Cooperative Groups. New York, Masson Publishing USA,
    Inc., 1980.
15. Mauer, H. M.: Current concepts in cancer: Solid tumors
    in children. N. Eng. J. Med. 299: 1345-1348, 1978.
16. Stonehill, E.H.: Impact of Cancer Therapy on Survival.
    Cancer 42: 1008-1014, 1978.
17. DeVita, V.T., Henney, J.E., and Stonehill, E.H.: Cancer
    Mortality: The Good News. In Adjuvant Therapy of
    Cancer II. S.E. Jones and S.E. Salmon (eds) New York
    Grune and Stratton, p. XV-XX, 1979.
18. Cancer facts & figures. American Cancer Society, Inc.,
    1977.
19. Axtell, L. M., Asire, A. J., and Myers, M. H. (Eds.):
    Cancer Patient Survival Report #5 - A report from the
    cancer surveillance, epidemiology, and end results
    (SEER) program, U.S. Dept. Health, Education & Welfare,
    Public Health Service HEW PHS, Publication No. National
    Institutes of Health (NIH) 77-992, Washington, D.C.,
    Govt. Printing Office (GPO), pp. 1-314, 1976.
20. Klein, E., Burgess, G.H., and Helm, F.: Neoplasms of
    the Skin. In Cancer Medicine. J. Holland and E. Frei
    (eds) Philadelphia, Lea and Febiger 1973, pp 1789-1822.
21. Kramer, S., Perez, C. A., Jenkins, R. D. T., and Cox,
    J.: Radiation therapy. In Cancer Research: Impact of
    the Cooperative Groups. In Hoogstraten, B. (Ed.).
    New York, Masson Publishing USA, Inc., 1980.
22. Hertz, R., Lewis, J., and Lipsett, M.: Five years
    experience with chemotherapy of metastatic chorio-
    carcinoma and related trophoblastic tumors in women.
    Am. J. Obstet. Gynecol. 82: 631-638, 1961.

23. Li, M. C.: Trophoblastic disease: Natural history, diagnosis and treatment. Ann. Int. Med. 74: 102-110, 1971.

24. Pinkel, D.: Treatment of acute lymphocytic leukemia. Cancer 43: 1128-1137, 1979.

25. George, S. L., Aur, R. J. A., Mauer, A. M., and Simone, J. V.: A reappraisal of the results of stopping therapy in childhood leukemia. N. Eng. J. Med. 300: 269-273, 1979.

26. Bonadonna, G., Zucali, R., Monfardini, S., Delena, M. and Uslenghi, C.: Cominbation chemotherapy of Hodgkin's disease with adriamycin, bleomycin, vincristine, and imidazole carboximide versus MOPP. Cancer 36: 252-262, 1975.

27. DeVita, V. T., Simon, R. M., Hubbard, S. M., Young, R. C., Berard, C. W., Moxely, J. H., Frei, E., III, Carbone, P. P., and Canellos, G. P.: Curability of advanced Hodgkin's disease with chemotherapy: Long-term follow-up of MOPP-treated patients at NCI. Ann. Intern. Med. 92(5): 587-595, 1980.

28. DeVita, V. T., Canellos, G. P., Schein, P., Hubbard, S. P. and Young, R. C.: Advanced diffused histiocytic lymphoma: a potentially curable disease. Lancet

29. Schein, P. S., Chabner, B. A., Canellos, G. P., Young, R. C., Berard, C., and DeVita, V. T.: Potential for prolonged disease-free survival following combination chemotherapy of non-Hodgkin's lymphoma. Blood 43: 181-189, 1974.

30. Skarin, A. T., Rosenthal, D. S., Moloney, W. C., Frei, E.: Combination chemotherapy of advanced non-Hodgkin's lymphoma with bleomycin, adriamycin, cyclophosphamide, vincristine, and prednisone (BACOP). Blood 49: 759-770, 1977.

31. Sweet, D. L., Golumb, H. M., Ultmann, J. E., Miller, J. B., Stein, R. S., Lester, E. P., Mintz, U., Bitran, J. B., Streuli, R. A., Daly, K., and Roth, N. O.: Cyclophosphamide, vincristine, methotrexate with leucovorn rescue and cytarabine (COMLA combination sequential chemotherapy for advanced diffuse histio-cytic lymphoma. Ann. Intern. Med. 92: 785-790, 1980.

32. Anderson, T., Bender, R. A., Fisher, R. I., DeVita, V. T., Chabner, B. A., Berard, C. W., Norton, L., and Young, R. C.: Combination chemotherapy in nonHodgkin's lymphoma: Results of long-term follow-up. Cancer Treat. Rep. 61: 1057-1066, 1977.

33. Ezdinli, E.Z., Costello, W. and Wasser, L.P.: Eastern cooperative oncology group experience with the Rappaport classification of non-Hodgkin's lymphoma. Cancer 43: 544-550, 1979.
34. Golumb, H. M. (Ed.): Non-Hodgkin's Lymphoma. Seminars in Oncology 7(3): September 1980.
35. Einhorn, L. H., Donohue, J.: Cis-diamminedichloro-platinum, vinblastine, and bleomycin combination chemo-therapy in disseminated testicular cancer. Ann. Inter. Med. 87: 293-298, 1977.
36. Young, R. C., Chabner, B. A., Hubbard, S. P., Fisher, R. I., Bender, R. A., Anderson, T., Simon, R. M., Canellos, G. P., and DeVita, V. T.: Advanced ovarian carcinoma: A prospective clinical trial of melphalan (L-PAM) versus combination chemotherapy (HEXA-CAF). N. Eng. J. Med. 299: 1261-1266, 1978.
37. Weinstein, H.J., Mayer, R.J., Rosenthal, D.S., Camitta, B.M., Coral, F.S., Nathan, DG. and Frei, E., III: Treatment of acute myelogenous leukemia in children and adults. N. Eng. J. Med. 303: 473-8, 1980.
38. D'Angio, G. J., Evans, A. Z., Breslow, N.: The treat-ment of Wilm's tumor: Results of the nation Wilm's tumor study. Cancer 38: 633-646, 1978.
39. Ziegler, J. L., Magrath, I. T., Olweny, C. L. M.: Cure of Burkitt's lymphoma: Ten year follow-up of 157 Ugandan patients. Lancet 2: 936-938, 1979.
40. Maurer, H. M., Donaldson, M., Gehan, E. A., et al: Rhabdomyosarcoma in childhood and adolescence. Curr. Probl. Cancer 2: 1-38, 1978.
41. Maurer, H. M., Moon, T., Donaldson, M., Fernandez, C., Gehan, E. A., Hammond, D., Hays, D. M., Lawrence, W., Newton, W., Ragat, A., Raney, B., Soule, E. H., Sutow, W. W., Teffo, M.: The intergroup Rhabdomyosar-coma study, a preliminary report. Cancer 40: 2015-2026, 1977.
42. Pomeroy, T. C., Johnson, R. E.: Combined modality therapy of Ewing's sarcoma. Cancer 35: 36-47, 1975.
43. Rosen, G., Caparros, B., Mosend, C., et al: Curability of Ewing's sarcoma and considerations for future therapeutic trials. Cancer 41: 888-889, 1978.
44. Perez, C. A., Razek, A., Teffo, M., et al: Analysis of local tumor control in Ewing's sarcoma: Preliminary results of a cooperative intergroup study. Cancer 40: 2864-2873, 1977.

45. Canellos, G.P., DeVita, V.T., Gold, G.L., Chabner, B.A.,
     Schein, P.S. and Young, R.C.: Cyclical combination
     chemotherapy for advanced breast carcinoma. Br Med J
     1: 218-220, 1974.
46. Bunn, P.A., Cohen, M.H., Ihde, D.C., Shackney, S.E.,
     Matthews, M.J., Fossieck, B.E. and Minna, J.D.: Review
     of Therapeutic Trials in Small Cell Brochogenic Car-
     cinoma of the Lung. In Lung Cancer Progress in Thera-
     peutic Research. F. Muggia and M. Rosenscweig. New
     York Raven Press 549-558, 1979.
47. Fisher B., Redmond, C., and Fisher, E.R. et al.: Con-
     tribution of recent NSABP clinical trials of primary
     breast cancer therapy to an understanding of tumor
     biology - An overview of findings. Cancer 46: 1009-
     1025, 1980.
48. Personal Communication - B. Fisher
49. Donehower, R.C., Erlichman, C., Schilsky, R. and
     Chabner, B.: Pharmacologic Considerations in Adjuvant
     Chemotherapy. In The Adjuvant Therapy of Cancer II.
     Salmon, S.E. and Jones, S.E. (eds) New York Grune and
     Stratton pp 37-46, 1979.
50. Rosenberg, S.A. and Sindelar, D.F.: Surgery and Adju-
     vant radiation-chemotherapy in soft tissue sarcomas:
     Results of treatment at the NCI. In Advances in the
     Treatment of Ovarian and Testicular Cancer and Sarcoma.
     A.T. van Oosterem (ed) New York, Academic Press,
     pp. 301-316, 1980.
51. Personal communication - R.I. Fisher.
52. Higgins, G.A., Dwight, R.W., Smith, J.V. and Keehn,
     R.J.: Fluorouracil as an adjuvant to surgery in car-
     cinoma of the colon. Arch Surg 1971; 102: 339-43.
53. Higgins, G.A., Lee, L.E., Dwight, R.W. and Keehn, R.J.:
     The case for adjuvant 5-fluorouracil in colorectal
     cancer. Cancer Clin Trials. 1978; 1: 35-41.
54. Grage, T.B., Metter, G.E. and Cornell, G.N., et al.:
     The role of 5 fluorouracil as an adjuvant to the surgi-
     cal treatment of large bowel cancer. In: Adjuvant
     Therapy of Cancer. Salmon, S.E., Jones, S.E., (eds).
     Amsterdam, North-Holland Publishing Co.; 1977 259-63.
55. Li, M.C. and Ross, S.T.: Chemoprophylaxis for patients
     with colorectal cancer: prospective study with five-
     year follow-up. J Am Med Assoc, 1976; 235: 2825-8.
56. Li, M.C., Whitmore, W.F., Golberg, R. and Grabstad.:
     Effects of combined drug therapy on metastatic cancer of
     the testes J Am Med Assoc, 174: 145-153, 1960.

57. Einhorn, L.H. and Williams, S.D.: The management of disseminated testicular cancer. In Testicular Tumors Management and Treatment. L.H. Einhorn (ed). New York Masson Publishing USA Inc. 1980 pp 117-149

58. DeVita, V.T., Oliverio, V.T., Muggia, F.M., Wiernik, P.W., Zeigler, J., Goldin, A., Rubin, D., Henney, J. and Schepartz, S.: The Drug Development and Clinical Trials Programs of the Division of Cancer Treatment NCI. Cancer Clin Trials 2: 195-216, 1979.

59. Santoro, A., Bonadonna, G., Bonfante, V. and Valagussa, P.: Non cross resistant regimens (MOPP and ABVD) vs. MOPP alone in Stage IV Hodgkin's disease. Proc. AACR and ASCO: Vol. 21: 1980, 470.

60. DeVita, V.T.: "Human models of human diseases; Breast cancer and the lymphomas. Intl J Rad Onc Biol Phys. 5: 1855-1867, 1979.

61. Dedrick, R.L., Myers, C.E., Burgay, P.M. and DeVita, V.T.: Pharmacokinetic rationale for peritoneal drug administration in the treatment of ovarian cancer. Cancer Treat Rep 62: 1-11, 1978.

62. Speyer, J.L., Sugarbaker, P.H., Collin, J.M., Dedrick, R.W., Klecker, R.W., DeVita, V.T. and Myers, C.E.: Portal uptake and hepatic metabolism of 5-fluorouracil administered by intraperitoneal dialysis. Cancer Research (in press).

63. Weinstein, J.M., Magin, R.L., Cysyk, R.L. and Zaharko, D.: Treatment of solid L210 murine tumors with local hyperthermia and temperature-sensitive liposomes containing methotrexate. Cancer Research 40: 1388-1396, 1980.

Promising Areas of Cancer Research

ROBERT A. GOOD

Vice President
Memorial Sloan-Kettering Cancer Center

NOORBIBI K. DAY

Head, Laboratory of Complement and Effector Biology

STEVEN S. WITKIN

Associate, Laboratory of Complement and Effector Biology

GABRIEL FERNANDES

Associate, Laboratory of Developmental Immunobiology
Sloan-Kettering Institute for Cancer Research
New York, New York

In accepting the challenge of this title, we must first recognize that it will not be possible to encompass all that it portends. For almost a week, beginning with Benno Schmidt's initial lecture on the aims of the conference, and encompassing multiple sessions from epidemiology to progress in chemotherapy, we have heard the descriptions of the best and most advanced cancer research extant. Indeed, we have been presented most of the promising leads in cancer research. As if that were not enough, we look forward next week to another international meeting in which we shall focus on cancer research in still another major perspective. Realizing that the greatest risk factor for cancer is aging, an entire international symposium will deal with the strides being made in biology, genetics and molecular biology which promise in the more remote future to provide understanding of the aging process and, with this understanding, insight into the diseases of aging, including cancer.

To try then to give a comprehensive overview of the promising areas for cancer research would not only be impossible,
it might seem absurd. There is no way we could even bring
highlights of the many areas of promise without being superficial. Consequently, we have chosen to describe areas of
cancer research we personally find most exciting, as evidenced
by the fact that these are some of the areas in which our
clinics and laboratories are working.

We will describe at the outset surging knowledge about how
the immune systems are organized and how the cells of these
complex systems work together to maintain the integrity and
uniqueness of the body in the sea of microorganisms chosen for
our ecological niche. We will try to appreciate the miracle
of immunology and analyze how current research is leading
rapidly to an explanation of this miracle in molecular genetic
terms. In this research, we see extraordinary achievement and
promise that lies at the very forefront of molecular biology.
We will emphasize the power and potential of monoclonal antibodies produced by the new hybridoma technology in which cancer cells are being trained for participation in the war on
cancer.

We will then consider breast cancer from both experimental
and clinical perspectives, focusing on exciting new evidence
which seems to be yielding information pertinent to ultimate
understanding of etiology, epidemiology, immunologically-
based treatment, and even prevention of breast cancer as a
representative of the most common forms of cancer. We will
also reflect on exciting relationships of cancer to aging and
the diseases of aging and consider briefly our new work which,
in certain experimental systems, has already made possible
the doubling or even tripling of the life-span in mice and
suppression of the development of the diseases of aging, including certain forms of cancer.

Finally, we will consider the achievements and promise from
both clinical and laboratory analysis of the approach to cellular engineering which we introduced 12 years ago by successfully carrying out the first allogeneic marrow transplant
to correct an inborn error of metabolism responsible for
severe combined immunodeficiency disease (Gatti et al,1968;
Good, 1971). This approach has now been applied as the most
effective treatment of some of the worst and most recalci-
trant forms of leukemia, as has been reviewed so ably by
Donnall Thomas elsewhere in this volume. This approach, indeed, is already working in the fight against both cancer and
genetically-determined diseases. Recent advances promise that
cellular engineering through bone marrow and other organ
transplantation will be very much extended in the immediate
future. In the laboratory, we are already able to transplant

across major histocompatibility barriers without causing
graft-vs-host reaction. The achievements of this form of
cellular engineering will lead naturally, perhaps even within
this decade, to genetic engineering, first at the somatic cell
level, and later perhaps even to manipulation of the germ
plasm to prevent both disease and the genetic transmission of
disease.

THE NEW VIEW OF THE IMMUNOLOGICAL SYSTEMS

Figure 1 illustrates how we now view the cellular basis of
immunity which underlies the specific immunological defenses
of the body. Whereas, at the start of this decade, it seemed
sufficient to talk of the two separate arms subserving two
distinct immunity functions, one must now think in terms of
two arms with two hands, fingers that work together to achieve
the delicate modulations, feedback controls and facilitations
of function essential to T and B cell-dependent immunities.
Thus the T-effector cells subserve the cellular immunities,
e.g., delayed allergy, defense against viruses and virus-
infected cells, fungi, intracellular bacterial pathogens and
tumor cells. B effector cells differentiate into the plasma
cell factories which produce the antibodies that are so

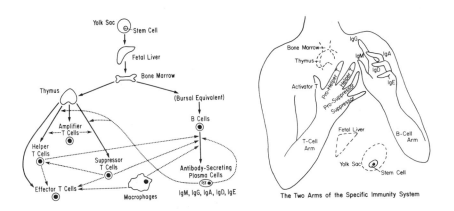

Figure 1. The specific immunity system: two schematic outlines.
Left: reprinted from Good RA, O'Reilly RJ, West A: Proc. of
Serono Symp. on Thymus, Thymic Hormones and T Lymphocytes,
Rome, 1979. New York, Academic Press, in press.
Right: reprinted from Gupta S, Good RA: Seminars Hematol 17:
1, 1980.

important in preventing infections and in defending us against
the high-grade encapsulated bacterial pathogens. The B cells
differentiate into numerous populations, each producing antibodies of different immunoglobulin classes that are differently distributed in the body and each of which has a specialized
function. One of the most challenging and most rapidly developing lines of investigation in immunology is the effort to
understand in genetic and molecular terms just how the B cells
differentiate--how they arrange and rearrange their genes to
make possible the miracle of immunology. To quote Sir Peter
Medawar, "We can affirm with complete confidence that a rabbit
not yet born will react specifically to a chemical not yet
synthesized" (Medawar, 1980).

Giants of modern molecular biology like Leder, Tonegawa,
Honjo and their associates (Perry et al, 1980; Maki et al,
1980; Miyata et al, 1980) have been analyzing the molecular
events which promise during this decade to permit full understanding of this miracle in relatively simple molecular terms.
Thus, focus on the B cells and plasma cells, and the events
involved in maturation to antibody secreting cells, continues
in the 80's to provide some of the most exciting fundamental
research in the cancer field. For the T cells at this junc-
ture, similar investigations are of promise, but may be more
difficult. Among the most important research in T cell biology is the analysis of differentiation of T cells into separate subclasses of cells, each with a distinct function. Figure 2 illustrates several steps in differentiation of mouse T
cells which occurs first within the thymus and then in the
peripheral lymphoid system, yielding subpopulations of T lymphocytes specialized as effector cells for different tasks.

The 70's have yielded evidence of specialization of T cell
function which permits the T cells to participate in the bodily defense through effector mechanisms and through communication with macrophages to contribute the defenses known as
cell-mediated immunities. Of utmost importance are the roles
of T lymphocytes which act as inducers and helpers of both T
and B cell function (the up-regulators of immunity) or T lymphocytes that act as suppressors (down-regulators) of both T
and B cell immunity. Each class of T cells in the mouse (the
best of all teachers of immunology) can now be recognized and
defined by antisera developed first by Old and Boyse, using
impeccable serological analyses over the past 20 years. Now
the displays of differentiation antigens which permit recognition, isolation of the cells and analysis of function of each
stage of development of T lymphocytes and which define crucial
developmental bifurcations into specialized sets can be recognized by monoclonal antibodies developed by the powerful
hybridoma technology. Thus, an area of intensive investigation and continuing great promise is to analyze in detail

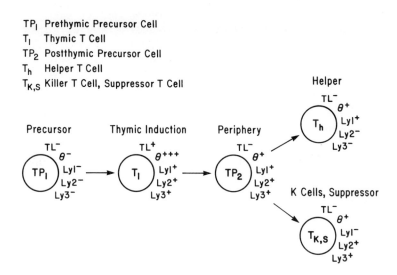

TP₁ Prethymic Precursor Cell
T₁ Thymic T Cell
TP₂ Postthymic Precursor Cell
Tₕ Helper T Cell
T_{K,S} Killer T Cell, Suppressor T Cell

Figure 2. Development of functional subclasses of T lympho-
cytes of the mouse. Reprinted from Alexander JW, Good RA:
Fundamentals of Clinical Immunology. Philadelphia, W.B.
Saunders Co., 1977, p 28.

not only the molecular basis of T cell specificity (still an
area of great uncertainty and controversy), but also the
molecular basis for the T cell signals that are involved in
inducer functions, as well as the specific helper, suppressor
and killer functions for which these emissaries of the thymus
are responsible.

   It seems extraordinary that the cellular organization of
the immunity system involves such complex circuitry and that
so much energy of immune function is devoted to regulation by
the T cells of the lymphocytes which are involved in immunity
function. However, similar complicated networks under the
same degree of tight function-mediated regulation are known
to subserve functions of the brain and endocrinological system.
The latter two major networks now seem also to relate intimately in their function to the complex immunological network.

   The promise of research on the complex circuitry involved
in regulation of immunity should progressively yield understanding of immunological development and involution, autoimmunities, viruses, effective immunity against viruses, fungi,
parasites and bacteria, and even immunity against cancer cells.
Someday, perhaps, all of this analysis will provide the basis
for effective immunotherapy and immunoprophylaxis against cancer. In the meantime, we already are obtaining better definition of the cells involved in the monoclonal expansions

represented by the leukemias and lymphomas and it seems certain that specific or non-specific immunotherapy directed
against residual cancer cells can be developed.

The development for man of monoclonal antibodies to define
the subpopulations of T and B cells, the steps involved in
their normal differentiation and the many different malignancies of the lymphoid system are advancing rapidly. On Figure
3 is illustrated a recent definition of these developmental
stages for human T cells, developed in Boston by Schlossman
and his group. Figure 4 shows some of the early interpreta-
tions of the definitions being undertaken with monoclonal antibodies produced by Evans et al (1980) in our laboratories.
One of the impressive consequences of this promising area for
cancer research is that the monoclonal antibodies which recognize stable differentiation antigens on the developing T and
B cells, the T and B-cell sets and leukemias and lymphomas, is
that uniform reagents can readily be made commercially so that
everyone can have identical reagents with which to analyze the
lymphocyte populations in health and disease.

MONOCLONAL ANTIBODIES AND THE HYBRIDOMA TECHNOLOGY

Rabbits, guinea pigs, horses and goats are being rendered
obsolete as factories for antibody production by the development of the powerful hybridoma technology. Basically, this
technology couples the immortality of a secretory cancer cell
(myeloma) with the genetic mechanisms of the normal antibody-
producing cell to generate hybrid cells which are immortal and
can produce large quantities of chemically and immunologically
uniform antibodies. After fusion of spleen cells of a mouse
stimulated with the cells or antigen one wants to recognize
and using careful selection procedures, the immunologist picks
the hybrid cells that are producing antibodies with the specificity he is seeking. Once a hybridoma is stabilized, the
clone of cells producing the uniform antibody can be grown in
culture or as a tumor in an immunologically deprived host.
Then, essentially unlimited amounts of the pure specific immunoglobulin can be produced. Application of this method promises
to develop into an industry already estimated in hundreds of
millions of dollars per year. It will provide the serological
basis for modern blood grouping, tissue typing, bacteriology,
virology, parasitology, mycology, cellular immunology, clinical and industrial biochemistry, and definition and identification of cancer cells and other aberrant cells from or within
the body.

At the present time, the hybridomas are prepared with a
mouse myeloma cell and the antibodies produced are mouse

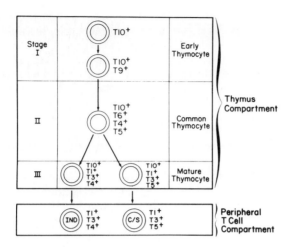

Figure 3. Stages of T-cell differentiation in human beings. Three discrete stages of thymic differentiation can be defined on the basis of reactivity with monoclonal antibodies. The most mature thymocyte population (Stage III) gives rise to the peripheral T-cell inducer (IND) and cytotoxic/suppressor (C/S) subsets. The cell-surface antigens expressed during T-cell ontogeny are shown. Reprinted from Reinherz EL, Schlossman SF: N Engl J. Med 303:370, 1980.

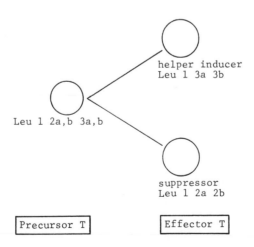

Figure 4. Lymphocyte phenotypes with SKI monoclonals. Evans et al: Proc Nat Acad Sci USA, in press.

proteins against which humans would react immunologically.
This research already is promising to generate human hybridomas. Two groups, one led by Kaplan at Stanford (this volume)
and the other by Nowinski at Seattle (Nowinski et al, in press)
have already announced their ability to produce hybridomas
that can make specific human immunoglobulins. This powerful
new methodology promises new approaches to detection of residual cancer cells after surgery, radiation or chemotherapy,
ability to destroy minimal residual tumors, effective anti-
metastatic therapy, and even capacity to deliver toxic chemicals directly to tumor cells.
    But the hybridoma technology need not stop with antibodies.
This same technique is being developed as an approach to production of lymphokines (those powerful molecules involved in
non-specific immunological mediation), peptide hormones, interferon, specific, non-specific and immunoglobulin class-
specific suppressor and helper factors. Indeed, fundamental
research on the specific immunity systems and on their intrinsic and extrinsic controls is a major approach to cancer
diagnosis, which will ultimately yield effective treatment
and prevention via the hybridoma technology.

THE THYMUS AND ITS HORMONES

    Major interest also continues to focus on the thymus and
its functions. This vital lymphoepithelial organ represents
the site for T cell development and differentiation. Further,
it produces a series of biologically active peptide hormones
which are involved in the differentiation, development and
maintenance of the T cell immunity, both within and outside of
the thymus. Exciting research is ongoing which has already
identified and defined the functions of some of these interesting peptide hormones. Already, the latter are being developed
as drugs to be used to correct certain immunodeficiencies, to
fortify the immune functions of the debilitated or aged and to
foster cell-mediated immunities as these are needed. Figure 5
represents 4 purified thymic hormones or peptides which have
been derived from thymus or are present in the blood but dependent on thymic epithelium for their presence. Thymosin α_1
and β_4 are hormones purified and fully sequenced by Allan
Goldstein and his associates (Goldstein et al, 1977). Thymopoietin II has been purified and sequenced by Gideon Goldstein
and collaborators (Schlesinger and Goldstein, 1975), and facteur thymique serique (FTS) purified, sequenced and analyzed
functionally by J.F. Bach and associates in Paris (Bach et al,
1977; Incefy et al, 1980).
    Since the greatest risk factor in cancer is aging, since
immunodeficiency and disordered immunologic function feature

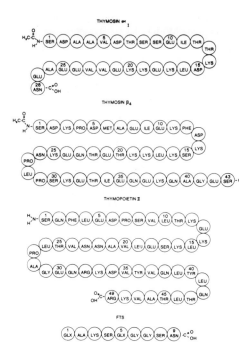

Figure 5. Sequence analysis of purified thymic factors. From Goldstein AL: Immunological Aspects of Cancer Therapeutics (ed. J. Mihich). New York, John Wiley & Sons, in press.

aging animals and man, and since one popular theory concerning the basis of aging involves defective immunity, it seems entirely pertinent to cancer research to study the thymic hormones, develop means for their assay and for their production and to investigate their influence on the functions of cells of thymus-deprived animals or aged man and animals.

Already Bach's hormone FTS can be synthesized and is available in early stages of clinical trials as a drug. A pentapeptide sequence of thymopoietin has been identified as representing an active site in thymopoietin II (G. Goldstein et al, 1979). It too has been synthesized and is available for clinical and experimental investigation. The genetic material coding for thymosin α_1 has been harnessed and cloned; coliform organisms are producing active thymosin α_1. Personal communication (A. Goldstein) reveals that such bacteria producing thymosin β_4 are being developed. Thus all four of these thymic hormones, each chemically distinct and unrelated to the others and each having different actions, will soon be available for clinical investigation. To illustrate the actions of these interesting biologically active peptides: thymosin β_4 in low concentrations induces the appearance of terminal deoxynucleotide transferase (TdT) in precursors of thymus cells. Thymosin α_1 in low concentration induces precursors of thymus

cells to lose their TdT and to take on certain other thymic
cell surface markers and functions. FTS at very low concentration has the capacity to induce the appearance of characteristic markers and functions on precursors of thymic cells in
bone marrow and spleen (Incefy et al, 1980).

Thymopoietin was the first of the thymic hormones shown to
be capable of inducing steps in thymic cell differentiation
(Komuro and Boyse, 1973). Its pentapeptide (32-36) is biologically active, being capable like the other hormones of inducing loss of certain markers found on thymic precursor cells,
gain in other markers characteristic of thymic cells, and even
gain of functions characteristic of thymic cells. In one
study, the peripheral blood lymphocytes of a child who had
been subjected to complete thymectomy were studied (Gupta et
al, 1979). The cells could be shown to be abnormal, having
some of the characteristics of lymphocytes normally found
within the thymus. These cells were different from those
normally found in the peripheral blood. When the child's abnormal peripheral blood lymphocytes were exposed to thymopoietin pentapeptide 32-36, the abnormal peripheral blood lymphocytes were promptly normalized. These findings illustrate
boldly the powerful biologic influence of this tiny segment of
the thymopoietin molecule.

In another important experiment, Weksler et al (1978) administered thymopoietin pentapeptide to thymectomized mice and
corrected abnormalities of affinities which characterize the
antibody produced by lymphocytes of aged mice. This isn't yet
the fountain of youth, but it may be a first step in developing a fountain of immunologic youth.

The importance of studying thymic hormones is also underscored when one considers the involution of immunologic function that occurs with aging in man and all vertebrates studied
thus far. It has long been known that the thymus involutes in
size and changes dramatically in morphology with aging (Good
et al, 1964). These changes in the thymus seem programmed in
the central nervous system and endocrine function but the details of its basis in molecular terms are obscure.

Perhaps reflecting the changes in size and morphology of
the thymus with aging are the changes in circulating thymic
hormone levels with aging. Using an assay for thymopoietin-
like activity in serum, thymectomy was shown to eliminate this
activity (Lewis et al, 1978). Thymopoietin-like activity was
found to be high at birth, to rise slightly during childhood
and to begin to decline in persons over 30. Indeed, a progressive decline occurs during the middle years and thymopoietin-like activity could not be measured in the blood of
persons older than 60. A similar decline in FTS levels has
been shown to follow sexual maturation in both humans and mice
using both functional and radioimmunoassays. Indeed, FTS

levels begin to decline even earlier .in life than thymopoietin
levels. Usually FTS levels become undetectable between 35 and
50 years of age (Bach et al, 1977; Iwata et al, 1979). Thymosin α_1 levels show quite a different pattern: radioimmunoassay
shows that maximum levels are present in humans at birth and
decline in early childhood. In most persons more than 15 years
old, thymosin α_1 is no longer measurable (Pahwa et al, in press).

Thus, promising areas of research on the thymus include
further definition of the thymic hormones, analysis of declining patterns with age, analysis of the relationship of declining hormone levels to loss or derangement of immunologic functions with age, and clinical and experimental studies of the
restoration and/or maintenance of immunologic function using
thymic hormone therapies or thymus transplantation. A further
area of much promise for research is the study of perturbations of thymic hormone levels that occur in diseases like mycosis fungoides (Safai et al, 1979), myasthenia gravis (Twomey
et al, 1979), benign and malignant thymic tumors, and in patients with immunodeficiency diseases (Iwata et al, unpublished).

THE BIOLOGIC AMPLIFICATION SYSTEMS

As with the specific immunologic systems and the thymus,
the biologic amplification systems, e.g., the complement system, have been extensively investigated and most successfully
defined over the past 20 years (Müller-Eberhard, 1975; Müller-
Eberhard and Schreiber, 1980). This research has led to the
virtually complete molecular definition of the complement system. This system comprises some 20 peptides or proteins which
interact in a cascade to generate a molecular attack that can
destroy bacterial cells and bodily cells that have been addressed by certain antibodies.

Functional, chemical and immunochemical definitions have
been applied to the identification and definition of each of
the individual components of this complex biologic amplification system. With full molecular definition of the complement
system and its functions, it has been possible to identify
diseases of man and animals in which one or another of the C
components has been left out or is defective. These fascinating immunodeficiencies are sometimes hereditary and sometimes
secondary to perturbations of the C system due to activation
and utilization in disease. The genetically-determined C deficiencies are regularly associated with increased susceptibility to certain infections and with mesenchymal or autoimmune diseases (Day et al, 1977). Further, some of these diseases can sometimes be corrected or prevented by administering
the component or inducing its production when it is missing or

abnormal (Miller and Nilsson, 1970; Gelfand et al, 1976). Future research will surely see some of these diseases corrected
by cellular or genetic engineering. One can also study perturbations of immunity in cancer and other diseases by seeking
evidence for activation of the C system and, in many patients
with cancer, evidence of ongoing immunity is revealed either
by activation of the C system or by the presence of circulating immune complexes (CIC) in which antigen and antibody are
coupled with complement components in the circulation.

EVIDENCE OF ONGOING IMMUNE RESPONSES IN CANCER PATIENTS

   Studies of the cells present within or adjacent to the
tumor tissue and studies of the histology of the regional
lymph nodes draining many different types of tumors have revealed evidence of immune responses in association with a
number of different human tumors. The nature of such immune
responses has remained enigmatic. Employing a number of different methods to quantify circulating immune complexes, Day
and her coworkers (Teshima et al, 1977), Theofilopoulos et al
(1976), and others (Rossen et al, 1972; Carpentier et al, 1977;
Samayoa et al, 1977) have obtained evidence that, in a high
proportion of patients with cancer, one can demonstrate circulating immune complexes in the blood. Indeed, in analyses
which now include studies of more than 5,000 cancer sera representing patients with almost every form of cancer, Day et al
have found evidence of circulating immune complexes in the
serum of more than 50% of the patients. Elevated levels of
CIC have been observed in every form of cancer studied.
Carpentier and coworkers have reported that, in patients with
leukemias, the quantity of CIC in the blood correlates with
the likelihood of obtaining complete remission with chemotherapy. Both Carpentier et al (1977) and Brandeis et al
(1978; 1980) showed that, in forms of cancer which can be
placed in remission by chemotherapy or surgery, CIC which are
present in the circulation in active disease disappear during
regression and remission and reappear upon exacerbation. The
number of patients with CIC in their blood and the levels of
CIC correlate with stage of disease and evidence of progression of the cancer in Hodgkin's disease and neuroblastoma of
childhood (Brandeis et al, 1978), as well as in colon cancer,
breast cancer, and in lung cancer in adults (Figure 6) (Day
et al, 1980a).
   One of the central issues in cancer immunology is to ascertain the composition of these CIC. This is more easily said
than done, since to define the antigens in the CIC is often
like trying to find a needle in a haystack. Nonetheless, immunoglobulins, especially IgG, and complement components have

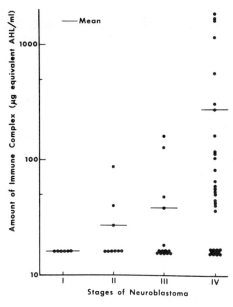

Figure 6. ICS levels in different stages of neuroblastoma. Each point represents the first sample of each patient. There is a close correlation with advanced stages of neuroblastoma and the mean of ICS levels. Reprinted from Brandeis WE, Helson L, Wang Y et al: J Clin Invest 62: 1201, 1978.

regularly been demonstrated in these CIC. In one case of chronic lymphatic leukemia (Day et al, 1976), the patient had marked perturbation of the complement system associated with circulating anti-lymphocyte antibody cryoglobulin. The cryoglobulin contained immunoglobulin, C-components and antibody against membrane components of both leukemic cells and normal lymphocytes. Much further research must be done to ascertain what antigens are involved in the CIC in patients with common cancers like breast, colon and lung cancer. It seems likely that study of the CIC with monoclonal antibodies prepared against the CIC will be revealing.

Studies of immune complexes in experimental systems may also be rewarding. Dogs, like humans, represent an outbred strain in which breast cancer occurs in high frequency. Bitches also have apparently benign fibrocystic disease of the breast in high frequency. Gordon et al. (1980) have recently shown that, in both breast cancer and benign cystic disease of the breast, elevated levels of CIC are often present in the blood. The composition of the CIC in these dogs is under intensive investigation in our laboratories at the present time. In cats with leukemia-lymphoma complex, CIC have recently been shown in a high frequency in these animals to contain IgG, C components and the specific reverse transcriptase of the virus known to transmit this disease horizontally (Day et al, 1980b).

INDUCTION OF REGRESSIONS OF BREAST CANCER IN DOGS
AND LEUKEMIA-LYMPHOMA COMPLEX IN CATS BY REMOVAL OF CIC

One promising area for further research in humans and experimental animals is to study the influence of removal of the
CIC on expression of immunity to cancer. Several years ago,
the Hellstroms discovered that serum in certain experimental
and human cancers could be made cytotoxic for the animal's own
tumor by removal of certain blocking substances (Hellstrom and
Hellstrom, 1969). These blocking factors interfered with the
cytotoxicity of the serum toward tumor cells. These same factors were later found by Sjogren et al (1971) and Baldwin and
Price (1976) to contain antigens and often to represent anti-
gen-antibody complexes. Using methods of extracorporeal filtration of the plasma introduced by Bansal et al (1978) which
removes CIC from the blood, Terman et al (1980) induced apparent clinical regression of breast cancer in dogs. These findings have now been confirmed by Holohan et al (1980) at the
NIH. Similarly, Jones, using repeated treatment of plasma by
filtration through staphylococcal paste which removes IgG and
certain immune complexes, also produced dramatic remissions of
the virus-based leukemia-lymphoma complex in cats (Jones et al,
1980). Prolonged treatment in the cats over several months
not only contributed sustained clinical improvement or remission in the cats but also appeared to eliminate cells from the
blood which possess immunologically detectable tracings of infection by feline leukemia virus. In a similar vein, Miller
et al (1980) reported that they can confirm the production of
remission of cat leukemia by repeated filtration of the cats'
serum with filters containing staphylococcal preparations. In
their studies, treatment of the cats' plasma in vitro with
staphylococcal filters that will remove CIC rendered the serum
cytotoxic for the leukemic cells.
    Some of these results in breast cancer in dogs and feline
leukemia in cats have been confirmed by Gordon et al and Jones,
working in Day's laboratory. A number of investigations of
the potential for immunomodulation by removal of CIC from the
blood of humans and animals with several forms of cancer are
underway. Already in the cat model, it has been shown that
treatment of cats with leukemia by staphylococcal filters can
lower the level of CIC and increase the level of circulating
hemolytic complement. This is certainly a promising line of
research on cancer that must be intensively pursued.

MuMTV ANTIGENS AND HUMAN BREAST CANCER

Over the past several years, evidence has been forthcoming
linking human breast cancer with the murine mammary tumor

virus (MuMTV). The observations have included disputed demonstration of viral-like particles in milk of patients prone to
breast cancer (Moore et al, 1971) and in breast cancer tissues
(Seman et al, 1971). In addition, evidence of enzymes thought
to be related to virus activity in breast cancer has appeared
(Ohno et al, 1977) and evidence of cell-mediated immunity to
purified MuMTV or to virus antigens has been presented (Black
et al, 1975). In more recent studies, Spiegelman's laboratory
prepared antibodies to a peptide component of the envelope
glycoprotein of MuMTV and, using an immunoperoxidase immuno-
histochemical assay, demonstrated antigens related to this
antigen in breast cancer tissue of nearly 50% of American
women with breast cancer (Ohno et al., 1979). All histological
forms of breast cancer were shown to contain this antigen, although those with invasive intraductal lesions showed the antigen most frequently. The antigen was not demonstrated in sections of a variety of other cancers, or in the tissues of patients with benign breast diseases. A fascinating epidemiological angle turned up when these investigators found the
antigen to be more readily demonstrable in breast cancers of
Tunisian women than in breast cancers of American women
(Levine et al, 1980) and less readily demonstrable in the
breast cancers of Japanese women than in those of Tunisian or
American women.

In complementary analyses, we have been studying antibodies
cross-reactive with antigens on MuMTV in the circulation of
patients with breast cancer. Witkin et al developed two reproducible methods for assaying for antibodies to antigens on
MuMTV. The first of these is a lytic assay in which the MuMTV
is lysed in the presence of antibody and complement, releasing
specific reverse transcriptase from the virus. The latter can
be quantified in the supernatant (Witkin et al, 1979). Type C
RNA tumor viruses are regularly lysed by complement as a consequence of activation of the alternative complement pathway
that does not require antibody. By contrast, the type B MuMTV
will not activate complement directly but is lysed by complement in the presence of antibody directed toward its envelope
glycoprotein (Witkin et al, 1979). Some women with breast
cancer and a smaller proportion of women with benign cystic
disease of the breast have antibodies against the MuMTV by
this virolytic assay.

An enzyme-linked immunosorbent assay that measures capacity
of antibody to bind to the MuMTV was then developed (Witkin et
al, 1980a). It was found that 18-25% of American patients
with breast cancer have elevated titers of antibodies to MuMTV
by either of these two methods. Further analysis revealed
antibodies in the blood of these patients to be reactive to
the GP-52 envelope glycoprotein or the GP-36 envelope protein
of the MuMTV (Witkin et al, 1980b). Careful absorption studies

of the antibodies revealed steep absorption curves when purified MuMTV was used as adsorbant. The antibody was also absorbed by the GP-52 envelope glycoprotein as well as by the
completely deglycosylated MuMTV. These findings indicate that
the antibody is reactive with the peptide moiety of the MuMTV
and is not a heterophile antibody. Such findings are concord-
ant with failure to block the antibody-virus interaction or to
absorb the antibody with a variety of sugars, red blood cells
and other retroviruses.
    We then studied sera of breast cancer patients from differ-
ent parts of the world to determine the frequency of these
antibodies in breast cancer patients of different populations.
In these studies, using the ELISA technique, we found that
elevated titers of the antibody to MuMTV were present in approximately 20% of American women with breast cancer, less
than 5% of Chinese women with breast cancer, more than 30% of
Indian breast cancer patients, and nearly 70% of East African
Black women with breast cancer (Day et al, 1980c; 1980d). The
antibody from representative sera of patients from each region
was absorbed with the MuMTV or the deglycosylated virus. These
exciting findings reveal that some but not all women with
breast cancer have antibodies to peptide antigens of the MuMTV
and that the frequency of this immune response varies among
breast cancer patients from different parts of the world. In
families with high frequency of breast cancer in both the US
and India, not only the breast cancer patients but many healthy
family members, including a few males, possessed these same
antibodies to the MuMTV. These findings, which must be ampli-
fied and more extensively analyzed, suggest that there exist
at least two different forms of breast cancer and that in one
form an intimate association with antigens present on and in
MuMTV exists. The essense of this relationship will have to
be established by further investigations. We submit, however,
that this is a most promising area of cancer research.

DIET AND BREAST CANCER OF MICE

    Another promising line of inquiry dates back to the early
and mid-40's when Tannenbaum (1940) and Vischer et al (1942)
linked diet to the development of breast cancer in mice. We
have more recently revived these inquiries and have begun correlative immunological and endocrinological analyses which may
shed light on the mechanism underlying this effective means of
preventing breast cancer in mice. Reduction of total food intake by approximately 1/3 from the time of weaning almost completely prevents the development of breast cancer in mice
(Fernandes et al, 1976a). Fat is a crucial variable since,
even with low calorie intake, when the proportion of dietary

fat is high, MuMTV-based breast cancer in mice occurs in high
incidence (Fernandes et al, 1979a). In C3H/Bi mice, breast
cancer occurs in some 90% of breeding females and 50-70% of
virgin females. This disease is genetically determined, caused
by the MuMTV and permitted by the endocrine make-up of the
host. Simply reducing calorie and fat intake from weaning
completely prevents the disease. Yet the mice on the low calorie intake experience normal oestrus cycles. Such putatively
underfed mice are sleek and healthy-appearing, are capable of
breeding, carrying a pregnancy to term, and even of lactating.
The ductular and glandular breast tissue develops normally in
the food-restricted mice as is revealed by studies of whole-
mount preparations of the breast tissue of C3H mice (Sarkar
et al, 1980).

In a fascinating recent analysis, we have further shown
with Dr. N. Sarkar that feeding restricted diets to C3H/Bi
mice decreases production of and inhibits maturation of virus
by the epithelial cells of the mammary gland. We have also
found from study of these animals that the diets that prevent
breast cancer produce rather dramatic immunological influences
as well (Day et al, 1980e; Fernandes et al, 1976a). Antibodies
against the MuMTV do not develop as they do in mice fed the
putatively normal diet (Day et al, 1980e), nor do these mice
develop the progressively increasing levels of circulating immune complexes which occur with mice on the normal diet (Day
NK, unpublished observations). Here then we see that inhibition of cancer development is associated with failure to develop antibodies and with low levels of CIC in the blood. Each
of these observations opens up promising areas of cancer research.

One must at the outset admit that problems of compliance,
which have plagued efforts to alter food intake in man, are
drastically limiting to any proposal to apply the influence of
diet to prevention or treatment of human cancer. The promise
of our investigations in mice and other small laboratory animals is that we feel certain we can define in cellular, endocrinological and molecular terms the fundamental influences of
the dietary manipulations we are studying.

As an example of the potential importance of this line of
inquiry, one can cite the investigations of Schwartz et al
(1979) in which dehydroepiandrosterone was administered to
mice, resulting in prevention of breast cancer. Schwartz was
aware of interesting findings of a group of scientists at
Lilly (Yen et al, 1977) which revealed that administration of
DHEA to mice prevented weight gain comparable to that of controls, even when the mice were eating the same ration of food.
Because breast cancer was preventable by low food intake,
Schwartz decided to use DHEA to try to prevent breast cancer
in mice. DHEA treatment did indeed prevent completely the

development of breast cancer in the mice while inhibiting growth of body weight to about the same degree that resulted when C3H mice were fed the low calorie, low fat diet which prevented breast cancer in our investigations.

These influences of diet are not unique to breast cancer but also hold for certain chemical carcinogen-induced cancers and many so-called spontaneous cancers of mice and rats. In a most promising investigation, Tucker and associates (1976) have shown that reducing calorie intake in mice and rats by only 25% inhibited the appearance of spontaneous tumors of many organs and tissues.

Illustrative of the lines of investigation which can be developed from studies such as these are investigations, still incomplete, which are being pursued by Sarkar and Karmali. In these investigations, using tissue culture cell lines, they have found that growing the breast cells in tissue culture in the presence of prolactin facilitates production of MuMTV. This influence can be inhibited by indomethacin and facilitated by prostaglandin. Thus, these experiments in vitro reveal a promising line for investigation of the basis for the dietary influence on production of the MuMTV-associated breast cancer in mice, and perhaps ultimately in humans.

THE INFLUENCE OF DIET ON LONGEVITY AND DEVELOPMENT OF THE DISEASES OF AGING OTHER THAN CANCER

Mice have in their genes the license to live between 3 and 4 years. For man, this genetic license appears to include the possibility of living at least 95-105 years. Many strains of mice and most humans do not realize this potential because diseases of aging develop and most people and mice succumb much earlier than the genetically-permitted life-span. We recognize several valid reasons for systematic study of immune systems and functions with aging in the hope of lessening the severity of the diseases of aging. One of the most promising approaches to delaying or preventing diseases of aging and also of interfering with the involution of the immune system which seems to be closely linked to the development of these diseases is by nutritional manipulation.

Beginning in the mid-thirties, McCay et al (1939) showed that life-span of long-lived mice and rats can be prolonged 20-25% by feeding low calorie intake from the time of weaning. Walford showed that calorie restriction from the time of weaning decreases immunological function slightly early in life but permits more prolonged maintenance of immunologic functions in older animals (Walford et al, 1974). Ross and Bras (1976) showed that calorie restriction from an early age inhibits development of certain of the diseases of aging in long-lived rats.

We have taken a slightly different tack. We chose to work with short-lived, autoimmune-prone strains of mice which develop early in life some, or even all, of the diseases we associate with aging. These mice may have life-spans as short as 300 days, as opposed to 1000-1200 days for mice of the longest-lived strains. Initially, we showed that life-span could be significantly lengthened and autoimmunity inhibited in the NZB mice by fat restriction (Fernandes et al, 1972). More recently, we have found that low calorie intake, especially when coupled with low fat intake, regularly doubles and sometimes even triples life-span of (NZB/NZW)F_1 hybrid B/W mice (Fernandes et al, 1976b). This treatment inhibited involution of immunity functions with age in this strain and prevented the manifestations of renal vascular disease and autoimmunities (Fernandes et al, 1978a). In similar studies with the MRL/lpr mice, which develop both autoimmune and striking lymphoproliferative disease (Fernandes and Good, 1979b), and the kd/kd mutant mice, that develop both autoimmunities and nephronophthesis, life-span can be more than doubled and their diseases prevented for long periods simply by restricting calorie intake from the time of weaning (Fernandes et al, 1978b).

By contrast, when B/W mice are fed a diet high in fat and containing the same total calories, they become obese and often develop cardiovascular lesions, coronary atherosclerosis and also arteriosclerosis involving the aorta and its major branches (Fernandes and Good, 1980). In this work we have developed a new model of vascular disease in which immune complexes and high fat diet both appear to contribute to the pathogenesis of the lesions. The question can, of course, be fairly asked as to whether these exciting observations on prolongation of health, prevention of diseases of aging, and maintenance of immunologic function and immunological balance with aging in mice are really relevant to man. Our answer to such a question must be philosophical but is based on long experience of scientific investigations involving both mice and humans. Whenever we have understood thoroughly anything about immunity in the mouse, the findings are directly relevant to man and require at most only slight modifications to make the interspecies conversion. Thus, perhaps from prejudice of past experience, we believe these findings will find their application in humans.

Supportive of this perspective are observations that lifestyles do pertain to human cancer. Females with extreme obesity have 8-10x the incidence of cancer of the endometrium as females of normal weight and extremely overweight females have a high incidence of breast cancer as well. Further, Boyd et al. (1980) have recently shown that the outcome of breast cancer in women is clearly a function of the presence or

absence of obesity. The promise for cancer research implicit
in the results of these studies is that life-span, cancer, and
other diseases of aging can be dramatically manipulated by diet
in mice where the possibility of investigating these influences in cellular, molecular, endocrinological and immunological
terms gives the best possible chance of further and ultimately
definitive analyses.

CONDITIONING THROUGH EXERCISE, RESISTANCE TO TUMORS
AND IMMUNOLOGICAL FUNCTION IN MICE

Recent studies carried out by two of us (Fernandes and Good,
unpublished observations) have opened another door to challenging immunological analysis. We have found that BALB/c mice
conditioned by daily running on a treadmill are better able to
resist progression of RLσ1 tumors than are unconditioned BALB/
c mice. These studies, still in their earliest phase of development, show truly dramatic differences in tumor progression
and metastases and readily demonstrable improvements in certain
immunological functions. The basis for these striking differences in resistance to cancer of conditioned and non-condi-
tioned mice is not clear, but our new model is currently under
intensive investigation in our laboratory.

BONE MARROW TRANSPLANTATION, CELLULAR ENGINEERING AND CANCER

In his dissertation presented earlier, Donnall Thomas most
ably summed up current status of the role of marrow transplantation in treatment of one form of acute malignancy, leukemia. I need not stress this further except to say, to my
view, bone marrow transplantation has become the treatment of
choice for some forms of leukemia in certain stages of their
management.
Twelve years ago, using for the first time a matched sibling donor, we performed the first successful allogeneic marrow transplantation to correct the inborn error of metabolism
represented by genetically determined severe combined immunodeficiency disease (SCID) (Gatti et al, 1968). In this instance, we had to use a marrow transplantation to correct for
the first time iatrogenic, immunologically based pancytopenia
(aplastic anemia) (Good et al, 1971). Since that time, bone
marrow transplantation has been used by us and others to cure,
at least sometimes, more than 20 diseases that are otherwise
regularly fatal. This has been an extraordinarily rewarding
development. Led by Parkman, the group at the Boston Children's Hospital pioneered in the full correction of Wiskott-
Aldrich (WA) syndrome, severe congenital neutropenia, and a

form of profound neutrophil malfunction (Parkman et al, 1978).
Using Busulfan to eliminate competing hematopoietic elements
and large-dose cyclophosphamide for immunosuppression, we too
have treated successfully 3 patients with WA syndrome (Kapoor
et al, unpublished), patients with osteopetrosis and severe
hematopoietic and immunological abnormalities associated with
cartilage hair hypoplasia (Sorell et al, 1979), and 5 genetically different forms of SCID including one associated with absence of adenosine deaminase (Good and Hansen, 1978). It has
been a most rewarding experience to virtually create life in
many of these patients for whom there would otherwise be no
hope. As Thomas also reported, we are only at a beginning in
using this form of cellular engineering to treat hematologic,
malignant and immunological disease. Many more diseases will
be correctable when we can prevent and control severe GVHD.
Already we can ask a $64,000 question relevant to cancer: Will
the correction of all hematological and immunological aspects
of WA syndrome, Fancani's anemia syndrome, and the several
forms of SCID (each of which predisposes to cancer in high frequency) prevent also the cancer complication of these genetically determined diseases? Only time will tell. We know that
some of these diseases are associated with chromosomal instability and it will be an outstanding achievement if marrow
transplantation can prevent cancer in these patients.

MARROW TRANSPLANTATION ACROSS MAJOR HISTOCOMPATIBILITY BARRIERS

Using pre-treatment of marrow cells in vitro with potent
anti-Thy-1 plus complement, Susan Krown and Coico in our laboratory have been able to transplant marrow across the strongest histocompatibility barriers from C57B1/6 mice to CBA mice
without producing GVHD. The requirement, it seems, is to eliminate from the marrow all post-thymic immunoincompetent as
well as immunocompetent lymphocytes. Even more successful has
been treatment of marrow prior to transplantation with a het-
erologous anti-Thy-1 antiserum without complement (Onoé et al,
1980). In this model, the elimination from the marrow of the
opsonized differentiated T cells of the donor was left to the
lytic mechanisms and reticuloendothelial system of the recipient. With this technique, long-lived chimerae have been produced in nearly 100% of cases and no evidence of either acute
or chronic GVHD was observed. Study of immunologic function
of such animals has been most encouraging. The only immunologic function tested in which the animals did not perform
well was the primary antibody response to sheep red blood cells
(SRBC), a T-dependent antigen. Even with this parameter, repeated exposure to the SRBC antigen resulted in apparent development of the capacity to make respectable amounts of

antibodies to both IgM and IgG classes. From our observations
we do not think that the genetic restrictions Zinkernagel and
coworkers (1979) have identified will place insurmountable barriers to marrow transplantation.   Indeed, we agree with Katz
that adaptive differentiation may be possible (Katz, 1979).

   Parallel to these observations in which thymus-differen-
tiated cells are removed with specific antibody are investigations using differential cell agglutination plus sedimentation by centrifugation which was introduced by Y. Reisner et al
(1978).   Reisner has come to work in our laboratories and,
with graduate student M. Hodes, has confirmed and extended his
original findings (Reisner et al, 1980).   They have shown in
mice that marrow or spleen cells can be fractionated by differential agglutination using peanut and soybean agglutinins
to separate the stem cells from the cells already differentiated by the thymus that can induce GVHR and GVHD.   The preparations of stem cells prepared by differential agglutination with
the plant lectins can be transplanted across major histocompatibility barriers and they do not induce GVHR.   Chimeric mice
prepared by transplantation of isolated stem cells live well
under conditions of reasonably good animal husbandry.   However,
the extensive immunologic analysis already completed for the
chimerae based on specific removal of Thy-1 lymphocytes from
the marrow has not yet been carried out for these chimerae.

   Already Reisner has developed effective differential agglutination methods for removing unwanted post-thymic T cells
from bone marrow of both monkeys and humans.   Marrow transplants which rapidly establish a state of full chimerism can
be achieved in monkeys following fatal irradiation plus transplantation with marrow across major histocompatibility barriers; no evidence of GVHR was seen.   Similar preparations of
marrow which do not respond by proliferation in mixed leukocyte
culture have been prepared with human marrow by the same differential agglutination procedures that are effective for the
monkey.   The first bone marrow transplantation using the marrow
preparation procedures from a haploidentical parent donor to
child with SCID has recently been performed at this Center.
It is still too early to evaluate this transplant.   There is
little question, however, that, using either T-specific cytotoxic monoclonal antibody techniques or the methods of differential agglutination, marrow transplantation crossing the major
histocompatibility barriers will be attempted for humans with
each of the several forms of SCID, leukemia, aplastic anemia,
congenital hematologic abnormalities, and even other cancers.
We predict success in extending the potentiality for effective
treatment using marrow transplantation in this way.

RESISTANCE GENES

In recent collaborative work with Tanaka et al (1979), we have studied the usefulness in fighting leukemia of introducing resistance genes by marrow transplantation. First, what do we mean by resistance genes? To think about this, let us consider the leukemia that develops in AKR mice. These animals are most susceptible to developing leukemia-lymphoma complex; this disease kills 95% of these animals by 14 months of age in most experiments. CBA/H mice have exceedingly low frequency of leukemia-lymphoma complex, as do C3H/Bi mice. When CBA/H mice are bred with AKR, the resultant (AKRxCBA)F_1 hybrids have a low frequency of leukemia. By contrast, when mice of the low leukemia C3H/Bi strain are crossed with AKR mice, the F_1 hybrid mice have a high incidence of leukemia-lymphoma complex. To explain these differences, we conclude that CBA/H mice have resistance genes which can interfere with expression of the susceptibility genes contributed by the AKR parent; C3H mice lack such resistance genes. The question is whether or not the resistance genes can be introduced by marrow transplantation following lethal irradiation.

Experiments have been launched which already show sufficient results to indicate that introduction of resistance genes by marrow transplantation is possible. AKR mice transplanted with CBA/H marrow cells resist development of leukemia and this resistance lasts longer than 2 years. By contrast, when AKR marrow cells are given to lethally irradiated AKR mice, the animals develop leukemia prior to 14 months, as do the control AKR mice kept in the same animal colony during the same period. In experiments not yet completed, it appears that lethally irradiated AKR mice given C3H/Bi marrow cells on the other hand develop leukemia between 9 and 14 months of age.

Another promising area for cancer research is to pursue these investigations to a cellular and humoral analysis of how these resistance genes actually work. Already we have evidence that they do not work by introducing immunity to the fully developed leukemia cells. Further, a chimeric state in which only 30% or so of the resistant cells are present in the thymus inhibits the development of the leukemia-lymphoma complex. The likelihood that we can learn from study of these resistance genes in mice how to recognize resistance genes in man and learn to use them to fight leukemia and other malignancies seems to us likely. Such an achievement should make possible much improved results in the treatment of certain forms of leukemia, which has the tendency to recur following bone marrow transplantation. This is surely a promising avenue of research.

SUMMARY

Knowledge of immunological systems is surging, thanks to
discovery of the biologic function of the thymus, definition
of the two major subpopulations of lymphocytes and identification of specialized subsets of fully differentiated T and B
cells. Cellular interactions represent a prime functional
process in immunity, but we are just beginning to understand
how these cellular interactions work in molecular terms. The
analysis of immunobiologic cells and functions is much facilitated by new technologies, including the best methods of molecular biology and the development of methods to directly analyze
the organization and reorganization of genes in the immunocompetent cells. Coupled with these powerful methods are the
equally powerful ones based on monoclonal antibodies produced
by the hybridoma technology. Together, these two approaches
should greatly improve our understanding of immunity. This new
knowledge can and is being translated into progressively improving capacity for analysis, manipulation and control of the
cellular basis of immunity in experimental systems. These approaches are facilitating immunological analyses and the development of immunotherapy of human disease, including diseases
featured by immunological susceptibility to cancer.

In breast cancer, as in so many other common cancers, there
is much evidence of ongoing immunities. In experimental cancers, e.g., breast cancer in out-bred dogs, feline lymphoma,
and leukemias in out-bred cats, immuno-manipulations have already altered the outcome of naturally occurring cancer. Much
new clinical research seems warranted from these prospectives.

In human breast cancer, complementary evidence from several
different directions continues to indicate that there is more
than one form of breast cancer and that some forms of breast
cancer express an important relationship to MuMTV which causes
breast cancer in mice.

Dietary restriction of calories and/or fat prevents experimental cancers caused by viruses, chemical carcinogens and also
the so-called spontaneous cancers in mice and rats. These influences are associated with immunological and endocrinological
consequences. We have already shown that dietary prevention of
breast cancer can be understood and analyzed from an immunologic perspective. Ultimately, immunological approaches may
contribute to treatment and even prevention of common cancers
like breast cancer.

We can show that immunodeficiencies associated with aging begin with evidence of thymic involution. We have found that in
short-lived mice, which develop early in life some or all of
the diseases of aging, it is possible in individual instances
to double and even triple life-span using only dietary manipulations. There seems no question that continued analysis

of the T and B cell responses and cellular and humoral immune responses at the surface and molecular levels in cancer and the diseases of aging will be most rewarding. Such studies can ultimately yield simplified treatments and preventions of many diseases which will be safe and appropriately deliverable.

REFERENCES

Bach FS, Dardenne M, Pleau JM: Nature 266:55, 1977

Baldwin RW, Price MR: Ann NY Acad Sci 276:3, 1976.

Bansal SC, Bansal BR, Thomas HC, et al: Cancer 42:1, 1978.

Black, MM, Zachran RE, Shore B, et al: Cancer 35:121, 1975.

Boyd NF, O'Sullivan B, Campbell J, et al: Clin Res 28:225A, 1980.

Brandeis WE, Helson L, Wang Y, et al: J Clin Invest 62:1201, 1978.

Brandeis WE, Tan C, Wang Y, et al: Clin Exp Immunol 39:551, 1980.

Carpentier NA, Gange GT, Fiere DM, et al: J Clin Invest 60:874, 1977.

Day NK, Winfield JB, Gee T, et al: Clin Exp Immunol 26:189, 1976.

Day NK, Moncada B, Good RA: In NK Day, RA Good, (Eds): Biological Amplification Systems in Immunology. New York, Plenum, 1977, pp. 229-245.

Day NK, Good RA, Witkin SS: In B Serrou, C Rosenfeld, (Eds): Human Cancer Immunology. New York, Elsevier/North-Holland Biomedical Press, 1980a, in press.

Day NK, O'Reilly RJ, Felice C, et al: J Immunol, in press, 1980b.

Day NK, Witkin SS, Sarkar NH, et al: Trans Assoc Am Phys, in press, 1980c.

Day NK, Witkin SS, Sarkar NH, et al: Proc Natl Acad Sci, in press, 1980d.

Day NK, Fernandes G, Witkin SS, et al: Int J Cancer, in press, 1980e.

Evans RL, Wall DW, Platsoucas CD, et al: Proc Natl Acad Sci, in press.

Fernandes G, Yunis EJ, Smith J, Good RA: Proc Soc Exp Biol Med 139:1189, 1972.

Fernandes G, Yunis EJ, Good RA: Nature 263:504, 1976a.

Fernandes G, Yunis EJ, Good RA: Proc Natl Acad Sci, 73:1279, 1976b.

Fernandes G, Friend P, Yunis EJ, Good RA: Proc Natl Acad Sci, 75:1500, 1978a.

Fernandes G, Yunis EJ, Miranda M, et al: Proc Natl Acad Sci, 75:2888, 1978b.

Fernandes G, West A, Good RA: Clin Bull (MSKCC) 9(3):91, 1979a.

Fernandes G, Good RA: Fed Proc 38:1370, 1979b.

Fernandes G, Good RA: Proc 4th Intl Cong Immunol, Paris, 1980.

Gatti RA, Meuwissen HJ, Allen HD, et al: Lancet 2:1366, 1968.

Gelfand JA, Sherins RJ, Alling DW, Frank MM: N Engl J Med 296: 1444, 1976.

Goldstein AL: personal communication.

Goldstein AL, Low TLK, MacAdoo M, et al: Proc Natl Acad Sci, 74:725, 1977.

Goldstein G, Scheid MP, Boyse EA, et al: Science 204:1309, 1979.

Good RA: In RA Good, DW Fisher (Eds): Immunobiology. Stamford, Conn., Sinauer Associates, 1971, pp. 230-238.

Good RA, Hansen MA: In Proceedings of the International Symposium on Immunodeficiency, Tokyo, 1976: Immunodeficiency: its Nature and Etiological Significance in Human Disease; Tokyo, University of Tokyo Press, 1978, pp. 93-132.

Good RA, Martinez C, Gabrielsen AE: In RA Good, Gabrielsen AE, (Eds.), The Thymus in Immunobiology. New York, Harper-Hoeber, 1964, pp. 3-48.

Gordon BR, Moroff S, Hurvitz AI, et al: Cancer Res 40, 1980, in press.

Gupta S, Kapoor N, Goldstein G, Good RA: Clin Immunol Immunopathol 12:404, 1979.

Hellstrom I, Hellstrom K: Int J Cancer 4:587, 1969.

Holahan T, Bowles C, Deisseroth A: Proc Am Ass Cancer Res 21:241, 1980.

Incefy GS, Mertelsmann R, Yata K, et al: Clin Exp Immunol 40:369-406, 1980.

Iwata T, Incefy GS, Cunningham-Rundles S, et al: Am J Med, submitted.

Iwata T, Incefy GS, Good RA: Biochem Biophys Res Comm 88: 1419-1427, 1979.

Jones FR, Yashida LH, Ladiges WC, Kenny MA: Cancer 46:675, 1980.

Kaplan HS: Progress in radiation therapy, This volume

Kapoor N, Kirkpatrick D, Blaese RM, et al: submitted.

Katz DH: Fed Proc 38:2065, 1979.

Komuro K, Boyse EA: J Exp Med 138:479, 1973.

Levine P, Mourali V, Tabbara F, et al: Proc Amer Assoc Cancer Res 21:170, 1980.

Lewis VM, Twomey JJ, Bealmear P, et al: J Clin Endocrinol Metabol 47:145, 1978.

Maki R, Traunecker A, Sakano H, et al: Proc Natl Acad Sci 77(4):2138, 1980.

McCay CM, Maynard LA, Sperling G, Barnes LL: J Nutrition 18:1, 1939.

Medawar PB, Review of EJ Steele et al: Somatic Selection and Adaptive Evolution. Toronto, Williams-Wallace Productions, 1980. Trends in Biological Sciences, 5(3): R 15, 1980.

Miller ME, Nilsson UR: N Engl J Med 282:354, 1970.

Miller WJ, Branda RF, Peacock TE, Jacob MS: Clin Res 28: 319A, 1980.

Miyata T, Yasunaga T, Yamawaki-Kataoka Y, et al: Proc Natl Acad Sci 77(4):2143, 1980.

Moore DH, Charney J, Kramarsky B, et al: Nature (London) 229: 611, 1971.

Müller-Eberhard HJ: Ann Rev Biochem 44:679, 1975.

Müller-Eberhard HJ, Schreiber RD: Adv Immunol 29:1, 1980.

Nowinski RC, et al: Science, in press.

Ohno T, Mesa-Tejada R, Keydar I, et al: Proc Natl Acad Sci 76:2460, 1979.

Ohno T, Sweet RW, Hu R, et al: Proc Natl Acad Sci 74:764, 1977.

Onoé K, Fernandes G, Good RA: J Exp Med 151:115, 1980.

Pahwa S, Pahwa R, Goldstein G, Good RA: Cell Immunol, in press.

Parkman R, Rappeport D, Geha R, et al: N Engl J Med 298:921, 1978.

Perry RP, Kelley DE, Coleclough C, et al: Proc Natl Acad Sci 77(4):1937, 1980.

Reisner Y, Ikehara S, Hodes MZ, Good RA: Proc Natl Acad Sci 77:1164, 1980.

Reisner Y, Itzicovitch L, Meshorer A, Sharon N: Proc Natl Acad Sci 75:2933, 1978.

Ross MH, Bras GJ: J Nutr 87:245, 1976.

Rossen RD, Reisberg MA, Hersh EM, Gutterman JN: J Natl Cancer Inst 58:1205, 1972.

Safai B, Good RA, Twomey JJ, et al: Blood 54:837, 1979.

Samayoa EA, McDuffie FC, Nelson AM, et al: Int J Cancer 19:12, 1977.

Sarkar NH, Fernandes G, Karande K, Good RA: In 12th Meeting

on Mammary Cancer in Experimental Animals & Man, Maastricht/ May 11-14, 1980. (Abstract).
Schlesinger DH, Goldstein G: Cell 5:361, 1975.
Schwartz AG: Cancer Res. 37:1129, 1979.
Seman G, Gallager HS, Lukeman JM, Dmochowski L: Cancer 28:1431, 1971.
Sjogren HO, Hellstrom I, Bansal SC, Hellstrom KE: Proc Natl Acad Sci 68:1372, 1971.
Sorell M, Kirkpatrick D, Kapoor N, et al: Pediatr. Res. 13: 455, 1979.
Tannenbaum A: Am J Cancer 38:335, 1940.
Terman DS, Yamamoto T, Mattiolo M, et al: J Immunol 124:795, 1980.
Teshima H, Wanebo H, PInsky C, Day NK: J Clin Invest 59:1134, 1977.
Theofilopoulos AN, Wilson CB, Dixon FJ: J Clin Invest 57:169, 1976.
Thomas ED: Bone marrow transplantation. This volume.
Tucker SM, Mason RL, Beauchine RE: Int J Cancer 23:803, 1979.
Twomey JJ, Lewis VM, Patten BM, et al: Am J Med 66:639, 1979.
Visscher MB, Ball ZB, Barnes RH, Sivertsen I: Surgery 11:48, 1942.
Walford RL, Liu RK, Gerbase-DeLima M, et al: Mech Aging Dev 2:447, 1974.
Weksler MC, Innes JD, Goldstein G: J Exp Med 148:996, 1978.
Witkin SS, Egeli RA, Sarkar NH, et al: Proc Natl Acad Sci 76:2984, 1979.
Witkin SS, Sarkar NH, Good RA, Day NK: J Immunol Meth 32:85, 1980a.
Witkin SS, Sarkar NH, Kinne DE, et al: Int J Cancer 25:721, 1980b.
Yen TT, Allen JV, Pearson DV, et al: Lipids 12:409, 1977.
Zinkernagel RM, Doherty PC: Adv Immunol 27:51, 1979.

Aided by USPHSR grants CA-19267, CA-17404, CA-23766, AI-11843, NS-11457, and AG-00541 from the National Institutes of Health, by the American Cancer Society, the Richard Molin Memorial Foundation, the Judith Harris Selig Memorial Fund, the Zelda R. Weintraub Cancer Fund, the Joseph and Helen Regenstein Foundation, and the MSKCC Special Projects Committee.

THE IMPACT OF THE NATIONAL CANCER PROGRAM

R. Lee Clark, M.D.

1980 International Symposium on Cancer

Memorial-Sloan Kettering

September 13-18, 1980

One of the major facets of the total positive impact the National Cancer Program has had in the United States has been the educational aspects of the cancer control activities. The initiation of these activities preceded the National Cancer Act of 1971, which spelled out the aims of the National Cancer Program.

The establishment of the National Cancer Institute in 1937 was the beginning of the first truly nationally organized effort to control cancer in the U. S. Although the emphasis of the new Institute was on research into the causes of cancer, which would lead to better treatment and eventually to prevention, it was acknowledged that education of a sufficient number of young physicians, dentists, and scientists in the current knowledge about cancer was essential to the success of any national program to control cancer.

Activities predating the creation of the National Cancer Institute had focussed national attention on the need for action. The American Society for the Control of Cancer (later renamed the American Cancer Society) had organized in 1913 and in conjunction with the American College of Surgeons began to educate the public and local practicing physicians regarding the importance of early detection of cancer. In 1931 the Committee on Cancer of the American College of Surgeons published minimal requirements for approved cancer clinics in community hospitals to enhance the education of practicing physicians and began a continuing program for accrediting cancer services.

But, during the Second World War, the members of the National Advisory Cancer Council (NACC) of the NCI became deeply concerned by the "lamentable ignorance" about cancer manifested by many graduates of U.S. medical schools. It was observed that many were poorly prepared for advanced training in their specialties as they pertained to oncology, and there was no recognized training in oncologic specialties. The NACC advocated revisions in medical undergraduate curricula that would foster multidisciplinary teaching.

After 2½ years of study, each medical school in the country was invited by the NACC and the NCI to review its educational approach to cancer and to submit a plan for improvement. The following year American schools of dentistry were invited to do the same. By the end of 1948, 72 of the 78 medical schools and 34 of the 40 dental schools had applied for the new Undergraduate Cancer Training (Education) Grants. The amount of each one-year grant was limited to $25,000 for each 4-year medical school and to $5000 for each dental school and 2-year medical school. By 1952, virtually all of the nation's medical, dental and osteopathic schools were receiving these grants. Schools of public health were invited to participate that year, also, but no applications were submitted. From 1961 to 1965, I was chairman of a committee of the National Advisory Cancer Council appointed to define the guidelines for clinical educational grants. This committee became a permanent one with Dr. Margaret Edwards acting as Executive Secretary. The Undergraduate Training (Education) Grants were replaced with Clinical Cancer Education Grants that were competitive, extended in scope to include graduate and continuing education, were extended to academically affiliated cancer centers, and contained no ceiling on funding. In 1966, 73 of the grants were funded and by 1972, 104 institutions were funded. Each institution receiving such grants was encouraged to appoint a professional person to coordinate the oncology teaching in that institution.

Actually, the NCI has supported clinical training since soon after its inception. Clinical traineeships and research fellowships were initiated in 1938, but in 1959 the clinical traineeships were transferred to the Division of Chronic Disease Control in the Bureau of Health

Services and remained available until 1968, when the Division was phased out.

In 1974, the National Research Service Award Act was enacted to replace legislative authority still another time. Awards may be made to individuals for research projects or to institutions that will select individuals for training in research. They support pre- and postdoctoral training but not M.D. residency training. In FY 1978 fellowship obligations totalled nearly $20 million, an increase of 83% since 1975. Pre- and postdoctoral candidates may also receive full-time research fellowship support grants through the Research Manpower Branch.

Research Career Awards had been initiated in 1961 and reached a maximum of 21 awards, but no new awards have been made since 1964, and 6 ongoing grants are being allowed to run their course. Research Career Development Awards were initiated at about the same time and, as of the beginning of FY 1980, there were 121 active awards. The annual number of graduate trainees has ranged from 55 to 205, but the goal for FY 1981 is to support 400 undergraduate and graduate trainees.

In 1975, Clinical Cancer Education grants were awarded to 51 institutions and in 1976 31 additional grants were awarded. In 1977, 84 institutions received these awards but 31 institutions, although approved, were not funded. In 1971, there had been fewer than a half dozen sections, divisions, or departments of oncology in the medical schools in the U.S., but currently, of the 115 medical schools in the country, 69 of them list a department, division or section of oncology and 8 others have oncology listed as a "specialty without organizational autonomy." Of 300 eligible institutions, 89 of them had Clinical Cancer Education Grants in 1980.

For approximately 40 years the American Cancer Society has encouraged efforts at cancer control by funding various professional educational activities, particularly to foster the earlier detection of cancer by privately practicing physicians. From 1948 to 1978 the ACS had awarded more than 4500 1-year Clinical Fellowships to institutions for advanced oncologic training in 8 medical and 4

dental specialties. In addition, Junior Faculty
Clinical Fellowships were funded, and occasionally,
local divisions of the Society funded additional
fellowships.

For a number of years the Leukemia Society
of America has funded   fellowships annually,
some of which are for clinical research on leukemia.
The Damon Runyon-Walter Winchell Cancer Fund
supports approximately 125 annual postdoctoral
research fellowships. Hospitals and medical
centers use funds derived from numerous local,
state, national, and private sources to support
training for interns, residents, and other advanced
medical trainees.

Without these training programs and funding
sources, many of which predated the passage of the
National Cancer Act of 1971 creating the National
Cancer Program, this Program would not have been
possible and the legislation would not have been so
strongly supported by taxpayers, the Congress, and
the President of the United States. It is because
of this staunch support and that of dedicated citizens that research and clinical professors have
been able to prepare the young minds that have
achieved the startlingly diverse advances on so
many biological fronts leading to progressively
better therapy and consequent better survival figures and strong expectations for the eventual prevention of many cancers.

When Senator Ralph Yarborough introduced
Resolution 376 in March 1970 creating the National
Panel of Consultants on the Conquest of Cancer, a
nationwide effort began that eventuated in input
from approximately 300 of the foremost clinical
oncologists and basic biological research
scientists in the country, delineating the
development of the national cancer effort to date,
outlining the then current state-of-the-art of
cancer therapy and scientific knowledge of carcinogenesis, and enumerating the scientific and
clinical areas ripe for immediate investigation
and exploitation. From this massive effort was
birthed the National Cancer Act of 1971 and an
annually updated 5-year National Cancer Plan.

December of this year will mark the 9th

anniversary of the signing of the legislation by President Nixon creating the National Cancer Program. In those short 9 years, the annual appropriations for the NCI rose from $190.4 million (1970) to $1 billion in 1980. In 1971, 1744 grant proposals were submitted and 1537 were funded. After the first 5 years of the National Cancer Program (1976), 3838 proposals were submitted and 2516 were funded. Four years later, in 1980, more grant applications than ever before are being submitted, a large percentage of them are approved for funding, but an increasingly smaller percentage of them are actually being funded. Knowledge has burgeoned so rapidly in the last 10 years (unfortunately so has inflation) that the billion dollars awarded for FY 1980 does not fund even 50% of the proposed cancer research and basic biological research with relevance to the malignant process. In 1979, 2569 RO1 and PO$_1$ grant proposals were submitted, 2191 were approved for funding as meritorious research, but only 901 were actually funded. Keep in mind that this figure does not include the 3- to 5-year grants that were not competing for funds but simply being renewed. Other types of grant applications would be for construction, training, clinical cooperative groups, and others. This year (1980) approximately the same number of grant proposals were submitted, 2559, slightly fewer were approved for funding than in 1979 (2082), but considerably fewer, 733, were actually funded. I also invite you to keep in mind that other true investigator-initiated grants are awarded through other programs; for instance, the organ site task forces, which include breast, bladder, large bowel, lung, pancreas, and prostate.

The percentages of the total FY 1980 NCI budget allocated to the major programs are prevention, 32%, treatment, 24%, and basic research, 44%. In round numbers, the dollar amounts allocated grants and contracts to four major categories of research -- cause/prevention, $290,000,000, detection/diagnosis, $57,000,000, treatment, $315,000,000, and biology, $141,000,000, for a total of $803,000,000. For resource development, the 1980 allocations in round numbers were cancer centers, $68,000,000, manpower training, $43,000,000, and construction, $15,000,000, for a total of $126,000,000. Funds allocated for cancer control totalled $70,000,000.

Here, listed briefly, are what I consider to be the 10 major accomplishments of the National Cancer Program:

(1)   acceptance of the concept of a comprehensive cancer center, acknowledgement of 3 already existing comprehensive centers, and the establishment of 18 new comprehensive cancer centers, at least 1/3 of which are not yet truly comprehensive but have the potential and the strong desire to be comprehensive;

(2)   funding of more cancer-related research and education than in the previous history of the NCI;

(3)   activation of the organ site task forces for breast, bladder, large bowel, lung, pancreas, and prostate;

(4)   reactivation and expansion of the Cancer Control Program;

(5)   establishment of the International Cancer Research Data Bank, with the invitation to scientists and physicians of the world to share cancer-related knowledge;

(6)   creation of the National Clearinghouse on Environmental Carcinogens, then later the National Toxicology Program;

(7)   development and expansion of new forms of therapy (chemotherapy, immunotherapy, hemotherapy, protected environments, nutritional and rehabilitation therapy, biological response modifiers)

(8)   coordination of all cancer-related organizations and activities in the country;

(9)   the freeing of the NCI from 7 tiers of bureaucracy to develop and defend its budget while remaining an integral part of the NIH;

(10) the appointment of the President's Cancer Panel to shepherd the new Cancer Program through difficult times that might cause it to founder and fail.

Activities of the program that we consider to have been of direct benefit to cancer patients are research results leading to the establishment of more protocol therapy, the establishment of more tumor clinics, organization of integrated cancer programs at every level, accreditation of hospital cancer programs, increased funding for research, greater interest in tumor registries, greater emphasis on and acceptance of continuing education, and the establishment of pilot clinical cancer patient data systems both in the United States and abroad.

During the 9 years of the National Cancer Program, certain trends have emerged, resulting from changes in emphasis as new knowledge was amassed, scientific perspectives shifted, and the public became better informed about causes of cancer and what they, collectively and as individuals, could do to help achieve the eventual control of cancer. Two changes occurred almost simultaneously -- the de-emphasis of contracts and an increasing emphasis on funding more investigator-initiated grant proposals that were subjected to peer review. In a similar vein, as the educational programs began to yield more adequately trained scientists and oncologists eager to conduct clinical research and to cooperate with basic scientists and pharmacologists, the intramural research programs of the NCI were scaled down in preference to more extensive peer-reviewed research throughout the growing oncologically oriented community of the nation.

In 1971 the greatest emphasis on any area of research was the attempt to solve the etiology of cancer with emphasis on the role of viruses. While this research was a potent factor in

establishing the value of molecular biology, it
failed to confirm the role of viruses in the
etiology of human cancers, although its role in
the etiology of experimental animal cancers was
demonstrated unequivocably. This research was
funded largely by contracts and was controlled in
its targeted phase as an extension of NCI intramural research. When these contracts had reached
a funded level of approximately $100,000,000
annually, the Zinder committee was asked by the
National Cancer Advisory Board and the President's
Cancer Panel to make an evaluation of methods and
goals of the viral research program of the NCI.
The Zinder report resulted in a reassignment of
viral research funds to a more appropriate
proportion of the NCI budget.

With the increase in multidisciplinary
comprehensive cancer centers and enhanced interest
of specialized institutions dedicated to more
discrete and intensive research into the mechanisms
of carcinogenesis, larger numbers of highly trained
and imaginative investigators were encouraged to
apply for the funds made available through the NCI,
which often, in turn, stimulated local financial
support for research and educational programs and
for expansion of facilities.

For instance, from 1972 to 1980, the NCI
awarded $208 million for construction of research
facilities. During those years, initially 25%
matching funds were required, later the percentage
was upped to 50%, so that a total of $82 million
was contributed by centers for construction. The
interesting figure, however, is that the $82
million contributed by centers also generated
another $123 million from various sources.
Consequently, $208 million of NCI money generated
$205 million of construction funds from multiple
outside sources.

One unanticipated difficulty arose for the
chronically under-staffed NCI group, and that was
the confusing administrative and organizational
variety of the cancer centers scattered throughout
the nation. It was difficult for the NCI staff
and site visitors to determine patterns of core

funding because of this variety, and many misunderstandings between the directors of cancer centers, NCI staff members, and site visitors arose (and still arise) because of the lack of "field experience" and the consequent enlightment of how many ways physicians, scientists, and administrators can "stack their blocks" to produce relevant cancer-oriented information.

There are three basic ways in which comprehensive cancer centers have been organized in this country -- as a free-standing entity; as an integral but independent entity within a university system and on a peer basis with a medical school; and as an integral part of a medical school. Considering this latter arrangement, I tend to agree with Dr. Palmer Saunders, who said recently in an address in Philadelphia that during the early days of NCI's attempt to establish clinical cancer centers "The medical school dean emerged as the most refractory of all administrative officials. With some very notable exceptions, the dean was the biggest enemy of the cancer center program."

As you all know by now, I consider absolutely crucial to the success of any comprehensive cancer center the autonomy of the director, who must have authority over program planning and execution; staff appointments (including faculty title); budget preparation, monitoring, and expenditure; space control and allocation; and patient control, including beds and the disposition of professional fees.

In addition to the essential cancer center roles of cancer research and patient care, education and the dissemination of new, verified information is crucial to its success and impact. Certainly all of the mechanisms of informational exchange have been greatly speeded and broadened with the many services made available to scientists and clinicians worldwide by the ICRDB, some of which are not yet being sufficiently utilized. Formalized, peer-reviewed publications are still an essential part of our permanent informational record and exchange, but ongoing progress reports and abstracted new findings keep the medical and

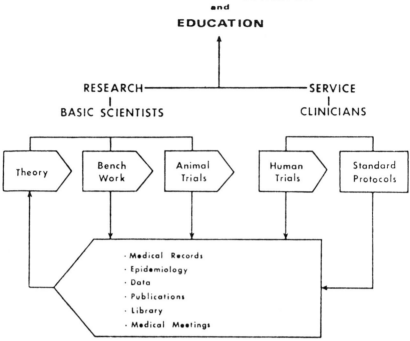

Figure 1. An example of flow of information within a Comprehensive Cancer Center. (From: Guidelines for Developing a Comprehensive Cancer Centre. International Union Against Cancer. Geneva, 1978.)

scientific communities more closely bound together
and functioning in greater scientific harmony and
economy than in the past. The ICRDB offers,
through the National Library of Medicine's
CANCERLINE, three major services to scientists and
clinicians interested in cancer - CANCERLIT, which
scans approximately 3000 journals and currently
contains approximately 225,000 citations, CLINPROT,
which contains approximately 2000 therapeutic
protocols, and CANCERPROJ, with 20,000 ongoing
research projects, 5000 of them contributed from
75 countries outside the United States. Each
institution can expedite the full use of these
systems by establishing, through their inhouse
libraries, an immediately available and responsive
search service which can provide on short notice,
not only searches of general interest covering a
wide field but also personalized searches targeting
very specialized information, which can be provided
on a routine monthly basis at minimal cost. Each
principal investigator is entitled to two CANCER-
GRAMS on specified topics without charge from the
International Bank. The EURONET system expedites
access to CANCERLINE for investigators throughout
Europe. The British Library, through a system
called Cancer Information Services for Developing
Countries, supplies CANCERLINE services to more
than 100 developing countries through a collaborative contract with the NCI, but unfortunately,
because of monetary constraints in the United
States, the NCI is able to honor this contract
only through 1980. With this International Data
Bank, it will become increasingly less likely that
a vital piece of the puzzle will lie fallow in
archives for 25 to 30 years, or that an isolated
individual or laboratory will labor for years on
a project only to find that the same techniques
and findings have already been reported elsewhere.

Additional trends that have evolved during
the National Cancer Program have been an increased
emphasis on defining the complexities of the human
immunologic system and its interactions with tumor
cells; a greater emphasis on the dual problems of
environmental carcinogenesis and prevention of
cancer by controlling predisposing environmental

agents, co-agents, or behavior; a recent greatly
enhanced interest in naturally occurring biological
response modifiers, such as interferon, and their
potential mass production with recombinant DNA
techniques derived from the expanded knowledge of
molecular biology and cytogenetics.

We are justified in claiming that the impact
of the National Cancer Program has been felt around
the world, not only through the worldwide informational dissemination of the ICRDB but also by
disseminating the increasingly popular concept of
the comprehensive cancer center and, through this
mechanism, a much more active interest and
participation from governmental structures
attempting to achieve better health and lifestyles for their citizens.

The NCI has, since 1972, had bilateral
agreements with other countries for mutual
exchange of biological scientific information and
personnel. The first one was initiated by
President Nixon and Mr. Breshnev in May 1972.
Currently there are 44 grants active in other
countries, totalling $2.4 million and 78 contracts,
totalling $8.8 million. Agreements were signed
between the U.S. and Japan in 1974, with Poland,
Egypt, and the Federal Republic of Germany in
1976, with France in 1977, with Italy and Hungary
in 1978, and with China in 1979.

Through the interactions of the NCI and
organizations such as the Association of American
Cancer Institutes, attempting to standardize
certain cancer-related activities for better
comparison of results and exchange of information
and personnel nationally, other nations and regions
around the world have been stimulated to form
national or regional organizations for cancer
institutes and to strive for similar goals.

Often members of the press, claiming
representation of "public" opinion and unrest,
accuse the NCI of defaulting on its "promise"
(never made) to find quick cures for all cancers.
If the critics were truly interested, they

would have found the real message contained in the 5/8-inch thick <u>Report of the National Panel of Consultants</u> to the Committee on Labor and Public Welfare of the U.S. Senate, which, as I previously mentioned, outlined the foundations already laid, upon which a plan and a program could be built and realized. Chemotherapy, for instance, which successfully cures 60% to 90% of eleven previously incurable cancers, had been the object of experimentation for approximately 15 years already, so that in the 5 years following gear-up of the program, survival figures were dramatically better than in any previous 5-year period in the history of medicine. The solid tumors, where no dramatic progress has been made, such as breast, colon-rectum, stomach, lung, pancreas, etc., have received greatly expanded protocol evaluation during the nine years of the National Cancer Program. Detection and diagnostic acumen have shown much technical advance and dissemination to the community level, such as mammography and use of computer-assisted tomography and other imaging techniques. Especially, the realization that systemic dissemination of these solid tumors requires combined therapy at an earlier stage and   more effective chemotherapeutic agents have set the goals for future research.

As for prevention, we physicians and scientists stand in amazement at the widespread disregard during the last 17 years of   the Surgeon General's report indicating   how to PREVENT lung cancer and other serious health problems by not inhaling tobacco smoke. We have watched the incidence of lung cancer in men sky-rocket, and triple since the 1960s for American women.

The scientists and physicians of this country have made remarkable progress toward bringing the diseases of cancer under better therapeutic control and are moving inexorably closer to laboratory definition of carcinogenesis and the consequent clinical manipulation of the mechanisms of initiation and promotion. We are finding agents that show evidence of arresting and

even reversing these mechanisms. We are defining
many more carcinogens, cocarcinogens, and carcinogenic metabolites of initially harmless or inactive
compounds. We are mapping, manipulating, and
learning about the functions of single genes and
their products. We are learning how DNA repairs
itself, once damaged, and how it fails to do so
under certain circumstances. We are testing and
probing the cell membrane with viral and immunologic tools to determine what normally closed
doors are opened in that membrane during the
processes of transformation and metastasis. Our
geneticists are mapping chromosome alterations to
define genetic susceptibility to cancer in
families. Biological assays are being developed
to assist us in still earlier detection of cancers,
for monitoring disease progress during therapy
and its absence during disease remission, for
prognosis, for sensitivity to new and old drugs
and combinations, and for early alert of re-
curring disease. We are learning ever more about
naturally protective mechanisms of our own
bodies and attempting to stimulate their more
active participation against tumor cells. We are
investigating alternative sources of energy, not
to solve our nation's fuel and industrial
constraints, but for detection of cancer by
attempting to use less or no ionizing radiation
but, instead, energy sources such as ultrasound,
thermography, and nuclear magnetic resonance.

     I could continue to catalog the numerous
types of basic and clinical research being
conducted, but others at this meeting have been
assigned this task. The National Cancer Program
of the National Cancer Institute has never been
nor ever could be perfectly satisfactory from all
points of view, retrospective or prospective.
Nevertheless, the American public has received
much more value for the tax dollars allocated to
cancer research than ever before. More scientists
have been supported for good basic biomedical
research that is yielding information of value for
the prevention or treatment of disease and for
better understanding of the life and aging
processes. Some of the detractors of the program

have been those who have eagerly accepted the
funding provided by the National Cancer Act to
enlarge their research contributions. Others have
criticized without offering better alternatives.
When criticism was valid, it was carefully weighed
by the National Cancer Advisory Board, the
President's Cancer Panel, and the heroic staff of
the NCI and its directors.

I would be remiss if I did not mention at
least a few names of people who have had major
roles in initiating and implementing the National
Cancer Act of 1971. These include Senator Ralph
Yarborough, President Richard Nixon, Senators
Warren Magnuson and Edward Kennedy, Congressman
Paul Rogers, the 3 directors of the NCI -- Dr. Carl
Baker, Dr. Frank Rauscher, and Dr. Arthur Upton --
Mrs. Mary Lasker, Mr. Elmer Bobst, the late Dr.
Sidney Farber, the members of the National Cancer
Advisory Board and its chairman Jonathan Rhoads,the
members of the President's Cancer Panel and
its indefatigable and judicious chairman
Benno Schmidt, the staffs of the NCI and the NIH,
the leaders of the American Cancer Society, and
those leaders of the Congress of the U.S.A. who
made it all possible by their unprecedented support.

We can be proud of what has been accomplished
in 9 years, because not only have we been helping
and are currently helping hundreds of thousands
of people who have cancer, but the scientific
legacy we are creating for people not yet born is
not even fully realized by us. We are in the
center of a biological evolution and revolution
that will far exceed in expected and unexpected
benefits those of any other planned program in
science and medicine in medical history.

I have participated this year in the unofficial
planning and evaluation of a budget for the NCI of
$1.5 billion and can assure you that it can be spent
wisely and effectively. We have gained the
knowledge necessary to justify this budget. Perhaps
the greatest impact of the National Cancer Act has
been the development of the medical and scientific
personnel and the teaching of oncology in all its
permutations   as an accepted area of expertise.

We now have the trained minds or the mechanisms
to train those needed for the future definitive
research required. We must strive to keep the
complex national and international effort and
momentum geared to maximum production for the
conquest of cancer.

Role of Government
in Cancer Research

PAUL G. ROGERS

Former Member of Congress
Currently Partner
Law Firm of Hogan & Hartson
Washington, D. C.

Today, this International Symposium on Cancer concludes
its week-long deliberations with reports from distinguished
scientists and men of medicine on progress in the fight
against cancer, and promising areas of cancer research, for
progress in the future.

The work product of each of you, along with your colleagues from all parts of this earth, give cause for all
men and women everywhere to praise the progress that has
been made and to have optimistic hope for the future!

The government of the United States joined in the fight
against cancer some years ago, and its support and efforts
also have seen progress in its programs. This symposium is
witness to this fact.

Forty-three years ago (1937) the National Cancer Institute was created as the Federal institution with exclusive
responsibility in cancer research. The priorities of that
day were largely focused on problems of treatment, with
little attention to prevention.

The support of the American people--expressed by Con-
gress--for substantial expenditures for cancer research has
been considerable. The first annual budget of the NCI was
$400,000. In 1958 - $56,000,000. In 1968 - $183,000,000.
In 1971 with the passage of the National Cancer Act -
$223,000,000. For fiscal year 1980 - $1,000,000,000.

The public support for cancer research has been steady
and firm.

No disease is so feared as cancer, and the concern for
an effective treatment and prevention program has made the

National Cancer Institute the most significantly funded
institute of all the National Institutes of Health.

As a beginning, much time and effort of scientists was
spent in the basic research of the disease itself--trying
to learn how cancer develops. These efforts continue as we
learn of the many types of cancers. In the earlier years
of cancer research, treatment was of course the most immediate concern of people stricken by cancer and by their
families and friends. This concern was transmitted by the
Congress to those setting the cancer program priorities.

As national policy on cancer research develops, we find
expression for different emphasis as our knowledge increases.

In the late 1960's and 1970's, as concern for the health
effect of pollutants mounted, chemical carcinogens became
overnight villains. Major laws to protect the environment
evolved. It was during this period that most landmark
legislation--such as the Clean Air Act, the Safe Drinking
Water Act, the Toxic Substances law, the Radiation Health
and Safety Act--were enacted. Health standards were the
basic bottom line for determinations made under their
provisions. Many of these standards are cancer related.

As the American public became more conscious of the
health effects of carcinogens and toxic substances, it
created agencies for research, for standards to be set and
for enforcement of laws to prevent these problems--the
Environmental Protection Agency, OSHA, the National Institute for Occupational Safety and Health. Research efforts
intensified, as demonstrated by the establishment of the
National Institute for Environmental Health Sciences, which
supports basic research on the toxic effects of environmental pollutants and ways to predict future crises. The
fruits of research conducted by these agencies has taught
us that the potential adverse health impact of environmental pollution is staggering. NIOSH's Registry of toxic
Effects of Chemical Substances in 1976 listed 25,000 different chemicals with about 2,000 suspect carcinogens.

One of the difficult areas being addressed by NIEHS is
the development of improved statistical methods for extrapolating from animal tests to humans and from high dose to
low dose. A continuing field of interest is to determine
threshold levels (if any) for carcinogens.

Cancer research, then, will be concerned not only with
human health problems, but with policy determinations for
major industries of the country--the chemical and food
industries in particular.

A quantum leap in the United States cancer program was taken in 1971, when the National Cancer Act was adopted by the Congress and signed into law by the President. And it is interesting that this initiative to increase the national commitment to fight cancer came from the Congress, not the executive branch of government. The efforts of Mary Lasker, Sid Farber, and of course Benno Schmidt who headed the Senate appointed Panel of Consultants, and has been an active force in the development of cancer activities by our government, sparked the Congress to pass the National Cancer Act 1971.

The main thrust of the law was to increase Federal support--tax dollars--for research, cut red tape for the Institute, and insure a better balance between basic and clinical research, to establish cancer centers for treatment and clinical research so that the research results could be spread around the country quickly, and the opportunity for community physicians to apply the latest knowledge to those who suffer.

Cancer control was given greater priority and certainly prevention was becoming an admitted goal accentuated by increased knowledge of environmental factors that could cause cancer.

1971 was indeed a watershed year for government's role in cancer research, not only because of the expanded role conferred upon the National Cancer Institute, but also-- and perhaps more importantly--because of the understanding of cancer research that the American public acquired as a result of the debate regarding the interplay of research and the proper relationship of the NCI and other research institutes. The debate was lengthy, well publicized, was of good quality and high intensity. During the debate, the public demand for increased funding of cancer research was demonstrated. A host of cancer researchers, many of them recipients of Nobel prizes, made the public aware that cancer research would produce no magic bullet--no total cure--but instead that the complexities of the disease itself demand a steady and continuous research effort, combining both basic and applied research. As a result of the debate, the Congress and the American public, in my judgment, have a more sophisticated understanding of what government can and must do to support cancer research. Equally important, I believe that the public understands that there are limitations--that the multi-faceted aspects of cancer and its causes are such that what must be expected is constant progress, and not a dramatic announcement that cancer has been cured.

The role of government in cancer research has been
principally to bring together the best scientific thought of
the times, support avenues of research that appear most
promising, using a peer review mechanism. Also, to provide
facilities' support and to create an arena for freedom of
thought and action for the best minds in our scientific
community has been an overall objective.

Through the legislative hearing process expressions of
disagreement come to the fore, emphasis on different
approaches and theories develop, and an accounting on
progress and failure is put on the record for the American
people. Policy judgments are then made.

For the 80's, governmental actions will be greatly
affected by the economy, inflation rate, the budget bal-
ancing efforts of the administration and the Congress.
Strict budgets will affect support for the biomedical
research programs of the nation. Already we have seen a
tightening up on appropriations for cancer research itself,
even though the Congress has been most generous with its
support of the National Cancer Institute above all others.

The current budget does not even provide for an increase
of the inflation factor in our economy resulting in a cut
in research programs. This means that harder judgments
will have to be made by administrators and particularly by
the scientific community to make sure that the most essential and promising research is not interrupted.

The support for cancer research will continue, but not
at the percentage of growth as in the last number of years.
Congressional oversight will increase, more talk of cost/
benefit ratio will be heard. This always becomes a dominant theme when budget tightening is required. Some in
Congress will question whether the outlays of money
resulting from the 1971 Cancer Act have brought sufficient
results to justify a continued billion dollar budget. On
the other hand, the government's role in cancer research
in the years ahead will be given impetus by the increasing
number of elderly citizens in our nation.

Life expectancy is greater than ever before. For those
born in 1980, average expectancy is 75 years--for men, 72
years--for women, 81.

At present the elderly comprise 11 percent of the
population; by 2030, that figure is expected to nearly
double, rising to 18 percent. The population of the very
old, those 80 and over, will increase especially rapidly.

The government will have to assume the burden for a
vast majority of these elderly citizens in their health

needs, and the incidence of cancer will increase in these age brackets unless answers through research are found to prevent, treat and cure cancer.

Thus, I do believe strongly that the American people understand the importance of cancer research and will continue to call for tax dollars to be spent for answers that come from this research.

It is well to make clear the progress that has been made in the fight against cancer, as you are doing at this conference, but the effort needs to be broadened.

Further, the public needs to be increasingly aware of the future possibility of the research efforts now in progress, the DNA research which will open untold knowledge for mankind, the research on hybridomas, immunology, and all that you have discussed at this meeting.

And finally, intelligent governmental policy will be fortified by constant reminders to the Congress and the American public that all research takes time, that an immediate payoff--a silver bullet--is not the expected course; that patience is required; that too much must not be expected too soon; that everyone involved is trying, as hard, as fast, and as effectively as is humanly possible to find the answer to the prevention, the treatment, and the cure of the dreaded cancer disease.

With public understanding of these factors, the governmental role in cancer research will be strong, realistic, and supportive of science's effort to conquer cancer.

Index

932

933

934

Laminar air flow (LAF) rooms, 699, 700
Laryngeal cancer, surgery and survival rate for, 812–816
Leukemia
  acute lymphocytic (lymphoblastic). *See* Acute lymphocytic (lymphoblastic) leukemia
  acute monoblastic, chemotherapy of, 279–281
  acute myelocytic (AML), chemotherapy of, 273–276
  acute nonlymphoblastic
    bone marrow transplantation in, 628
    in children, 328–330
  acute promyelocytic, chemotherapy of, 276–279
  bone marrow transplantation in. *See* Bone marrow transplantation— in leukemia
  chemotherapy of. *See* Chemotherapy—of leukemia
  chronic granulocytic, 331–332
  chronic lymphocytic, 332–334
  chronic myelocytic, 251–252
  etiology of, 250–251
  feline, 894
  in vitro studies of, 264–265
  L1210
    imidazole triazenes in treatment of, 73
    nitrosoureas in treatment of, 71–72
    resistance to chemotherapy, 56–59, 62
  as lymphoma treatment consequence, 467–470
  markers for, 263–264
  meningeal, 257–258
  murine, collateral sensitivity in, 62–63
  myelocytic (granulocytic), 271–285
    classification of, 271–273
  overview of, 249–266
  prognostic factors in acute leukemia, 291–298
  prospects for research on, 265–266

T cell
  nude mice xenografts, studies in, 49–50
Leukemia-associated inhibitory activity (LIA), 264–266
Leukemia-lymphoma complex in cats, 894
Leukemia Society of America, 912
Liposome-encapsulated macrophage-activating agents, 77–87
Liver, biotransformation of drugs in, 97, 100
Liver cancer, surgery and survival rate for, 816, 818
Longevity, diet and, 898–900
L-2 protocol for acute lymphoblastic leukemia, 302–315
L-10 (or L-10M) protocol for acute lymphoblastic leukemia, 302–315
Lung cancer, 539–550
  chemotherapy of, 575–576
  nonsmall cell, 545–549
  prospects for treatment of, 549–550
  PEPA program in, 707–708
  small cell anaplastic carcinoma (SCCL), 540–545
  surgery for, 801–806
Lungs, drug injury to, 167–168
Lymphomas, 419–471. *See also* Hodgkin's disease
  chemotherapy of. *See also* Late effects of treatment of
    in animals, 21
    diffuse lymphomas, 437–438
    future prospects, 438–439
    nodular (follicular) lymphoma, 436–437
  classifications of, 419–421, 427–429
  diagnosis of, 422–423
  diffuse, chemotherapy of, 437–438
  future challenges in treatment of, 424–425
  interdisciplinary research and patient care groups, 424
  late effects of treament of, 459–471

941

a
b
c
d
e
f
g
h
1 i
8 2 j